T0142281

Advances in Intelligent Systems and Computing

Volume 762

Series editor

Janusz Kacprzyk, Polish Academy of Sciences, Warsaw, Poland
e-mail: kacprzyk@ibspan.waw.pl

The series "Advances in Intelligent Systems and Computing" contains publications on theory, applications, and design methods of Intelligent Systems and Intelligent Computing. Virtually all disciplines such as engineering, natural sciences, computer and information science, ICT, economics, business, e-commerce, environment, healthcare, life science are covered. The list of topics spans all the areas of modern intelligent systems and computing such as: computational intelligence, soft computing including neural networks, fuzzy systems, evolutionary computing and the fusion of these paradigms, social intelligence, ambient intelligence, computational neuroscience, artificial life, virtual worlds and society, cognitive science and systems, Perception and Vision, DNA and immune based systems, self-organizing and adaptive systems, e-Learning and teaching, human-centered and human-centric computing, recommender systems, intelligent control, robotics and mechatronics including human-machine teaming, knowledge-based paradigms, learning paradigms, machine ethics, intelligent data analysis, knowledge management, intelligent agents, intelligent decision making and support, intelligent network security, trust management, interactive entertainment, Web intelligence and multimedia.

The publications within "Advances in Intelligent Systems and Computing" are primarily proceedings of important conferences, symposia and congresses. They cover significant recent developments in the field, both of a foundational and applicable character. An important characteristic feature of the series is the short publication time and world-wide distribution. This permits a rapid and broad dissemination of research results.

Advisory Board

Chairman

Nikhil R. Pal, Indian Statistical Institute, Kolkata, India
e-mail: nikhil@isical.ac.in

Members

Rafael Bello Perez, Universidad Central "Marta Abreu" de Las Villas, Santa Clara, Cuba
e-mail: rbellop@uclv.edu.cu

Emilio S. Corchado, University of Salamanca, Salamanca, Spain
e-mail: escorchado@usal.es

Hani Hagras, University of Essex, Colchester, UK
e-mail: hani@essex.ac.uk

László T. Kóczy, Széchenyi István University, Győr, Hungary
e-mail: koczy@sze.hu

Vladik Kreinovich, University of Texas at El Paso, El Paso, USA
e-mail: vladik@utep.edu

Chin-Teng Lin, National Chiao Tung University, Hsinchu, Taiwan
e-mail: ctlin@mail.nctu.edu.tw

Jie Lu, University of Technology, Sydney, Australia
e-mail: Jie.Lu@uts.edu.au

Patricia Melin, Tijuana Institute of Technology, Tijuana, Mexico
e-mail: epmelin@hafsamx.org

Nadia Nedjah, State University of Rio de Janeiro, Rio de Janeiro, Brazil
e-mail: nadia@eng.uerj.br

Ngoc Thanh Nguyen, Wroclaw University of Technology, Wroclaw, Poland
e-mail: Ngoc-Thanh.Nguyen@pwr.edu.pl

Jun Wang, The Chinese University of Hong Kong, Shatin, Hong Kong
e-mail: jwang@mae.cuhk.edu.hk

More information about this series at http://www.springer.com/series/11156

Ewa Pietka · Pawel Badura
Jacek Kawa · Wojciech Wieclawek
Editors

Information Technology in Biomedicine

Proceedings 6th International
Conference, ITIB'2018, Kamień Śląski,
Poland, June 18–20, 2018

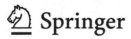 Springer

Editors
Ewa Pietka
Faculty of Biomedical Engineering
Silesian University of Technology
Zabrze
Poland

Jacek Kawa
Faculty of Biomedical Engineering
Silesian University of Technology
Zabrze
Poland

Pawel Badura
Faculty of Biomedical Engineering
Silesian University of Technology
Zabrze
Poland

Wojciech Wieclawek
Faculty of Biomedical Engineering
Silesian University of Technology
Zabrze
Poland

ISSN 2194-5357   ISSN 2194-5365   (electronic)
Advances in Intelligent Systems and Computing
ISBN 978-3-319-91210-3   ISBN 978-3-319-91211-0   (eBook)
https://doi.org/10.1007/978-3-319-91211-0

Library of Congress Control Number: Applied for

© Springer International Publishing AG, part of Springer Nature 2019
This work is subject to copyright. All rights are reserved by the Publisher, whether the whole or part of the material is concerned, specifically the rights of translation, reprinting, reuse of illustrations, recitation, broadcasting, reproduction on microfilms or in any other physical way, and transmission or information storage and retrieval, electronic adaptation, computer software, or by similar or dissimilar methodology now known or hereafter developed.
The use of general descriptive names, registered names, trademarks, service marks, etc. in this publication does not imply, even in the absence of a specific statement, that such names are exempt from the relevant protective laws and regulations and therefore free for general use.
The publisher, the authors and the editors are safe to assume that the advice and information in this book are believed to be true and accurate at the date of publication. Neither the publisher nor the authors or the editors give a warranty, express or implied, with respect to the material contained herein or for any errors or omissions that may have been made. The publisher remains neutral with regard to jurisdictional claims in published maps and institutional affiliations.

Printed on acid-free paper

This Springer imprint is published by the registered company Springer International Publishing AG part of Springer Nature
The registered company address is: Gewerbestrasse 11, 6330 Cham, Switzerland

Preface

Continuous growth of the amount of medical information and the variety of multimodal content necessitates the demand for a fast and reliable technology able to process data and deliver results in a user-friendly manner at the time and place the information is needed. The requirements can be met through the cooperation of three specific partners. Patient needs are recognized by experienced physicians who collaborate with scientists and engineers and define the goal of the research that should satisfy the functional requirements of authorized medical staff as well as the overall healthcare system for the benefit of the patients. Many of these areas are recognized as research and development frontiers in employing new technology in a clinical environment. Technological assistance can be found in prevention, diagnosis, treatment, and rehabilitation. Homecare support in any type of disability may improve the standard of living and make it safer and more comfortable.

We give back to the readers the conference proceedings, which include papers written by members of academic society and vendors who develop products applied in biocybernetics. The volume is divided into eight parts.

The first two parts contain papers that present image processing approaches and their implementation in computer-aided surgery. The analysis is carried out in 2- or 3-dimensional space depending on further clinical implementation. Part 3 addresses a precisely defined implementation of data analysis in computer-assisted diagnosis. Part 4 undertakes mostly cardiac problems and presents new approaches to ECG analysis with local and remote access to the results. Part 5 discusses processing methods applied to microscopic images of tissue samples taken during the biopsy procedure as well as tools for genotyping. The analysis of complex anatomical structures and biomedical processes often requires various experimental setups to investigate the sensitivity of these structures to various external or internal conditions. Modeling and simulation of these processes are introduced in Part 6.

Two special sessions are given at the meeting. Unstructured data analysis on sources including written text as well as speech signals is becoming more and more popular. The text analysis detects the content similarity of medical records, and the speech signal processing recognizes the speaker emotions. These issues are presented in Part 7. Recognition of disability, objective measurement of disability level in all age groups including children and the elderly, and assistance during medical procedures are introduced in Part 8.

I would like to express my gratitude to the authors who have submitted their original research papers as well as all the reviewers for their valuable comments. Your effort has contributed to the high quality of the proceedings that we pass on to our readers.

Ewa Pietka

Organization

Scientific Committee Members

M. Akay, USA
P. Augustyniak, Poland
A. Bargieła, Great Britain
R. Brűck, Germany
K. Cápová, Slovakia
M. Černý, Czech Republic
S. Czudek, Czech Republic
A. Drygajło, Switzerland
M. Dyvak, Ukraine
P. Forczmański, Poland
A. Gertych, USA
D. Greenhalgh, Great Britain
M. Grzegorzek, Germany
M. Gzik, Poland
A. Hajdasiński, Netherlands
J. Haueisen, Germany
Z. Hippe, Poland
M. Juszczyk, Germany
E. Krupinski, USA
M. Kurzyński, Poland
M. Last, Israel
C. Li, China
A. Liebert, Poland
R. Maniewski, Poland
J. Marciniak, Poland
M. McNitt-Gray, USA
A. Mitas, Poland

A. Napieralski, Poland
E. Neri, Italy
A. Nowakowski, Poland
D. Paulus, Germany
T. Pałko, Poland
Z. Paszenda, Poland
W. Pedrycz, Canada
M. Penhaker, Czech Republic
E. Pietka, Poland
I. Provaznik, Czech Republic
A. Przelaskowski, Poland
K. Shirahama, Japan
P. Słomka, USA
D. Spinczyk, Poland
B. Stasiak, Poland
P. Strumiłło, Poland
E. Supriyanto, Malaysia
P. Szczepaniak, Poland
A. Świerniak, Poland
R. Tadeusiewicz, Poland
E. Tkacz, Poland
M. Vozňák, Czech Republic
H. Witte, Germany
A. Wojciechowski, Poland
S. Wong, USA
Z. Wróbel, Poland

Contents

Multimodal Imaging and Computer-Aided Surgery

Computer-Aided Diagnosis

Signal Processing and Medical Devices

Contents

Image Processing

A Brief Review for Content-Based Microorganism Image Analysis Using Classical and Deep Neural Networks

Chen Li[1], Ning Xu[2], Tao Jiang[3], Shouliang Qi[1], Fangfang Han[1], Wei Qian[1], and Xin Zhao[1(✉)]

[1] Northeastern University, Shenyang, China
zhaoxin@mail.neu.edu.cn
[2] Liaoning Shihua University, Fushun, China
[3] Chengdu University of Information Technology, Chengdu, China

Abstract. Microorganisms play very important roles in people's daily life. To discover the information of them is a fundamental work in microbiological studies, which can assist microbiologists and related scientists to get to know more properties, habits and characteristics of these tiny but obbligato living beings. To this end, effective *Content-based Microorganism Image Analysis* (CBMIA) approaches using *Artificial Neural Networks* (ANNs) are introduced to microbiological fields from the 1990s. In order to clarify the development history and find the developing trend of ANNs in the CBMIA field, we briefly survey around 60 related works in this paper, including classical ANNs, deep ANNs and methodology analysis.

Keywords: Content-based image analysis · Deep learning
Artificial Neural Networks · Feature extraction · Classification

1 Introduction

Microorganisms are very tiny, but they play significant roles in human's daily life and development. For example, 'beneficial' microorganisms, like *Rhizobium leguminosarum*, can help soybean to fix nitrogen and supply food to human beings; and 'harmful' microorganisms, like *Mycobacterium tuberculosis*, can lead to disease and death. Hence, in order to discover more useful information of them, effective *Content-based Microorganism Image Analysis* (CBMIA) techniques are introduced to assist microbiologists in recent decades. In our previous work [36], related works are surveyed from different application points of microorganisms, so it is more suitable for microbiological researchers to refer to. In contrast, we propose this paper to review the related works from the technical points, and specially focus on the development history of *Artificial Neural Network* (ANN) methods in this domain. So, this paper is more suitable for computer scientists to consult. In Fig. 1, an example of different microorganisms is shown.

© Springer International Publishing AG, part of Springer Nature 2019
E. Pietka et al. (Eds.): ITIB 2018, AISC 762, pp. 3–14, 2019.
https://doi.org/10.1007/978-3-319-91211-0_1

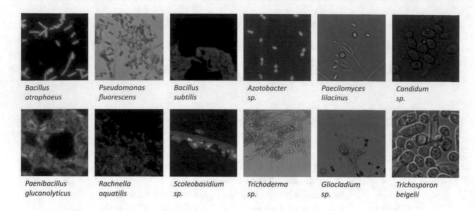

Fig. 1. The examples of images of the investigated classes of microorganisms [34]

Traditionally, microorganism analysis is done by chemical, physical, molecular biological, and morphological methods. These methods have different working mechanisms and results, but mainly suffer from three respects: Secondary pollution, expensive equipment and long duration time. In order to solve problems of the mentioned traditional methods, CBMIA approaches are applied to support a cleaner, cheaper, and more rapid way for microorganism analysis tasks [35].

Because CBMIA systems only need visual information for analysis, they do not create any chemical pollution. Furthermore, because CBMIA systems are usually semi- or full-automatic, they are effective and can save a lot of human resource. In addition, CBMIA approaches only need some cheap equipment, like microscopes and computers, the above analysis work can reduce many financial investments. Hence, CBMIA can help people to obtain useful microcosmic

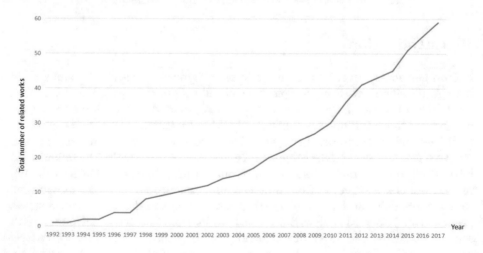

Fig. 2. The total number of related works using ANN methods for CBMIA tasks

information effectively, and it is widely used in many research and production fields [44]. Especially, because ANN methods, including both classical and deep neural networks, are a kind of very effective artificial intelligence algorithms [43], they are widely used in the CBMIA fields for image segmentation, feature extraction and classification tasks. The development trend is shown in Fig. 2.

To clarify the CBMIA work using ANN approaches in recent years, we propose this brief review paper with the following structure: In Sect. 2, the CBMIA work using classical ANN methods are introduced; in Sect. 3, state-of-the-art deep ANN methods are summarized; in Sect. 4, reasons of the effectiveness of the ANNs in the CBMIA are explained; and Sect. 5 closes this paper with a short conclusion.

2 CBMIA Using Classical Neural Networks

2.1 Classification Tasks

In the 1990s: In [3], a CBMIA method is proposed to classify eight classes of microorganisms, where shape features and an ANN classifier are used. The work in [11] introduces a system to classify five microorganism categories. In this work, Fourier transform features and an ANN classifier are applied. As a further work of [11], they compare the classification performance of two ANNs in [10,12], including a multi-layer ANN and a radial basis function (RBF) network, and the RBF network shows a better classification performance.

In [52,56], a self-tuning vision system is proposed to classify two main forms of yeast-like fungus in a fermentation process, where image segmentation is first done, then shape features are extracted, lastly ANN and fuzzy logic approaches are combined for classification. In [62], six categories of yeasts and bacteria are classified by a three layer ANN classifier, where the original images are used as input data first, and then 9-by-9 pixel size filters are used to map the local shape features into 92 neurons in a hidden layer. In [58], edge detection, shape feature extraction and different classifiers, including a multi-layered ANN, are applied to distinguish one class of medical microorganisms from other objects. Finally, the best classification result is obtained by the ANN classifier. A microorganism classification method is introduced in [5], where edge detection, shape feature extraction and an ANN classifier are used. In [29], three classes of *Gyrodactylus salaris* are semi-automatically identified by a CBMIA system, where original microscopic images are first interactively analysed by biological experts for extracting ten shape features, then four classifiers are designed, including an ANN (feed-forward neural network).

In the 2000s: In [15], a classification approach is used to classify four classes of microorganisms. In this work, image segmentation, shape features, textural features, and an ANN classifier are used for classifying them. In [4], 11 Pleistocene taxa during routine work are classified using a five layer ANN classifier.

In [61], an medical microorganism classification system is built up using a dither filter, shape and textural features, and an ANN classifier. In [27,28,32], a dual-classification strategy is applied to do the plankton classification task. In the first step, shape features and an ANN classifier are applied; in the second step, texture features and a support vector machine (SVM) classifier are used. In [19], a preliminary semi-automatic system for multi-class classification is developed to recognise several groups of protozoa and metazoa in aeration tanks, where shape features are extracted first, then an ANN classifiers is built for the classification.

In [60], two three-layer ANN classifiers are used in a multi-class aquatic microorganism classification task. The first ANN is a back propagation (BP) neural network, and the second is a RBF neural network. In [1], a semi-automatic multi-class classification method is proposed to identify seven protozoa species in wastwater treatment, where image segmentation and shape feature extraction approaches are first applied, then an ANN classifier is built to classify the microorganisms. In [63], a unary-class classification approach is introduced to distinguish fluorescently stained bacteria, where spatially invariant estimators are used as features to represent the microorganisms first, and then an ANN classifier is designed.

In a serial work [7,37–40], a global and local feature fusion technique is used to classify multi-class microorganisms in different datasets, where a shape feature is used as the global feature and a spatial feature is used as the local feature. Then, an ANN (BP network) is used for classification. In another serial work [21–26], three types of spiral bacteria are classified using image segmentation, five shape features and ANN classifiers.

In the 2010s: In [30], a CBMIA system is proposed to classify micro-alike images of macroinvertebrate, where multiple global, local, shape, colour, pair-wise, texture features are extracted using a third party toolbox (ImageJ [16]), and then ANN classifiers are used for classification. In [53], image segmentation, shape features and an ANN classifier are used in a two-class medical microorganism classification task. In [45–47], different types of tuberculosis are classified using a CBMIA approach, where image segmentation is first applied, then six affine moments are extracted to describe shape characteristics, lastly an ANN (hybrid multi-layered perceptron network) is built to classify the medical microorganism styles. In [41], a CBMIA approach is proposed to classify five classes of algae in freshwater, where object detection, image processing, segmentation, shape feature extraction, feature selection and an ANN classifier are used. In [54], the performance of discriminant analysis and ANN classifiers are compared in an algae classification task using shape features.

In [59], a one-class classification system is developed to detect powdery mildew spores, where multiple CBMIA methods are applied, including image enhancing, segmentation, shape feature extraction, and ANN classifier design. In [55], a multi-class classification system is introduced to classify ten categories of phytoplankton, where image segmentation, shape and texture feature extraction, and ANN classification methods are used. In [2], a unary classification system is introduced to distinguish tuberculosis and other objects in a microscopic image, where image segmentation, shape feature extraction, and an ANN classifier are used. In [8,9], a CBMIA system is proposed to classify 24 different microalgae in fresh and salt water bodies, where image segmentation, shape and colour feature extraction, pigment signature determination and ANN grouping are used for this task.

In [17], a CBMIA approach is proposed to identify tuberculosis mycobacterium, where image segmentation is first done, then 30 colour features are extracted from four colour spaces, thirdly three filters are used to separate the aim medical microorganisms, including a size filter, a geometric filter and a rule-based filter, lastly an ANN classifier is designed to solve the classification problem. In [33,34], a multi-class classification system is proposed to identify 12 microorganism categories, where image segmentation is first done, then various shape and colour features are extracted, thirdly a fast correlation-based filter is applied to select 21 the most important features, lastly the classification result is obtained by an ANN classifier.

2.2 Other Tasks

In the 1990s: In [18], a CBMIA system is introduced to detect *Aspergillus awamori*, where six shape features, cluster analysis and an ANN classifier are used.

In the 2010s: In [49,50], a CBMIA system is proposed to detect tuberculosis from a microscopic image, where an ANN and a neuro fuzzy inference methods are applied jointly to enhance the classification performance. Furthermore, in [51], based on image segmentation, shape feature extraction and feature selection results, a new classification method using multi layer perceptron neural network activated by SVM learning algorithm is proposed. This new approach can do image classification and object segmentation jointly.

2.3 Summary

From the review above, we can find that since the 1990s till the early years of the 2010s, most of the usages of the classical ANNs in the CBMIA domain concentrate on the classification tasks, without any feature extraction or image segmentation functions like the current deep ANNs. This situation is mainly because of the limitation of hardware during these decades, where the computational ability of computers are not high enough to do large scale calculation to extract effective image features. Furthermore, because properties of microorganism images are highly various, complicated and unpredictable, it is difficult for simple classification algorithms to handle, but suitable for the ANNs which are able to work in a parallel and adaptive way. Hence, many CBMIA works choose ANNs due to their robust classification performance.

3 CBMIA Using Deep Neural Networks

3.1 CBMIA Tasks

In [42], a unary classification method is proposed to detect bacteria in different environmental conditions, where a convolutional deep belief network and a SVM classifier are used to segment possible objects first, then a six layers convolutional neural network (CNN) is applied to predict the positive microorganism class.

In [13], a deep CNN frame work is designed to classify microscopic images of 121 plankton categories with around 30000 examples. In this work, because the data size is too small to train a good performance deep learning system, an effective data augmentation approach is applied to solve the small dataset problem, where rotation, translation, rescaling, flipping, shearing and stretching operations are used. This data augmentation approach observably improves the effectiveness of the deep ANN approach. Finally, this deep ANN framework is built, including ten convolutional layers, three fully connected layers and four spatial pooling layers.

In [14,48], both classical and novel machine vision methods are used in a diatom classification task, where a deep CNN framework is designed based on Caffe and LeNet resources.

In [31], the labeling of environmental microorganisms is proposed by an engine that can automatically analyze microscopic images using conditional random fields (CRF) and deep CNN methods. First, to effectively represent scarce training images, a deep CNN pre-trained for image classification using a large amount of data is re-purposed to the feature extractor that distils pixel-level features in microscopic images. In addition, pixel-level classification results by such features can be refined using global features that describe the whole image *in toto*. Finally, the CRF model localizes and classifies the microorganisms by considering the spatial relations among deep CNN-based features, and their relations to global features. Furthermore, the original image dataset, ground truth images and codes are released as open sources for academic purposes[1]. In Fig. 3, the workflow of this multifunctional work is shown.

3.2 Summary

From the survey above, we can find that the deep ANN techniques are used more and more since the middle of the 2010s, where, nearly all pattern analysis tasks can be solved by them, including image pre-processing, feature extraction, post-processing and classifier design. This development trend is mainly caused by the powerful ability of the fast evolution of hardware, which supports a high feasibility to implement the high computational complexity deep ANN algorithms. In addition, in contrast to the traditional manual craft feature extraction methods, the deep ANNs support a kind of full-automatic feature extraction approaches, which are more robust to describe complex morphological characteristics and structures of microorganisms. Therefore, the deep ANNs show a very huge potential in the CBMIA domain.

---

[1] DGM LIB: Semantic Image Segmentation with Conditional Random Fields. 2018, Available at: http://research.project-10.de/dgm/.

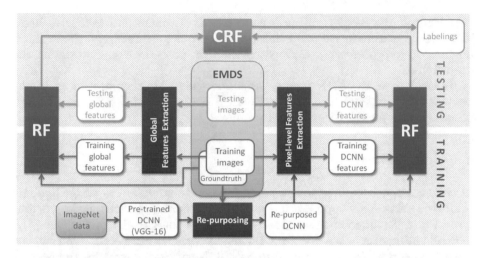

Fig. 3. An overview of the CRF-based environmental microorganism classification and segmentation framework [31]. In the CRF framework, global and pixel-level features (DCNN features) are first extracted. Then, the extracted features together with the ground truth data are used to train random forest classifiers, where the trained classifiers are used as unary potentials in the CRF model. Finally, together with the pairwise potentials, the CRF model is applied to segment (pixel-level labelling) and classify (image-level labelling) microorganisms in test images

4 Methodology Analysis

There are many classification methods used in CBMIA tasks, like Bayesian and SVM classifiers. In contrast to other classifiers, the ANN classifiers have a very stable developing history and a very huge potential in the future [43].

Compared to similarity-based classifiers, ANNs are good at working in a high-dimensional feature space. Because of many irrelevant dimensions, similarity-based classifiers fail to appropriately measure similarities in high-dimensional feature spaces. In contrast to probability-based classifiers, ANNs are able to solve small dataset problem much better. Probability-based classifiers need a large number of image examples to appropriately estimate probabilistic distributions in high-dimensional feature spaces [20]. However, due to the practical CBMIA tasks, it is usually difficult to collect a large and statistically relevant number of data for training. For these reasons, weight-based classifiers can train different weights (parameters) for different components in a feature vector and construct a decision boundary between images of different data classes based on the margin maximisation principle. Due to this principle, the generalisation error of the ANN is theoretically independent of the number of feature dimensions [57]. Furthermore, a complex (non-linear) decision boundary can be extracted using a non-linear ANN to enhance the classification performance [6,43]. Hence, ANN classifiers are chosen and applied in many CBMIA works in the past periods for classification tasks.

Although the SVMs are also weight-based classifiers and can solve high-dimensional feature space and small dataset problems effectively, they cannot do image pre-processing, feature extraction or post-processing works as the deep ANNs.

In conclusion, the ANN approaches support not only classification methods, but also other pattern analysis functions. Hence, ANNs are very effective and potential ways for the CBMIA applications.

5   Conclusion

In this paper, a brief overview of content-based microorganism image analysis (CBMIA) using ANN approaches is proposed. In Sect. 1, an introduction is first given to clarify the motivation of using ANNs for the CBMIA tasks. Then, the methods using classical ANNs for CBMIA are reviewed in Sect. 2. Thirdly, the usages of deep ANNs are surveyed in Sect. 3. Next, Sect. 4 explains the reasons of the wide use of ANNs in the CBMIA. By this brief review, finally we find that because of the fast development of hardware in recent years, deep ANNs are able to do many pattern analysis work for the CBMIA tasks, which shows a very hopeful developing trend in the future.

Acknowledgement. We thank our previous cooperators in related works: Prof. Dr.-Ing. Marcin Grzegorzek, Dr.-Ing. Kimiaki Shirahama, Dr.-Ing. Joanna Czajkowska, M.Sc. Sergey Kosov, Dr.-Ing. Fangshu Ma, Prof. Yanling Zou and Prof. Dr. Beihai Zhou. We also thank the 'Double Top Construction' funding supported by the North-eastern University, China.

References

1. Amaral, A.L., Ginoris, Y.P., Nicolau, A., Coelho, M.A.Z., Ferreira, E.C.: Stalked protozoa identification by image analysis and multivariable statistical techniques. Anal. Bioanal. Chem. **319**(4), 1321–1325 (2008)
2. Ayas, S., Ekinci, M.: Random forest-based tuberculosis bacteria classification in images of ZN-stained sputum smear samples. SIViP **8**(1), 49–61 (2014)
3. Balfoort, H.W., Snoek, J., Smits, J.R.M., Breedveld, L.W., Hofstraat, J.W., Ringelberg, J.: Automatic identification of algae: neural network analysis of flow cytometric data. J. Plankton Res. **14**(4), 575–589 (1992)
4. Beaufort, L., Dollfus, D.: Automatic recognition of coccoliths by dynamical neural networks. Mar. Micropaleontol. **51**(1–2), 57–73 (2004)
5. Blackburn, N., Hagstrom, A., Wikner, J., Cuadros-Hansson, R., Bjornsen, P.K.: Rapid determination of bacterial abundance, biovolume, morphology, and growth by neural network-based image analysis. Appl. Environ. Microbiol. **64**(9), 3246–3255 (1998)
6. Chang, C., Lin, C.: LIBSVM: a library for support vector machines. ACM Trans. Intell. Syst. Technol. **3**(2), 1–27 (2011)
7. Chen, C., Li, X.: A new wastewater bacteria classification with microscopic image analysis. In: WSEAS International Conference on Computers, pp. 915–921 (2008)

8. Coltelli, P., Barsanti, L., Evangelista, V., Frassanito, A.M., Gualtieri, P.: Water monitoring: automated and real time identification and classification of algae using digital microscopy. Environ. Sci. Process. Impacts **16**(11), 2656–2665 (2014)
9. Coltelli, P., Barsanti, L., Evangelista, V., Frassanito, A.M., Gualtieri, P.: Reconstruction of the absorption spectrum of an object spot from the colour values of the corresponding pixel(s) in its digital image: the challenge of algal colours. J. Microsc. **264**(3), 311–320 (2016)
10. Culverhouse, P., Herry, V., Parisini, T., Williams, R., Reguera, B., Gonzalez-Gil, S., Fonda, S., Cabrini, M.: DiCANN: a machine vision solution to biological specimen categorisation. In: Proceedings of the EurOCEAN 2000 Conference, pp. 239–240 (2000)
11. Culverhouse, P.F., Ellis, R., Simpson, R.G., Williams, R., Pierce, R.W., Turner, J.T.: Automatic categorisation of five species of cymatocylis (protozoa, tintinnida) by artificial neural network. Mar. Ecol. Prog. Ser. **107**, 273–280 (1994)
12. Culverhouse, P.F., Simpson, R.G., Ellis, R., Lindley, J.A., Williams, R., Parsini, T., Reguera, B., Bravo, I., Zoppoli, R., Earnshaw, G., McCall, H., Smith, G.C.: Automatic classification of field-collected dinoflagellates by artificial neural network. Mar. Ecol. Prog. Ser. **139**(1–3), 281–287 (1996)
13. Dieleman, S.: Classifying plankton with deep neural networks (2015). https://benanne.github.io/2015/03/17/plankton.html
14. Dorado, A.P.: Automatic recognition of diatoms and its applications to the study of water quality. Ph.D. Dissertation in the Universidad de Castilla-La Mancha (2016)
15. Embleton, K.V., Gibson, C.E., Heaney, S.I.: Automated counting of phytoplankton by pattern recognition: a comparison with a manual counting method. J. Plankton Res. **25**(6), 669–681 (2003)
16. Ferreira, T., Rasband, W.: Image user guide (2012). https://imagej.nih.gov/ij/docs/guide/user-guide-USbooklet.pdf
17. Filho, C.F.F.C., Levy, P.C., Xavier, C.D.M., Fujimoto, L.B.M., Costa, M.G.F.: Automatic identification of tuberculosis mycobacterium. Res. Biomed. Eng. **31**(1), 33–43 (2015)
18. Gerlach, S.R., Siedenberg, D., Gerlach, D., Schtigerl, K., Giuseppin, M.L.F., Hunik, J.: Influence of reactor systems on the morphology of aspergillus awamori. application of neural network and cluster analysis for characterization of fungal morphology. ProceAs Biochem. **33**(6), 601–615 (1998)
19. Ginoris, Y.P., Amaral, A.L., Nicolau, A., Ferreira, E.C., Coelho, M.A.Z.: Recognition of protozoa and metazoa using image analysis tools, discriminant analysis and neural network. In: International Conference on Chemometrics in Analytical Chemistry, p. 1 (2006)
20. Guo, G., Dyer, C.R.: Learning from examples in the small sample case: face expression recognition. Syst. Man Cybern. Part B: Cybern. **35**(3), 477–488 (2005)
21. Hiremath, P.S., Bannigidad, P.: Automatic classification of bacterial cells in digital microscopic images. Int. J. Eng. Technol. **2**(4), 9–15 (2009)
22. Hiremath, P.S., Bannigidad, P.: Automatic identification and classification of bacilli bacterial cell growth phases. Int. J. Comput. Appl. **1**, 48–52 (2010). Special Issue on RTIPPR
23. Hiremath, P.S., Bannigidad, P.: Digital image analysis of Cocci bacterial cells using active contour method. In: International Conference on Signal and Image Processing, pp. 163–168 (2010)
24. Hiremath, P.S., Bannigidad, P.: Digital microscopic image analysis of spiral bacterial cell groups. In: International Conference on Intelligent Systems & Data Processing, pp. 209–213 (2011)

25. Hiremath, P.S., Bannigidad, P.: Identification and classification of cocci bacterial cells in digital microscopic images. Int. J. Comput. Biol. Drug Des. **4**(3), 262–273 (2011)
26. Hiremath, P.S., Bannigidad, P.: Spiral bacterial cell image analysis using active contour method. Int. J. Comput. Appl. **37**(8), 5–9 (2012)
27. Hu, Q.: Application of statistical learning theory to plankton image analysis. Ph.D. Dissertation in the Massachusetts Institute of Technology and the Woods Hole Oceanographic Institution (2006)
28. Hu, Q., Davis, C.: Accurate automatic quantification of taxa-specific plankton abundance using dual classification with correction. Mar. Ecol. Prog. Ser. **306**, 51–61 (2006)
29. Kay, J.W., Shinn, A.P., Sommerville, C.: Towards an automated system for the identification of notifiable pathogens: using gyrodactylus salaris as an example. Parasitol. Today **15**(5), 201–206 (1999)
30. Kiranyaz, S., Ince, T., Pulkkinen, J., Gabbouj, M., Arje, J., Karkkainen, S., Tirronen, V., Juhola, M., Turpeinen, T., Meissner, K.: Classification and retrieval on macroinvertebrate image databases. Comput. Biol. Med. **41**(7), 463–472 (2011)
31. Kosov, S., Shirahama, K., Li, C., Grzegorzek, M.: Environmental microorganism classification using conditional random fields and deep convolutional neural networks. Pattern Recogn. p (2017)
32. Kramer, K.A.: Identifying plankton from grayscale silhouette images. Master thesis in University of South Florida (2005)
33. Kruk, M., Kozera, R., Osowski, S., Trzcinski, P., Paszt, L.S., Sumorok, B., Borkowski, B.: Computerized classification system for the identification of soil microorganisms. AIP Conf. Proc. **1648**(660018), 1–4 (2015)
34. Kruk, M., Kozera, R., Osowski, S., Trzcinski, P., Sas-Paszt, L., Sumorok, B., Borkowski, B.: Computerized classification systemfor the identification of soil microorganisms. Appl. Mathe. Inf. Sci. **10**(1), 21–31 (2016)
35. Li, C.: Content-Based Microscopic Image Analysis. Logos Verlag Berlin GmbH, Berlin (2016)
36. Li, C., Wang, K., Xu, N.: A survey for the applications of content-based microscopic image analysis in microorganism classification domains. Artif. Intell. Rev. p (2017)
37. Li, X., Chen, C.: A novel bacteria recognition method based on microscopic image analysis. New Zealand J. Agric. Res. **50**(5), 697–703 (2007)
38. Li, X., Chen, C.: A novel wastewater bacteria recognition method based on microscopic image analysis. In: WSEAS International Conference on Circuits, Systems, Electronics, Control and Signal Processing, pp. 265–271 (2008)
39. Li, X., Chen, C.: An improved BP neural network for wastewater bacteria recognition based on microscopic image analysis. WSEAS Trans. Comput. **8**(2), 237–247 (2009)
40. Li, X., Chen, C., Yv, Z.: A novel bacteria classification scheme based on microscopic image analysis. In: WSEAS International Conference on Applied Computer Science, pp. 447–451 (2007)
41. Mosleh, M.A., Manssor, H., Malek, S., Milow, P., Salleh, A.: A preliminary study on automated freshwater algae recognition and classification system. BMC Bioinf. **13**(Suppl 17), 1–13 (2012)
42. Nie, D., Shank, E.A., Jojic, V.: A deep framework for bacterial image segmentation and classification. In: ACM Conference on Bioinformatics, Computational Biology and Health Informatics, pp. 306–314 (2015)
43. Nielsen, M.A.: Neural Networks and Deep Learning. Determination Press (2015)

44. Orlov, N., Johnston, J., Macura, T., Shamir, L., Goldberg, I.: Computer vision for microscopy applications. In: Obinata, G., Dutta, A. (eds.) Vision Systems: Segmentation and Pattern Recognition, pp. 222–242. I-Tech, Austria (2007)
45. Osman, M.K., Mashor, M.Y., Jaafar, H.: Hybrid multilayered perceptron network trained by modified recursive prediction error-extreme learning machine for tuberculosis bacilli detection. In: Kuala Lumpur International Conference on Biomedical Engineering, pp. 667–673 (2011)
46. Osman, M.K., Mashor, M.Y., Jaafar, H.: Tuberculosis bacilli detection in Ziehl-Neelsen-stained tissue using affine moment invariants and extreme learning machine. In: IEEE International Colloquium on Signal Processing and Its Applications, pp. 232–236 (2011)
47. Osman, M.K., Mashor, M.Y., Jaafar, H.: Online sequential extreme learning machine for classification of *Mycobacterium tuberculosis* in Ziehl-Neelsen stained tissue. In: International Conference on Biomedical Engineering, pp. 139–143 (2012)
48. Pedraza, A., Bueno, G., Deniz, O., Cristobal, G., Blanco, S., Borrego-Ramos, M.: Automated diatom classification (Part B): a deep learning approach. Appl. Sci. **7**(5), 1–25 (2017)
49. Priya, E., Srinivasan, S.: Automated identification of tuberculosis objects in digital images using neural network and neuro fuzzy inference systems. J. Med. Imag. Health Inf. **5**(3), 506–512 (2015)
50. Priya, E., Srinivasan, S.: Separation of overlapping bacilli in microscopic digital TB images. Biocybern. Biomed. Eng. **35**(2), 87–99 (2015)
51. Priya, E., Srinivasan, S.: Automated object and image level classification of TB images using support vector neural network classifier. Biocybern. Biomed. Eng. **36**(4), 670–678 (2016)
52. Ronen, M., Guterman, H., Shabtai, Y.: Monitoring and control of pullulan production using vision sensor. J. Biochem. Biophys. Methods **51**(3), 243–249 (2002)
53. Rulaningtyas, R., Suksmono, A.B., Mengko, T.L.R.: Automatic classification of tuberculosis bacteria using neural network. In: International Conference on Electrical Engineering and Informatics, pp. 1–4 (2011)
54. Schaap, A., Rohrlack, T., Bellouard, Y.: Optofluidic microdevice for algae classification: a comparison of results from discriminant analysis and neural network pattern recognition. In: Proceedings SPIE 8251, Microfluidics, BioMEMS, and Medical Microsystems X, pp. 825,104-1–825,104-10 (2012)
55. Schulze, K., Tillich, U.M., Dandekar, T., Frohme, M.: PlanktoVision-an automated analysis system for the identification of phytoplankton. BMC Bioinf. **14**(115), 1–10 (2013)
56. Shabtai, Y., Ronen, M., Muknenev, I., Guterman, H.: Monitoring micorbial morphogenetic changes in a fermentation process by a self-tuning vision system (STVS). Pergamon **20**(1), 321–326 (1996)
57. Vapnik, V.N.: Statistical Learning Theory. Wiley-Interscience, New York (1998)
58. Veropoulos, K., Campbell, C., Learmonth, G.: Image processing and neural computing used in the diagnosis of tuberculosis. In: IEEE Colloquium on Intelligent Methods in Healthcare and Medical Applications, pp. 8/1–8/4 (1998)
59. Wang, D., Wang, B., Yan, Y.: The identification of powdery mildew spores image based on the integration of intelligent spore image sequence capture device. In: International Conference on Intelligent Information Hiding and Multimedia Signal Processing, pp. 177–180 (2013)
60. Weller, A.F., Harris, A.J., Ware, J.A.: Two supervised neural networks for classification of sedimentary organic matter images from palynological preparations. Math. Geol. **39**(7), 657–671 (2007)

14   C. Li et al.

61. Widmer, K.W., Srikumar, D., Pillai, S.D.: Use of artificial neural networks to accurately identify cryptosporidium oocyst and giardia cyst images. Appl. Environ. Microbiol. **71**(1), 80–84 (2005)
62. Wit, P., Busscher, H.J.: Application of an artificial neural network in the enumeration of yeasts and bacteria adhering to solid substrata. J. Microbiol. Methods **32**(3), 281–290 (1998)
63. Zeder, M., Kohler, E., Pernthaler, J.: Automated quality assessment of autonomously acquired microscopic images of fluorescently stained bacteria. Cytometry Part A **77(A)**, 76–85 (2010)

On the Influence of Image Features Wordlength Reduction on Texture Classification

Michał Strzelecki$^{(\boxtimes)}$, Marcin Kociołek, and Andrzej Materka

Institute of Electronics, Lodz University of Technology,
ul. Wolczanska 211/215, 90-924 Lodz, Poland
michal.strzelecki@p.lodz.pl
http://eletel.p.lodz.pl/mstrzel

Abstract. Texture is present in a large number of medical images. Its structure codes selected properties of visualized organ and tissues so texture can be rich source of information regarding their condition. Quantitative texture analysis plays significant role in imaging diagnosis support systems, enabling segmentation of analyzed organs, detection of lesions, and assessment of the degree of their pathological change. Unfortunately, medical images are often corrupted by noise which affect texture based image features. One of the steps of texture feature extraction is reduction of gray levels number which is performed after a normalization of pixel intensities inside a region of interest. This reduces the noise effect on texture feature values. We demonstrated, based on analysis of natural and MR images, that such reduction improves classification accuracy while reducing the computational costs.

Keywords: Texture features · Image processing

1 Introduction

Texture is present in a large number of medical images. Its structure codes selected properties of visualized organ and tissues. In tomographic images, texture describes cross-section of internal structures being a rich source of information regarding their condition. Thus, quantitative texture analysis plays significant role in imaging diagnosis support systems, enabling segmentation of analyzed organs, detection of lesions, and assessment of the degree of their pathological change. Unfortunately, medical images are mostly corrupted by noise and affected by artifacts that are specific for a given imaging modality. For example, in MRI noise is produced by the stochastic motion of free electrons in radio frequency receiver coils and by eddy current loses in the patient [2]. In Ultrasound images the superposition of acoustical echoes coming witch random phases and amplitudes produces speckle noise [13]. In CT Poisson noise is caused statistical error of low photon counts in detectors [3]. Noise, beside of degrading the image quality, influences also analysis results by distorting estimated values of

© Springer International Publishing AG, part of Springer Nature 2019
E. Pietka et al. (Eds.): ITIB 2018, AISC 762, pp. 15–26, 2019.
https://doi.org/10.1007/978-3-319-91211-0_2

texture parameters [5]. There are multiple research paper dealing with noise reduction in medical images below some examples are shown. In [6] median filters with weighted central elements are applied for impulse noise removal. In [22] adaptive anisotropic filtering is used for removing noise in cone beam computed tomography (CBCT) images. A speckle-reduction method based on soft thresholding of the wavelet coefficients of a logarithmically transformed medical ultrasound image is described in [9]. An application of partial differential equations for noise removal in MRI images is shown in [11]. There also multiple reviews of noise reduction techniques eg. [16,17] or [14]. Generally, noise removal techniques are tedious (especially in the case of the multiplicative noise present in MR images) [15], moreover their implementation often lead to the change of the image content which may reduce important diagnostic information, e.g. due to granular effects caused by local estimation of non-stationary noise parameters in some MR parallel sequences [1]. Texture feature estimation consists of four major steps:

1. image intensity normalization, usually performed independently for each separate region of interest,
2. reduction of gray levels number,
3. linear or nonlinear image transform (wavelet, Gray Level Co-occurrence Matrix, Run Length Matrix),
4. calculation of statistical parameters from a given transform, which result in textural features.

Reduction of gray levels number reduces the noise effect on texture feature values. We demonstrated, based on analysis of natural and MR images, that such reduction improves classification accuracy while reducing the computational costs. This can be viewed as optimization of feature estimation parameters. The experiments were performed for three texture parameter groups widely used in medical image analysis, i.e. gray level co-occurrence matrix (GLCM), run-length matrix (RLM) and Haar wavelet transform based.

2   Materials and Methods

Ten image textures from Brodatz album [4] were considered for analysis (Fig. 1). There were 256 gray level images with dimensions 512×512 pixels.

These images were corrupted by additive Gaussian noise for two values of standard deviation, $\sigma_1 = 0.01$ and $\sigma_2 = 0.02$ (scaled to $[0 \ldots 1]$ pixel intensity range). Also, MR liver images were analyzed. They represent healthy control and patients with liver fibrosis. They were imaged with breath-hold respiration motion artifact reduction technique, using a 3T MRI device (Philips Achieva) and a T1 weighted pulse sequence (THRIVE iso: ultra-fast gradient echo, $TR/TE = 2.76/1.36$ ms, $a = 10°$, $FOV = 400 \times 400$ mm^2, matrix size $= 192 \times 192$, isotropic voxel $= 2.08 \times 2.08 \times 2.08$ mm^3). For analysis, 13 cross-sections of each case representing middle part of the liver were considered. Sample cross-sections are presented in Fig. 2.

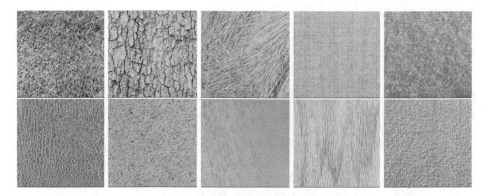

Fig. 1. Analyzed textures from Brodatz album [4]; from top left: 'Grass' (D9), 'Bark' (D12), 'Straw' (D15), 'Herringbone weave' (D15), 'Woolen cloth' (D19), 'Pressed calf leather' (D24), 'Beach sand' (D29), 'Water' (D38), 'Wood grain' (D68), 'Raffia' (D84)

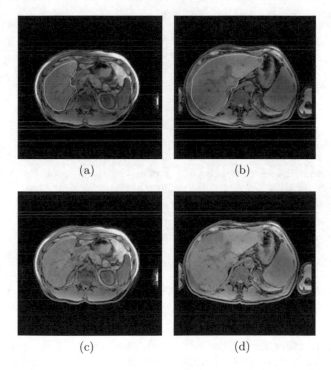

(a)   (b)

(c)   (d)

Fig. 2. Sample slices of 192 × 192-pixel MR liver images; lines delimit ROIs of: (a) healthy and (b) fibrotic liver; corresponding images after ROI inhomogeneity correction using the multiplicative model, healthy (c) and fibrotic (d)

The liver disease was diagnosed based on liver biopsy. The images of each type were acquired for a patient and a healthy volunteer with their informed consent, approved by a local ethics committee (courtesy of Dr Jacques de Certaines, within the framework of EU COST B21 action [18]).

The steps of image analysis include ROI definition, feature extraction, feature selection and classification. For Brodatz textures, there 16 non-overlapping square ROIs (square side equal to 60 pixels) were defined while ROIs for liver images were manually delineated by the expert. Before analysis, each ROI was normalized by calculating mean value (m) and standard deviation (σ) of its gray levels. Normalization involved ROI mean value subtraction and division of the difference by the standard deviation. Subsequently, the ROI gray levels were quantized in the range of $m \pm 3\sigma$ [21]. Next, for each ROI the texture features were estimated for standard images (8 bit coded) and after gray level reduction to 6 bits and 4 bits per pixel, respectively, as shown in Fig. 3. For better visualization of the influence of number of gray-level reduction to the texture the color map was used to visualize sample ROIs in Fig. 3.

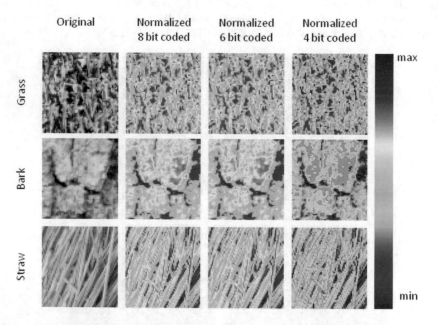

Fig. 3. Examples of analyzed ROIs (60 × 60 pixels) for three Brodatz textures; original image and three normalized images coded witch 8, 6 and 4 bits shown in pseudocolors

The texture parameters were estimated based on the following approaches: co-occurrence matrix, run-length matrix, and Haar wavelet transform. A detailed definition of these features is described in [10, 20]. To reduce the number of texture features to most significant ones, the Fisher criterion was applied. SVM classifier was used for Brodatz textures whereas 1-nearest neighbor classifier $(1 - NN)$ in the case of liver images. Only selected parameters with the highest Fisher coefficient were used (three features for natural textures and two for MR images).

Before analysis of the liver images, they background nonuniformity was corrected. Such artifact in the case of MRI has source is in spatial variation of the measured RF signal power (e.g. related to B_0 magnetic field or RF receiver coils nonuniformities) [19]. Such intensity variations are of multiplicative nature, and it was demonstrated in [20] that they can strongly influence image classification. No noise reduction was performed for the analyzed data. For the multiplicative model, the corrected image was obtained through

$$f_m(x, y) = f(x, y) f_s(x, y, a_{opt}) \qquad (1)$$

where f_s is the background image intensity inside ROI modeled by a 3rd order polynomial

$$f_s(x, y) = 1 + a_0 + a_1 x + a_2 y + a_3 x^2 + a_4 xy + a_5 y^2 + a_6 x^3 + a_7 x^2 y + a_8 xy^2 + a_9 y^3 \qquad (2)$$

The parameter vector $a = [a_0, a_1, \ldots, a_9]$ of the surface (2) is used to represent the multiplicative artifacts. a_{opt} represent optimal parameters of (2) computed through minimization of error function defined as a difference between the background image intensity and its model defined by (2). Details of the background nonuniformity correction are provided in [12].

3   Results

Classification results of textures from Fig. 1 are shown in Table 1. Misclassification errors were evaluated as average values obtained as a result of 5-fold cross validation testing applied for SVM classifiers. Experiments were performed separately for three texture features groups (GLCM, RLM, Haar wavelets). The parameters were estimated for original images as well for corrupted by additive Gaussian noise with two different standard deviation values, $\sigma - 0.01$ and $\sigma = 0.02$, respectively. For all types of images, the parameters were evaluated for image coded by 8, 6, and 4 bits per pixel.

Table 1. Classification errors [%] for Brodatz textures evaluated for different texture parameter groups, number of bits per pixel, for original and noisy images

	Bits/Pixel	GLCM	Run length	Wavelet
No noise	8	18.8	27.5	14.4
	6	21.9	30.6	11.9
	4	25.0	28.7	14.4
$\sigma = 0.01$	8	28.1	52.5	17.5
	6	22.5	44.4	16.9
	4	21.2	45.6	16.2
$\sigma = 0.02$	8	46.9	57.5	19.4
	6	42.1	55.6	19.4
	4	30.6	55.0	16.2

As can be observed from Table 1, in case of GLCM based features for noiseless images the classification error is increasing with reduced number of image grey levels. It is rather obvious since decreasing of image bits/pixel eliminates some texture details reducing total amount of information in the image. Obtained results are also in line with these presented in [7] where influence of grey level quantization on the classification of various datasets with use of GLCM features were investigated Similarly, in the case of Run Length matrix based features the lowest classification error exists for 8 bits per pixel. For those features the maximum error was observed for 6 bits per pixel. A different situation happens for wavelet based features. This time the lowest error was for 6 bits per pixel. However, in the presence of noise the opposite effect is noticed - for all groups of texture features the classification error is reduced when number of bit per pixel is getting smaller. It is worth to notice that wavelet based features are noticeable less sensitive for the noise and change of number of bits used for pixel intensity coding.

Distributions of two features selected for liver classification (according to Fisher criterion) along with obtained error is presented in Fig. 4. Again, experiments were performed for three texture feature groups (GLCM, RLM and Haar wavelet) and three values of image gray levels (8, 6, and 4 bits/pixel). Convention of wavelet feature names will be explained in Discussion Section.

As in the case of natural textures, the classification error is decreasing with reduced number of image bit per pixel. Also, better separation between healthy and fibrotic liver classes is observed. This agrees with classification results of ultrasound breast images presented in [8]. There, analysis of GLCM features as a function of gray level quantization was performed. Moreover, a change of number of bits coding the intensity has marginal influence on discrimination capabilities of wavelet based texture features.

4   Discussion

The reduction of classification error observed for smaller number of image grey levels for GLCM features and noisy textures can be explained by analyzing how the noise influences the GLCM structure. It is illustrated in Fig. 5, where such matrices for 'Beach sand' texture (original and noisy with $\sigma = 0.01$) are presented for various image bits/pixel rates (matrices obtained for 6 and 4 bits per pixel were reshaped to the size of GLCM estimated for 8 bits/pixel). It can be noticed that noise added to the image 'blurs' the GLCM resulting in wider distribution of its elements (Fig. 5(d) versus Fig. 5(a) where GLCM for an original texture is shown). These additional matrix entries modify values of estimated parameters, making their values different from these characterizing original texture, which in consequence leads to worse classification results. For reduced number of image gray levels the 'blurring' effect becomes less significant. There, a noise is partly suppressed which results in removing of some GLCM entries (see Fig. 5(e) where GLCM for 6 bits/pixel is shown). For example, the 'tail' visible in top left part of Fig. 5(d) is lost in 5(e), making the GLCM

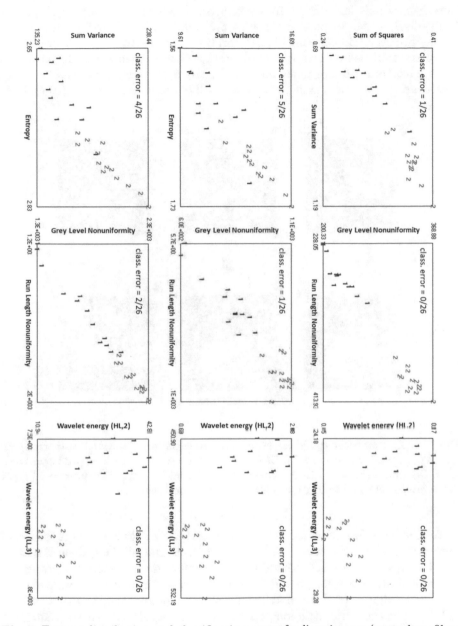

Fig. 4. Feature distribution and classification errors for liver images (control vs. fibrosis); analysis performed for 8 bit (left column), 6 bit (middle column), and 4 bit (right column) images; top row represents GLCM features, middle row – RLM features, bottom – wavelet transform based features; '1' indicates samples of healthy liver, '2' represents fibrotic ones; all GLCM features were calculated for matrices build for horizontal direction and interpixel distance 1

more like its noiseless version from Fig. 5(b). This similarity is even bigger for 4 bits/pixel, as can be observed in Figs. 5(c) and (f). The blurring effect is still visible, however GLCM from Fig. 5(f) probably preserves most salient properties of the analyzed texture while lacks majority of elements introduced by the noise. Therefore, texture parameters evaluated from this matrix enable better classification than those estimated from GLCMs presented in Figs. 5(d) and (e).

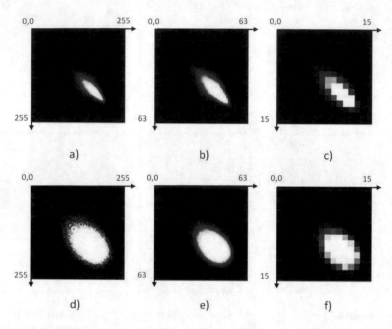

Fig. 5. GLCM matrices (build for horizontal direction and interpixel distance 1) for 'Beach sand' texture; top row: GLCM for original texture, image bits/pixel equal to 8 (a), 6 (b), and 4 (c), respectively; bottom row: GLCM for noisy texture $\sigma = 0.01$), of image bits/pixel equal to 8 (d), 6 (e), and 4 (f), respectively

A different effect of added noise is observed on RL matrix. There, shape of noise distribution influences distribution of texture runs making them Gaussian like. This is shown in Fig. 6, where RL matrices for 'grass' texture are presented, for original and noisy image and for various image bits per pixel values. Only three first columns of these matrices are shown (for run lengths equal to 1, 2, and 3), since there are little longer runs in the image. Thus, all the remaining RL matrix columns are sparse. Additive Gaussian noise is reflected in RL matrix by normal-like distribution of first column elements (which codes distribution of runs with length 1, corresponding to the pixels whose neighbors have different values from them), as shown in Figs. 6(d)–(f). This effect occurs independently of the texture type, thus making discrimination of textures based on RLM features not very efficient. This is reflected in classification errors values that are lower for GLCM features than RLM ones. For original 8 bit textures this difference is less than 9% while for noisy images is increased in the favor of GLCM parameters and varies from 12% to 25%, depending of the noise variance. Reduction of image gray levels smoothes distribution of runs (see Figs. 6(d) and (e)), increasing the similarity between matrices estimated for original and noisy texture. Thus for 4 bits/pixel estimated features are less noise dependent which results in slightly decrease of classification error. Also, number of longer runs is increasing, as can be observed in distribution of columns 2 and 3 (Figs. 6(b),(c) and (e),(f)).

As this was shown in Table 1, noise has a reduced influence on discriminative power of wavelet based features. This is due the way how the features are derived. In our case a Harr wavelet is used because it has the smallest kernel, which allows for simple calculation of features in arbitrary shaped ROIs. Simplifying, rectangular part of the image containing arbitrary region of interest is filtered by means of four filters with kernels shown below.

$$\mathbf{LL} = \begin{bmatrix} 0.25 & 0.25 \\ 0.25 & 0.25 \end{bmatrix}, \mathbf{LH} = \begin{bmatrix} 0.5 & -0.5 \\ 0.5 & -0.5 \end{bmatrix}, \mathbf{HL} = \begin{bmatrix} 0.5 & 0.5 \\ -0.5 & -0.5 \end{bmatrix}, \mathbf{LH} = \begin{bmatrix} 0.5 & -0.5 \\ -0.5 & 0.5 \end{bmatrix}$$

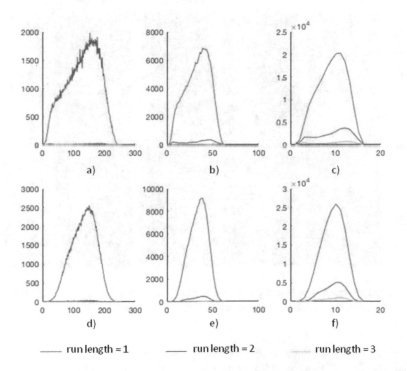

Fig. 6. Three first rows of RL matrices (build for horizontal direction) for 'Grass' texture; top row: original texture, number of image bits/pixel equal to 8 (a), 6 (b), and 4 (c), respectively; bottom row: noisy texture ($\sigma = 0.01$), number of image bits/pixel equal to 8 (d), 6 (e), and 4 (f), respectively

Results of those filters are called images of wavelet coefficients for four bands: **LL**, **LH**, **HL** and **HH** for the first scale of 2D wavelet decomposition. The band **LL** is decimated by four and acts as input for the next scale of the decomposition. In this way one can obtain images of wavelet coefficients calculated at multiple scales. The wavelet based features are mean pixel energies (sum of squared pixel values divided by the number of pixels) of wavelet coefficient images calculated in the ROI fitted to the given scale. For given ROI there are four wavelet energies calculated at each scale (The naming scheme is as follow: Wavelet energy, band, scale). For first scale there is averaging of 4 pixels in **LL** band and averaging of two pairs of pixels in other bands. Because of cascaded algorithm on the second scale 16 pixels values are averaged during **LL** band calculation and two times 8 pixels for other bands. Due to averaging the noise is attenuated, especially for the larger scales of the wavelet decomposition. Figure 7 shows pixel energies of wavelet coefficient images for scale 2 and band **LH**.

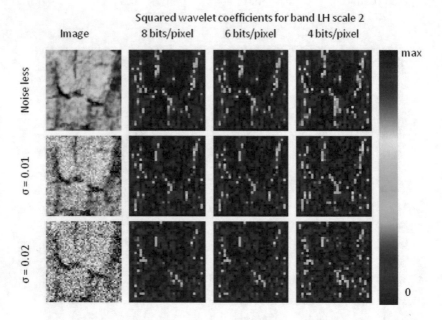

Fig. 7. Pixel energies of wavelet coefficient images for scale 2 and band LH derived for one of investigated regions of interest from Brodatz texture 'bark'

As it can be easy seen on Fig. 7 noise have limited influence on energies of wavelet coefficient images. Moreover wordlength reduction causes that images of wavelet coefficient energies for noisy images are more similar to the ones calculated for non-distorted ones. This can be explained by the fact that low count of quantization levels exposes basic structure of the texture. Summarizing, mean energies of wavelet coefficient images gives quite stable classification results noise and bit per pixel invariant.

5   Conclusion

It was demonstrated for selected textures that limitation of gray level image bits/pixel reduces the noise effect on feature values derived from the image. Based on analysis of Brodatz textures and MR liver images, such approach improved classification accuracy. These preliminary results are promising. However, the experiments must be repeated for much wider class of biomedical data. Also, other popular texture parameters, like Local Binary Pattern or Gabor filters will be investigated in the forthcoming studies. Moreover, the effect of image normalization on classification of noisy textures will be also analyzed.

References

1. Aja-Fernández, S., Tristán-Vega, A., Alberola-López, C.: Noise estimation in single- and multiple-coil magnetic resonance data based on statistical models. Magn. Reson. Imaging **27**(10), 1397–1409 (2009). https://doi.org/10.1016/J.MRI.2009. 05.025. http://www.sciencedirect.com/science/article/pii/S0730725X09001404? via%3Dihub
2. Aja-Fernández, S., Vegas-Sánchez-Ferrero, G.: Statistical Analysis of Noise in MRI: Modeling, Filtering and Estimation, 1st edn. Springer International Publishing, Cham (2016). https://doi.org/10.1007/978-3-319-39934-8
3. Boas, F.E., Fleischmann, D.: Imaging in medicine. Future Med. **4**. http://www. openaccessjournals.com/articles/ct-artifacts-causes-and-reduction-techniques. html
4. Brodatz, P.: Textures: a photographic album for artists and designers. Dover Publications, New York (1966)
5. Brynolfsson, P., Nilsson, D., Torheim, T., Asklund, T., Karlsson, C.T., Trygg, J., Nyholm, T., Garpebring, A.: Haralick texture features from apparent diffusion coefficient (ADC) MRI images depend on imaging and pre-processing parameters. Sci. Rep. **7**(1), 1–11 (2017). https://doi.org/10.1038/s41598-017-04151-4
6. Chervyakov, N., Lyakhov, P., Orazaev, A., Valueva, M.: Efficiency analysis of the image impulse noise cleaning using median filters with weighted central element. In: 2017 International Multi-Conference on Engineering, Computer and Information Sciences (SIBIRCON), pp. 141–146. IEEE (2017). https://doi.org/10.1109/ SIBIRCON.2017.8109856. http://ieeexplore.ieee.org/document/8109856/
7. Clausi, D.A.: An analysis of co-occurrence texture statistics as a function of grey level quantization. Can. J. Remote Sens. **28**(1), 45–62 (2002). https://doi.org/10. 5589/m02-004
8. Gómez, W., Pereira, W.C., Infantosi, A.F.: Analysis of co-occurrence texture statistics as a function of gray-level quantization for classifying breast ultrasound. IEEE Trans. Med. Imaging **31**(10), 1889–1899 (2012). https://doi.org/10.1109/ TMI.2012.2206398
9. Gupta, S., Chauhan, R.C., Sexana, S.C.: Wavelet-based statistical approach for speckle reduction in medical ultrasound images. Med. Biol. Eng. Comput. **42**, 189–192 (2004). https://doi.org/10.1007/BF02344630
10. Kociolek, M., Materka, A., Strzelecki, M., Szczypinski, P.: Discrete wavelet transform - derived features for digital image texture analysis. In: International Conference on Signals and Electronic Systems, September, Lodz, pp. 163–168 (2001)

11. Lysaker, M., Lundervold, A., Tai, X.-C.: Noise removal using fourth-order partial differential equation with applications to medical magnetic resonance images in space and time. IEEE Trans. Image Proces. **12**(12), 1579–1590 (2003). https://doi.org/10.1109/TIP.2003.819229. http://ieeexplore.ieee.org/document/1257394/
12. Materka, A., Strzelecki, M.: On the importance of MRI nonuniformity correction for texture analysis. In: 2013 Conference on Processing Algorithms Architectures Arrangements and Application (ISPA), pp. 118–123. IEEE (2013)
13. Michailovich, O., Tannenbaum, A.: Despeckling of medical ultrasound images. IEEE Trans. Ultrason. Ferroelectr. Freq. Control **53**(1), 64–78 (2006). https://doi.org/10.1109/TUFFC.2006.1588392. http://ieeexplore.ieee.org/document/1588392/
14. Ouahabi, A.: A review of wavelet denoising in medical imaging. In: 2013 8th International Workshop on Systems, Signal Processing and their Applications (WoSSPA), pp. 19–26. IEEE (2013). https://doi.org/10.1109/WoSSPA.2013.6602330. http://ieeexplore.ieee.org/document/6602330/
15. Pieciak, T., Aja-Fernandez, S., Vegas-Sanchez-Ferrero, G.: Non-stationary rician noise estimation in parallel MRI using a single image: a variance-stabilizing approach. IEEE Trans. Patt. Anal. Mach. Intell. **39**(10), 2015–2029 (2017). https://doi.org/10.1109/TPAMI.2016.2625789. http://ieeexplore.ieee.org/document/7736984/
16. Priya, D.K., Sam, B.B., Lavanya, S., Sajin, A.P.: A survey on medical image denoising using optimisation technique and classification. In: 2017 International Conference on Information Communication and Embedded Systems (ICICES), pp. 1–6. IEEE (2017). https://doi.org/10.1109/ICICES.2017.8070729. http://ieeexplore.ieee.org/document/8070729/
17. Somkuwar, A., Bhargava, S.: Noise reduction techniques in medical imaging data-a review. In: 2nd International Conference on Mechanical, Electronics and Mechatronics Engineering (ICMEME 2013), vol. 1, 17–18 June 2013, London, UK, pp. 115–119 (2013)
18. Strzelecki, M., de Certaines, J., Ko, S.: Segmentation of 3D MR liver images using synchronised oscillators network. In: 2007 International Symposium on Information Technology Convergence (ISITC 2007), pp. 259–263. IEEE (2007). https://doi.org/10.1109/ISITC.2007.13. http://ieeexplore.ieee.org/document/4410646/
19. Styner, M., Leemput, K.V.: Retrospective evaluation and correction of intensity inhomogeneity. In: Landini, L., Positano, V., Santarelli, M. (eds.) Advanced Image Processing in Magnetic Resonance Imaging, pp. 145–186. CRC Press, Boca Raton (2005)
20. Szczypinski, P., Kociolek, M., Materka, A., Strzelecki, M.: Computer program for image texture analysis in Ph.D. students laboratory. In: Proceedings International Conference Signals and Electronic Systems, pp. 255–261 (2001)
21. Szczypinski, P.M., Strzelecki, M., Materka, A., Klepaczko, A.: MaZda-a software package for image texture analysis. Comput. Methods Programs Biomed. **94**(1), 66–76 (2009). https://doi.org/10.1016/j.cmpb.2008.08.005
22. Yilmaz, E., Kayikcioglu, T., Kayipmaz, S.: Noise removal of CBCT images using an adaptive anisotropic diffusion filter. In: 2017 40th International Conference on Telecommunications and Signal Processing (TSP), pp. 650–653 (2017). https://doi.org/10.1109/TSP.2017.8076067. http://ieeexplore.ieee.org/document/8076067/

Application of Fuzzy Image Concept
to Medical Images Matching

Piotr Zarychta[(✉)]

Faculty of Biomedical Engineering, Silesian University of Technology,
Roosevlta 40, Zabrze, Poland
piotr.zarychta@polsl.pl

Abstract. The main aim of this research is presenting an automated image matching methodology being used in the field of medicine for inter- and intraobjectional image matching. This paper shows a different approach avoiding the standard procedures associated with performing four main steps of the registration process: feature detection, feature matching, mapping function design and image transformation with resampling, and replacing them with the fuzzy image concept combined with the use of similarity measures. This methodology has been implemented in MATLAB and tested on clinical T1- and T2-weighted magnetic resonance imaging (MRI) slices of the knee joint in coronal and sagittal plane.

Keywords: Entropy measure of fuzziness · Similarity measures
Medical image matching · Knee joint · Cruciate ligament

1 Introduction

The developments in medical imaging techniques have made it possible that at present clinical diagnosis and then treatment verification are to a large extent based on medical imaging. Nowadays the most popular techniques for medical imaging are: X-ray Imaging, MRI-Magnetic Resonance Imaging, CT-Computed Tomography, USG-Ultrasonography and also MRS-Magnetic Resonance Spectroscopy, PET-Positron Emission Tomography and SPECT-Single Photon Emission Computed Tomography. These techniques provide functional information – about metabolic processes of the human body (PET, SPECT, MRS) and anatomical information – about the anatomic structure of the human body (MRI, USG, X-ray, CT). In many cases, the patient needs to perform various medical tests in different places (hospitals, clinics, medical laboratories, etc.). It is often necessary to integrate the information obtained from two or more medical imaging studies for the same patient, but at different points in time (for example before and after medical treatment). The differences in patient positioning and different image acquisition parameters require registration of these images to be performed before overlapping them. The literature review shows that medical image registration is a key problem [11, 27]. It is a highly complex

© Springer International Publishing AG, part of Springer Nature 2019
E. Pietka et al. (Eds.): ITIB 2018, AISC 762, pp. 27–38, 2019.
https://doi.org/10.1007/978-3-319-91211-0_3

and absolutely crucial problem especially in medical application [18, 19], where the registration process should be automatic and reliable.

The literature review shows that over the last twenty years the medical image registration has been developed significantly for many organs of the human body [18]. Image registration can be performed for both soft- and hard- tissues on internal and external organs of the human body. Below there are some examples of image registration for different organs of the human body. The most popular in this respect are: brain [14, 17], heart [12], lung [16, 20], retina [15], breast [13], bones [9, 10] and knee [22, 25].

The aim of the paper is to show a different approach avoiding the standard procedures associated with the performance of four main steps of the registration process: feature detection, feature matching, mapping function design and image transformation with resampling [27], and replacing them with the fuzzy image concept combined with the use of similarity measures. Secondly, this article demonstrates the use of this methodology for inter- and intraobjectional image matching.

Fuzzy logic applied to the cruciate ligaments analysis allows a comprehensive knee joint computer aided diagnosis tool to be developed. The classical methods are useful in the case of artificial image analysis, but unfortunately do not give correct results in biomedical use. In the case of the biomedical images two important problems are faced:the first concerns inaccuracy (lack of possibility of precise description of the segmented structures) and the second concerns data uncertainty (identical results are difficult to obtain especially for the cruciate ligaments of the knee joint). Therefore, in many practical applications fuzzy methods are used (fuzzy c-means, fuzzy connectedness) [1, 8, 21, 24].

2   Methodology

Many years ago in 1972, Deluca and Termini introduced a definition of non-probabilistic entropy in the setting of fuzzy set theory [6]. And 25 years later, Czogala and Leski used this concept to the ECG signal processing [4]. In 2006 the fuzzy image concept based on the entropy measure of fuzziness, after extension to two dimensions and combined with the use of similarity measures, has been implemented to medical images matching. First, these were MRIs of the knee joint, and then also MRIs of the brain [25]. The preliminary results of pilot studies met with positive opinions of reviewers and led the author of this paper to test this methodology for inter- and intraobjectional image matching in various planes of MRI.

Generally the entropy measure of fuzziness may be expressed as highlighting the parts of the image with a significant difference in the intensity of the neighbouring pixels.

In this paper the methodology of finding the entropy measure of fuzziness is not described in detail. An exhaustive description hereof can be found in [25].

The next step in the procedure of image matching (especially for medical images used in diagnostics), is the assessment of similarity (usually the assessment of similarity of slices in whole series). For this purpose similarity measures are used. In practice, there are two main groups of similarity measures based on the features and the intensities, respectively [18, 19, 25].

Feature-based measures may use the information about the objects obtained in the image processing. This information can be used for the evaluation of similarity. Extracted features should be chosen in order to reflect the essential elements of differentiation for the compared images, i.e. the location of control points, parameters describing the size and shape of the selected structures included in the image etc.

Intensity-based measures use the information determined on the basis of gray levels in two medical images. The analysis may concern the entire image, or (exceptionally in order to omit non-relevant image parts) separate regions of interest. The advantage of this group of measures (especially when they are used for the entire image) is the option to skip the phase of features extraction. The latter is often complicated, time-consuming, and the results may be subject to errors. The disadvantage of the intensity-based measures is their being less sensitive to small differences in the compared images, especially when these differences concern rather the shape of the image structures that do not translate into a global change in intensity (hence there is often the need to analyze only selected regions of interests).

In the research described in this article only the following intensity-based measures have been taken into consideration: NCC, GC and GD. Normalized cross-correlation is defined by the equation:

$$
NCC = \frac{\sum_{\substack{m,n \in I_1 \\ m,n \in I_2}} \left[I_1(m,n) - \overline{I}_1\right] \left[I_2(m,n) - \overline{I}_2\right]}{\sqrt{\sum_{m,n \in I_1} \left[I_1(m,n) - \overline{I}_1\right]^2} \sqrt{\sum_{m,n \in I_2} \left[I_2(m,n) - \overline{I}_2\right]^2}}, \tag{1}
$$

where $\overline{I}_1$ and $\overline{I}_2$ are the mean intensity values in the images I_1 and I_2, respectively. From a practical point of view it is very desirable, in the case of normalized cross-correlation, that neither of the different values of contrast and brightness, respectively, should affect the similarity measure.

Gradient correlation (GC) is a form of the gradient of normalized cross-correlation (1), in which the gradient images $\frac{dI_1}{dm}, \frac{dI_1}{dn}, \frac{dI_2}{dm}$ i $\frac{dI_2}{dn}$ are used. These images can be obtained by horizontal $H_{3\times3}$ and vertical $V_{3\times3}$ Sobel templates.

GC is then calculated as NCC between $\frac{dI_1}{dm}$ and $\frac{dI_2}{dm}$ as well as $\frac{dI_1}{dn}$ and $\frac{dI_2}{dn}$. The final value of this measure is equal to the average of the two normalized cross correlations.

GD is defined by the equation as follows:

$$
GD = \sum_{m,n \in I} \frac{A_H}{A_H + \left[I_{difH}(m,n)\right]^2} + \sum_{m,n \in I} \frac{A_V}{A_V + \left[I_{difV}(m,n)\right]^2}, \tag{2}
$$

where A_H and A_V are constant values determining the variance of the reference image. Gradient difference evaluates two differential images

$$I_{difH} = \frac{dI_1}{dm} - s\frac{dI_2}{dm} \tag{3}$$

and

$$I_{difV} = \frac{dI_1}{dn} - s\frac{dI_2}{dn}, \tag{4}$$

which are calculated on the basis of the image gradients.

3   Discussion and Results

The methodology has been tested on 107 clinical T1- and T2-weighted MRI studies of the knee joint (Fig. 1). This group consists of 62 normal and 45 pathological cases of posterior cruciate ligaments as well as 33 normal and 74 pathological cases of anterior cruciate ligaments. The application of fuzzy image concept to the matching of the MRI slices of the knee joint has been tested in coronal and sagittal planes of these images.

In the case of the interobject matching, on the basis of the reference slice containing ACL or PCL structures in one subject (Fig. 2(a)) slices containing the same anatomical structures were sought in the MRI study of the knee joint of another subject (Fig. 2(b)).

Figure 3 shows the results of the matching process for two slices containing ACL and PCL structures (Fig. 3). For slices no. 11 and no. 12 of the 1st group (first subject) the similarity measure value is the highest for slices no. 12 and no. 13 of the 2nd group (another subject), respectively. In both cases the highest value of the similarity measure indicates the most similar slice from the 2nd group.

The proposed method of using fuzzy image for finding the most similar MRI slices in the interobject matching (slices containing ACL and PCL structures) has been tested on 107 clinical T1-weighted MR studies of the knee joint in the coronal plane. The correct results have been yielded in 88 cases, and the accuracy of the method equals 82.24%.

In the next stage of the study the concept of the fuzzy image has been tested in order to find a selected pathology of the ACLs or PCLs. In this way, on the basis of a reference slice containing the pathological structures of ACL or PCL (ligament rupture of the 'shaving brush' type) in one subject (Fig. 4(a)) slices were sought containing the same pathological structures in the MRI study of the knee joint of another subject (Fig. 4(b)). The ligament rupture of the 'shaving brush' type is characterized in the MRI study by massive swelling and fraying ligament fibers over their entire length [2,3,5,7].

The proposed method of finding a selected pathology (rupture of the 'shaving brush' type) has been tested on 14 pathological cases of PCLs and 27 pathological cases of ACLs containing the rupture of the 'shaving brush' type (Table 1). In 9 cases of PCLs and 18 cases of ACLs the proposed method gave a correct result

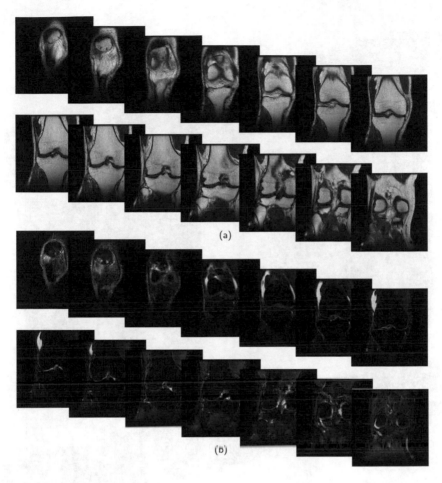

Fig. 1. MRI slices of the knee joint in the coronal plane (a) T1-weighted (b) T2-weighted

(the accuracy of the method equals 64.29% and 66.67%, respectively). In other cases (mainly due to different sizes of the knee joint) it was necessary to modify the algorithm. This modification consisted, firstly, in finding regions of interest which include the ligaments structures [22, 23] in both groups (in the 1st group – including the reference slice and in the 2nd group – including the test slices), and, secondly, transferring a larger region for both series and finally performing calculations only for this region of interest. This way by 2D ROI finding can significantly reduce the computational complexity and the analysed region is reduced by over 6 times (2D ROI: 100 × 100 pixels, entire slice: 256 × 256 pixels). In this case, the proposed approach allowed proper identification of the rupture of the 'shaving brush' type in both cases of ligaments, and the accuracy of the method is equal to 92.86% for PCL and 96.29% for ACL.

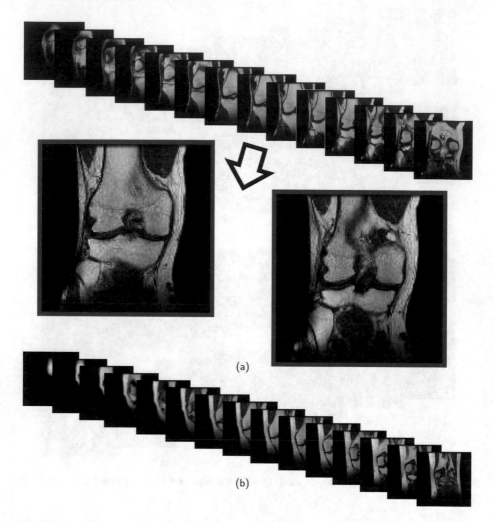

Fig. 2. T1-weighted MRI slices of the knee joint in the coronal plane (a) reference series (slices containing ACL or PCL structures appear in the frame) (b) tested series

Table 1. Obtained results for the image matching containing the pathological structures of ACL or PCL (ligament rupture of the 'shaving brush' type)

Type of ligament	All cases	Correct matching for entire slice	Matching accuracy [%]	Correct matching for 2D ROI	Matching accuracy [%]
PCL	14	9	64.29	13	92.86
ACL	27	18	66.67	26	96.29

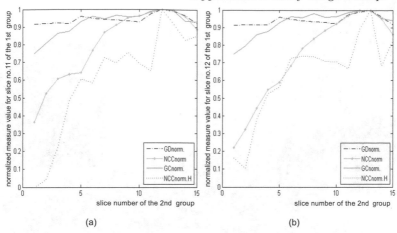

Fig. 3. Similarity measures for slice (a) no. 11 and (b) no. 12 of the reference series (slices containing ACL or PCL structures (1st group) and tested series (2nd group)

In the research described in this article only the intensity-based measures have been considered because they use the information determined on the basis of gray levels, and their main advantage (particularly when applied to the entire image) is the option to skip the phase of features extraction, which can be complicated and time-consuming, and the results may be affected by errors.

In the case of the interobjectional image matching, it can be proved, taking into account the performed examination, that on the basis of the slice containing the structures of the cruciate ligaments it is possible to identify the slice that contains the same anatomical structures of the knee MRI of another patient. The application of the fuzzy image concept combined with the use of similarity measures in order to match the MRI slices of the knee joint, returns correct results under the condition of a similar number of information pixels in both compared images. On the basis of the examination performed on 107 clinical T1- and T2-weighted MRI studies of the knee joint in the coronal and sagittal plane, the threshold of acceptable difference has been determined at the level of 11%. In other cases it was necessary to find regions of interest containing the ligaments structures [22, 23] in both compared groups of slices (in the 1st group – containing the reference slice and in the 2nd group – containing the test slices) in the first step, and transfer, in the second step, a larger region for both series and then perform calculations only for this region of interest in the next step. In this way the correct results have been yielded in 101 cases, and the accuracy of the method equals 94.39%.

On the basis of the received results, it can be proved that when the process of finding a selected pathology of both kinds of ligaments ended in success and a slice has been found containing the same kind of pathology of the ACL or PCL in the MRI study of the knee joint of another patient (Fig. 4(b)), all implemented similarity measures suggested just one (the same) slice of the test group (Fig. 5(a)).

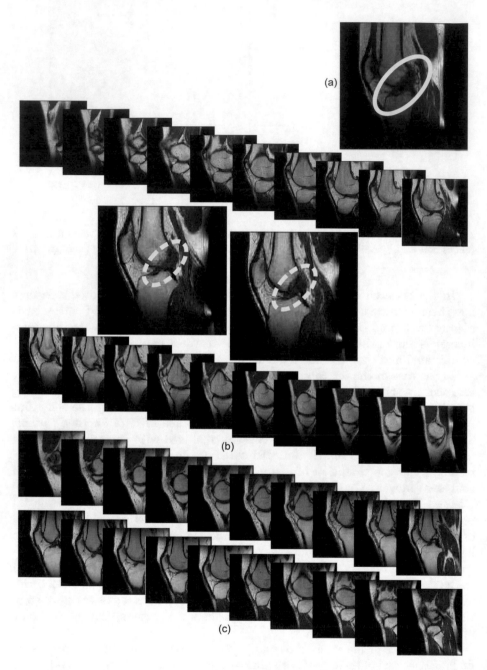

Fig. 4. T1-weighted MRI slices of the knee joint in the sagittal plane (a) reference slice showing ACL rupture of the 'shaving brush' type, tested series (b) containing the same kind of pathology and (c) another kind of pathology

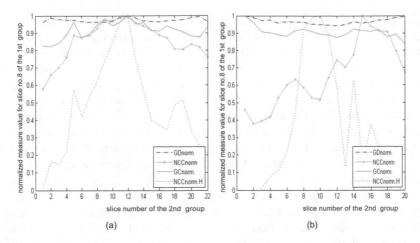

Fig. 5. Similarity measures for slice no. 8 of the reference series showing ACL rupture of the 'shaving brush' type (1st group) and tested series (2nd group) containing (a) the same and (b) another kind of pathology

Usually in this type of pathology, in the typical MRI study of the knee joint in the sagittal plane, in T1-weighted series there are two slices visible containing the rupture of the 'shaving brush' type (slices no. 11 and 12 in Fig. 4(b)). The analysis of the results received confirms this thesis. Figure 4(c) shows, that for slice no. 12 of the 2nd group the similarity measures value is equal to 1 and for slice no. 11 these values are very close to the highest value.

In the absence of a slice containing the rupture of the 'shaving brush' type (Fig. 4(c)), the implemented similarity measures suggested different slices of the test group (Fig. 5(b)) as the most similar.

The proposed method of finding a selected pathology (rupture of the 'shaving brush' type) has been tested on 14 pathological cases of PCLs and 27 pathological cases of ACLs containing the rupture of the 'shaving brush' type. In 9 cases of PCLs and 18 cases of ACLs the proposed method gave a correct result. In other cases (mainly due to different sizes of the knee joint) it was necessary to modify the algorithm. This modification consisted, firstly, in finding regions of interest which include the ligaments structures in both groups (in the 1st group – including the reference slice and in the 2nd group – including the test slices), and, secondly, transferring a larger region for both series and finally performing calculations only for this region of interest. This approach allowed proper identification of the rupture of the 'shaving brush' type in both cases of ligaments.

The obtained results have been verified by two independent experts (radiologist and orthopaedist). In the case of interobject matching of the whole slices containing the ACL and PCL structures, the indications of the experts were consistent with the results obtained by computer simulations in 86 cases (about 80%). However, in this situation is important the fact that experts did not have any problem with an indication of the most similar slices in both groups. Analysis of the results of computer simulations show that the interobject matching of the slices containing the ACL and PCL structures in the coronal plane is the small problem (Fig. 3). This is related to the fact that the two highest values of the implemented measures of similarity ($GD_{norm.}$, $NCC_{norm.}$, $GC_{norm.}$) are different less than 1%. The situation looks much better in the case of $NCC_{norm.H}$ where the above mentioned difference is much greater than 10%, which immunizes the process of finding the most similar MRI slices in the interobject matching from potential interference. A better solution (than interobject matching of the whole slices) is to find regions of interest containing the ligaments structures in both compared groups of slices in the first step, and transfer, in the second step, a larger region for both series and then perform calculations only for this region of interest in the next step. This modification results in a significant improvement of the efficiency of the method. Then the indications of the experts were consistent with the results obtained by computer simulations in 101 cases (about 94%).

In the case of interobject matching of the parts (region of interest containing the ligaments structures) of slices containing a selected pathology (rupture of the 'shaving brush' type) the indications of the experts were consistent in the 32 cases (about 78%) with the result obtained on the basis of computer simulations. The differences in the indication of the experts in the remaining cases were related to the selection (as the most similar slice) of the neighboring slice. From a medical point of view, this solution is acceptable, since the rupture of the 'shaving brush' type is usually visible in 2–3 MRI slices of the knee joint in the sagittal plane.

4   Conclusions

The described automated image matching methodology based on the fuzzy image concept seems to be very effective and promising. In the opinion of experts, each additional element supporting the diagnostics is important. Such is the role of the proposed image matching methodology. On the basis of the described methodology a software application has been built, which is the next stage in computer aided diagnostics of the knee joint [21] and in the diagnosis of pathologies of the lower limb, especially in the alloarthroplasty of the knee joint [24, 26].

The fact that this method of image matching is automatic, is based on the features of the images themselves, and the application of entropy measure of fuzziness for the similarity assessment of the MRI slices, makes it a reliable and fast computational method, which leads all to the conclusion that this method is useful in medical applications.

Acknowledgement. This research was supported by Silesian University of Technology, Faculty of Biomedical Engineering statutory financial support No. BK-209/RIB1/2018 (07/010/BK_18/0021).

References

1. Badura, P., Kawa, J., Czajkowska, J., Rudzki, M., Pietka, E.: Fuzzy connectedness in segmentation of medical images. In: Proceedings of the International Conference on Evolutionary Computation Theory and Applications and International Conference on Fuzzy Computation Theory and Applications ECTA 2011/FCTA 2011, pp. 486–492 (2011)
2. Bochenek, A., Reicher, M.: The Human Anatomy. PZWL, Warsaw (1990)
3. Ciszkowska-Lyson, B.: The anatomy of the cruciate ligament in the MRI study. Acta Clin. **4**(1), 321–330 (2001)
4. Czogala, E., Leski, J.: Application of entropy and energy measures of fuzziness to processing of ECG signal. Fuzzy Sets Syst., 9–18 (1997)
5. Czyrny, Z.: Diagnostics of the injuries cruciate ligaments in the MRI study. Acta Clin. **4**(1), 331–339 (2001)
6. Deluca, A., Termini, S.: A definition of non-probabilistic entropy in the setting of fuzzy set theory. Inf. Control **20**, 301–312 (1972)
7. Dziak, A.: Injuries of the cruciate ligaments of the knee joint. Acta Clin. **4**(1), 271–274 (2001)
8. Galinska, M., Ogieglo, W., Wijata, A., Juszczyk, J., Czajkowska, J.: Breast cancer segmentation method in ultrasound images. In: Gzik, M., Tkacz, E., Paszenda, Z., Pietka, E. (eds.) Innovations in Biomedical Engineering IBE 2017. AISC, vol. 623, pp. 23–31. Springer (2018)
9. Heger, S., Portheine, F., Ohnsorge, J., Schkommodau, E., Radermacher, K.: User-interactive registration of bone with A-mode ultrasound. IEEE Eng. Med. Biol. Mag. **24**(2), 85–95 (2005)
10. Hurvitz, A., Joskowicz, L.: Registration of a CT-like atlas to fluoroscopic X-ray images using intensity correspondences. Int. J. Comput. Assist. Radiol. Surg. **3**, 493–504 (2008)
11. Goshtasby, A.: Image Registration: Principles, Tools and Methods. Springer, New York (2012)
12. Huang, X., Ren, J., Guiraudon, G., Boughner, D., Peters, T.M.: Rapid dynamic image registration of the beating heart for diagnosis and surgical navigation. IEEE Trans. Med. Imaging **28**(11), 1802–1814 (2009)
13. Karacali, B.: Information theoretic deformable registration using local image information. Int. J. Comput. Vision **72**(3), 219–237 (2007)
14. Liao, Y.L., Sun, Y.N., Guo, W.Y., Chou, Y.H., Hsieh, J.C., Wu, Y.T.: A hybrid strategy to integrate surface-based and mutual-information-based methods for co-registering brain SPECT and MR images. Med. Biolog. Eng. Comput. **49**, 671–685 (2011)
15. Lin, Y., Medioni, G.: Retinal image registration from 2D to 3D. In: Proceedings of the IEEE Conference on Computer Vision and Pattern Recognition, CVPR, Anchorage, Alaska, USA, pp. 1–8 (2008)
16. Mattes, D., Haynor, D., Vesselle, H., Lewellen, T., Eubank, W.: PET-CT image registration in the chest using free-form deformations. IEEE Trans. Med. Imaging **22**(1), 120–128 (2003)
17. Mayer, A., Zimmerman-Moreno, G., Shadmi, R., Batikoff, A., Greenspan, H.: A supervised framework for the registration and segmentation of white matter fiber tracts. IEEE Trans. Med. Imaging **30**(1), 131–145 (2011)
18. Oliveira, F., Tavares, J.: Medical image registration: a review. Comput. Methods Biomech. Biomed. Eng. **17**(2), 73–93 (2014)

19. Sotiras, A., Davatzikos, Ch., Paragios, N.: Deformable medical image registration: a survey. IEEE Trans. Med. Imaging **32**(7) (2013)
20. Spinczyk, D., Karwan, A., Copik, M.: Methods for abdominal respiratory motion tracking. Comput. Aided Surg. **19**(1–3), 34–47 (2014)
21. Zarychta, P.: Features extraction in anterior and posterior cruciate ligaments analysis. Comput. Med. Imaging Graph. **46**, 108–20 (2015)
22. Zarychta, P.: Posterior cruciate ligament - 3D visualization. In: Kurzynski, M., et al. (eds.) Conference on Computer Recognition Systems. AISC, vol. 45, pp. 695–702. Springer, Heidelberg (2007)
23. Zarychta, P., Zarychta-Bargiela, A.: Anterior and posterior cruciate ligament-extraction and 3D visualization. In: Pietka, E., Kawa, J. (eds.) Information Technologies in Biomedicine. AISC, vol. 69, pp. 115–122. Springer (2010)
24. Zarychta, P., Konik, H., Zarychta-Bargiela, A.: Computer assisted location of the lower limb mechanical axis. In: Pietka, E., Kawa, J. (eds.) Information Technologies in Biomedicine. Lecture Notes in Bioinformatics, vol. 7339, pp. 93–100. Springer (2012)
25. Zarychta, P.: Automatic registration of the medical images T1- and T2-weighted MR knee images. In: Napieralski, A. (ed.) International Conference Mixed Design of Integrated Circuits and Systems, MIXDES 2006, pp. 741–745 (2006)
26. Zarychta, P.: A new approach to knee joint arthroplasty. Comput. Med. Imaging Graph. (2017). https://doi.org/10.1016/j.compmedimag.2017.07.002
27. Zitova, B., Flusser, J.: Image registration methods: a survey. Image Vis. Comput. **21**(11), 977–1000 (2003)

High Dynamic Range in X-ray Imaging

Przemysław Skurowski[1]([⊠]) and Kamila Wicher[2]

[1] Institute of Informatics, Silesian University of Technology, Gliwice, Poland
przemyslaw.skurowski@polsl.pl
[2] Silesian Veterinary Center, Chorzów, Poland
http://inf.polsl.pl

Abstract. The article demonstrates the usability of HDR techniques applied to the X-ray images. It is intended for the improvement of diagnostic abilities of the X-ray imaging through the fusion of different exposures obtained with different photon energies (kVp). The article comprises background analysis, proof-of-concept using the generic exposure fusion through the Laplace pyramid and a broad survey of tone mapping techniques. The results of the survey were obtained through the experts systematic quality assessment using an adjective-numerical scale.

Keywords: High dynamic range · X-ray · Medical imaging
Tone mapping

1 Introduction

High Dynamic Range (HDR) [18] imaging is nowadays an important topic in research and engineering on imaging and photography, although its roots date in the 19th century. Contemporary HDR is mature technology present in numerous software and hardware appliances. The general idea behind all the HDR techniques is to bring to the machines the human capability to adapt pupil size to the viewing conditions. That goal is commonly achieved by fusion of several low dynamic range (LDR) images taken with bracketing – different exposures (times/apertures) that reveal scene contents in shadows, mid-tones and lights partially separately.

The contribution in the article is several-fold. First, we present a proof-of-concept (PoC) demonstrating that even generic exposure fusion can be applied to the X-ray images, to obtain improved visibility of anatomic parts. Then, we propose how to fabricate HDR of Xray images. Finally, we propose methodology and evaluate pool of actual methods, verifying feasibility of tone mapping operators (TMO). It is noteworthy that TMOs need no special adoption to the data developed for the general photography, other than tonal range scaling. In the article, we reviewed 27 different TMOs, which were systematically evaluated for the visual quality by a group of experts.

The paper is organized as follows. Section 1 brings introduction and basics of X-ray and HDR imaging. Section 2 provides the rationales and overall idea. Section 3 contains experimental part comprising two stages – proof-of-concept and TMO evaluation. Finally, Sect. 4 contains conclusions and summary.

© Springer International Publishing AG, part of Springer Nature 2019
E. Pietka et al. (Eds.): ITIB 2018, AISC 762, pp. 39–51, 2019.
https://doi.org/10.1007/978-3-319-91211-0_4

1.1   Basics of X-ray Image Formation

The fundamental property of X-rays, that makes it imaging diagnostic tool [27] is their varying penetration abilities, depending on the tissue density. The more dense material the stronger attenuation is observed, so the tissues and structures can be observed. Although, the difference in attenuation changes with varying energy of radiation (see Fig. 1(b)), this makes X-rays with variable photon energy applicable for the different tissue imaging purposes.

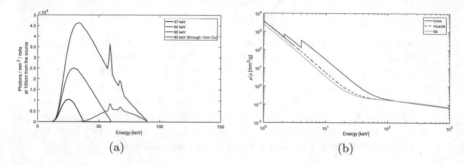

(a)   (b)

Fig. 1. X-ray imaging physical characteristics for different energies (wavelengths): (a) tube emissions spectra (as used in the paper), (b) attenuation of different tissues

Assuming typical design of X-ray imaging device with a tube as a radiation source, there are two factors to be considered by a radiologist:

- amount of radiation (mAs), which is governed by the current in the tube and exposure time, which is adjusted to the patient body mass or thickness;
- peak photon energy (kVp), controlled by the acceleration voltage applied to the tube as in numerical model [21] of radiation used in this research in Fig. 1(a), it is adjusted according to the tissues which are intended to be visible.

1.2   HDR Techniques Overview

Pipeline. High dynamic range techniques are intended to reveal the observer all the contents of the scene regardless they are dim or light. This goal is simply achieved by humans with adaptation to the visual conditions or the observed fragment of scene, alas, it is not so simple for the most of contemporary image acquisition devices. Overall HDR pipeline [2,18] comprises following stages:

1. Acquisition – several LDR images – a stack – with different exposures (aperture, shutter speed, or sensitivity) are fused into floating point image representing Luminance. It is achieved with following steps:
   (a) If it is necessary the images should be processed for motion distortions occurring between taken exposures – aligning appearing due to camera egomotion and deghosting canceling motion in an acquired scene.
   (b) Due to nonlinearity of cameras this step requires to linearize LDR images with camera response function (CRF) – there are various methods proposed to recover CRF from the image stack [7].

(c) Component values are summed with appropriate weights.
2. Storing – in-memory requires floating point representation (12 bytes per pixel), but efficient file representations are proposed as well such, these are RGBE, XYZE, LogLuv, or OpenEXR.
3. Visualization – because of the limited availability of native HDR displays the output phase requires the adoption of HDR contents to the LDR image by tone mapping. This operation called tone map operator (TMO) and is a crucial step for visual plausibility and fidelity of the results. It is ongoing research and numerous TMOs were proposed.

Tone Mapping Operators. TMOs are pivotal HDR processing stage in this study, these algorithms intended to adapt HDR images to approximate them when displaying on ordinary LDR screens. There are numerous proposals based on different rationales, that result in various outcomes. What is important, the TMOs operate mainly on the achromatic Luminance component, leaving the chromatic information intact. Typically TMO can be denoted as:

$$f(I) : \mathbb{R}^C \Rightarrow [0..255]^C, \tag{1}$$

where: f – denotes TMO, I is an image, C number of color channels. Individual TMOs differ in the overall approach and the intent in their design. In the systematic approach the first taxonomy criterion is the principle of the computation, Banterle [3] distinguished four types of computations involved (although some authors mention just first two of them):

- global (G) – point operators where the same mathematical operation is applied to all pixels in an image,
- local (L) – where tonal remapping depends on a pixel and its neighborhood,
- frequency (F) – based on the image division into low and high (details) frequency bands, where the tonal mapping is applied to low bands and details remain intact,
- segmentation (S) – based on segmenting the images into relatively large regions and individual mapping of each of them.

The other, very important, aspect is the design intent of the TMO or its intended application area, according to Banterle two main classes for static images and one additional for videos can be noted:

- perceptual (P) – this class of TMOs is based on modeling properties of human visual system (HVS) to achieve minimal perceptual difference (according to that model) between real scene and reproduced image,
- empirical (E) – where certain heuristics are considered for similarity to original scene appearance as an objective criterion, usually they employ well-motivated objectives such as contrast, brightness, colors, noise, or amount of details. This class of TMOs is further subdivided by other authors [10],
- temporal – suitable for HDR video and animations – out of scope of this work (Table 1).

Table 1. Taxonomy of used TMOs (updated version of [3])

	Empirical	Perceptual
Global	Exponential, Logarithmic, Schlick [26], WardGlobal [31], Kim-Kautz [13], Normalize, Gamma	Ferwerda [12], Pattanaik [20], Tumblin [28], VanHateren [29], Drago [8], WardHistAdj [16], ReinhardDevlin [24]
Local	Chiu [6], Reinhard [25], BruceExpoBlend [4]	Ashikimin [1]
Frequency	Durand [9], Fattal [11], Raman [22]	Kuang [15]
Segmentation	Lischinski [17], Mertens [19]	Banterle [3], Krawczyk [14], Yee [32]

2 The Concept

The idea follows everyday experience of a photography interested reader, that several images of different exposure (time or amount of radiation), can be merged into HDR images and then using TMO it is adopted backward to display with LDR, yet bringing more visual information. Although, we propose slightly modified approach – to use variable wavelengths instead of exposures. It conforms the tutorial guidelines in radiology [27], where operating the exposure as current multiplied by time (mAs) is adopted to the body mass and acceleration voltage is tuned for obtaining visibility of certain tissues.

Proposed approach could be compared to taking photos in the visible range with different colors of illumination. Similar idea is also behind the spectral CT [34], although the main visualization is focused on showing how the tissues would look like with different voltages [23]. In the proposed approach we try to include visual information fro all the composing images. The acquiring of HDR from composing images is a bit tricky in our case, due to lack of formal background. The HDR construction requires knowledge of exposure value (EV), which are not relevant as we do not operate on actual exposure. They need to be set up artificially in order to mimic shadows/midtones/lights interpretation.

The ability to render X-ray images with TMOs is a corollary of two rationales:

- In the X-ray images, the visible contents depends on the photon energy. The images obtained using different photon energies exhibit variable visibility of different tissues. These images reveal the images that are somewhat complementary – some show better bones, the others soft tissues.
- The general principle of TMOs – to deliver within a single image as much visual information as possible from the different images of the same scene.

3   Experiments

Experimental part comprises two stages – proof-of-concept and TMO analysis. For the test purposes, a chicken wing from the grocery store was used as a model. Three images were acquired using different peak photon voltages. Next, the HDR image was produced, then tone mapped back into LDR. The most generic approach was shown as a PoC, whereas in the review stage different state of the art TMOs were used. Finally, the outcomes were evaluated by a group of expert veterinarians judging visibility of the body parts.

3.1   Acquiring Images

The source of images was pretty old X-ray imaging device TDv 6545/016-15 with frame: 12×12 cm of 768×776 px resolution, tube: COMET Type: DO 10– 150, current: 320 mA/2mA (fluoroscopy). The X-ray device outputs fluoroscopic images, provided as the analog video signal which is then converted to the digital form using Matrix-II/Y/C FrameGrabber. Images were captured at 5 Hz for 16 s, totaling 80 frames and then averaged out. Pictures were taken at a constant current of 2 mA and at three acceleration voltages: 37, 60 and 90 keV, with an acrylic plate used as a support for the object and additional copper plate in case of 90 keV. For each of the settings, the signal visual amplification was adjusted visually by an experienced operator (Fig. 2).

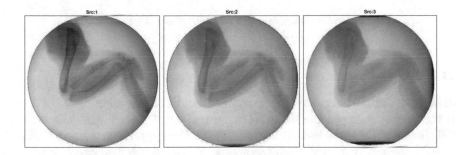

Fig. 2. Source images obtained with 37, 60 and 90 keV

3.2   Proof-of-Concept

In order, to verify the ability to improve visibility of object details, we employed the most generic operator used for that purpose [19,35] – fusion by Laplacian pyramid [5]. Laplacian pyramid (band-pass) decompose input images into multi-resolution representation comprising the base and detail layers (bands) by consecutive low-pass filtering, sub-sampling and obtaining the difference of adjacent layers for all but last (base) layer, which is just a low resolution representation. Then pyramids are combined and the output image is reconstructed in reverse process – pyramid expanding. The fusion of Laplacian pyramids (L) of N images at K-th level pyramid maximizes local (x, y) image variance, it is described as:

$$L_{out}^{k=1..K-1}(x,y) = \max\left(L_1^{k=1..K-1}(x,y), ..., L_N^{k=1..K-1}(x,y)\right), \qquad (2)$$
$$L_{out}^K(x,y) = \left(L_1^K(x,y) + ... + L_N^K(x,y)\right)/N.$$

The resulting image with one of source images and their difference is presented in Fig. 3. Visual inspection reveals enhanced contrasts in bones, visible outline of soft tissues, fat tissue gap, and augmented shadows of muscles. None of the source images contains all the details. It proves that one can obtain more visual information from exposure fusion, despite fact that the Laplacian operator is the most generic one. We can suppose that more sophisticated operators, involving observer models, can bring notably better visual image quality.

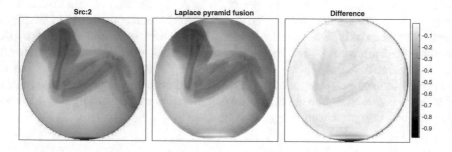

Fig. 3. Result of Laplace pyramid fusion of the test images

3.3   TMO Analysis

An objective of the next step in this research was to review a large pool of TMOs for their performance in the X-ray HDR. In this stage, we artificially created the HDR image of the three test source images and then applied numerous TMOs to get LDR images backward. Finally, quality of images was evaluated by a group of experts using systematic quality assessment. Whole the processing of HDR images, including the relatively large pool of TMOs, was performed in Matlab environment with HDR Toolbox created by Francesco Banterle [2].

Building HDR Image. We assumed sRGB color space for the building of the HDR image, as the source images were adjusted during the acquisition to display on relatively common CRT monitor. Using sRGB involves the assumption of the 2.2 gamma function as CRF for the HDR build. That was a reasonable choice as obtaining CRF estimation using Debevec and Malik [7] or other algorithms makes not much sense and results in unpredictable outcomes. The HDR image was built using artificial exposure values (EV_i). They were obtained as a solution of the optimization problem, looking for the EV values maximizing an objective function – consistency between the HDR and the best (K) of LDR images measured as one minus Spearman Rank Order Correlation Coefficient (SROCC):

$$[EV_1, \ldots, EV_N] = \underset{EV_1, \ldots, EV_N}{\arg\min} \ (1 - SROCC(HDR, \ LDR_K), \qquad (3)$$

$$\text{where:} \quad HDR = f(LDR_1, \ldots LDR_N, EV_1, \ldots, EV_N).$$

Quality Assessment Problem. The resulting images are quite numerous and usually similar to each other, therefore the pivotal aspect of this research is to propose reliable quality evaluation. The objective methods such as SSIM [30] or others are focused on the similarity of resulting image to the source one, so all image modifications are measured as imperfections, including also improvements such as contrast enhancement or deblurring. Moreover, HDR oriented variant of SSIM – TMQI [33] additionally employs a measure of *naturalness*, which is quality aspect not relevant to the medical images.

Hence, we propose subjective quality assessment by a group of experts, which was supported with questionnaire table providing systematic criteria of evaluation for each of the images – certain parts and tissues are distinguished in Table 3. The images were presented to the experts on NEC SpectraView Reference 242 monitor, which was calibrated using Xrite i1 Photo spectrophotometer.

The assessment procedure was as follows. The full set of source and resulting images (see Fig. 4) was demonstrated individually to the members of a group of 6 expert veterinarians for free viewing. They could then point each of the images and see them individually with free zooming. Next, using a random order of images, for each of the distinguished body parts, they were asked to judge in numerical scale the visible quality of images. The resulting values are averaged for each of the TMOs and for each of the body parts indicating respectively performance of the tone mapping and difficulty to reproduce these body parts. Additionally, we asked experts to evaluate the visibility of the same body parts in source images, using the same scale to get the quality of the source material (Table 2).

Table 2. Quality scale adjective-numerical mapping

Quality adjective	Bad	Poor	Moderate	Fair	Good
Numerical scale	-2	-1	0	1	2

Results. The results are presented in Table 3. For each of the anatomic segments (columns) versus different TMOs (row) the averaged experts responses are stored in respective array cells. Additionally same evaluations are also provided source images. Additionally, For each row (source or TMOs image) the table provides also three row-wise average values of evaluation scores of anatomic segments – separate for bones, soft tissues and overall average. The average evaluation scores

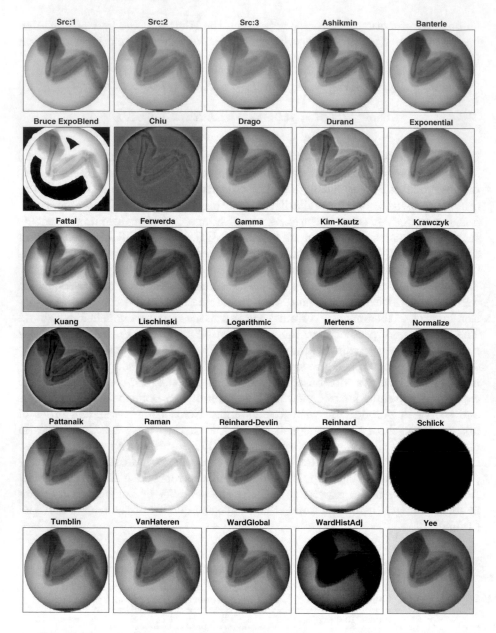

Fig. 4. The set of source and TMO resulting images presented to the experts

are then summarized in a form of ranking, sorted according to overall average values. It is shown in Fig. 5, it includes both tone-mapped and source images. Such a ranking allows to compare how much, according to experts, the source images were improved (or degraded).

Table 3. Averaged expert evaluations of source LDR and HDR tonemapped images for each anatomic segment (columns) visibility versus different TMOs (rows), with additional three columns containing averaged scores (bones/soft tissues/overall) for each TMO

	humerus	ulna	d. radius	radius	ulnare	metacarpals	phalanx 1	phalanx 2	phalanx 3	muscles	skin	bones	soft tiss.	overall
src:1	1.1667	0.6667	0.0000	0.6667	-0.1667	0.3333	-0.3333	-0.6667	-0.6667	-0.1667	-0.3333	0.1111	-0.2500	0.0455
src:2	1.0000	0.3333	0.6667	0.8333	-0.1667	-0.3333	-0.6667	-0.6667	-0.8333	-0.1667	-0.1667	0.0185	-0.1667	-0.0152
src:3	-0.1667	-1.0000	-1.1667	-1.0000	-1.5000	-1.3333	-1.5000	-1.5000	-1.5000	-0.8333	-1.0000	-1.1852	-0.9167	-1.1364
Ashikmin	0.8333	0.8333	0.8333	1.0000	0.3333	0.1667	-0.3333	-0.1667	-0.3333	0.1667	0.3333	0.3519	0.2500	0.3333
Banterle	1.6667	1.3333	0.8333	1.1667	0.5000	0.6667	0.1667	0.0000	-0.5000	0.8333	0.1667	0.6481	0.5000	0.6212
BruceExpoBlend	0.5000	0.1667	0.1667	0.3333	0.0000	-0.6667	-0.6667	-0.5000	-1.0000	-0.6667	-1.6667	-0.1852	-1.1667	-0.3636
Chiu	1.0000	0.5000	0.3333	0.6667	0.1667	0.3333	-0.3333	-0.5000	-0.6667	0.0000	0.0000	0.1667	0.0000	0.1364
Drago	1.1667	0.8333	0.3333	1.0000	0.6667	0.8333	-0.5000	-0.6667	-1.1667	0.1667	0.3333	0.2778	0.2500	0.2727
Durand	1.3333	1.3333	1.0000	1.0000	1.0000	0.3333	-0.1667	-0.5000	-0.6667	0.8333	0.6667	0.5185	0.7500	0.5606
Exponential	1.1667	1.0000	0.8333	1.0000	0.1667	0.3333	-0.3333	-0.5000	-0.8333	0.5000	0.0000	0.3148	0.2500	0.3030
Fattal	1.1667	1.3333	1.0000	1.1667	1.0000	0.5000	-0.1667	0.0000	-0.3333	1.1667	0.8333	0.6296	0.2500	0.6970
Ferwerda	1.0000	1.3333	1.0000	1.1667	1.0000	0.6667	-0.1667	-0.3333	-0.5000	0.6667	0.6667	0.5741	0.6667	0.5909
Gamma	0.6667	0.5000	0.5000	0.6667	0.0000	-0.1667	-1.0000	-1.1667	-1.1667	0.3333	-0.1667	-0.1296	0.0833	-0.0909
Kim-Kautz	0.3333	0.8333	0.0000	0.6667	-0.1667	0.1667	-0.5000	-0.6667	-0.8333	0.1667	0.1667	-0.0185	0.1667	0.0152
Krawczyk	0.5000	0.6667	0.1667	0.3333	0.0000	-0.1667	-0.8333	-0.8333	-1.1667	0.1667	0.1667	-0.1481	0.1667	-0.0909
Kuang	1.8333	1.6667	1.6667	1.6657	1.3333	1.3333	1.0000	0.8333	0.6667	1.6667	1.8333	1.3333	1.7500	1.4091
Lischinski	0.5000	0.6667	0.8333	0.6657	0.5000	0.8333	-0.1667	0.1667	-0.1667	-0.1667	-0.5000	0.4259	-0.3333	0.2879
Logarithmic	0.3333	0.6667	0.1667	0.3333	0.5000	0.0000	-0.5000	-0.8333	-0.8333	0.1667	0.0000	-0.0185	0.0833	-0.0000
Mertens	-0.1667	-0.6667	-0.8333	-0.6667	-1.3335	-1.1667	-1.8333	-1.8333	-1.8333	-1.5000	-1.8333	-1.1481	-1.6667	-1.2424
Normalize	0.6667	0.6667	0.5000	0.6667	0.3335	0.3000	-0.5000	-0.5000	-0.6667	0.3333	-0.1667	0.1296	0.0833	0.1212
Pattanaik	0.8333	0.8333	0.5000	0.6667	0.0000	0.3000	-0.6667	-0.6667	-0.8333	0.3333	0.1667	0.0741	0.2500	0.1061
Raman	0.1667	-0.1667	-0.6667	-0.1667	-1.1667	-1.5000	-1.5000	-1.5000	-1.5000	-1.1667	-1.5000	-0.8889	-1.3333	-0.9697
Reinhard-Devlin	1.0000	0.8333	0.3333	0.8333	0.0000	0.0000	-0.6667	-0.8333	-0.8333	0.6667	0.3333	0.0741	0.5000	0.1515
Reinhard	1.0000	1.3333	1.0000	1.1667	0.8333	0.3333	-0.1667	-0.1667	-0.3333	0.3333	0.0000	0.6111	0.1667	0.5303
Schlick	-2.0000	-2.0000	-2.0000	-2.0000	-2.0000	-2.0000	-2.0000	-2.0000	-2.0000	-2.0000	-2.0000	-2.0000	-2.0000	-2.0000
Tumblin	0.8333	0.6667	0.1667	0.6667	-0.1667	-0.3333	-0.6667	-1.0000	-1.0000	-0.1667	-0.3333	-0.0926	-0.2500	-0.1212
VanHateren	1.3333	1.0000	1.0000	1.1667	0.5000	0.5000	-0.3333	-0.3333	-0.5000	0.1667	0.1667	0.4815	0.1667	0.4242
Ward Global	1.3333	1.0000	0.8333	1.3333	0.3333	0.5000	-0.1667	-0.1667	-0.1667	-0.1667	-0.5000	0.5370	-0.3333	0.3788
WardHistAdj	-2.0000	-2.0000	-2.0000	-2.0000	-2.0000	-2.0000	-2.0000	-2.0000	-2.0000	-2.0000	-2.0000	-2.0000	-2.0000	-2.0000
Yee	1.0000	0.5000	0.5000	0.6667	0.0000	-0.3333	-1.0000	-1.0000	-1.0000	-0.3333	-0.3333	-0.0741	-0.3333	-0.1212

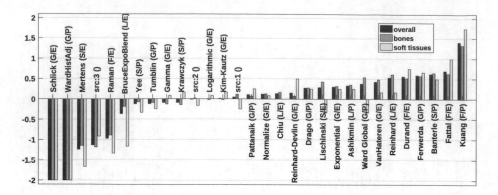

Fig. 5. TMO ranking according to the averaged experts assessment, with annotated taxonomy (type/intent)

3.4   Discussion

The most of the TMO resulting images offer improved quality, when compared to any of the source images (denoted in the Figure as *src*). Considering the ranking in Fig. 5, the Kuang TMO appears to be the indisputable winner, offering fair or good visibility of all bones and soft tissues. Fattal, Banterle, Ferwerda, and Durand are ranked on further positions.

All the best ranked operators augmented contrasts of the edges, although, diagnostic quality of observed of output images does not rely directly on the image fidelity. The best ranked operators enhanced the visibility of contents (such as muscles, skin or cartilage) which is barely visible in all any of the source images. Additionally, most of the top ranked operators introduced slight halos around the bones (especially arm). It improves visibility of these, but in conventional HDR photography halos are considered to be distorting phenomenon, which degrades image quality.

Looking into the ranking, the frequency based operators outperformed the other ones. We could not observe any other notable discriminants – it relates to both design intent and computation type. Perceptually and empirically designed TMOs are equally distributed in rank list. Also TMOs other than based on frequency computation techniques do not exhibit any notable superiority.

Aside, the main evaluation procedure, we noted also free comments of the experts on the specific images. They pointed out the following:

– visibility of the cartilage bone heads in the best TMOs,
– variable visibility of different parts is caused by their nonuniform thickness, some of TMOs allow to omit that problem.

The resulting images of the best TMOs appeared to be independent of the tissue thickness to a certain degree. It means that the very thin structures are visible together with thicker ones, which is the situation requiring tuning of the exposition in conventional X-ray imaging.

Prospectively, usage of the HDR techniques in the X-ray imaging may give more sharp scenes with better visibility on details than standard projections. Thanks to the improved images, usually hard to notice changes such as Osteomalacia, Osteolysis and Osteosclerosis could have good visibility and it may improve further diagnostic, although it would require further testing on the actual pathological samples.

4   Summary

In the article, it was verified that the HDR techniques can be effectively employed to obtain images containing visible different tissues. A simple proof-of-concept proves that even the simplest HDR exposure fusion by Laplacian pyramid is able to improve visibility of the details in the X-ray images. Next, a systematic review brings the proposal how to create an artificial HDR image of X-ray images and analyzes numerous tone mapping operators for their efficiency in the adopting HDR to the display. The latter allowed us to identify a pool of effective TMOs, capable to visualize hard and soft tissues jointly.

Further works in this area should include verification of the TMOs efficiency using different objects (preferably mammals) and X-ray imaging devices of a high quality. For formalities, also dosimetry aspects should be taken into consideration, although, taking several (or hundreds in tomography) images in one session is nothing unusual so the doses of an HDR X-ray session in a living patient should be also on an acceptable level.

Acknowledgement. The authors would like to thank Dr. J. Ihnatowicz, and D. Bednorz for help in acquiring images. Thanks also go to Dr. R. Fabisz, J. Karel, M. Ksoll, A. Balica, M. Stefanek for evaluation of images. The evaluation was done with the hardware purchased within the Motorola Solutions Foundation grant realized by Institute of Computer Science at Silesian University of Technology, no ZZD/1/Rau2/2015/507. We also acknowledge the support of Silesian University of Technology grant BK-213/RAu2/2018.

References

1. Ashikhmin, M.: A tone mapping algorithm for high contrast images. In: Proceedings of the 13th Eurographics Workshop on Rendering, EGRW 2002, pp. 145–156. Eurographics Association (2002)
2. Banterle, F., et al.: Advanced High Dynamic Range Imaging: Theory and Practice. CRC Press, Natick (2011)
3. Banterle, F., et al.: Dynamic range compression by differential zone mapping based on psychophysical experiments. In: Proceedings of the ACM Symposium on Applied Perception, SAP 2012, pp. 39–46. ACM (2012)
4. Bruce, N.D.B.: ExpoBlend: information preserving exposure blending based on normalized log-domain entropy. Comput. Graph. **39**, 12–23 (2014)
5. Burt, P., Adelson, E.: The Laplacian pyramid as a compact image code. IEEE Trans. Commun. **31**(4), 532–540 (1983)

6. Chiu, K., et al.: Spatially nonuniform scaling functions for high contrast images. In: Graphics Interface, pp. 245–245. CANADIAN INF. PROC. SOC. (1993)
7. Debevec, P.E., Malik, J.: Recovering high dynamic range radiance maps from photographs. In: SIGGRAPH 1997, pp. 369–378. ACM (1997)
8. Drago, F., et al.: Adaptive logarithmic mapping for displaying high contrast scenes. Comput. Graph. Forum **22**(3), 419–426 (2003)
9. Durand, F., Dorsey, J.: Fast bilateral filtering for the display of high-dynamic-range images. In: SIGGRAPH 2002, pp. 257–266. ACM (2002)
10. Eilertsen, G., et al.: Evaluation of tone mapping operators for HDR-video. Comput. Graph. Forum **32**(7), 275–284 (2013)
11. Fattal, R., Lischinski, D., Werman, M.: Gradient domain high dynamic range compression. In: SIGGRAPH 2002, pp. 249–256. ACM (2002)
12. Ferwerda, J.A., et al.: A model of visual adaptation for realistic image synthesis. In: SIGGRAPH 1996, pp. 249–258. ACM (1996)
13. Kim, M.H., Kautz, J.: Consistent tone reproduction. In: Proceedings of the 10th IASTED International Conference on Computer Graphics and Imaging, pp. 152–159. ACTA Press (2008)
14. Krawczyk, G., Myszkowski, K., Seidel, H.P.: Lightness perception in tone reproduction for high dynamic range images. Comput. Graph. Forum **24**(3), 635–645 (2005)
15. Kuang, J., Johnson, G.M., Fairchild, M.D.: iCAM06: a refined image appearance model for HDR image rendering. J. Vis. Commun. Image Represent. **18**(5), 406–414 (2007)
16. Larson, G.W., Rushmeier, H., Piatko, C.: A visibility matching tone reproduction operator for high dynamic range scenes. IEEE Trans. Vis. Comput. Graph. **3**(4), 291–306 (1997)
17. Lischinski, D., et al.: Interactive local adjustment of tonal values. In: SIGGRAPH 2006, pp. 646–653. ACM (2006)
18. Mantiuk, R.K., Myszkowski, K., Seidel, H.P.: High dynamic range imaging. In: Wiley Encyclopedia of Electrical and Electronics Engineering, pp. 1–42. Wiley (2015)
19. Mertens, T., Kautz, J., Reeth, F.V.: Exposure fusion. In: 15th Pacific Conference on Computer Graphics and Applications, PG 2007, pp. 382–390 (2007)
20. Pattanaik, S.N., et al.: Time-dependent visual adaptation for fast realistic image display. In: SIGGRAPH 2000, pp. 47–54. ACM (2000)
21. Punnoose, J., et al.: Technical note: spektr 3.0: a computational tool for x-ray spectrum modeling and analysis. Med. Phys. **43**(8), 4711–4717 (2016)
22. Raman, S., Chaudhuri, S.: Bilateral filter based compositing for variable exposure photography. In: Alliez, P., Magnor, M. (eds.) Eurographics 2009 - Short Papers. The Eurographics Association (2009)
23. Rassouli, N., et al.: Detector-based spectral CT with a novel dual-layer technology: principles and applications. Insights Imaging **8**(6), 589–598 (2017)
24. Reinhard, E., Devlin, K.: Dynamic range reduction inspired by photoreceptor physiology. IEEE Trans. Vis. Comput. Graph. **11**(1), 13–24 (2005)
25. Reinhard, E., Stark, M., Shirley, P., Ferwerda, J.: Photographic tone reproduction for digital images. In: SIGGRAPH 2002, pp. 267–276. ACM (2002)
26. Schlick, C.: Quantization techniques for visualization of high dynamic range pictures. In: Photorealistic Rendering Techniques. Focus on Computer Graphics, pp. 7–20. Springer, Heidelberg (1995)
27. Thrall, D.E. (ed.): Textbook of Veterinary Diagnostic Radiology, 6th edn. Elsevier, St. Louis (2013)

28. Tumblin, J., Hodgins, J.K., Guenter, B.K.: Two methods for display of high contrast images. ACM Trans. Graph. **18**(1), 56–94 (1999)
29. Van Hateren, J.H.: Encoding of high dynamic range video with a model of human cones. ACM Trans. Graph. **25**(4), 1380–1399 (2006)
30. Wang, Z., et al.: Image quality assessment: from error visibility to structural similarity. IEEE Trans. Image Process. **13**(4), 600–612 (2004)
31. Ward, G.: A contrast-based scalefactor for luminance display, pp. 415–421. Academic Press Professional, Inc., San Diego (1994)
32. Yee, Y.H., Pattanaik, S.: Segmentation and adaptive assimilation for detail-preserving display of high-dynamic range images. Vis. Comput. **19**(7–8), 457–466 (2003)
33. Yeganeh, H., Wang, Z.: Objective quality assessment of tone-mapped images. IEEE Trans. Image Process. **22**(2), 657–667 (2013)
34. Zagoudis, J.: Spectral Imaging Brings New Light to CT. Imaging Technology News (2015)
35. Zheng, Y.: Multi-scale fusion algorithm comparisons: pyramid, DWT and iterative DWT. In: 2009 12th International Conference on Information Fusion, pp. 1060–1067 (2009)

Analysis of the Possibility
of Doppler Tomography Imaging
in Circular Geometry

Tomasz Świetlik$^{(\boxtimes)}$ and Krzysztof J. Opieliński

Faculty of Electronics, Wroclaw University of Science and Technology,
Wybrzeze Wyspianskiego 27, 50-370 Wroclaw, Poland
tomasz.swietlik@pwr.edu.pl

Abstract. Doppler Tomography (DT) is an innovative method that can
be used for imaging the internal structure of tissue immersed in water. In
order to reconstruct the image, the Doppler signal is necessary, recorded
by a two-transducer ultrasonic probe. This method can be used in *in
vivo* medical diagnostics. In this paper, in order to analyse the possibility of DT imaging in circular geometry, a simulation-based method
for determining the Doppler signal has been developed. Additionally, an
algorithm determining the frequency value for particular inclusions at a
given moment of rotation of the probe was developed. For the purposes
of reconstructing the cross-sectional area of the examined object, a fast
tomographic algorithm was used. On the basis of the results obtained,
analyses were made and a discussion was conducted on the possibilities
and limitations in imaging the structure of objects using this method,
depending on the way of acquiring the Doppler signal.

Keywords: Doppler tomography
Continuous Wave Ultrasonic Tomography · Calculation model
Doppler signal

1 Introduction

Continuous Wave Ultrasonic Tomography (CWUT) or Doppler Tomography
(DT) uses the continuous wave and Doppler effect for imaging the cross-sections
of objects. Two acquisition geometries are possible here [3,4]. The first one is
linear geometry, in which the two-transducer ultrasonic probe moves along the
examined object [4] (Fig. 1(a)). The second is circular geometry, in which the
probe rotates around the imaged tissue [4] (Fig. 1(b)). In both cases, a moving
source (the probe) generates a continuous ultrasonic wave of frequency f_T. As
soon as the wave encounters an inclusion (the scatterer) it returns to the probe
with a changed frequency f_R. The difference between these two frequencies at a
given probe angle and for a particular inclusion is Doppler frequency f_d.

The method of Doppler tomography in circular geometry has been used and
discussed in this paper. One of its advantages is its potential use in *in vivo*

© Springer International Publishing AG, part of Springer Nature 2019
E. Pietka et al. (Eds.): ITIB 2018, AISC 762, pp. 52–63, 2019.
https://doi.org/10.1007/978-3-319-91211-0_5

diagnostics of women's breasts or limb bones. If the source is in motion and the scatterer is stationary as well as in the reverse situation, f_d is the same.

One of DT's main advantages is the use of only one two-transducer ultrasonic probe for imaging the tissue, which will significantly reduce the cost of building a device based on this method. It should also be mentioned that the ultrasonic wave itself, in contrast to X-rays, allows for multiple and safe imaging. DT is a relatively new method for imaging tissue cross sections *in vivo* and very sparsely presented in literature [3,4]. Nowadays there is no device available on the market based on this method.

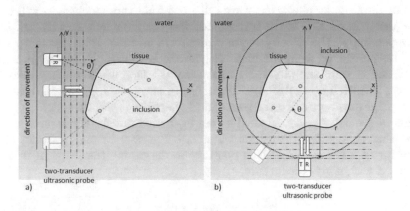

Fig. 1. The basic data acquisition way for Doppler tomography: (a) in the linear geometry, (b) in the circular geometry

Since it is much easier to explain the nature of Doppler tomography for circular geometry in the case of the rotation of scatters, for the purposes of this paper it was assumed in this paper that the ultrasonic probe is stationary, whereas the object under examination rotates.

2   Doppler Tomography Method for Circular Geometry

2.1   Methodology of Measurement Data Acquisition

The idea of imaging in Doppler tomography method is to record Doppler frequencies coming from objects scattering the ultrasonic wave. In order to determine these frequencies for a particular scatterer, one should use formula (1) where: f_T – ultrasonic wave frequency generated by the probe, v – linear component of the scatterer velocity moving toward the ultrasonic wave propagation, θ – rotation angle, c – ultrasonic wave velocity in the tissue (the cross-section of the examined object).

$$f_d = \frac{2 \cdot f_T \cdot v \cdot \cos(\theta)}{c}. \tag{1}$$

The formula (1) is identical to the formula determining Doppler frequency in classical blood flow velocity testing using ultrasonic directional blood flow meter [7]. It should be remembered, however, that DT differs significantly from this method because it illustrates the structure of the cross-section of an object and not the particles moving in it.

An example of the measurement data acquisition in Doppler tomography is shown in Fig. 2(a), where there are three stationary inclusions (scatterers) a, b, c inside the cross-section of an object. At a given rotation angle $\theta=0$ of this cross-section, the linear components of motion velocities for individual scatterers, in the direction of ultrasonic wave propagation, are v_a, v_b and v_c respectively. As a result of the Doppler effect, the wave reflected from these inclusions will change its frequency in relation to the transmitted frequency f_T by respectively f_{da}, f_{db}, f_{dc}. Depending on the velocity vector direction, a given Doppler frequency will be added or subtracted from the basic frequency. For example, inclusion a moves in a direction from the ultrasonic probe, so the Doppler frequency associated with it will initially be subtracted from f_T. In turn, f_{dc} frequency is associated with a point moving toward the probe, and therefore it will be added to f_T. The process of acquisition the reflected signal is carried out for subsequent rotation angles that change by a constant value $\Delta\theta$. By transforming formula (1), we obtain formula (2) by which it is possible to determine the Doppler frequency associated with a given inclusion:

$$f_d = 2 \cdot f_T \cdot \omega_{turn} \cdot r \cdot \frac{\cos(\theta)}{c}. \qquad (2)$$

In formula (2) ω_{turn} is the rotation pulsation of the object under examination (the cross section of the tissue), r is the distance between the inclusion and the centre of rotation, and θ is the rotation angle of the object.

An in-depth explanation of the principle of imaging by means of the DT method requires the observation of two facts concerning the distribution of the velocity components in the direction of ultrasonic wave propagation of moving scatterers within the imaging zone. This distribution is shown in Fig. 2(b). Firstly, on each line parallel to the direction of wave propagation, the velocity components of the scatterers located on it have the same values (cf. velocity v_c in Fig. 2(b)). However, for parallel lines, starting from the centre of rotation, the velocity components increase from zero to their maximum value v_{max} (Fig. 2(b)). On the basis of formula (1) we can unequivocally state that the linear component of velocity v and Doppler frequency are directly proportional. Thus, it can be noted that the frequency distribution f_d in the imaging zone is the same as for velocity v.

From the previous considerations it can be concluded that in order to determine the position of the scatterers in a given zone, it is necessary to record a signal containing Doppler frequencies generated by inclusions. This signal is called Doppler signal and can be determined on the basis of the signal reflected and transmitted by the ultrasonic probe.

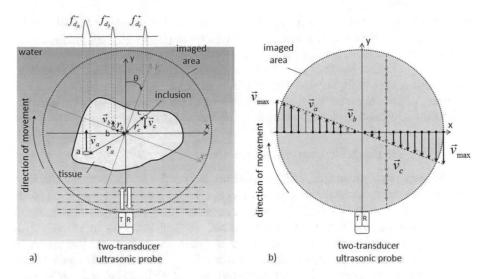

Fig. 2. The measurement data acquisition way for the DT method (a) and the distribution of shift velocity components of scatterers in the direction of propagation of the ultrasonic wave in the imaged zone (b)

To this end, these two signals should be multiplied and the range above the maximum Doppler frequency, correlated with velocity v_{max}, should be filtered out. Using formula (2), we obtain the following formula:

$$f_{dmax} - 2 \cdot f_{T} \cdot \omega_{turn} \cdot r_0 \cdot \frac{1}{c}, \tag{3}$$

where: r_0 – diameter of the zone under examination.

The first step required by the image reconstruction algorithm for Doppler tomography in circular geometry is to record the reflected signal by means of a two-transducer ultrasonic probe for all rotation angles. On the basis of this signal and the transmitting signal, the Doppler signal is determined. These data can be treated as complex, where amplitude and phase are involved (coherent method) or as real (incoherent method) [4,6]. In the incoherent method, which will be discussed later in the paper, it is possible to apply fast image reconstruction algorithms used in X-ray tomography [2].

The next step is to determine the maximum Doppler frequency on the basis of formula (3). It is now necessary to specify the range $[-f_{dmax}; f_{dmax}]$. This range shall be divided into subdivisions of equal length Δf_d. The resulting ranges are called Doppler bands. It should be remembered that on each of the lines along the propagation of the ultrasonic wave (vertical lines), the values of Doppler frequencies are the same. Thus, at a given rotation angle, the sums of Doppler frequency amplitudes derived from the Doppler signal spectrum are recorded for each band from the range $[-f_{dmax}; f_{dmax}]$. At this stage it is possible to create a matrix which in lines contains the mentioned sums of frequency amplitudes for the range from $-f_{dmax}$ to $+f_{dmax}$ by Δf_d. The columns of this matrix change subsequent rotation angles. This matrix is called tomographic sinogram. It is used to reconstruct the image in X-ray tomography [8]. At this stage it is possible to use one of the fastest algorithms, which is Filtered Back Projection (FBP) [8]. As a result of such image reconstruction of the object's (tissue's) cross-section, we obtain the distribution of local amplitude values of Doppler frequencies, which characterize in this way the position and the estimated amount of dispersion caused by inclusions inside the investigated object.

2.2   Filtered Back Projection Algorithm

The filtered back projection (FBP) method is based on the assumption that the measurements made for one projection can be treated as a two-dimensional filtering operation in the field of spatial frequency ($\xi = 1/\lambda$) [2]. In the general case, the measurement data shall be treated as a continuous function $p_\theta(s)$, where $s \,\epsilon\,(-1,1)$ is the normalized distance between the probe and the centre of the rotation axis for the object under examination (centre of the imaged zone). When Fourier's transformation is completed, the $p_\theta(s)$ function will be defined in the field of so-called spatial frequency. This transformation is described by formula:

$$P_\theta(\xi) = \int_{-1}^{1} p_\theta(s) \cdot e^{-j\xi s} d\xi, \tag{4}$$

where $\xi = [-\xi_m, ..., \xi_m]$, with $\xi_m = 1/\Delta\lambda$ being the maximum value of the spatial frequency that appears in the measurement data in the geometry of the parallel-radial projections ($\Delta\lambda$ - shift change). $P_\theta(\xi)$ is a complex-valued function.

Filtration is obtained by multiplying the modules of the functional arguments $P_\theta(\xi)$ by the so-called filtering function. This procedure gives a number of possibilities of using different functions of this type, which in effect allows optimal reconstruction of the image from the noisy data.

$$\widetilde{P}_\theta(\xi) = |P_\theta(\xi)| \cdot W(\xi) \cdot e^{j \, \arg(P_\theta(\xi))}, \tag{5}$$

where the filtering function is as follows:

$$W(\xi) = \begin{cases} \left| \frac{\xi}{2\xi_m} \right| & \text{for} \quad |\xi| \leq \xi_m, \\ 0 & \text{for} \quad |\xi| > \xi_m. \end{cases} \tag{6}$$

The last step in the filtration procedure is to apply Fourier's reverse transformation:

$$\widetilde{p}_\theta(s) = \frac{1}{2\pi} \int_{-\xi_m}^{\xi_m} \widetilde{P}_\theta(\xi) \cdot e^{j\xi t} d\xi. \tag{7}$$

The image is then reconstructed after back projection operation:

$$f(x,y) = \int_{0}^{\pi} p(x \cdot \cos\theta + y \cdot \sin\theta) d\theta. \tag{8}$$

The value of each image pixel $f(x, y)$ is the sum of the measuring rays passing through the pixel area.

The Doppler tomography method uses discrete measurement data. It is therefore necessary to use Fourier's discrete transformation in the FBP algorithm [2]. In addition, the maximum discrete frequency of Doppler frequency amplitude variation, marked as W, should be determined. The number of projections N_p and M_p rays should also be determined. In the DT method, the number of projections corresponds to the number of angles of rotation for the object or probe under examination, while the rays are the number of Doppler bands with a fixed width Δf_d is the number of rays. According to Nyquist's criterion on sampling, projection values $p_\theta(mT)$ should be measured with a period $T = 1/(2W)$, where $m = -N/2, ..., 0, ..., N/2 - 1$, for a sufficiently large N value. In Doppler tomography, the T period is associated with the bandwidth Δf_d. In the image reconstruction, first of all, for each projection using formula (9) an approximation of Fourier transform $S_\theta(w)$ is calculated. For Doppler tomography, $S_\theta(w)$ is a discrete function of the Doppler frequency amplitude variation frequency at a given rotation angle θ:

$$S_\theta(w) \approx S_\theta\left(m\frac{2W}{N}\right) = \frac{1}{2W} \sum_{k=-N/2}^{N/2-1} p_\theta\left(\frac{k}{2W}\right) \cdot e^{j2\pi(mk/N)}, \qquad (9)$$

where N – number of projection samples is usually equal to the number of M_p measurement rays (equal to the number of Doppler frequency bands in the DT method), supplemented by zeroes in such a way that the number N is a power of 2 (due to the use of FFT).

In the next step, each projection is filtered with regard to frequency and multiplied by a window function (e.g. Hammings window) to eliminate noise in the reconstructed image [1], according to formula:

$$Q_\theta\left(\frac{k}{2W}\right) \approx \left(\frac{2W}{N}\right) \sum_{m=-N/2}^{N/2} S_\theta\left(m\frac{2W}{N}\right) \cdot \left|m\frac{2W}{N}\right| \cdot H\left(m\frac{2W}{N}\right) \cdot e^{j2\pi(mk/N)},$$

$$(10)$$

where $k = -N/2, ..., 0, ..., N/2$, while $H(m(2W/N)$ means the window function.

In the final step, the reconstruction is made by means of the back projection method, as presented in formula:

$$f(x, y) = \frac{\pi}{K} \sum_{i=1}^{K} Q_{\theta_i}(x \cdot \cos\theta_i + y \cdot \sin\theta_i), \qquad (11)$$

where $K = N_p/2$, which means that the use of the π range for the θ_i angle is sufficient.

Graphical interpretation of the image reconstruction using the FBP algorithm is shown in Fig. 3. Figure 3(a) shows the image zone divided into pixels, together with the results of calculation of Q projection values for three selected rotation angles θ_i, θ_j, θ_k. The Q results are set at appropriate angles.

Figure 3(b) shows that for a given angle θ_j the value of the projection that passes through the pixel is searched for.

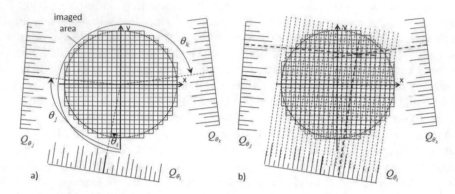

Fig. 3. Graphical interpretation of image reconstruction using a filtered back projection algorithm. Position of the projection results for three selected angles θ_i, θ_j, θ_k (a), determining the value for the selected pixel (b)

In the next step, the values of subsequent projections which pass through by a given pixel are summed up, thus determining its value.

3   Analysis of the Influence of Doppler Signal Acquisition on DT Imaging

3.1   Doppler Signal Simulation

The Doppler signal has the greatest influence on the reconstructed image in the Doppler tomography method. That is why it is so important to be able to simulate this signal.

In the calculations performed, it was assumed that in the examined cross-section of the object there is a finite number of pin-type scatterers of an infinitely small diameter which scatter the ultrasonic wave in each direction in the same way. They are attached to a 10 cm swivel platform, placed in distilled water. The signal from the two-transducer ultrasonic probe is recorded by an ultrasound blood flow meter. This device has the ability to simultaneously determine the Doppler signal for positions in which a given scatterer moves in the direction of the probe (channel A) and in the opposite direction (channel B). This is an important property which, when reconstructing the image, makes it possible to determine which Doppler frequencies should be placed in the range $[-f_{dmax}; 0]$ and which in the range $[0; f_{dmax}]$. The difference between the values of the signal from these two channels (A − B) results in a Doppler signal for one rotation. In the real case it can be registered with an oscilloscopic card installed on the computer. In addition, taking into account current measurement capabilities it is assumed that the transmitted wave frequency is $f_T = 4.7\,\text{MHz}$, the platform rotation frequency is 2 times per second, the number of registration angles equals 400 and the ultrasonic wave velocity in water calculated from empirical formula [5] at 20 °C is 1482.38 m/s.

The Doppler signal is of the *chirp* type. For a single scatterer placed at a distance r_0 from the centre of rotation and an angle α_0, the change in frequency of the signal during rotation must be carried out according to formula (12). It was derived from formula (2):

$$f(t) = \frac{2 \cdot f_T \cdot f_{rot} \cdot 2 \cdot \pi \cdot r_0 \cdot \cos(2 \cdot \pi \cdot f_{rot} \cdot t + \alpha_0)}{c}, \tag{12}$$

where f_{rot} is the rotation frequency of the object. The Doppler signal can be presented in the form of $s(t) = A \cdot \sin(\phi(t))$, where $\phi(t)$ is a sought-after modulating function, and A is a signal amplitude. It should be noted that the equation which allows the determination of $\phi(t)$ is as follows:

$$f(t) = \frac{1}{2\pi} \frac{d\phi(t)}{dt}. \tag{13}$$

After the necessary calculations based on formula (12) and (13), function $s(t)$ takes the following form:

$$s(t) = A \sin\left(\frac{4 \cdot \pi \cdot f_T \cdot r_0}{c} \cdot (\sin(2\pi \cdot f_{rot} \cdot t + \alpha_0) - \sin \alpha_0)\right). \tag{14}$$

In case of a scatterer layout, function $s(t)$ should be generated for each of them separately and summed up. Figure 4(b) shows an example illustrating a normalized Doppler signal generated by means of formula (14) for a full rotation, coming from a scatterer located in coordinates $r_0 = 4\,\text{cm}$, $\alpha_0 = 0°$.

It can be observed that the frequency of this signal near the 90° and 270° angles oscillates around zero (Fig. 4(a) and (b)).

3.2 The Influence of Doppler Signal on Imaging

Image reconstruction algorithm for Doppler tomography method requires the acquisition of Doppler signal values for each rotation angle of the object under examination. On this basis, Doppler frequencies are determined. Sums of the amplitudes of these frequencies are recorded in the appropriate Doppler bands. However, the method does not specify what length of the Doppler signal should be recorded for particular angles of rotation. The simplest solution seems to be to record a part of the signal between two successive angles of rotation and to assign the Doppler frequency calculation result and its amplitude, for example to the smaller one from the angles. It should be noted that the image reconstruction with satisfactory resolution requires a large number of acquisition angles. This would mean that a small time range of the signal is available for calculation. Since the Doppler signal spectrum is determined using FFT, the ratio of the f_s sampling frequency to number of samples N has the greatest influence on the accuracy of Doppler frequencies and their amplitudes determination.

60　　T. Świetlik and K. J. Opieliński

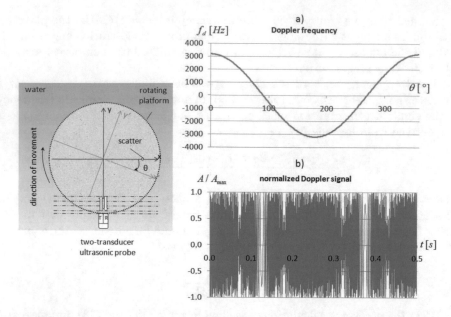

Fig. 4. Dependence of Doppler frequency value, generated by the scatterer, on its rotation angle (a) and Doppler signal simulation for one scatterer for a full rotation (b)

For example, consider a case when we have one pin-type object located in coordinates $r_0 = 4\,\mathrm{cm}$, $\alpha_0 = 0°$, the number of acquisition angles is equal to 400 and the number of archived samples per half rotation is 25 000.

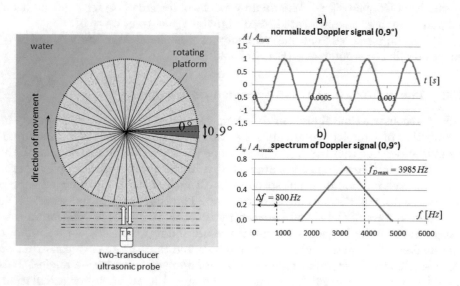

Fig. 5. Normalized Doppler signal at the acquisition angle width of 0.9° (a), Doppler normalized signal spectrum at the acquisition angle width of 0.9°(b)

Considering the assumptions made in Sect. 3.1, regarding f_T, f_{rot}, c and the diameter of the image zone, it can be calculated that the maximum frequency $f_{dmax} = 3984.27\,Hz$. The value of the spectrum calculation for a $0°$ rotation angle is shown in Fig. 5(b).

In this case, the spectral resolution is $\Delta f = 800\,Hz$ and the Doppler signal length used to calculate the spectrum equals the rotation angle width of $0.9°$ (Fig. 5(b)). It is clear that the accuracy of the assigned spectrum is far from sufficient to determine the Doppler frequency, which in this case is $f_d = 3187.40\,Hz$. It should be noted that increasing the sampling rate will not increase the resolution of Δf because the number of samples N increases at the same time. The solution to this problem may be an increase in the length of the Doppler signal used to determine the spectrum for individual angles of rotation, while at the same time keeping their number at a constant (400). In this case, it is necessary to register a continuous Doppler signal for a full rotation. Increasing the angle width (the length of the Doppler signal) to $27°$ will significantly improve the resolution of the spectrum, as shown in Fig. 6(a). In this case, the spectral resolution is $\Delta f = 26.66\,Hz$. Further increasing of the Doppler signal angle width will improve the resolution of Δf, but then unwanted frequencies appear in the spectrum. This is illustrated in Fig. 6(b). After determining the optimum Doppler signal acquisition width for a single object, it should be used to reconstruct more complex structures.

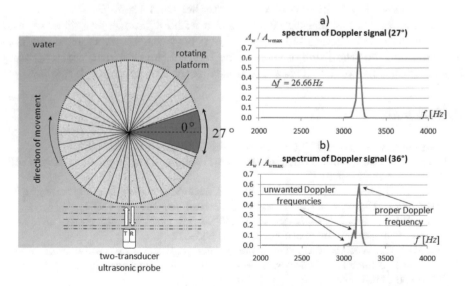

Fig. 6. Spectrum of normalized Doppler signal at the acquisition angle of $27°$ (a), spectrum of normalized Doppler signal at the acquisition angle of $36°$ (b)

4   Conclusions

The Doppler tomography method for circular geometry can be used to the examination and creation of images of the internal tissue structure. In combination with a fast and accurate image reconstruction algorithm such as a Filtered Back Projection, high quality images can be expected. However, it should be remembered that in its classic form this method has certain limitations. One of such cases is the Doppler frequency determination at a given rotation angle. Necessary changes in the method of the Doppler signal acquisition should be made here.

First of all, the Doppler signal acquisition should not be selected during measurements for each rotation angle separately. It was determined that it is more efficient to register it for a full rotation of the examined object (or the probe) and to reconstruct the image with access to all data at a given time. This is particularly important due to the resolution of Doppler signal spectra determination, on the basis of which Doppler frequencies and their amplitudes are determined. Determining these frequencies with a major error will result in major errors in object imaging. As shown in Sect. 3.2, with the Doppler signal time interval resulting from its even division according to the number of acquisition angles, the resolution Δf is far too high. In order to correct it, it is necessary to use a wider signal time interval, however, it has to be selected in such a way that no faulty frequencies appear. It is also worth noting that for the examined acquisition angle width of $27°$, one can detect slightly below 300 Doppler bands. This gives the possibility to image objects not smaller than 1 mm [9].

On the basis of Doppler signal simulation without interference, it was found that it is possible to determine Doppler frequency with an error below one percent (Sect. 3.2) for the Doppler signal time interval (angle width) corresponding to a rotation angle of $27°$. This translates directly into good image quality.

References

1. Hamming, R.W.: Digital Filters. Prentice-Hall, Englewood Cliffs (1977)
2. Kak, A.C., Slaney, M.: Principles of Computerized Tomographic Imaging. IEEE Press, New York (1988)
3. Liang, H.-D., Halliwell, M., Wells, P.N.T.: Continuous wave ultrasonic tomography. IEEE Trans. Ultrason. Ferroelectr. Freq. Control **48**, 285–292 (2001)
4. Liang, H.-D., Tsui, C.S.L., Halliwell, M., Wells, P.N.T.: Continuous wave ultrasonic Doppler tomography. Interface Focus **1**(4), 665–672 (2011)
5. Marczak, W.: Woda jako wzorzec w pomiarach prędkości propagacji ultradźwięków w cieczach. Akustyka Molekularna i Kwantowa (Mol. Quantum Acoust.) **17**, 191–197 (1996). (in Polish)
6. Nagain, K., Greenleaf, J.F.: Ultrasonic imaging using the Doppler effect caused by a moving transduser. Opt. Eng. **29**(10), 1249–1254 (1990)
7. Nowicki, A.: Podstawy ultrasonografii dopplerowskiej. Wydawnictwa Naukowe PWN, Warszawa (1995). (in Polish)

8. Opieliński, K.J., Gudra, T.: Ultrasonic transmission tomography. In: Sikora, J., Wojtowicz, S. (eds.) Electrotechnical Institute, Warsaw (2010)
9. Świetlik, T., Opieliński, K.J.: The use of Doppler effect for tomographic tissue imaging with omnidirectional acoustic data acquisition. In: Piętka, E., et al. (eds.) Information Technologies in Medicine, Advances in Intelligent Systems and Computing, vol. 471. Springer, Switzerland (2016)

Efficient Genetic Algorithm for Breast Cancer Diagnosis

Lukasz Chomatek[✉] and Agnieszka Duraj

Lodz University of Technology, Lodz, Poland
lukasz.chomatek@p.lodz.pl

Abstract. In almost all datasets some number of abnormal observations is present. Such outliers may affect the process of data analysis. However several methods of outlier detection already exist, there is still a need to look for a new, more effective ones. In this paper we propose a set of objectives that allows to efficiently identify outliers with the use of multiobjective genetic algorithm. Conducted research shown that such a method can be successfully used with the most common genetic algorithms designed for multiobjective optimization. The results of tests, which were conducted on the set of medical data from the repository, indicate that our method can be successfully applied to the medical problem.

Keywords: Genetic algoritms · Multiobjective optimization
Outlier detection

1 Introduction

In almost all datasets some number of abnormal observations is present. Such outliers may affect the process of data analysis.

The variety of methods and applications of outlier detection demonstrates the importance of outliers in the retrieving information from databases. Distinction is made between statistical models, methods based on distance and density. Statistical methods are used mainly for quantitative data, the processing of data sets with quantitative, real, continuous values, or at least qualitative data with ordinal values. At present there is a great need for processing non-ordinal data. We have to deal with the multidimensionality of data (variables). Distance-based methods can be found in the literature. One of the most frequently used and modified methods is the k-nearest neighbors method [17–19]. This is a nonparametric approximation method which uses measures such as Euclid, Manhatan, cosinus, Chebyshev, and other to calculate the distance between neighbors, and in our case the distance between outliers and neighbors. There are also various modifications to the k-nn algorithm with the aim of outlier detection. See e.g. work [3]. Most of the methods, which are based on the distance, in relation to the number of elements in the dataset. However, there may be a problem if the data set is very large or changes dynamically. Statistical methods generally focus on

© Springer International Publishing AG, part of Springer Nature 2019
E. Pietka et al. (Eds.): ITIB 2018, AISC 762, pp. 64–76, 2019.
https://doi.org/10.1007/978-3-319-91211-0_6

detecting outliers among single data variables. They require a priori knowledge on data distribution. In such cases, the user must first define the data model using the statistical distribution. Outliers are therefore detected in the context of a predetermined model. The basic problem that may arise in this case is the lack of sufficient knowledge of the user about the distribution of the data and thus incorrectly determined model and then incorrectly detected outliers.

Most often the detection of outliers is performed according to methods based on distributions [30], depth [28], distance [3,19], density [24], clusters [13,14] and carrier vectors [23]. There are works detecting outliers on the basis of approximate sets theory [16], as well as there are outlier detection procedures combining different algorithms into one. See for example [16,27].

Works on the detection of outliers are also based on artificial intelligence methods [4], and machine learning techniques. In [4], we find a very complete compilation of the most outstanding outlier detection methods. An overview of outlier detection methods is also found in [1,2,15].

In our previous works [5,9], we proposed a method of evolutionary detection of outliers. The novelty of this approach is that we utilized a set of criteria to decide whether an object is an outlier or not. In this paper, we propose a new objectives for the fitness function which allow to obtain better and more stable results.

This paper is organized as follows: at first, we present selected methods of outlier detection. Next we describe our method for solving this problem with us of genetic algorithms. In Sect. 4, we present the results of performed experiments. The last section includes summary and proposals of future research.

2   Related Work

The detection of outliers is an important issue in machine learning, in knowledge discovery from databases or even in preliminary data processing. The concept of an outlier is defined in various ways.

The Local Outlier Factor algorithm assigns each object a degree of its uniqueness according to the formula (1) and defines the so-called local outlier. If the value of the coefficient for a given object changes abruptly in relation to its local neighbors, then the object is an outlier.

$$LOF_{M_{int}}(x) = \frac{\sum_{o \in N}^{max} \frac{lgo_{Mint}(o)}{lgo_{Mint}(x)}}{|N_{MMint}(x)|} \tag{1}$$

where lgo means the local density of the object x defined by (2) and $obr - dM(x,o)$ denotes the achievable distance of the object x from the object o.

$$lgo_M(x) = \frac{|N_{Mint}(x)|}{\sum_{o \in N}^{max} obr - d_M(x,o)} \tag{2}$$

It should be noted that the higher the degree of uniqueness of an object is, the more likely it is that the object is an outlier.

Connectivity Outlier Factor (COF) is a modification of LOF. This algorithm is based on the distance between objects, including the density of objects in the set. For each object, it determines the so-called COF isolation factor defined by Eq. (3). This coefficient determines to what extent a given object is isolated from the whole set, where SCP is called the average distance of connection or the average cost of connection.

$$COF_k(x) = \frac{|N_k(x)| \cdot SCP_{Nk(x)}(x)}{\sum_{o \in N_k(x)}^{max} SCP_{Nk(o)}(o)} \qquad (3)$$

An object is considered an outlier if the value of the determined coefficient $COFk(x)$ for this object is greater than the accepted threshold of isolation Pr, i.e. $COFk(x) > Pr$.

Most often, objects are considered outliers if $COF > 1$. In addition, in some studies, the uniqueness index, defined as (4), is introduced. An object o is an outlier if it satisfies Eq. (4).

$$COF(o) > COF_{max} - \frac{COF_{max} - 1}{WW} \qquad (4)$$

where $WW \neq 0$ is an indicator of uniqueness, and $COF_{max} = max\{COF(o_1), COF(o_2), ..., COF(o_k)\}$

It is important that the smaller the uniqueness index WW is, the more outliers COF algorithm can indicate. For $WW = 1$, objects whose $COF > 1$ will be outliers. Another algorithm for detecting outliers in a data set is the Density Based Spatial Clustering of Applications with Noise (DBSCAN) density. It performs the classification of objects into basic objects, limit objects and outliers based on two parameters: the maximum radius of the neighborhood Eps and the minimum number of points in the Eps-neighborhood MinPts. The outlier, in this algorithm, are points that have not been assigned to any of the clusters. Undoubtedly, the advantage of DBSCAN is the ability to detect clusters (areas) of irregular shapes. The difficulty concerns the proper selection of input parameters.

Outlier detection in medical data was discussed in more detail in [8]. Duraj and Szczepaniak in [10] proposed an outlier detection method based on linguistic summaries. See also [22,25].

3   Proposed Method

Most of the deterministic algorithms for outlier detection are parameterized. Proper tuning of such algorithms is very time consuming. What is more, actual performance of these methods depends on the shape of the dataset. It is hard to determine, which method is the best one for the dataset, for which we do not have any knowledge, so that all of the methods should be treated equally. This leads to the multiobjective optimization problem, where different methods of identification of outliers are the objectives. Iterative heuristic optimization tools, such as genetic algorithms, are widely used in the multiobjective optimization problems. In such optimization problems, one have to find non-dominated solutions, where the domination relation defined as follows:

The solution $f(x_1) \in \mathbb{R}^n$ dominates $f(x_2) \in \mathbb{R}^n$ iff

$$\forall_{i \in 1,...,n} f_i(x_i) \leq f_i(x_2) \tag{5}$$

and

$$\exists_{i \in 1,...,n} f_i(x_1) < f_i(x_2) \tag{6}$$

where $f_i(x)$ is the i-th value of the fitness function f, and n is the number of objectives.

The most popular approaches in this domain are [20]:

- SPEA2, proposed by Zitzler et al. [31]. This algorithm ranks the solutions by the number of other individuals they dominate and utilize the concept of archive to protect the best solutions.
- NSGA-II [7], which also favors non-dominated solutions and ensures that individuals are genetically diversified.
- PESA-II [6] which divides the search space into some number of hypercubes. In each region of the search space, the independent optimization process is performed.

3.1 Encoding and Initial Population

Each chromosome, denoted as ch, consists of some number of genes. Each gene contains an identifier of observation which is supposed to be treated as an outlier. Number of genes in the chromosome is not fixed – it can vary between the chromosomes and can be changed by crossover and mutation.

Number of individuals is constant in the whole simulation. In the initial population, each individual's chromosome consist of the specified number of genes g, which is a parameter of the algorithm. Identifiers of observations in the chromosome are chosen randomly, without repetitions.

3.2 Genetic Operators

The mutation operator has three parameters:

- p_m probability of changing the value of each gene in each chromosome,
- p_{mr} probability of removing a random sample identifier from a chromosome,
- p_{ma} probability of adding a random sample to the chromosome.

We assumed, that a sample can be removed/added once in each iteration, with the probability p_{mr} and p_{ma} respectively. During the addition of gene, we ensure that its value is distinct from the genes currently present in the chromosome.

In our algorithms we utilize well known concept of uniform crossover, which is adapted to the chromosomes of possibly different lengths. For each parent chromosome we choose a crossover point and substitute the parts of the chromosome, which is located after that point. Before we can calculate the fitness function, we have to ensure, that there are no repetitions of genes in the offspring chromosomes. If so, we substitute the repetitions with randomly chosen values.

3.3 Fitness Function

The most significant component of the algorithm is a fitness function. As it was mentioned in the previous sections, there are numerous deterministic methods for identification, which of the observations are outliers. Some of them can be directly used as the components of fitness function in genetic algorithms. In our former research we used three kinds of such measures:

– average k-nearest distance of the outliers from the non-outlier observations,
– average distance of outliers from the centroid of the dataset,
– overall number of outliers.

Let us denote as x_{ch} a set of observations identified as outliers by an individual with chromosome ch. Moreover, we denote as x'_{ch} a set of observations which are not in x_{ch}.

The first objective is the average distance of the samples in x_{ch} from the k nearest samples in x'_{ch}. It is denoted as $d_k(ch)$. To get the value for this measure, one need to:

– calculate the distances from the samples in x'_{ch} for each sample $s \in x_{ch}$,
– sort the samples and take the k-th value,
– add the values obtained in the previous step and divide them between the number of elements in x_{ch}.

The second type of objective in the fitness function is the average distance of the samples in x_{ch} to the centroid of the x'_{ch} dataset. Centroid is actually an average position of the samples in x'_{ch}:

$$c(x'_{ch}) = \frac{\sum_{s' \in x'_{ch}} s'}{|x'_{ch}|} \tag{7}$$

The actual value of this objective is calculated as follows:

$$dc(ch) = \frac{\sum_{s \in x_{ch}} s - c(x'_{ch})}{|x_{ch}|} \tag{8}$$

where $|x_{ch}|$ is the number of elements in the set x_{ch}.

As it is supposed that the number of outliers should be much smaller than the number of samples in the whole dataset, the last type of objective is the number of the identified outliers (denoted as $no(ch)$).

In our former experiments we used the fitness function composed of five objectives: d_1, d_2, d_3, dc and no (Eq. (9)).

$$fitness(ch) = [-d_1(ch), -d_2(ch), -d_3(ch), -dc(ch), no(ch)] \tag{9}$$

In Eq. (9), d_k distances and dc are taken with '$-$', because we expect all of the criteria to be minimized (Eqs. (5) and (6)).

However the results obtained with use of fitness function in the form given in Eq. (9) were promising [5], we decided to introduce new types of objectives to improve the stability of the optimization process. In this paper we propose two new measures and use them to substitute these, which are based on the k-nearest distance.

The first new measure, denoted as $non_t(ch)$, is the average number of outliers, that are in the neighborhood of size t, of each observation $o' \in x'_{ch}$. While calculating the neighborhood of o' we use the Euclidean distance.

The second new measure, denoted as sno, is the difference between desired number of observations to be marked as outliers (denoted as d) and actual number of such observations:

$$sno(ch, d) = |d - |x_{ch}||$$ (10)

The final form of the fitness function is

$$fitness(ch, t, d) = [-dc(ch), non_t(ch), sno(ch, d)]$$ (11)

Obviously, there can be more than one individual in the Pareto-set found by genetic algorithms. In this case we decided to introduce the accuracy factor for each sample s (denoted as $acc(s)$). Let X denote the set of individuals that are on the Pareto front. Value of $acc(s)$ is calculated as follows:

$$acc(s) = \frac{\sum\limits_{ch \in X} p(s, ch)}{|X|}$$ (12)

where:

$$p(s, ch) = \begin{cases} 1 & \text{for } s \in x_{ch} \\ 0 & \text{otherwise} \end{cases}$$ (13)

4 Results

We conducted our experiments in jMetal environment [11,12]. JMetal is a framework written in Java, that supports computations with use of multiobjective heuristic methods. As a dataset for this paper we used broadly examined Wisconsin Breast Cancer data [26,29]. There are 699 samples in the dataset. Each sample consists of 9 attributes describing the results of examination and one attribute classifying the disease (malignant or benign). The attributes describing the disease are [26]:

- clump thickness,
- uniformity of cell size,
- uniformity of cell shape,
- marginal adhesion,
- single epithelial cell size,
- bare nuclei,
- bland chromatin,
- normal nucleoli,
- mitoses.

Due to the fact, that some samples contains attributes with missing values, we decided not to take them into account during the computations. For our experiments, we took first 100 samples with no missing values. Such a dataset contained 82 benign samples and 18 malignant samples, which were supposed to be treated as outliers.

We performed two series of experiments. In the first experiment, we have taken into account all nine attributes describing the disease. In the second experiment we considered only first four attributes. The attribute identifying the type of disease was never included in the computations, but only used for checking whether obtained results were correct.

In our research we used three different genetic algorithms: NSGA-II, PESA2, SPEA-2. Parameters of the algorithms were set as follows:

- crossover probability: 60%,
- mutation probability for each gene (p_m): 1%, equal probabilities p_{ma} and p_{mr}: 2%,
- archive size: 20,
- number of bisections: 5 (only for PESA2 algorithm),
- tournament selection with two competitors,
- initial number of genes: 20,
- desired number of outliers: 20,
- threshold size for the observations marked as outliers: 10.

In both experiments we examined different sizes of the population (10, 20 or 50 individuals) and different number of fitness function evaluations (2000, 3000, 4000, 5000).

As the results of our experiments we present:

- percent of correctly identified outliers (denoted as CO),
- average accuracy for correctly identified outliers (denoted as COAcc),
- percent of correct observations identified as outliers (denoted as FO),
- average accuracy for incorrectly identified outliers (denoted as FOAcc).

For each set of parameters we performed 20 runs of all three algorithms. The values of CO and FO presented in this paper are the most frequent values from these runs.

4.1   Full Feature Set

In the Tables 1, 2 and 3 we gathered the results of the first experiment. We observed, that even for the lowest size of the population, obtained results are satisfying. What is more, all of the algorithms found a solution with relatively small number of fitness function evaluations. Obtained results do not vary significantly while comparing the algorithms, however for the NSGA-II we observed the smallest values of the accuracy for false outliers. Actual number of incorrectly identified outliers does not differ depending on the algorithm as well.

Table 1. Performance of the SPEA2 algorithm on the full feature set

Population	Evaluations	CO [%]	COAcc	FO [%]	FOAcc
10	2000	88.88	0.89	3.65	0.66
10	3000	83.33	0.89	4.87	0.64
10	4000	77.77	0.92	8.53	0.41
10	5000	83.33	0.93	3.65	0.66
20	2000	72.22	0.92	7.31	0.80
20	3000	72.22	0.98	8.53	0.62
20	4000	88.88	0.9	2.43	1.00
20	5000	88.88	0.82	4.87	0.50
50	2000	83.33	0.93	6.09	0.61
50	3000	72.22	0.88	12.19	0.49
50	4000	77.77	0.93	6.09	0.63
50	5000	83.33	0.86	3.65	1.00

4.2   Limited Feature Set

Results obtained for the limited feature set are gathered in the Tables 4, 5 and 6. Actual values of CO and COAcc does not differ significantly from those obtained for the full feature set. As in the previous case, we observed that there is no need to use a big number of individuals in the population, as well as big number of evaluations. As one can see, values of FO are higher for the lower number of fitness function evaluations. This can be caused by the fact, that in the limited

Table 2. Performance of the PESA2 algorithm on the full feature set

Population	Evaluations	CO [%]	COAcc	FO [%]	FOAcc
10	2000	83.33	0.92	7.31	0.51
10	3000	83.33	0.90	4.87	0.92
10	4000	72.22	0.97	7.31	0.58
10	5000	77.77	0.96	4.87	0.57
20	2000	83.33	0.99	3.65	0.63
20	3000	77.77	0.92	3.65	0.73
20	4000	72.22	1.0	6.09	0.72
20	5000	83.33	0.88	3.65	0.62
50	2000	83.33	0.85	7.31	0.60
50	3000	77.77	0.97	6.09	0.42
50	4000	88.88	0.81	4.87	0.52
50	5000	88.88	0.92	4.87	0.49

Table 3. Performance of the NSGA-II algorithm on the full feature set

Population	Evaluations	CO [%]	COAcc	FO [%]	FOAcc
10	2000	72.22	0.96	10.97	0.46
10	3000	83.33	0.82	7.31	0.61
10	4000	83.33	0.80	6.09	0.52
10	5000	88.88	0.80	4.87	0.35
20	2000	77.77	0.91	8.53	0.54
20	3000	88.88	0.84	4.87	0.65
20	4000	94.44	0.84	3.65	0.73
20	5000	83.33	0.92	4.87	0.42
50	2000	77.77	0.84	14.63	0.37
50	3000	77.77	0.99	4.87	0.61
50	4000	88.88	0.78	3.65	0.81
50	5000	83.33	0.90	3.65	0.71

Table 4. Performance of the SPEA2 algorithm on the limited feature set

Population	Evaluations	CO [%]	COAcc	FO [%]	FOAcc
10	2000	83.33	0.85	4.87	0.42
10	3000	77.77	0.85	13.41	0.39
10	4000	83.33	0.84	10.97	0.38
10	5000	83.33	0.85	8.53	0.21
20	2000	83.33	0.97	3.65	0.78
20	3000	88.88	0.86	3.65	0.71
20	4000	83.33	0.83	4.87	0.62
20	5000	88.88	0.88	3.65	0.53
50	2000	83.33	0.97	8.53	0.4
50	3000	72.22	0.96	6.09	0.52
50	4000	88.88	0.89	4.87	0.48
50	5000	77.77	0.93	4.87	0.51

feature space, the outliers are closer to the real observations. On the other hand, after 5000 evaluations, values of FO does not differ from those obtained for the full feature set.

Table 5. Performance of the PESA2 algorithm on the limited feature set

Population	Evaluations	CO [%]	COAcc	FO [%]	FOAcc
10	2000	83.33	0.93	6.09	0.66
10	3000	77.77	0.91	7.31	0.56
10	4000	88.88	0.93	2.43	0.67
10	5000	94.44	0.83	3.65	0.70
20	2000	66.66	1.00	7.31	0.63
20	3000	66.66	0.95	7.31	0.56
20	4000	83.33	0.78	3.65	0.41
20	5000	88.88	0.86	3.65	0.66
50	2000	72.22	0.93	8.53	0.52
50	3000	77.77	0.98	6.09	0.60
50	4000	77.77	0.93	7.31	0.45
50	5000	83.33	0.93	3.65	0.46

Table 6. Performance of the NSGA-II algorithm on the limited feature set

Population	Evaluations	CO [%]	COAcc	FO [%]	FOAcc
10	2000	77.77	0.97	4.87	0.59
10	3000	83.33	0.92	4.87	0.39
10	4000	72.22	0.76	9.75	0.33
10	5000	88.88	0.88	2.43	0.79
20	2000	72.22	0.94	6.09	0.74
20	3000	83.33	0.88	9.75	0.25
20	4000	83.33	0.93	4.87	0.37
20	5000	94.44	0.83	3.65	0.65
50	2000	72.22	0.85	8.53	0.37
50	3000	88.88	0.75	10.97	0.26
50	4000	83.33	0.82	4.87	0.50
50	5000	83.33	0.92	3.65	0.70

5 Conclusion

In this paper we proposed new measures for identifying outliers. First of them represents the difference between the number of samples actually marked as outliers and desired number of such observations. However it can be relatively hard to choose a desired number correctly, in some cases it can be based on the expert's knowledge.

The second measure, we proposed determines how many observations from the dataset are close to the observations marked as outliers. Conducted experiments revealed that such an objective can be successfully applied in the fitness function for the multiobjective genetic algorithm. Such a measure cannot be directly applied to the deterministic algorithms, because they are not iterative.

Obtained results shown that proposed fitness function and the method for acquiring the accuracy can be used with all of the most popular genetic algorithms. In all the cases, most of the outliers were identified correctly with the high value of the accuracy coefficient. On the other hand, the number of false outliers was relatively small (3–4 cases of the 82) and the accuracy coefficient for these observations was usually significantly lower than one obtained for the real outliers.

Actual performance of all investigated algorithms was similar – even for the small population and low number of evaluations of the fitness function, the percentage of correctly identified outliers was satisfying. The higher number of evaluations allowed to decrease the number of incorrectly identified outliers.

As it was mentioned before, there is a need to set the values of two parameters (desired number of outliers and the size of threshold for outliers) to calculate value of the fitness function. Finding optimal values of these parameters can be hard. In our future works we will try to mitigate this phenomenon and propose the method that allows automatic selection of the parameters' values.

Acknowledgement. This work was supported by a grant of the Dean of the Faculty of Technical Physics, Information Technology and Applied Mathematics, Lodz University of Technology. The dataset used in our research was taken from the UCI Machine Learning Repository [21].

References

1. Aggarwal, C.C.: Outlier detection in categorical, text and mixed attribute data. In: Outlier Analysis, pp. 199–223. Springer (2013)
2. Aggarwal, C.C., Yu, P.S.: Outlier detection for high dimensional data. ACM SIGMOD Rec. **30**, 37–46 (2001)
3. Bay, S.D., Schwabacher, M.: Mining distance-based outliers in near linear time with randomization and a simple pruning rule. In: Proceedings of the Ninth ACM SIGKDD International Conference on Knowledge Discovery and Data Mining, pp. 29–38. ACM (2003)
4. Chandola, V., Banerjee, A., Kumar, V.: Anomaly detection: a survey. ACM Comput. Surv. (CSUR) **41**(3), 15 (2009)
5. Chomatek, L., Duraj, A.: Multiobjective genetic algorithm for outliers detection. In: 2017 IEEE International Conference on Innovations in Intelligent SysTems and Applications (INISTA), pp. 379–384. IEEE (2017)
6. Corne, D.W., Jerram, N.R., Knowles, J.D., Oates, M.J.: PESA-II: region-based selection in evolutionary multiobjective optimization. In: Proceedings of the 3rd Annual Conference on Genetic and Evolutionary Computation, pp. 283–290. Morgan Kaufmann Publishers Inc. (2001)

7. Deb, K., Pratap, A., Agarwal, S., Meyarivan, T.: A fast and elitist multiobjective genetic algorithm: NSGA-II. IEEE Trans. Evol. Comput. **6**(2), 182–197 (2002)
8. Duraj, A., Krawczyk, A.: Finding outliers for large medical datasets. Przeglad Elektrotechniczny **86**, 188–191 (2010)
9. Duraj, A., Chomatek, L.: Supporting breast cancer diagnosis with multi-objective genetic algorithm for outlier detection. In: International Conference on Diagnostics of Processes and Systems, pp. 304–315. Springer (2017)
10. Duraj, A., Szczepaniak, P.S.: Information outliers and their detection. In: Information Studies and the Quest for Transdisciplinarity, pp. 413–437. World Scientific Publishing Company (2017)
11. Durillo, J.J., Nebro, A.J.: jMetal: a java framework for multi-objective optimization. Adv. Eng. Softw. **42**(10), 760–771 (2011)
12. Durillo, J.J., Nebro, A.J., Alba, E.: The jMetal framework for multi-objective optimization: design and architecture. In: 2010 IEEE Congress on Evolutionary Computation (CEC), pp. 1–8. IEEE (2010)
13. He, Z., Deng, S., Xu, X.: Outlier detection integrating semantic knowledge. In: International Conference on Web-Age Information Management, pp. 126–131. Springer (2002)
14. He, Z., Xu, X., Deng, S.: Discovering cluster-based local outliers. Pattern Recogn. Lett. **24**(9), 1641–1650 (2003)
15. Hodge, V.J., Austin, J.: A survey of outlier detection methodologies. Artif. Intell. Rev. **22**(2), 85–126 (2004)
16. Jiang, F., Sui, Y., Cao, C.: Outlier detection using rough set theory. In: Rough Sets, Fuzzy Sets, Data Mining, and Granular Computing, pp. 79–87 (2005)
17. Knorr, E.M., Ng, R.T.: Finding intensional knowledge of distance-based outliers. In: VLDB, vol. 99, pp. 211–222 (1999)
18. Knorr, E.M., Ng, R.T., Tucakov, V.: Distance-based outliers: algorithms and applications. Int. J. Very Large Data Bases (VLDB) **8**(3–4), 237–253 (2000)
19. Knox, E.M., Ng, R.T.: Algorithms for mining distance-based outliers in large datasets. In: Proceedings of the International Conference on Very Large Data Bases, pp. 392–403. Citeseer (1998)
20. Konak, A., Coit, D.W., Smith, A.E.: Multi-objective optimization using genetic algorithms: a tutorial. Reliab. Eng. Syst. Saf. **91**(9), 992–1007 (2006)
21. Lichman, M.: UCI machine learning repository (2013). http://archive.ics.uci.edu/ml
22. Lilford, R., Mohammed, M.A., Spiegelhalter, D., Thomson, R.: Use and misuse of process and outcome data in managing performance of acute medical care: avoiding institutional stigma. Lancet **363**(9415), 1147–1154 (2004)
23. Petrovskiy, M.: A hybrid method for patterns mining and outliers detection in the web usage log. In: Advances in Web Intelligence, pp. 954–954 (2003)
24. Ren, D., Wang, B., Perrizo, W.: Rdf: A density-based outlier detection method using vertical data representation. In: 2004 Fourth IEEE International Conference on Data Mining, ICDM 2004, pp. 503–506. IEEE (2004)
25. Shaari, F., Bakar, A.A., Hamdan, A.R.: A predictive analysis on medical data based on outlier detection method using non-reduct computation. In: International Conference on Advanced Data Mining and Applications. pp. 603–610. Springer (2009)
26. Street, W.N., Wolberg, W.H., Mangasarian, O.L.: Nuclear feature extraction for breast tumor diagnosis. In: IS & T/SPIE's Symposium on Electronic Imaging: Science and Technology, pp. 861–870. International Society for Optics and Photonics (1993)

27. Tang, J., Chen, Z., Fu, A.W.C., Cheung, D.: A robust outlier detection scheme for large data sets. In: 6th Pacific-Asia Conference on Knowledge Discovery and Data Mining. Citeseer (2001)
28. Theodore, J., Ivy, K., Raymong, T.: Fast computation of 2D depth contours. ACM SIG KDD, pp. 224–228 (1998)
29. Wolberg, W.H., Street, W.N., Mangasarian, O.: Machine learning techniques to diagnose breast cancer from image-processed nuclear features of fine needle aspirates. Cancer Lett. **77**(2–3), 163–171 (1994)
30. Yamanishi, K., Takeuchi, J.i.: Discovering outlier filtering rules from unlabeled data: combining a supervised learner with an unsupervised learner. In: Proceedings of the seventh ACM SIGKDD International Conference on Knowledge Discovery and Data Mining, pp. 389–394. ACM (2001)
31. Zitzler, E., Laumanns, M., Thiele, L., et al.: Spea2: Improving the strength pareto evolutionary algorithm (2001)

Preliminary Development of an Automatic Breast Tumour Segmentation Algorithm from Ultrasound Volumetric Images

Wojciech Wieclawek[✉], Marcin Rudzki, Agata Wijata, and Marta Galinska

Faculty of Biomedical Engineering, Silesian University of Technology,
Roosevelta 40, 41-800 Zabrze, Poland
wojciech.wieclawek@polsl.pl
http://ib.polsl.pl

Abstract. Breast tumour is a leading cause for woman mortality. While cancer screening is mostly performed by the use of mammography, 3D ultrasound seems better suited for the purpose. It gives 3D view of the breast structure, is less painful and can be considered less invasive, as the patient is not exposed to x-ray radiation. Therefore, the development of automatic algorithms that remove from the diagnostician the tedious and time consuming task of finding suspicious regions in large volumetric images is of key importance. The paper concludes a preliminary study for the development of an automatic method for breast tumour segmentation in ultrasound volumetric images. The method is based on multi-scale blob detector, watershed transform with the final precise segmentation performed by an active contour approach. The method has been evaluated using 16 volumes acquired from a breast phantom containing nodules. The obtained results reached up to 94.68% sensitivity, 100.00% specificity, 92.63% Dice index, 99.95% Accuracy, 92.61% Cohen's Kappa index and 86.28% Jaccard index.

Keywords: Breast tumour · Ultrasonography
Automatic segmentation · Image processing

1 Introduction

Breast cancer is the second most common cancer overall and the fifth most common cause of death from cancer. In women it is the most common type of cancer with 1.67 million new cases and 0.52 million casualties worldwide estimated for the year 2012 [1]. Breast Ultrasound (BUS) is becoming an important method for breast tumour diagnosis. Ultrasound (US) can be considered less invasive than mammography as it does not expose the patient to x-ray radiation. Also it is less painful, yet the acquisition protocol is more operator dependent. With the availability of 3D transducers or tracking systems together with volumetric image reconstruction methods, the obtained image datasets enable diagnosticians to perform more precise measurements than using just planar imaging.

© Springer International Publishing AG, part of Springer Nature 2019
E. Pietka et al. (Eds.): ITIB 2018, AISC 762, pp. 77–88, 2019.
https://doi.org/10.1007/978-3-319-91211-0_7

However, manual analysis of image volumes containing hundreds of slices is a timely and tedious work. Thus the development of automatic methods for detection of suspicious regions is of key importance.

Breast tumours appear as hypointensive (hypoechoic) areas in BUS images. Frequently they are also accompanied with echo shadows that highly influence the perceived tumour borders within the image. US images also exhibit multiplicative speckle noise that further makes the detection and segmentation task much more difficult. The subject of tumour segmentation is widely represented in the literature. Some segmentation approaches have been summarized in Table 1. Most of the approaches use planar 2D images, hence can utilize very complex processing algorithms including machine learning classifiers due to relatively small image size when comparing to volumetric data. Some approaches are semiautomatic that require the operator to select at least a rectangular region around the lesion. Numerical results of the literature methods are summarised in Table 2. However, in many cases the tumour segmentation itself was not of concern, as the method was aimed at classification of cases/images as benign or malignant and only those results were reported. Therefore, direct comparison of just the segmentation approaches is limited.

Despite the reported results reach up to over 90% sensitivity and almost 100% specificity, the tumour segmentation task is still considered a non-trivial task, thus motivating various research groups to accept the challenge.

This paper concludes a preliminary study that is a direct follow-up of [8] and is aimed at the development of a fully automatic method for breast tumour segmentation in volumetric BUS images. The method has been validated on a set of 16 volumetric images, that come from a phantom of breast tumour composed of a hydrogel ball immersed *ex vivo* in animal muscular tissue. Due to the acquisition method (described in the next section) the BUS images also contain additional content, that the automatic segmentation method should ignore.

2   Materials

A measurement station consists of an ultrasound machine Philips iU22 with linear transducer Philips L12-5 operating at Small Parts Breast Advanced preset. The transducer was equipped with markers for tracking its position and orientation in 3D space. NDI Polaris Vicra was used as a tracking system and it was calibrated with the use of *Public software Library for UltraSound imaging research* (PLUS) Toolkit [15]. Image data was acquired using Epiphan DVI2USB3.0 frame grabber at 10 frames per second. Frames were captured directly from the US scanner's video output, thus contain additional content, not only the US image itself. Each acquired image frame has been supplemented with affine transformation matrix specifying the 3D position and orientation data provided by the tracking system. The PLUS Toolkit was also used for volumetric reconstruction of the acquired planar images into a single volumetric image. The voxel size of the reconstructed volumes was 0.1 mm in each direction and typical image size was $550 \times 630 \times 500$ voxels.

Table 1. Summary of BUS segmentation approaches – used methods

Ref. year	Dim	Preprocessing	Candidate region	Final segmentation
[4] 2003	3D	Histogram equalization, 3D stick filter	Automatic threshold, Morphology	3D snake
[11] 2004	2D	Filters selected by neural network based on texture analysis	Gray level and connectivity based	Marker-based Watershed
[3] 2005	2D	Anisotropic diffusion, stick filter, Otsu threshold	Manual	Level-Set
[21] 2010	2D	Multi-peak Generalized Histogram Equalization	Manual	Markov Random Field with Metropolis sampler
[16] 2010	2D	Intensity membership determined by maximum fuzzy entropy	16 × 16 pixel lattice to be classified	Kernelized Support Vector Machine on texture descriptors
[12] 2012	2D	Not stated	AdaBoost with Haar-like features, Support Vector Machine on intensity features	Random Walk algorithm
[18] 2012	2D	Gaussian smoothing, anisotropic diffusion	Manual	Active contour
[19] 2013	3D	Anisotropic diffusion, sigma filter	Hessian based blob detector	Regression models in feature space, threshold
[20] 2013	2D	Lee, Frost, Kuan edge preserving smoothing	Hierarchical fuzzy C-means	Generalized Gradient Vector Flow snake
[13] 2014	2D	Boundary removal, morphology, averaging	Modified Otsu threshold, morphology	Region size and location constraints
[22] 2015	2D	Gaussian smoothing, adaptive non-linear intensity remapping	Anatomy-based seeds, morphological reconstruction, Otsu threshold	Max-flow min-cut graph optimization with spatial and frequency constraints
[10] 2015	2D	Total-variation model	Robust Graph-Based grouping, Support Vector Machine classification using intensity, gradient and shape features	Active contour
[9] 2016	3D	Morphological reconstruction	Sobel edge detector	2D watershed, intensity and size threshold criteria
[8] 2017	2D	Anisotropic diffusion	Manual contour points selection	Active contour

Table 2. Summary of BUS segmentation approaches – reported results

Ref. year	Dim.	Number of images used	Measure	Value
			Quantitative Results	
[4] 2003	3D	8	match rate	90.2% – 99.6%
[11] 2004	2D	60 (40 training,	match rate	83.11% – 99.44%
		20 validation)	precision ratio	67.56% – 88.80%
[3] 2005	2D	210	accuracy	90.95%
segmentation results not stated,			Sensitivity	88.89%
numerical results only for			specificity	92.5%
classification benign/malignant			positive predictive value	89.89%
			negative predictive value	91.74%
[21] 2010	2D	87	area under curve	0.964
segmentation results not stated,			accuracy	94.25%
numerical results only for			sensitivity	91.67%
classification benign/malignant			specificity	96.08%
			positive predictive value	94.29%
			negative predictive value	94.23%
[16] 2010	2D	112	precision ratio	82.33%
			recall ratio	83.81%
[12] 2012	2D	112	accuracy	87.5%
segmentation results not stated,			sensitivity	88.8%
results only for tumour/healthy			specificity	84.4%
[18] 2012	2D	100	area under curve	0.88
segmentation results not stated,			sensitivity	92.7%
results only for tumour/healthy			specificity	90.3%
[19] 2013	3D	159	sensitivity	100%
			false positive per pass	17.4
			sensitivity	90%
			false positive per pass	8.8
			sensitivity	70%
			false positive per pass	2.7
[20] 2013	2D	195 synthetic	true positives	97.47% – 99.89%
			Hausdorff distance	6.40 – 4.59
		48 real	true positives	87.58% – 92.06%
			Hausdorff distance	11.59 – 5.17
[13] 2014	2D	89	sensitivity for benign	90.47%
			sensitivity for malignant	92.59%
[22] 2015	2D	184	true positive ratio	91.23%
			false positive ratio	9.97%
			similarity ratio	83.73%
			average Hausdorff error	20.43%
			average mean absolute error	4.93%
[10] 2015	2D	46	true positives	85.01%
			false positives	1.78%
			false negatives	14.99%
			average radial error	9.08
[9] 2016	3D	21	overlap ratio	85.7%
			Jaccard similarity index	70.3% – 80.6%
			segmentation error	10.2% – 5.1%
[8] 2017	2D	6 synthetic	Dice index	78% – 92%
			Hausdorff distance	6.26 – 4.89
		6 real	Dice index	64% – 87%
			Hausdorff distance	14.18 – 6.86

All experiments were performed on a breast phantom with an 11 mm diameter hydrogel sphere immersed in poultry meat slices [8]. The hydrogel may simulate a cyst because of its similarity to water echogenicity. The meat around the sphere acted as healthy breast tissue. All datasets were recorded in the same manner: first frames contain images of meat without visible hydrogel, next the probe was moved, and area of the sphere was scanned with straight linear freehand motion with an average speed of 1 mm/s. Last frames contain images behind the inserted sphere. This method of data acquisition together with volume reconstruction gives volumetric images of the simulated tumor and its environment. The experiment was repeated 16 times and each case was subject to further analysis. All volumes have been supplied with expert manual delineations providing ground truth for the assessment of the automatic segmentation results obtained within this study.

3   Methods

3.1   Image Processing

The developed segmentation method is summarized in the Fig. 1 and consists of two fundamental parts: candidate region determination and proper tumour segmentation. The determination of candidate region is a crucial part of the segmentation algorithm influencing the final segmentation results.

First, the input image Fig. 1a is despeckle using median filter. In order to reduce the required resources (processing time and memory) for the proposed method, the first part is performed on images 3-times downsampled using bicubic interpolation. Intermediate results are then resized and in the final stage the input image is analysed in its original resolution.

In order to detect initial tumour regions a Hessian based dark blob detector [19] (that is based on Frangi's multiscale vesselness filter [7]) together with watershed transform [17] are used. The blobness filter produces a relatively large positive peak in the candidate regions (Fig. 1b). After intensity inversion a topographic area with a very deep basin is formed at the place of the blob, that is further subject to watershed transform. Additionally, the blobness result is binarized (Fig. 1c) and used as marker to select watershed basins. In this way neighbouring regions of high blobness are separated by watershed dams (Fig. 1d). Next, the region having the largest volume is assumed to be the candidate tumour region (Fig. 1e). Using this candidate region as an initial contour and median-filtered downsampled BUS image the candidate region is expanded (Fig. 1f) to enable faster proper segmentation in the last stage of the algorithm where images in original resolution are processed. For this purpose the Chan-Vese [2] active contour algorithm is used.

The final stage is responsible for precise segmentation in the native image resolution, hence, the previously obtained candidate regions are accordingly upsampled. These regions are then used as a starting contour for the Chan-Vese active contour approach, where the feature input of the active contour is median-filtered input BUS image. Finally the precise delineation is obtained (Fig. 1g).

82   W. Wieclawek et al.

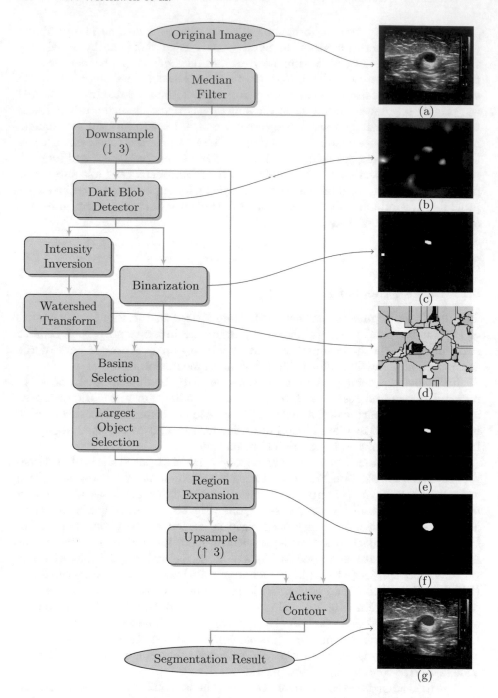

Fig. 1. The proposed automatic tumour segmentation algorithm

3.2   Quality Measures

The segmentation quality was assessed based on sensitivity:

$$Sens = \frac{TP}{TP + FN}, \tag{1}$$

and the specificity:

$$Spec = \frac{TN}{TN + FP} \tag{2}$$

coefficients. TP, TN, FP, FN denote the number of True Positive, True Negative, False Positive and False Negative voxel detections, respectively. In the following section of the paper, both measures (sensitivity and specificity) are presented as percentage.

The results are also quantified by the use of Dice index:

$$D = \frac{2 \cdot TP}{2 \cdot TP + FP + FN}, \tag{3}$$

and the Jaccard index:

$$J = \frac{D}{2 - D}. \tag{4}$$

Both the Dice index and Jaccard index are considered in the percentage scale.

Finally, the dispersion between manual and automatic delineations and segmentation results is evaluated by Cohen's Kappa [6] measure defined as:

$$\kappa = \frac{Acc - randAcc}{1 - randAcc} \tag{5}$$

where accuracy (Acc) is an observational probability of agreement and random accuracy ($randAcc$) is a hypothetical expected probability of agreement under an appropriate set of baseline constraints [14]. Accuracy can be written as:

$$Acc = \frac{TP + TN}{TP + TN + FP + FN}, \tag{6}$$

while random accuracy as:

$$randAcc = \frac{(TN + FP) \cdot (TN + FN) + (FN + TP) \cdot (FP + TP)}{(TP + TN + FP + FN)^2}. \tag{7}$$

4   Results

To evaluate the proposed automatic approach with expert delineations typical segmentation quality indices were computed. Numerical values and their aggregates of the quality measures for all BUS examinations are presented in Table 3.

These values are also presented in the box plot (Fig. 2) which graphically illustrates the obtained results. The asterisk (*) symbol is used to mark the mean value.

Table 3. Segmentation quality measures for the proposed algorithm

BUS series	Sens	Spec	Dice	Acc	Kappa	Jaccard
1	62.96	100.00	76.99	99.79	76.89	62.58
2	86.94	99.93	87.35	99.86	87.29	77.55
3	89.42	99.96	90.98	99.91	90.93	83.45
4	65.35	100.00	78.97	99.81	78.88	62.25
5	80.32	99.97	85.62	99.87	85.56	74.86
6	69.81	99.95	77.17	99.80	77.07	62.83
7	94.68	99.97	92.63	99.95	92.61	86.28
8	71.44	99.96	80.08	99.82	79.99	66.78
9	86.55	99.95	87.81	99.89	87.75	78.26
10	68.89	99.96	78.03	99.80	77.93	63.98
11	78.90	99.98	85.70	99.90	85.65	74.98
12	68.29	99.95	76.58	99.78	76.47	62.05
13	87.85	99.95	88.32	99.90	88.26	79.08
14	83.99	99.95	85.11	99.89	85.05	74.07
15	77.17	99.98	84.24	99.88	84.18	72.77
16	88.58	99.96	89.05	99.91	89.01	80.27
Max	94.68	100.00	92.63	99.95	92.61	86.28
Median	79.61	99.96	85.37	99.88	85.31	74.47
Mean	78.82	99.96	84.04	99.86	83.97	72.63
Min	62.96	99.93	76.58	99.78	76.47	62.05

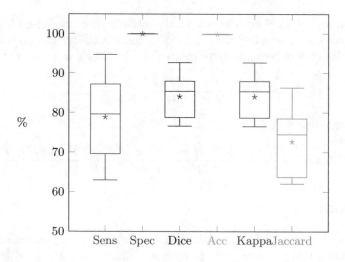

Fig. 2. The segmentation quality measures for all BUS cases

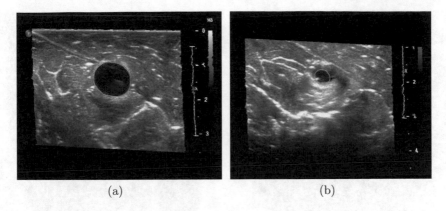

(a)   (b)

Fig. 3. Delineations comparison for case No. 1: (a) middle slice and (b) outer slice (green – gold standard, red – segmentation result)

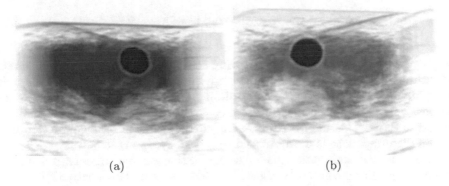

(a)   (b)

Fig. 4. 3D visualization of the segmentation results, cases: (a) No. 11 and (b) No. 13

The visual comparison of the segmentation result (red contour) with gold standard (green delineation) on a 2D view for two exemplary slices is shown in Fig. 3. Additionally, the volumetric presentation of the segmentation results is shown in Fig. 4. Due to the relatively small differences between the automatic segmentation results and the gold standard, the reference delineation is not shown.

At the preliminary stage of the evaluation, the method was also tested on several clinical images available to the authors. As can be seen in Fig. 5 the method gives promising results in terms of identification of suspected image regions. However, the evaluation over a larger dataset with numerical validation of the method will be carried out in the next phase of the project.

5 Discussion

One can observe that the input images are disturbed what can be easily noticed on non-US image content (especially axes and legend). This is mainly caused

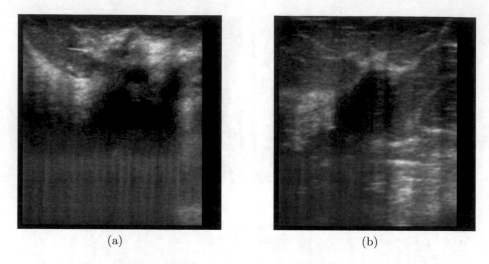

(a)   (b)

Fig. 5. Segmentation results for clinical data

by the used acquisition scheme involving tracking device and reconstruction algorithm. However, in clinical use the environment will not be as repeatable as in laboratory, thus the only way to limit its influence is to use more precise devices. This, on the other hand generates cost, thus the final solution may not be cost-effective. Developing a processing method that is capable of operation also on disturbed data is a way to reduce overall system cost.

The proposed automatic tumour segmentation method undersegments the image, i.e. resulting contour is situated inside gold standard contour. This can be considered a safer option, however geometric parameters (e.g. volume, minor and major axis) estimation also become understated. The method is also robust enough to ignore the non US image content despite presence of large dark areas also indicated by blob detector. Tests of the presented method performed on clinical data indicate its usefulness for large datasets, where automatic detection of potentially pathological regions can significantly reduce time needed for the diagnosis. The method is to be further developed as more clinical images will become available.

To the best knowledge of the authors, there is still no publicly available benchmark database of BUS images (still unresolved issue indicated by e.g. [5]) that would allow various methods and CAD systems to be easily compared. Due to heavy dependence on acquisition setup and operator experience image databases used in various research groups may not be comparable and so the obtained results. An approach using a cheap and easy to prepare phantom seems to be an idea worth following, however, it still does not resolve the issue of image variability between studies.

The used phantom (hydrogel spheres *ex vivo* immersed in animal muscular tissue) does not ideally reflect the breast tissue, however it allows for a more controllable acquisition protocol to be developed. The resulting images do not differ significantly from real BUS images. The development of the phantom itself is also an interesting research area.

6 Summary

In this paper an automatic algorithm for breast tumour segmentation in volumetric BUS images has been presented. The method was validated using phantom-based volumetric images acquired using a standard US protocol and transducer additionally equipped with tracking system that allowed volumetric image reconstruction. Obtained results are promising, but further research is required. Obtaining clinical BUS images in order to assess and further develop the method is of main concern for the near future.

Acknowledgement. This research was supported by the Polish National Centre for Research and Development (NCBR), grant no. STRATEGMED2/267398/3/NCBR/2015. The authors would also like to thank Andre Woloshuk for his English language corrections.

References

1. Cancer fact sheets: Breast cancer. http://gco.iarc.fr/today/fact-sheets-cancers?cancer=15&type=0&sex=2
2. Chan, T.F., Vese, L.A.: Active contours without edges. Trans. Img. Proc. **10**(2), 266–277 (2001). https://doi.org/10.1109/83.902291
3. Chang, R.F., Wu, W.J., Moon, W.K., Chen, D.R.: Automatic ultrasound segmentation and morphology based diagnosis of solid breast tumors. Breast Cancer Res. Treat. **80**(2), 179 (2005). https://doi.org/10.1007/s10549-004-2049-z
4. Chang, R.F., Wu, W.J., Moon, W.K., Chen, W.M., Lee, W., Chen, D.R.: Segmentation of breast tumor in three-dimensional ultrasound images using three-dimensional discrete active contour model. Ultrasound Med. Biol. **29**(11), 1571–1581 (2003). https://doi.org/10.1016/S0301-5629(03)00992-X
5. Cheng, H., Shan, J., Ju, W., Guo, Y., Zhang, L.: Automated breast cancer detection and classification using ultrasound images: a survey. Patt. Recogn. **43**(1), 299–317 (2010). https://doi.org/10.1016/j.patcog.2009.05.012
6. Cohen, J.: A coefficient of agreement for nominal scale. Educ. Psychol. Measur. **20**, 37–46 (1960)
7. Frangi, A.F., Niessen, W.J., Vincken, K.L., Viergever, M.A.: Multiscale vessel enhancement filtering. In: Wells, W.M., Colchester, A., Delp, S. (eds.) Medical Image Computing and Computer-Assisted Intervention – MICCAI 1998, pp. 130–137. Springer, Heidelberg (1998)
8. Galińska, M., Ogiegło, W., Wijata, A., Juszczyk, J., Czajkowska, J.: Breast cancer segmentation method in ultrasound images. In: Gzik, M., Tkacz, E., Paszenda, Z., Piętka, E. (eds.) Innovations in Biomedical Engineering, pp. 23–31. Springer, Cham (2018)
9. Gu, P., Lee, W.M., Roubidoux, M.A., Yuan, J., Wang, X., Carson, P.L.: Automated 3D ultrasound image segmentation to aid breast cancer image interpretation. Ultrasonics **65**, 51–58 (2016). https://doi.org/10.1016/j.ultras.2015.10.023

10. Huang, Q., Yang, F., Liu, L., Li, X.: Automatic segmentation of breast lesions for interaction in ultrasonic computer-aided diagnosis. Inf. Sci. **314**, 293–310 (2015). https://doi.org/10.1016/j.ins.2014.08.021
11. Huang, Y.L., Chen, D.R.: Watershed segmentation for breast tumor in 2-D sonography. Ultrasound Med. Biol. **30**(5), 625–632 (2004). https://doi.org/10.1016/j.ultrasmedbio.2003.12.001
12. Jiang, P., Peng, J., Zhang, G., Cheng, E., Megalooikonomou, V., Ling, H.: Learning-based automatic breast tumor detection and segmentation in ultrasound images. In: 2012 9th IEEE International Symposium on Biomedical Imaging (ISBI), pp. 1587–1590 (2012). https://doi.org/10.1109/ISBI.2012.6235878
13. Kim, J.H., Cha, J.H., Kim, N., Chang, Y., Ko, M.S., Choi, Y.W., Kim, H.H.: Computer-aided detection system for masses in automated whole breast ultrasonography: development and evaluation of the effectiveness. Ultrasonography **33**(2), 105–115 (2014). https://doi.org/10.14366/usg.13023
14. Landis, J., Koch, G.: The measurement of observer agreement for categorical data. Biometrics **33**(1), 159–174 (1977)
15. Lasso, A., Heffter, T., Rankin, A., Pinter, C., Ungi, T., Fichtinger, G.: PLUS: Open-source toolkit for ultrasound-guided intervention systems. IEEE Trans. Biomed. Eng. **61**(10), 2527–2537 (2014). https://doi.org/10.1109/TBME.2014.2322864
16. Liu, B., Cheng, H., Huang, J., Tian, J., Tang, X., Liu, J.: Fully automatic and segmentation-robust classification of breast tumors based on local texture analysis of ultrasound images. Patt. Recogn. **43**(1), 280–298 (2010). https://doi.org/10.1016/j.patcog.2009.06.002
17. Meyer, F.: Topographic distance and watershed lines. Sig. Process. **38**(1), 113–125 (1994). https://doi.org/10.1016/0165-1684(94)90060-4
18. Minavathi, M., Murali, S., Dinesh, M.S.: Classification of mass in breast ultrasound images using image processing techniques. Int. J. Comput. Appl. **42**(10), 29–36 (2012). Full text available
19. Moon, W.K., Shen, Y.W., Bae, M.S., Huang, C.S., Chen, J.H., Chang, R.F.: Computer-aided tumor detection based on multi-scale blob detection algorithm in automated breast ultrasound images. IEEE Trans. Med. Imaging **32**(7), 1191–1200 (2013). https://doi.org/10.1109/TMI.2012.2230403
20. Rodtook, A., Makhanov, S.S.: Multi-feature gradient vector flow snakes for adaptive segmentation of the ultrasound images of breast cancer. J. Vis. Commun. Image Representation **24**(8), 1414–1430 (2013). https://doi.org/10.1016/j.jvcir.2013.09.009
21. Shi, X., Cheng, H., Hu, L., Ju, W., Tian, J.: Detection and classification of masses in breast ultrasound images. Dig. Sig. Process. **20**(3), 824–836 (2010). https://doi.org/10.1016/j.dsp.2009.10.010
22. Xian, M., Zhang, Y., Cheng, H.: Fully automatic segmentation of breast ultrasound images based on breast characteristics in space and frequency domains. Patt. Recogn. **48**(2), 485–497 (2015). https://doi.org/10.1016/j.patcog.2014.07.026

A Preliminary Evaluation
of a Basic Fluorescence Image Processing
in MentorEye System Using Artificially
Prepared Phantoms

Marcin Majak[✉], Magdalena Wojtków, Matylda Żmudzińska,
Wojciech Macherzyński, Zbigniew Kulas, Michał Popek,
Ewelina Świątek-Najwer, and Magdalena Żuk

Wroclaw University of Science and Technology, Wrocław, Poland
marcin.majak@pwr.edu.pl

Abstract. This paper presents preliminary results for fluorescence image processing implemented in MentorEye computer-aided surgery system. For this purpose we have prepared some artificial phantoms enabling fluorescence excitation with different properties. In this study, we have used basic algorithms for image segmentation with some modifications for noise removal and transparency mask generation. MentorEye system comprises of few modules for planning, virtual plan realization and finally validation phase. Apart from well-known CT DICOM data, we have enriched intraoperative module with a fluorescence visualization. MentorEye uses near-infrared (NIR) fluorescent light for better tumor identification inside operating room.

Keywords: Image segmentation · Fluorescence imaging
Computer-aided surgery

1 Introduction

Computer aided surgery systems are constantly developed and used in many real-life medical problems. Advancement in image processing techniques and better hardware design allows to significantly improve medical treatment in various aspects. Currently, whole procedure is divided into three main phases: virtual planning, intraoperative plan realization under the control of a navigation system, postoperative verification [11,12]. This approach is more complex than single and direct surgery intervention, but is specially adjusted for individual patient's needs. Moreover, recent improvements in technology resulted in merging new image modalities into systems apart from well-know Computed Tomography (CT) or Magnetic Resonance Imaging (MRI). Another important aspect worth mentioning is related to head mounted displays (HMD) which gradually replace commonly used external monitors. This technology still has

© Springer International Publishing AG, part of Springer Nature 2019
E. Pietka et al. (Eds.): ITIB 2018, AISC 762, pp. 89–100, 2019.
https://doi.org/10.1007/978-3-319-91211-0_8

some limitations due to relatively low resolution and necessity for personalized calibration [18], but rapid development in this area gives promising perspectives for the future.

The recent years have witnessed an extensive development in the optical imaging which exploits invisible near-infrared fluorescent (NIR) light and fluorescent contrast agents. These techniques have a huge potential to improve cancer surgery and treatment, because intraoperatively we can observe positions of blood veins and tumors. Current study is a part of a wide project which aims at developing a new computer and fluorescence-guided system for both: planning and aiding oncological treatment. General idea of such a system was presented in paper [14]. Generally, one of the main purposes of this project is to develop hardware and software for intraoperative fluorescence imaging to indicate a melanoma area. Schematic description for MentorEye intraoperative modules is presented in Fig. 1.

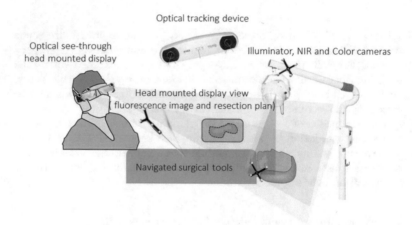

Fig. 1. Schematic description for MentorEye intraoperative modules

The purpose of a current study is to preliminary evaluate basic fluorescence image processing in MentorEye system, as well as a design of artificial phantoms for qualitative and quantitative validation of various image processing methods. Although, commercially available intraoperative near-infrared fluorescence imaging systems allow for qualitative visualization of fluorescence response, quantitative metric for decision-making is still in its infancy [15]. Furthermore, fusion of fluorescence images with video images, preoperative plan and data from optical navigation system is still posing a challenge. Such system calibration and assessment requires specially prepared fluorescence phantoms.

The organization of this paper is as follows. Section 2 describes fluorescence phenomena and its application to computer aided surgery. In Sect. 3 artificial phantoms for fluorescence imaging are presented. Fluorescence device, phantoms and image processing algorithms used in this study are included in Sect. 4, while image segmentation results are located in Sect. 5. Whole paper is concluded in Sect. 6 together with some plans for future improvements.

2   Fluorescence Phenomena and Fluorescence Imaging Devices in Medical Applications

Proper tumor visualization is crucial for differentiating malignant from healthy tissues during surgery. MentorEye uses near-infrared (NIR) fluorescent light (700 nm–900 nm) for a tumor identification. In short, fluorescence is the emission of light by a substance that absorbed electromagnetic radiation and cease to glow immediately when the radiation source is switched off. The emitted wavelength is usually longer than the fluorescent excitation wave. In our case a fluorescence occurs under the influence of NIR LED (Light Emitting Diode) light.

Intraoperative fluorescence imaging depends on the availability of contrast agent and imaging system to visualize the invisible emission of contrast agent. Indocyanine green (ICG) is the only NIR fluorescent contrast that is approved for clinical indication. Also, sufficiently diluted, methylene blue (MB) has recently been applied clinically in NIR fluorescence (NIRF) clinical studies [16]. MB was introduced in an era when no formal approval was needed and it is still widely used. It should be noted that in this study we have used ICG. NIR light has many advantages over visible light: can travel up to centimeters through tissue (typically millimetres) [2], signal-to-background ratio is high because tissue exhibits almost no autofluorescence [5]. NIR light also does not use ionizing radiation unlike other intraoperative techniques (e.g. X-ray fluoroscopy technique) and is invisible which means that it does not alter the look of the surgical field. What is more, NIR fluorescent contrast can be visualized with acquisition times in the millisecond enabling real-time analysis during surgery - emission of fluorescence stops almost immediately (10^{-8} s).

The near-infrared fluorescence imaging technique using ICG is becoming more and more popular among surgeons of various specialties: open surgery, laparoscopy, thoracoscopy, robotic surgery, to name only a few [15]. NIR using ICG has been developed for cancer cells [10], sentinel lymph nodes [8] mapping during lymphadenectomy in the assessment of cancer process advancement in general surgery, urology and gynecology or neurological diseases [1].

3   Artificial Phantoms for Fluorescence Imaging

Phantoms containing fluorescent tumor-simulating inclusion are used for NIRF imaging as a tool for simulating both pre- and intraoperative tumor localization, tumor resection prepared using real-time NIRF system or assessment of the tumor margin localization. In general, phantoms are composed of liquids, hydrogels or polymers (eg. polydimethylsiloxane and epoxy). However, due to the applications presented above, phantoms used for NIRF imaging should hold specified requirements which correspond with the properties of the human tissue such as elastic or optical properties (scattering and absorption). The most popular type of phantoms used for NIRF imaging are gelatinous or agarose phantoms, which are characterized by similar elastic properties to human tissue and can be cut using conventional surgical instruments [4, 13]. Moreover, epoxy resin phantoms are described as a good tool in context to the tissue-like scattering and absorption properties [9]. Furthermore, such phantoms can be made by straight capillaries embedded in silicone [3], resin or polyurethane. A promising approach is represented also by three-dimensional printing which has a potential to become a widespread, practical method for fabrication of complex biomimetic phantoms. In NIRF imaging contexts, especially stereolithography (SLA) is characterized as a useful technique for creating phantoms with a high precision and proper optical properties [6]. Another research direction is related with biodegradable markers which can be visualized in both: X-ray imaging and intraoperatively using NIR fluorescence imaging [7].

4   Proposed Material and Method

4.1   Fluorescence Imaging Device

The basic components of a NIR fluorescence system (Fig. 2) are:

- NIR and visible light sources,
- light collection optics (filters),
- cameras (for visible and NIR light),
- instrument control and acquisition (PC with a dedicated software),
- display for surgeon.

Excitation light source must fulfill some requirements: spectral bandwidth, output efficiency and the ability to control. Commonly used sources are filtered lamps, laser diodes and light emitting diode (LED). In our system NIR and white LED diodes have been used. To ensure homogenity of the excitation field, LEDs have been combined into an array. Collection optics was equipped in variable magnification for various operating distance that enables to operate and illuminates surgical field. Emission filter design was critical to maximize detection sensitivity by limiting background light. Color and NIR cameras have been applied simultaneously for optimal imaging. Visible (white) illumination of the surgical field was merged with NIR fluorescence images in specially designed software.

4.2   Phantoms

For the needs of the research, we decided to test 5 different types of phantoms presented in Figs. 3, 4, 5, 6 and 7. In each case we present also an intensity profile generated along selected one image row. X axis in this chart describes sample number, while Y axis describes pixel's intensity.

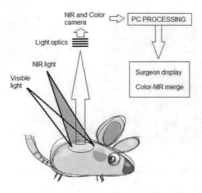

Fig. 2. The schematic of NIR fluorescence imaging in MentorEye system

1. Gelatinous phantom (Fig. 3) – phantom was created to evaluate fluorescent response of a tumor depending on the thickness of the soft tissue layer above its surface, and the fluorescent response depending on tumor thickness. 3D printed mold (SLS, Sinterit LISA) was filled with solution of gelatine, dimethyl sulfoxide (DMSO) and indocyanine green (ICG). After solidification of the gelatine, the mold was immersed in a solution imitating optical and mechanical properties of soft tissues, prepared following the recipe by [13]. As a result, the phantom with fluorescent inclusions under a layer of respectively 0 mm, 5 mm, 10 mm, 15 mm and 20 mm of tissue imitating substance, was obtained.
2. Tubes embedded in silicone (Fig. 4) – phantom was created by embedded PVC (polyvinyl chloride) hoses with 3 different diameters (3, 4 and 6 mm) in silicone (Silicone 45 clear, Kauposil). Hoses were embedded at two different depth according to the surface of phantom- 1 and 7 mm, respectively. To ensure the proper position of hoses (parallel to the surface) special mold for suffusing was created. Used silicone is characterized by shore hardness scale as 45A.

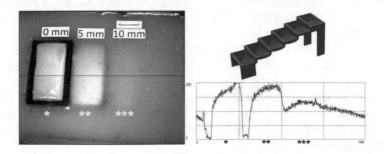

Fig. 3. Gelatinous phantom

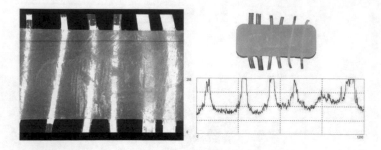

Fig. 4. Tubes embedded in silicone

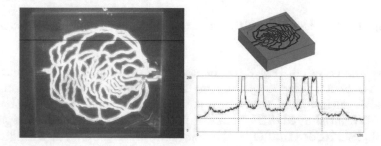

Fig. 5. PolyJet phantom (3D printing)

3. PolyJet phantom (3D printing) (Fig. 5) – prepared phantom represents anatomical human retinal vasculature system [6]. A PolyJet 3D printer (Objet30 Prime, Stratasys) was used to fabricate phantom– PolyJet is one of the most precise 3D printing technology (accuracy down to 0.1 mm) which uses the liquid photopolymers which are cured by UV light. PolyJet phantom was printed using transparent material (VeroClear, Stratasys) which simulates PMMA. Due to complicated geometry of the retinal vasculature-irregular, sinuous and thin channels (with a diameter approx. 2 mm), model was divided into 2 parts (the division plane passes through the channels symmetry axis in the transverse plane). Both parts of the model had different thicknesses, which simulates different system localization depth of 1 mm and 7 mm, respectively.

4. Phantom with active infrared markers (Fig. 6) – the active infrared marker was built using four appropriately arranged infrared diodes emitting a 935 nm wave. This is the wavelength detected by the NIR camera. Due to the invisible range of calibration diodes, one diode in the visible range was added to indicate that the device was turned on – this is important because of the battery power supply. The device also includes potentiometers to adjust the intensity of lighting.

5. Animal heart (Fig. 7) – a fresh porcine heart with solution of indocyanine green injected into coronary vessels was used as a phantom.

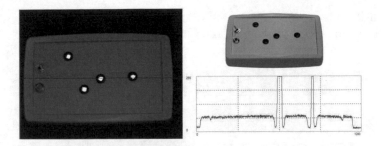

Fig. 6. Phantom with active infrared markers

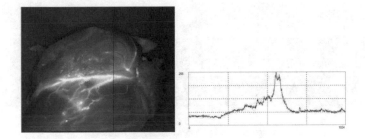

Fig. 7. Animal heart

In case of phantoms: 1–3 and 5, tumor-simulating inclusions, containing indocyanine green (ICG), were used. Fluorescent inclusions were prepared as $14\,\mu\mathrm{M}$ ICG solution in DMSO.

4.3   Image Processing of Fluorescence Images

The basic problem with images captured by infrared camera used in the project is relatively low image dynamics, as well as uneven lighting. Therefore, normalization of the image is required to provide the same thresholding conditions for all pictures. The most commonly used approach is histogram alignment, however, in the case of fluorescence imaging, it may lead to strong saturation of certain areas causing improper binarization results. Due to this reason, a better approach is to apply local contrast correction – Contrast-limited Adaptive Histogram Equalization CLAHE algorithm [17]. During testing, the contrast threshold in the filter was set to 4, while the processing area was determined as 9×9 box.

When detecting the phenomenon of fluorescence in the image, one should pay attention to two very important aspects. First of all, one should properly binarize the image with an appropriate threshold, and then apply generated mask into final image. It should be also noted, that the brightness or transparency of the pixel in the mask should depend on the brightness of the pixel in the input image, as opposed to the standard mask after thresholding. Basing on the initial

tests which were carried out, the following image processing sequence with the
fluorescence phenomenon was proposed in Fig. 8.

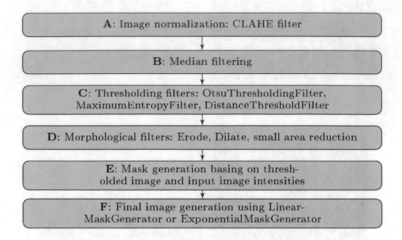

Fig. 8. Image processing pipeline

In this paragraph, we will shortly describe each step from processing pipeline.
After CLAHE filter, median filtering is used to remove noise from an image. During tests, we have configured this filter with 5×5 kernel. Image from step **B** is
ready for thresholding. The main goal of step **C** is to generate binarized image
which indicates areas for potential fluorescence phenomenon. In this paper, we
have chosen three standard filters for thresholding: Otsu thresholding with modified threshold value, Maximum Entropy filter and Distance Threshold filter.
Internal parameters for each filter were selected independently after initial tests.
Step **D** was introduced in processing pipeline to remove false detection. We have
noticed that very often thresholded image contained single binarized pixels or
small areas. To overcome this problem morphological operations were added such
as: Morphological Open, Morphological Close. Kernel for these filters was set as
3×3 with cross shape. What is more, Connected component filter was applied
and components with size equal to or lower than 5 were removed. Last two
steps: **E** and **F** are devoted to the final image generation. At first, mask image
with different pixels transparency is created. This transparency is dependent on
pixel intensities in the image from step **B**. For this purpose we have to define
transformation mapping pixel's intensity into proper transparency. Two implementations were prepared for tests presented in this paper. The first is based
on the linear transformation and the second one on the non-linear (exponential)
transformation.

5   Results

Image segmentation results for five phantoms are presented in Figs. 9, 10, 11, 12 and 13. In each case, the order of images is as follows (from the left): an original image, segmentation with DistanceThresholdFilter, OtsuThresholdFilter, MaximumEntrophyFilter. For all presented results CLAHE filter was used as an initial preprocessing step and Linear transformation was applied as a method for pixel's transparency mapping. Each input image also manually segmented by expert. This allows to calculate Dice coefficient between ground truth segmentation and algorithm result and finally, to choose the best segmentation algorithm.

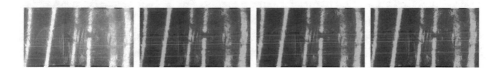

Fig. 9. Image segmentation results for Gelatinous phantom. Dice coefficients are as follows: 0.58, 0.55, 0.74

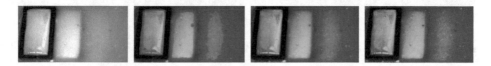

Fig. 10. Image segmentation results for Tubes embedded in silicone. Dice coefficients are as follows: 0.80, 0.78, 0.79

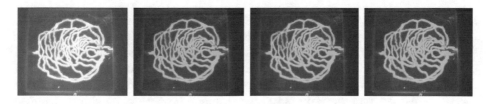

Fig. 11. Image segmentation results for PolyJet phantom (3D printing). Dice coefficients are as follows: 0.87, 0.86, 0.83

According to presented tests, satisfactory segmentation results can be obtained by version with DistanceThreshold filtering. Another two solutions tend to enlarge segmentation area too much. It should be noted that proper segmentation for fluorescence phenomenon is a complex task. We should pay more attention to the preprocessing steps when input image is normalized and

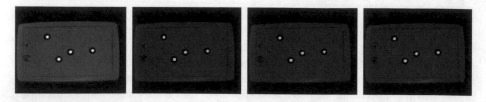

Fig. 12. Image segmentation results for Phantom with active infrared markers. Dice coefficients are as follows: 0.95, 0.95, 0.98

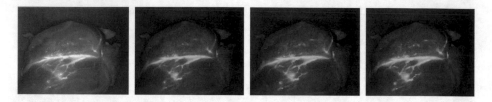

Fig. 13. Image segmentation result for Animal heart phantom. Dice coefficients are as follows: 0.49, 0.49, 0.46

different lightning conditions are compensated. Filters settings and image processing pipeline should be carefully chosen depending on the material properties where fluorescence phenomenon is supposed to be excited. Currently, our software allows to check various filter's settings and configurations and selects the best suited for environment in the operating room. In this study we have tested segmentation algorithm using five prepared phantoms. They have simulated fluorescence excitation in controlled conditions. Five phantoms allowed to check how material properties and depth influence the final fluorescence response.

6   Conclusions

In this paper we have presented a preliminary results for a basic fluorescence image processing implemented in MentorEye system. For this purpose, five different artificial phantoms were prepared. Each of them had different material properties and what is more fluorescence excitation was designed at selected depth. For fluorescence simulation, inclusions containing indocyanine green was used. In this paper we have proposed basic image processing pipeline for image segmentation. At the beginning, this involved input image normalization using CLAHE and median filtering. Later, three algorithms for automatic segmentation were proposed along with morphological filters for removing false, noise segmentation. Final step was connected with proper mask generation determining pixel's transparency. In the future we would like to improve image segmentation with the help of machine learning algorithms. To accomplish this task we have to collect more training images along with manual segmentation masks.

It is worth mentioning that several different phantoms for fluorescence imaging have been proposed. Fluorescence phenomenon has been observed and compared for all proposed phantoms. The main advantage of these artificial phantoms is known, long lasted or easily identified geometry of fluorescence response area, which is useful during preliminary validation or calibration procedures, because manual segmentation of a fluorescence response for biological materials could be time consuming and erroneous. However, such conditions are commonly met in clinical practice and should also be considered. Gelatin phantom, which simulates optical properties of biological tissues and animal tissues will be appropriate to overall assessment of a level of fluorescence response before in-vivo tests. These phantoms have limited shelf life, while 3D printed PolyJet, silicon phantom and active infrared markers are reusable. 3D printed PolyJet and silicon phantoms require preparing ICG solution, which is totally unnecessary in case of active infrared phantom. The active infrared marker seems to be appropriate for fast system tests and for calibration procedures due to very high identification level. 3D printing using liquid photopolymer enables complex, biologically inspired, very accurate geometry. However, such printing service is still quite expensive. Further development of silicone phantoms using molding method instead tubes is quite promising due to low costs and high availability.

Acknowledgement. The work is supported by National Centre of Research and Development in Poland, in frames of the project: 'Development of Polish complementary system of molecular surgical navigation for tumor treatment', STRATEGMED1/233624/4/NCBR/2014.

References

1. Belykh, E., Martirosyan, N., Yagmurlu, K., Miller, E.J., Eschbacher, J., Izadyyazdanabadi, M., Bardonova, L.A., Byvaltsev, V.A., Nakaji, P., Preul, M.C.: Intraoperative fluorescence imaging for personalized brain tumor resection: current state and future directions. Front. Surg. (2016)
2. Chance, B.: Near-infrared images using continuous, phase-modulated, and pulsed light with quantitation of blood and blood oxygenation. Ann. New York Acad. Sci. **838**, 29 45 (1998)
3. Chen, C., Klämpfl, F., Knipfer, C., Riemann, M., Kanawade, R., Stelzle, F., Schmidt, M.: Preparation of a skin equivalent phantom with interior micronscale vessel structures for optical imaging experiments. Biomed. Opt. Express **5**(9), 3140–3149 (2014). https://doi.org/10.1364/BOE.5.003140
4. Fathima, A.: Selective sensitivity of mueller imaging for tissue scattering over absorption changes in cancer mimicking phantoms. Opt. Lasers Eng. **102**(Supplement C), 112–118 (2018). https://doi.org/10.1016/j.optlaseng.2017.10.016
5. Frangioni, J.V.: In vivo near-infrared fluorescence imaging. Curr. Opin. Chem. Biol. **7**(5), 626–634 (2003). https://doi.org/10.1016/j.cbpa.2003.08.007
6. Ghassemi, P., Wang, J., Melchiorri, A., Ramella-Roman, J., Mathews, S., Coburn, J., Sorg, B., Chen, Y., Pfefer, T.: Rapid prototyping of biomimetic vascular phantoms for hyperspectral reflectance imaging. J. Biomed. Opt. **20**(12) (2015). https://doi.org/10.1117/1.JBO.20.12.121312

7. Gorecka, Z., Teichmann, J., Nitschke, M., Chlanda, A., Choinska, E., Werner, C., Swieszkowski, W.: Biodegradable fiducial markers for x-ray imaging - soft tissue integration and biocompatibility. J. Mater. Chem. B **4**, 5700–5712 (2016). https://doi.org/10.1039/C6TB01001F

8. Mondal, B.S., Gao, S., Zhu, N., Sudlow, G.P., Liang, K., Som, A., Akers, W.J., Fields, R.C., Margenthaler, J., Liang, R., Gruev, V., Achilefu, S.: Binocular goggle augmented imaging and navigation system provides real-time fluorescence image guidance for tumor resection and sentinel lymph node mapping. Technical report (2015). https://doi.org/10.1038/srep12117

9. Netz, U.J., Toelsner, J., Bindig, U.: Calibration standards and phantoms for fluorescence optical measurements. Med. Laser Appl. **26**(3), 101–108 (2011). https://doi.org/10.1016/j.mla.2011.05.002. Basic Investigations for diagnostic purposes

10. Onda, N., Kimura, M., Yoshida, T., Shibutani, M.: Preferential tumor cellular uptake and retention of indocyanine green for in vivo tumor imaging. Int. J. Cancer **139**(3), 673–682 (2016). https://doi.org/10.1002/ijc.30102

11. Pietruski, P., Majak, M., Świątek-Najwer, E., Popek, M., Jaworowski, J., Żuk, M., Nowakowski, F.: Image-guided bone resection as a prospective alternative to cutting templates-A preliminary study. J. Crano-Maxillo-Facial Surg. **43**(7), 1021–1027 (2015). https://doi.org/10.1016/j.jcms.2015.06.012

12. Pietruski, P., Majak, M., Świątek-Najwer, E., Popek, M., Szram, D., Żuk, M., Jaworowski, J.: Accuracy of experimental mandibular osteotomy using the image-guided sagittal saw. Int. J. Oral Maxillofacial Surg. **45**(6), 793–800 (2016). https://doi.org/10.1016/j.ijom.2015.12.018

13. Pleijhuis, R., Timmermans, A., De Jong, J., De Boer, E., Ntziachristos, V., Van Dam, G.: Tissue-simulating phantoms for assessing potential near-infrared fluorescence imaging applications in breast cancer surgery. J. Visualized Exp. JoVE **91**, 112–118 (2014). https://doi.org/10.3791/51776

14. Świątek-Najwer, E., Majak, M., Żuk, M., Popek, M., Kulas, Z., Jaworowski, J., Pietruski, P.: The new computer and fluorescence-guided system for planning and aiding oncological treatment. In: CARS 2017–Computer Assisted Radiology and Surgery–Proceedings of the 31–st International Congress and Exhibition, vol. 2, pp. S1–S286 (2017)

15. Vahrmeijer, A.L., Hutteman, M., van der Vorst, J.R., van de Velde, C.J.H., Frangioni, J.V.: Image-guided cancer surgery using near-infrared fluorescence. Nat. Rev. Clin. Oncol. **10**, 507–518 (2013). https://doi.org/10.1038/nrclinonc.2013.123

16. Verbeek, F.P., van der Vorst, J.R., Schaafsma, B.E., Swijnenburg, R.J., Gaarenstroom, K.N., Elzevier, H.W., van de Velde, C.J., Frangioni, J.V., Vahrmeijer, A.L.: Intraoperative near infrared fluorescence guided identification of the ureters using low dose methylene blue: a first in human experience. J. Urol. **190**(2), 574–579 (2013). https://doi.org/10.1016/j.juro.2013.02.3187

17. Zuiderveld, K.: Graphics Gems iv. Chapter Contrast Limited Adaptive Histogram Equalization, pp. 474–485. Academic Press Professional, Inc., San Diego (1994)

18. Żuk, M., Majak, M., Świątek-Najwer, E., Popek, M., Kulas, Z.: Evaluation of calibration procedure for stereoscopic visualization using optical see-through head mounted displays for a complex oncological treatment. In: VipIMAGE 2017: Proceedings of the VI ECCOMAS Thematic Conference on Computational Vision and Medical Image Processing Porto, pp. 354–359. Springer, Cham (2018). https://doi.org/10.1007/978-3-319-68195-5_39

Reconstruction of Gigapixel Stereometric Maps of Ceramic Surfaces

Marcin Płatek, Wiktoria Sapota$^{(\boxtimes)}$, Sebastian Stach, and Zygmunt Wróbel

Faculty of Computer Science and Material Science, Institute of Computer Science,
University of Silesia in Katowice, Katowice, Poland
wiktoria.sapota@us.edu.pl
http://ii.us.edu.pl

Abstract. For the purposes of the paper, a three-dimensional geometric structure of a biomaterial surface was reconstructed well above an individual field of view using a laser confocal microscope and systematic scanning. The entire analysed area was divided using a square grid with regular component fields in both columns and rows. Adjacent sub-surfaces were measured in such a way as to retain a 20% overlapping area. Individual sub-images were always measured with the same resolution of 4096×4096 pixels. The resulting image, after stitching sub-images, was a multiple of this size. The procedure resulted in a gigapixel map of surface topography, which enabled three-dimensional observation of the material surface geometry as well as measurements and additional analyses of the surface morphology.

Keywords: Ceramic surfaces · Gigapixel stereometric map
Surface reconstruction · Stitching method

1 Introduction

The development of methods for a quantitative description of a material microstructure and surface is an essential tool for quantitative materials analysis. It is implemented to modernize the manufacturing technology of biomaterials, to improve their design and properties. Research methods enable to characterize a material microstructure by using a comprehensive description including geometric and statistical distributions as well as a full range of indicators and stereological parameters [1]. Morphological analysis of several dozen of geometric characteristics of a surface structure allows inferences about the effectiveness of the preparation of a surface layer to work in the kinematic system or about surface morphology changes resulting from its operation and the possibility of its further use. For this purpose, computer analysis of a microscopic image is used, as high magnification usually narrows the field of view [2]. The operation of connecting surfaces (stitching) is ideal if the measuring equipment, such as a confocal microscope or a scanning electron microscope, does not enable thorough examination of a sample surface due to the limited field of view. Nowadays,

© Springer International Publishing AG, part of Springer Nature 2019
E. Pietka et al. (Eds.): ITIB 2018, AISC 762, pp. 101–110, 2019.
https://doi.org/10.1007/978-3-319-91211-0_9

there are many computer programs that allow to combine partial stereometric data to create one large size surface image. Surfaces must be measured using scanning in a rectangular grid with regular spacing between rows and columns. Each area should have the same width, length and resolution. Surrounding areas must have an area of overlap (recommended overlap is 20%) [3]. The operating principle of the method is shown in Fig. 1. An observation area of a fixed side moves across the analysed area in accordance with the principle of systematic scanning. Edges of the observation area are oriented parallel and perpendicular to the direction of the microscope table movement. Observation areas completely cover the stitched range in such a way that the position of the next area with respect to the previous measurement results in an overlapped area. In every location of the observation area, the surface geometric structure is reconstructed by scanning it with the same data acquisition settings. It results in a square matrix of scanned sub-surfaces which are then subjected to stitching, using the appropriate software, into a single stitched image corresponding to the stitched range.

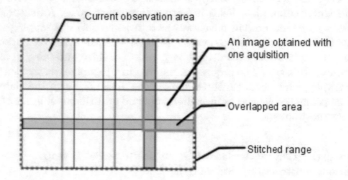

Fig. 1. Diagram showing operating principle of stitching [3]

2   Tools and Research Methods

2.1   Measuring Devices

Analyses of Al_2O_3 ceramic surface were made on a non-worn hip joint implant using the Olympus LEXT OLS4000 confocal laser microscope. This microscope is designed for imaging the surface of tested materials with nanometer scale detail, studying their roughness, and creating 3D projection. The zoom range from 108× to 17280× satisfies high research needs [4]. Objective lenses with a high numerical aperture and an optical system which uses laser light with a wavelength of 405 nm are dedicated to this microscope. They enable to achieve maximum performance and study surfaces of samples whose geometric structure components have slopes at an angle of up to 85°. The LEXT OLS4000 system has a newly developed dual confocal system capable of capturing a clear image of a sample consisting of materials with different levels of reflectivity (Fig. 2). The advantage of the LEXT OLS4000 microscope is the ability to perform non-contact analyses of samples with large surface areas. There is no need for special preparation of a sample, which enables to conduct research continuously and obtain the results quickly during the successive modifications of the measured elements [4, 5].

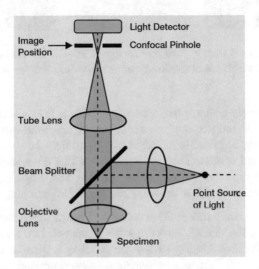

Fig. 2. Diagram showing the operating principle of the confocal optical system

The manufacturer informs that the Olympus LEXT OLS4000 [3], supporting wide-field observation. Higher-magnification imaging generally narrows the visual field range. The advanced stitching function of the OLS4000 enables to stitch up to 500 images together to create a high-resolution, wide-field image. In addition, 3D display and 3D measurements are available on the stitched image (Fig. 3) [4].

The microscope allows to create one image out of 529 combined images (23 × 23 images). In addition, the resulting image can be represented in 3D visualization. The overlap area between images is normally set at 10%. This value can be freely configured. Scanning of all the sub-surfaces is automatically followed by stitching. This option can be disabled and users can decide which of the scanned images are to be combined.

2.2 Software

LEXT Application Software from Olympus. LEXT Application Software version 2.2.3 (Microscope control 2.2.3.1) is a comprehensive software bundled by Olympus, the manufacturer of the LEXT OLS4000 microscope. It is primarily used to operate the microscope and to define the measurements to be made using a microscope. It is used primarily to operate the microscope and define the measurements to be performed with it. It also allows a series of transformations

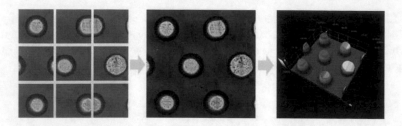

Fig. 3. Stitching several images into one image: first – brightness of the image before stitching; second – brightness of the image after stitching; third – stitched 3D image [6]

of the resulting surface and appropriate calculations. It enables to obtain parameters such as height, length, surface area, levels, line and surface roughness in accordance with the applicable standards [1], particle analysis, edge detection, layer thicknesses and others. The new formula of the advanced, but easy to use, software allows its users to customize the profile, the scope of the research and analysis of the results [6]. This software also enables stitching.

topoStitch^{TM} 2 from Image Metrology. The topoStitch^{TM} 2 is one of the newest software on the market for connecting images. It uses an easy and accurate method of stitching. Owing to the file reading engine from SPIP^{TM}, which enables to read over 90 different extensions, images needed for this process can come from all kinds of test equipment, such as confocal microscopes, interferometers, profilometers, AFM (atomic force microscope), SPM (Scanning Probe Microscope). This program has a number of useful features and technologies that make it easier to work in its environment. The software automatically arranges images in the right way, provided that it has information about their position, otherwise the grid wizard helps to arrange them manually within a few seconds. The interactive grid layout tool enables to easily adjust the overlap and tilt of images relative to each other, and advanced drag and semitransparent rendering make it easy to set and adjust them manually. With sub-pixel correlation algorithms, the program automatically rotates and aligns images during the process of joining them. Owing to the advanced memory support and performance optimization, any number of images, without any limitations, can be used to create very high resolution images. The effects can be exported to both the topographic (.bcrf) and graphic (.tiff) formats. In order to learn to use the software, a new user is instructed by the topoStitch^{TM} tutorial program: what options and in what order they should be selected to perform the procedure of stitching [7]. On August 15, 2013, Image Metrology company released version 2 of the software that enables to stitch hundreds or even thousands of 3D images also in grayscale [7,8].

2.3   Research Methodology

Image stitching or photo stitching is the process of combining multiple images with overlapping fields of view to produce a segmented panorama or high-resolution image. Commonly performed through the use of computer software, most approaches to image stitching require nearly exact overlaps between images and identical exposures to produce seamless results. Stitching refers to the technique of using a computer to merge images together to create a large image, preferably without it being at all noticeable that the generated image has been created by computer. Algorithms for aligning images and stitching them into seamless photo-mosaics are among the oldest and most widely used in computer vision [9].

The samples were scanned using the MPLAPON100XLEXT objective lens which is dedicated to laser light. The observed surface areas were $128 \times 128\,\mu\text{m}$. Thus, a sampling step of 31.3 nm in both X and Y axes was obtained. The distance between confocal planes was always $0.06\,\mu\text{m}$. In this way, the analysis time of one image, including data saving on the hard drive, was about 8 min. The option of stitching the scanned sub-surfaces was disabled after the completion of the stitching procedure. In the microscope software, there is certain convenience which allows to define the table settings. The option of stage coordinates enables to define the grid of coordinates of previously specified table movement in the X and Y axes (Fig. 4). The initial coordinates were defined and then 10×10 grid of coordinates of the table settings was specified with the $102\,\mu$ step of its movement along the X and Y axes ($128\,\mu\text{m} - 20\%$ overlap).

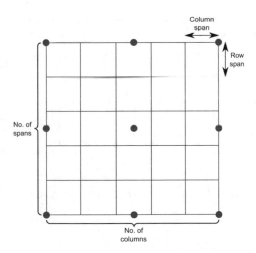

Fig. 4. Schematic diagram showing the principle of defining stage coordinates

The basic premise of the study was to make a gigapixel topographic surface map of the best possible quality made up of high quality sub-images. Therefore, scanning of the observation areas in the Fine mode and in the resolution of 4096 dots × 4096 lines was selected. It was also assumed that the overlap area will be 20%. Preliminary calculations were made based on the diagram (Fig. 5) to find out how many sub-images with the set parameters should be scanned in order to obtain a comprehensive topography map of the scanned surface consisting of at least a billion pixels (Table 1).

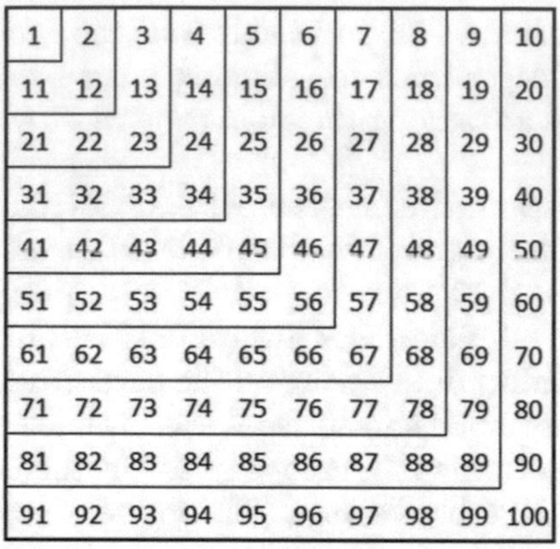

1	2	3	4	5	6	7	8	9	10
11	12	13	14	15	16	17	18	19	20
21	22	23	24	25	26	27	28	29	30
31	32	33	34	35	36	37	38	39	40
41	42	43	44	45	46	47	48	49	50
51	52	53	54	55	56	57	58	59	60
61	62	63	64	65	66	67	68	69	70
71	72	73	74	75	76	77	78	79	80
81	82	83	84	85	86	87	88	89	90
91	92	93	94	95	96	97	98	99	100

Fig. 5. Diagram of the stitched image

Table 1. Theoretical parameters of the stitched image assuming 4096×4096 sub-image size and the overlap of 20%

Size of the stitched [image]	Number of stitched [image]	Image size after stitching		Pixel density $[px/\mu m^2]$	Number of pixels [Gpx]
		[px]	[μm]		
1×1	1	4096×4096	128×128	1024	0.02
2×2	4	7373×7373	230×230	1024	0.05
3×3	9	10650×10650	333×333	1024	0.11
4×4	16	13926×13926	435×435	1024	0.19
5×5	25	17203×17203	538×538	1024	0.3
6×6	36	20480×20480	640×640	1024	0.42
7×7	49	23757×23757	742×742	1024	0.56
8×8	64	27034×27034	845×845	1024	0.73
9×9	81	30310×30310	947×947	1024	0.92
10×10	100	33587×33587	1050×1050	1024	1.13

With such a scanning configuration, the examined area should be scanned in the mode of 10×10 images in order to obtain an overall image consisting of a billion pixels (Fig. 6).

3   Results

A scan of the entire area of the surface scan was carried out each time the table settings were changed after the measurement was completed. As a result,

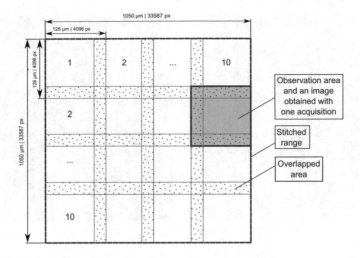

Fig. 6. Diagram of surface analysis using stitching

100 partial images were obtained, which in the next stage were joined by the stitching method in the topoStitch^{TM} 2 program. Using the program is very intuitive. The user has full control of the stitched image from loading the images via their respective sorting and defining overlap settings (Figs. 7 and 8(a), (b)), until the final procedure of stitching (Fig. 9).

Full details of the procedure for stitching images is presented in (Table 2).

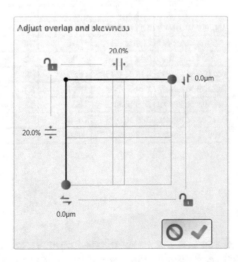

Fig. 7. Overlap configuration window for stitched images

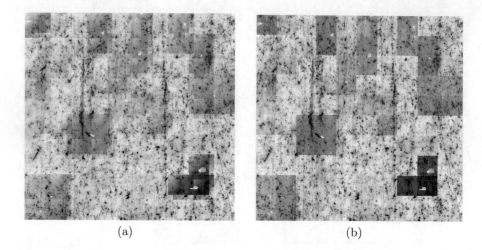

(a)   (b)

Fig. 8. Pre-stitched images: (a) image with a schematic view of the stitched surface with the visible overlap defined in Fig. 7; (b) image with a schematic view of the stitched surface

Table 2. Parameters of images obtained by stitching from sub-surfaces sized 4096 × 4096 measuring points, 20% overlap, topoStitch^{TM} program

Size of the stitched [image]	Number of stitched [image]	Image size after stitching		Pixel density [px/μm²]	Spacing [nm]	File size [GB]	Number of pixels [Gpx]
		[px]	[μm]				
1 × 1	1	4096 × 4096	129 × 129	1008	32	0.06	0.02
2 × 2	4	7326 × 7374	231 × 232	1008	32	0.21	0.05
3 × 3	9	10537 × 10625	333 × 335	1004	32	0.43	0.11
4 × 4	16	13730 × 13871	434 × 437	1004	32	0.73	0.19
5 × 5	25	16923 × 17145	534 × 540	1006	32	1.08	0.29
6 × 6	36	20179 × 20452	636 × 645	1006	32	1.53	0.41
7 × 7	49	23403 × 23697	739 × 748	1004	32	2.06	0.55
8 × 8	64	26595 × 26972	839 × 851	1004	32	2.67	0.73
9 × 9	81	29774 × 30235	939 × 953	1006	32	3.35	0.90
10 × 10	100	32931 × 33679	1038 × 1062	1006	32	4.13	1.11

4   Discussion

The study carried out for the purposes of the paper involved stitching of sub-surfaces analysed with a confocal microscope in order to obtain a large area of research in the form of a topographic map. The procedure was performed using the topoStitch^{TM} commercial software. In order to be able to carry out the stitching operation, it was first necessary to obtain partial images of 100 fields of the surface under investigation by systematic scanning. It was assumed

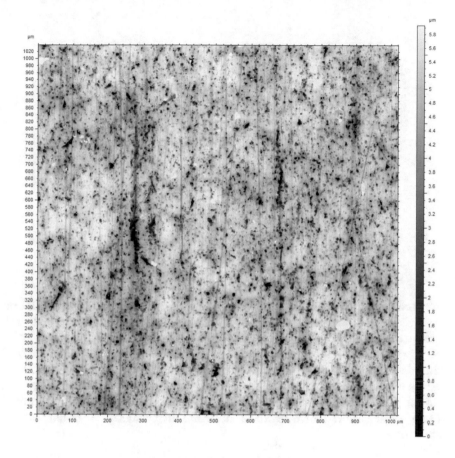

Fig. 9. Resulting image after the stitching procedure

that the resulting images stitched in accordance with the described procedure (Table 1) will have invariably the same parameters like the distance between the scan points and pixel density, whereas their size in pixels will change, being a multiple of the stitched sub-images. During the implementation of the stitching process, it was noticed that the time needed to carry out this procedure increases in proportion to the number of folded images. It is completely understandable and results from the complicated procedure of matching images of surfaces whose stereometric data are distributed in 3D space. Several areas from the merged surface were selected to demonstrate an image obtained by this method and its level of detail (Fig. 10).

Full details of the procedure for stitching images is presented in (Table 2).

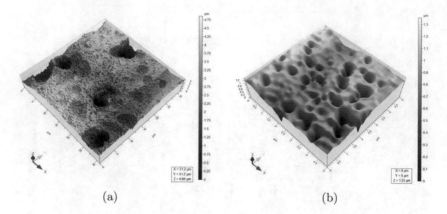

(a)   (b)

Fig. 10. Two magnifications of the central part of an image after stitching

5   Conclusion

topoStitch™ 2 software that allowed the stitching procedure to be carried out correctly. The automatic assembly of overlapping multiple measurements into one large area is particularly useful for stitching topographic photos from AFM, SPM microscopes, profilometers, interferometers and confocal microscopes with a limited field of view. The software also made it possible to record stereometric data in a format that allows their subsequent analysis of surface morphology. The use of topoStitch™ all assumptions of this research could be easily implemented, and the results are a source of many information presented in numerical and visual form.

References

1. ISO 25178-2, Geometrical product specifications (GPS) – Surface texture: Areal – Part 2: Terms, definitions and surface texture parameters. http://www.iso.org
2. Ward, G.: Hiding seams in high dynamic range panoramas. In: Proceedings of the 3rd Symposium on Applied Perception in Graphics and Visualization. In: ACM International Conference Proceeding, vol. 153 (2006). ISBN 1-59593-429-4
3. http://www.digitalsurf.fr
4. http://www.olympus-ims.com
5. Matuszewski, M., Styp-Rekowski, M.: Konfokalny laserowy mikroskop skaningowy w badaniach tribologicznych. Tribologia **1**, 157–165 (2010). (in Polish)
6. LEXT Application Software (additional help files)
7. http://www.topostitch.com
8. Fathimaa A.A., Karthikb R., Vaidehic V.: Image stitching with combined moment invariants and sift features. In: The 4th International Conference on Ambient Systems, Networks and Technologies, Procedia Computer Science, vol. 19, pp. 420–427 (2013)
9. Mehta, J.D., Bhirud, S.G.: Image stitching techniques. In: Conference paper on ThinkQuest 2010: Proceedings of the First International Conference on Contours of Computing Technology, pp. 74–80 (2010)

Segmentation of Three-Dimensional Images of the Butterfly Wing Surface

Żaneta Garczyk[1(✉)], Sebastian Stach[1], Ştefan Tălu[2], Sobola Dinara[3], and Zygmunt Wróbel[1]

[1] Faculty of Computer Science and Materials Science, Institute of Computer Science, University of Silesia in Katowice, Będzińska 39, 41-205 Sosnowiec, Poland
zaneta.garczyk@us.edu.pl
[2] Faculty of Mechanical Engineering, Department of AET, Discipline of Descriptive Geometry and Engineering Graphics, Technical University of Cluj-Napoca, 103-105 B-dul Muncii Street, 400641 Cluj-Napoca, Cluj, Romania
[3] Faculty of Electrical Engineering and Communication, Physics Department, Brno University of Technology, Technická 8, 616 00 Brno, Czech Republic

Abstract. The main objective was to develop a script in Matlab which would allow for the segmentation of the three-dimensional surface images of the samples. The motifs of peaks and pits were segmented on surface images of test samples using a watershed segmentation algorithm implemented in Matlab. The same software was also used to calculate the values of parameters characterizing the individual motifs. A summary of the determined parameters made it possible to compare the test sample surfaces. In order to verify the obtained results and correctness, and thus verify the suitability of the developed script, segmentation was performed using MountainsMap Premium. The software was also used to generate a set of parameters relating to separated motifs, which were compared with the calculations made using the script. This stereometric analysis proves to be an effective method that can be successfully used for estimation of micro- and nano- topography by processing of stereometric data.

Keywords: Image segmentation · Surface motifs
Stereometric data analysis · Matlab

1 Introduction

Properties of materials largely depend on the shape of the surface. The stereometric shape, known as surface geometric structure, is a collection of existing irregularities thereon or topographical elements such as peaks, pits, valleys, ridges [1,6].

A surface point higher than its surrounding area is called a peak. The peak neighbourhood is called a hill. From any point on a hill there is an upward path that ends at a unique peak. If the upward path from a point ends at another

© Springer International Publishing AG, part of Springer Nature 2019
E. Pietka et al. (Eds.): ITIB 2018, AISC 762, pp. 111–121, 2019.
https://doi.org/10.1007/978-3-319-91211-0_10

peak, then this point belongs to another hill. All point belonging to a hill are enclosed by a course line. A surface point that is lower than its surrounding area is called a pit. The pit neighbourhood is called a dale. From any point on a dale there is a downward path that ends at a unique pit and the dale defines a catchment basin: a drop of water starting from any point in the basin (dale) will run down to the pit. If the downward path from a point ends at another pit, it means that this point belongs to another dale. All point belonging to dale are enclosed by ridge line (Fig. 1). Saddle points are at the intersection point of ridge lines and course lines. They correspond to a maximum on a course line, and a minimum on a ridge line (Fig. 2) [5].

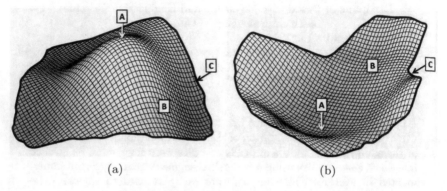

(a)   (b)

Fig. 1. (a) A: peak, B: reprezentation of a hill, C: course line; (b) A: pit, B: reprezentation of a dale, C: ridge line [5]

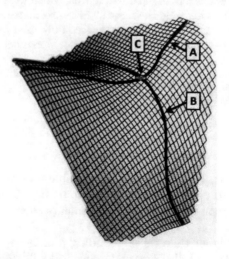

Fig. 2. A: ridge line, B: course line, C: saddle point [5]

The relationship between material surface structure and its properties is the reason for carrying out measurements and stereometric analysis of the surface. An important element of the measurements is the selection of a proper method and measurement tools. They should allow for the best possible reproduction of the actual topography. One of the tools used during stereometric measurements is an atomic force microscope (AFM). The microscope enables to create three-dimensional maps of the surface topography, which are the basis for analysis. Stereometric data obtained by means of AFM provide information on the shape and size of the structures present on the surface. The resolving power of the device allows for the display of details whose size is comparable to the size of an atom [3, 4].

Analysis of the structures present on the test surface, called motifs (pits, peaks), requires the use of specific image processing techniques such as segmentation. The process of segmentation enables to separate individual motifs. The algorithm most commonly used for this purpose and giving good effects is the watershed segmentation algorithm [9]. The segmented motifs may be then subjected to statistical analysis by determining their characteristic parameters which enable to describe and compare the test surfaces.

Surface analysis is an important and inseparable part of the development of materials in all areas and allows for the development of materials with novel properties [1, 6]. The development of materials engineering is associated with the development of research methods, measuring instruments as well as modern information technologies cooperating with research equipment.

The main objective was to develop a script in Matlab which would allow for the segmentation of the three-dimensional surface images of the samples.

2   Materials and Methods

2.1   Research Material

The research material was three samples reflecting the wing surfaces of two butterfly species exhibiting strong dependence of the wing colour on the angle of incidence of light. This is structural coloration and it depends on the surface topography.

2.2   Research Tool

Research tool, which provided stereometric data of the analysed samples, was an atomic force microscope (AFM). The microscope is one of the scanning probe microscopes (SPM).

2.3   Software

Matlab R2012 released by MathWorks was used to implement the script, by means of which three-dimensional images of the sample surfaces were segmented and the motifs located on them were analysed.

Simultaneous analysis was performed using MountainsMap Premium version 6.2.7487 released by Digital Surf. The analysis was to verify the results obtained using the script developed in Matlab.

2.4   Research Method

The stereometric data of the analysed samples were uploaded into the Matlab workspace. The input images can be treated as 2D intensity. To avoid over-segmentation, the local maxima were pre-determined by creating the extended-maxima transform. For this purpose, the function *imextendedmax* supplied by Matlab were used. The transform eliminates the maxima lower than or equal to the specified value of the input parameter. The local minima were designated for the completed input data, at points where the extended-maxima transform was non-zero, i.e. the points corresponding to the local maxima. For this purpose, the function *imimposemin* supplied by Matlab were used. Then, the watershed transformation was carried out, which determined the watershed lines and identified individual areas created around the local minima. For this purpose, the function supplied by Matlab performing watershed transforms were used. The transformation result is a label matrix with values greater than or equal to 0. The zero-valued elements are the watershed lines separating the individual regions [2,7].

The use of the watershed transformation allowed for the segmentation of images of the sample surfaces, and as a result they were divided into the motifs of significant peaks (Fig. 3).

In order to detect surface pits, the local minima were first determined by creating the extended-minima transform. For this purpose, the function *imextendedmin* supplied by Matlab were used. Then, at the points where the extended-minima transform was non-zero (corresponding to the local minima), the local minima were determined for the input data. The watershed transformation result was segmentation of surface images of the analysed samples and separation of the motifs of significant surface pits (Fig. 4) [2].

To characterize the segmented motifs, the parameters related to all the peaks, and then pits, were calculated, such as the number of motifs, mean height, mean perimeter, mean area, mean of minimum and maximum diameters, mean of mean diameters, mean of minimum and maximum diameter angles, mean orientation.

The height of the peak is the distance between the peak and the highest saddle point on the course line of the motif. For surface pits, the height is defined as the distance between the pit and the lowest saddle point on the ridge line of the motif. The motif area is a horizontal surface bounded by the course line in the case of peaks and the ridge line for pits. The radii of the motif, both in the case of surface peaks and pits, are drawn from its centre of gravity to particular points on its perimeter. The minimum diameter of the motif is equal to the doubled radius of the shortest length, whereas the maximum diameter is the doubled radius of the longest length. The mean angle of the smallest and largest diameter of the motif is measured from its centre of gravity [5,10].

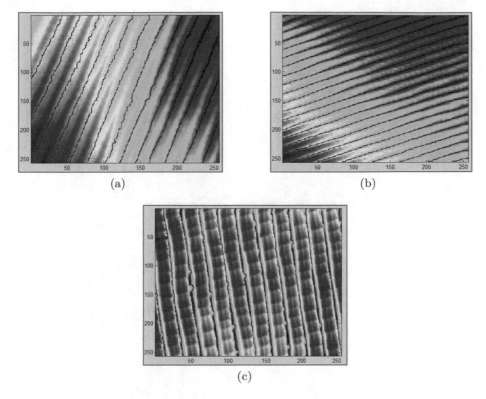

Fig. 3. Results of segmentation of surface peaks – watershed lines shown on the input stereometric data: (a) first sample, (b) second sample, (c) third sample

To characterize motifs, treated as a flat shape on the horizontal plane, a set of morphological parameters, such as an equivalent diameter, aspect ratio, elongation, roundness, compactness, were also determined.

The equivalent diameter of the motif is defined as the diameter of the circle, whose surface area is equal to the surface area of the motif (1) [5].

$$M_{ED} = \sqrt{\frac{4A}{\pi}} \qquad (1)$$

where: M_{ED} – equivalent diameter of the motif; A – surface area of the motif.

The aspect ratio of the motif is the ratio of the surface area of the motif to the square of the perimeter (2) [5].

$$M_{FF} = \frac{4\pi A}{\prod^2}. \qquad (2)$$

where: M_{FF} – aspect ratio of the motif; A – surface area of the motif; $\prod$ – perimeter of the motif.

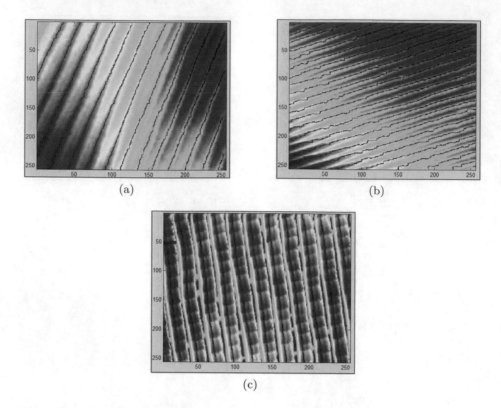

Fig. 4. Results of segmentation of surface pits – watershed lines shown on the input stereometric data: (a) first sample, (b) second sample, (c) third sample

The ratio of the maximum diameter to the minimum diameter is the elongation of the motif (3) [5].

$$M_{AR} = \frac{D_{max}}{D_{min}} \qquad (3)$$

where: M_{AR} – elongation of the motif; D_{max} – maximum diameter of the motif; D_{min} – minimum diameter of the motif.

The roundness of the motif is defined as the ratio of the surface area of the motif to the area of the circle, whose diameter is equal to the maximum diameter of the motif (4) [5].

$$M_{RN} = \frac{4A}{\pi D_{max}^{2}} \qquad (4)$$

where: M_{RN} – roundness of the motif; A – surface area of the motif; D_{max} – maximum diameter of the motif.

The ratio of the equivalent diameter to the maximum diameter is the compactness of the motif [5].

The morphological parameters determine the shape and were calculated for individual motifs. Next, their mean values for peaks and then pits were calculated.

3 Results

Using a script implemented in the programming environment of the Matlab package, the images of the test surfaces were segmented. As a result, they were divided into motifs of peaks and then pits. In the case of peaks, the boundary of the motif was marked out with the course line. The ridge line, however, determined the boundaries of the surface peaks. Using the script, the parameters for all the segmented peaks and pits were also calculated.

3.1 Method of Result Verification

In order to verify the correctness of the results obtained by means of the developed script, segmentation with the use of MountainsMap Premium was performed. This software is also used by the watershed segmentation algorithm to determine motifs. The software allows for surface analysis both in graphic form and by means of generated values of parameters relating to motifs.

Analysis of the motifs on the first sample allowed for segmentation of peaks and pits present on its surface. To avoid detection of too local motifs, which may result from noise, a smoothing filter sized 3×3 was used and a minimum height of the motifs was set at 3% of the maximum height of the surface [8]. The parameters of all the motifs were also generated (Fig. 5).

Similarly to the first sample, segmentation was also performed for the second and third sample using analysis of motifs and taking into account the adopted filtering and thresholding. At the same time, the parameters of all the segmented motifs were determined.

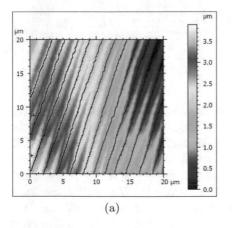
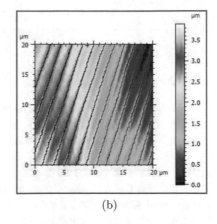

(a)   (b)

Fig. 5. Result of segmentation performed to detect the surface motifs of the first sample: (a) surface peaks, (b) surface pits

3.2   Summary of Results

In order to compare the surfaces of individual samples and check the correctness of the results obtained, a summary of parameters describing the segmented motifs of these surfaces was prepared. The summary includes the values of parameters calculated using the script and MountainsMap Premium (Tables 1 and 2).

Table 1. Mean values of values of parameters relating to the surface peaks of individual samples obtained using the script developed in Matlab and MountainsMap Premium (MMP)

Parameter	Software					
	Matlab			MMP		
	S-1	S-2	S-3	S-1	S-2	S-3
Number of motifs	14	24	12	14	24	12
Height [μm]	0.46	0.72	1.13	0.43	0.62	0.97
Perimeter [μm]	41.2	35.25	43.35	41.12	35.41	43.58
Area [μm²]	28.2	16.24	33.17	28.8	16.8	33.6
Minimum diameters [μm]	1.56	0.94	1.58	1.57	0.94	1.65
Maximum diameters [μm]	19.31	16.48	20.39	17.82	15.51	19.14
Mean diameters [μm]	9.85	8.4	10.71	4.12	2.74	4.42
Min. diameter angles [°]	20.44	57.49	−7.77	16.36	56.29	−20.5
Max. diameter angles [°]	−71.82	−20.32	80.66	−72.29	−20.13	81.17
Equivalent diameters [μm]	5.86	4.31	6.38	5.77	4.22	6.26
Aspect ratio	0.22	0.19	0.21	0.21	0.19	0.2
Elongation	12.51	17.08	13.63	11.66	15.96	11.67
Roundness	0.1	0.08	0.1	0.12	0.11	0.11
Compactness	0.31	0.28	0.31	0.34	0.31	0.32
Orientation [°]	71.82	20.32	99.34	72.76	21.21	95.57

3.3   Analysis of Results

The analysis of parameters determined by means of the script showed that on the surface of the second sample the number of motifs, both peaks and pits, is the largest. The third sample is characterized by the smallest number of motifs of all the analysed samples. However, their mean height is the greatest. The smallest mean height of the motifs is characteristic of the first sample. Both the mean length of the perimeter and the mean surface area are the highest for the third sample and the smallest for the second sample. The third sample also has the highest mean value of minimum diameters, maximum diameters, mean diameters and equivalent diameters, in contrast to the second sample, for which these parameters have the smallest values. Among the analysed samples, the second

Table 2. Mean values of values of parameters relating to the surface pits of individual samples obtained using the script developed in Matlab and MountainsMap Premium (MMP)

Parameter	Software					
	Matlab			MMP		
	S-1	S-2	S-3	S-1	S-2	S-3
Number of motifs	15	24	12	15	24	12
Height [μm]	0.53	0.63	1.55	0.49	0.59	1.44
Perimeter [μm]	38.68	35.92	42.24	39.1	36.12	43.47
Area [μm²]	26.33	16.27	33.18	26.88	16.8	33.6
Minimum diameters [μm]	1.46	0.94	1.65	1.5	0.92	1.68
Maximum diameters [μm]	17.98	16.26	19.6	16.89	15.56	18.85
Mean diameters [μm]	9.28	8.35	10.43	3.9	2.72	4.43
Min. diameter angles [°]	19.81	66.45	−6.52	15.27	57.33	−13.92
Max. diameter angles [°]	−71.92	−20.5	80.38	−72.67	−20.75	80.83
Equivalent diameters [μm]	5.56	4.31	6.38	5.47	4.22	6.27
Aspect ratio	0.24	0.19	0.23	0.22	0.18	0.21
Elongation	11.99	16.94	12.03	11.08	16.46	11.26
Roundness	0.11	0.09	0.11	0.12	0.11	0.11
Compactness	0.32	0.29	0.33	0.35	0.32	0.34
Orientation [°]	71.92	20.5	99.62	73.34	21.23	95.65

sample has the smallest mean value of the angles of the largest diameters of the motif, but also the largest mean value of the angles of the smallest diameters of the motif, in contrast to the third sample, which has the largest mean of the maximum angles of diameters and the smallest mean of the minimum angles of diameters.

The parameters such as aspect ratio, elongation, roundness and compactness are used to determine the horizontal shape of motifs. The motifs whose values of aspect ratio, roundness and compactness are close to one have a round shape. On the other hand, the values of these parameters for elongated motifs are close to 0. The largest value of the mean aspect ratio is characteristic of the first sample. The third sample has a similar value of the mean aspect ratio, and also the highest mean roundness and compactness. However, the values of these parameters are not close to 1. Therefore, it is impossible to talk about disc-shaped motifs. The lowest mean aspect ratio, roundness and compactness characterize the second sample, and thus the most elongated motifs exist on its surface. It is also confirmed by the fact that this sample has the highest mean elongation. The first sample is characterized by the lowest mean elongation. Therefore, there are the least elongated motifs on its surface. The last parameter is mean orientation. The largest value of this parameter is characteristic of the third sample, whereas its value for the second sample is the lowest.

4   Discussion

The segmentation was performed using the watershed transform, proceeded by extended-maxima or extended-minima transform. The extended-maxima and extended-minima transforms helped to avoid oversegmentation. After the segmentation the images were divided into areas localized around local maxima or minima of the surface. The values of parameters characterizing individual motifs were also calculated, which made it possible to analyse the motifs in terms of their size and shape. The script was implemented in a Matlab programming environment. The commercial software MountainsMap Premium was used for the results verification. The parameters relating to the segmented motifs, which were determined using the script implemented in Matlab and those generated by means of MountainsMap Premium, have similar values.

It was found that the script accomplishes its purpose and could be helpful to measure properties of the 3D surface. The possibility of presenting the results of the script enables practical application. However, the watershed lines, which form boundaries of the motifs, are limited by the boundaries of the image. Therefore, exclusion the objects that are limited by the frame can be considered in the case of another representation of the input images.

5   Conclusions

The main objective was to develop a script in Matlab which would allow for segmentation of three-dimensional surface images of the samples. The three-dimensional images were divided into motifs of peaks and pits. The values of individual parameters describing the segmented motifs were also determined.

The correctness of the segmentation results and calculated values of parameters were verified using MountainsMap Premium. The comparison of the values calculated using the developed script and those generated using the software enables to conclude that the segmentation method used in the script has yielded very good results. Verification of the results demonstrated their correctness, and therefore the usefulness of the implemented script, which is a functional tool for the analysis of surface motifs.

Segmentation of surface motifs and determination of their parameters allow for the analysis and characterization of the motifs with regard to their size, shape, etc. Analysis of motifs is related to the determination of the stereometric shape of the surface, which is closely related to material properties. Therefore, it is an important step in the work of scientists as it helps them to create materials with properly shaped surface topography, which enables to achieve better material properties.

Acknowledgement. The research leading to these results has received funding from the Ministry of Science and Higher Education from the budget for science in the years 2016–2020 in context of the 'Diamentowy Grant' project (grant number: DI2015 019045).

References

1. Dobrzański, L.: Shaping the Structure and Surface Properties of Engineering and Biomedical Materials. OCSCO, Gliwice (2009)
2. Garczyk, Ż., Stach, S., Tălu, Ş., Sobola, D., Wróbel, Z.: Stereometric parameters of butterfly wings. J. Biomimetics Biomaterials Biomed. Eng. **31**, 1–10 (2017). https://doi.org/10.4028/www.scientific.net/JBBBE.31.1
3. Jóźwiak, G., Gotszalk, T.: Analysis of surface images in the microscopy of close interactions. PAK **56**(1), 46–47 (2010)
4. Kruk, T.: Atomic Force Microscopy (AFM). LAB **18**(1), 46–50 (2013)
5. Leach, R.: Characterisation of Areal Surface Texture. Springer, Berlin (2013)
6. Mateuszewski, M., Styp-Rekowski, M.: Confocal laser scanning microscope in tribological tests. Tribologia **229**(1), 157–165 (2010)
7. MathWorks documentation for Matlab. http://www.mathworks.com/help
8. Stach, S., Garczyk, Ż., Tălu, Ş., Solaymani, S., Ghaderi, A., Moradian, R., Nezafat, N.B., Elahi, S.M., Gholamali, H.: Stereometric parameters of the Cu/Fe NPs thin films. J. Phys. Chem. C **119**(31), 17887–17898 (2015). https://doi.org/10.1021/acs.jpcc.5b04676
9. Tadeusiewicz, R., Korohoda, P.: Computer Image Analysis and Processing. Publisher of the Progress of Telecommunications Foundation, Kraków (1997)
10. Tălu, Ş., Stach, S., Solaymani, S., Moradian, R., Ghaderi, A., Hantehzadeh, M.R., Elahi, S.M., Garczyk, Ż., Izadyar, S.: Multifractal spectra of atomic force microscope images of Cu/Fe nanoparticles based films thickness. J. Electroanal. Chem. **749**, 31–41 (2015). https://doi.org/10.1016/j.jelechem.2015.04.009

Multimodal Imaging and Computer-Aided Surgery

Algorithm for the Fusion of Ultrasound Tomography Breast Images Allowing Automatic Discrimination Between Benign and Malignant Tumors in Screening Tests

Krzysztof J. Opieliński[1]([✉]), Piotr Pruchnicki[1], Andrzej Wiktorowicz[2], and Marcin Jóźwik[3,4]

[1] Faculty of Electronics, Wroclaw University of Science and Technology, Wroclaw, Poland
krzysztof.opielinski@pwr.edu.pl
[2] Dramiński S.A. Ultrasound Scanners, Olsztyn, Poland
[3] Faculty of Medicine, Collegium Medicum, University of Warmia and Mazury in Olsztyn, Olsztyn, Poland
[4] Gyneka Center for Woman's Health, Krakow, Poland

Abstract. This paper presents an algorithm which allows a multi-parameter *in vivo* visualization of a breast structure by fusing two quantitative ultrasound tomography images and by automatically identifying areas of fat and glandular tissue, as well as areas of benign or malignant lesions, with the background of the reflection ultrasound tomography image of structures scattering ultrasonic waves. The threshold values for identifying particular tissue areas in quantitative images were adjusted to patient age using empirical linear functions. The viability of the algorithm was confirmed in preliminary *in vivo* breast ultrasound tomography screening tests. The obtained results allow a prediction that the ultrasound tomography scanner, which uses the here-presented algorithm to fuse the reconstructed images, and which is currently deployed by the private investor in cooperation with the authors of this paper, will provide a new standard in breast cancer diagnostics through fast and cheap screening tests.

Keywords: Ultrasound tomography · Breast diagnostics
Screening test · Ultrasound image fusion · Cancer recognition

1 Introduction

'Nowadays, hospitals and health-care providers are moving from their current heavy reliance on diagnostic tools like X-rays, CT scans and MRIs to a health-care system that leans more on digital imaging, genetics, apps and artificial intelligence for both diagnosis and treatment. Few believe computers will replace

© Springer International Publishing AG, part of Springer Nature 2019
E. Pietka et al. (Eds.): ITIB 2018, AISC 762, pp. 125–137, 2019.
https://doi.org/10.1007/978-3-319-91211-0_11

doctors anytime soon, but they already can scan millions of images in seconds to help them identify specific illnesses and rule out others' [3]. Ultrasound methods, which offer an increasing number of realtime modalities, belong to the most interesting methods for non-invasive imaging of the human body. Apart from the standard ultrasound imaging of tissue structures in the so-called B-mode (Brightness Mode), these methods also enable the estimation of tissue hardness in the ultrasound elastography (USE) mode [6]. In effect, ultrasound diagnostic tools cover a broad range of applications, such as detecting breast cancer [13,24], which is the most frequently diagnosed type of malignant tumor with women and the second most frequent cause of death among women, after bronchial cancer [15]. Also, unlike X-ray and nuclear techniques, which make use of ionizing radiation, ultrasound methods are not hazardous to the health of patients. Moreover, the costs related to ultrasound diagnostics are relatively low. The above advantages encourage researchers to pursue new, advanced methods for parametric ultrasound imaging to enable improved breast cancer detectability and characterization [5,11,27]. Ultrasound parametric imaging constitutes an attempt to extract quantitative information on the distribution of local ultrasound wave attenuation and velocity values from ultrasound signals reflected in the tissue structure (the so-called echoes) [16,19]. According to current research results, ultrasound speed is found to be greater in breast tissue affected by tumor than in healthy tissue [4,9], and the speed characteristics allow differentiating between fat, healthy tissue and concentrated masses. Increased scattering and absorption of ultrasound in malignant lesions, on the other hand, causes ultrasound wave attenuation to increase [7,9,25]. Therefore, the combination of ultrasound attenuation distribution with ultrasound speed distribution may provide an effective method for the discrimination between benign and malignant tumors. No current solution offers a sufficiently precise and mathematically efficient reconstruction of ultrasound speed and attenuation distribution based on ultrasound signals reflected in the tissue structure and obtained with ultrasound B-mode scanners. The problem lies in the excessive calculation complexity of such methods, which renders realtime imaging impossible in practice [16,19].

Quick reconstruction of ultrasound speed and attenuation distribution in the breast tissue is possible with the use of ultrasound wave transmission in the tomographic system of scanning coronal sections, the so-called ultrasound tomography (UST). This is a perfectly safe, painless and noninvasive hybrid method, which combines the diagnostic potential of mammography (MMG), conventional ultrasound imaging (US) and magnetic resonance tomography (MRT) [2,8,20–22,26]. The innovative hybrid ultrasound tomography scanner is currently deployed by the private investor in cooperation with the authors of this paper [10,22]. The device enables simultaneous production of quantitative and qualitative *in vivo* images, which represent breast tissue with the use of several various acoustic parameters in coronal sections covering the whole breast submerged in water. The scanning procedure lasts between 3 and 5 min.

This paper presents an algorithm which allows a multi-parameter *in vivo* visualization of a breast structure by fusing two reconstructed, quantitative, transmission ultrasound tomography images, and by automatically identifying areas of fat and glandular tissue, as well as areas of benign or malignant lesions. The background of that fusion image is reflection ultrasound tomography image of structures scattering ultrasonic waves, such as vessels, milk ducts, ligaments, septa and fibers. The viability of the algorithm was confirmed in preliminary *in vivo* breast ultrasound tomography screening tests performed on 50 patients aged between 20 and 73. Clinical diagnosis for each patient was made by a doctor on the basis of a conventional breast ultrasound imaging (US). All malignant tumors were identified on the basis of histopathological examination. Ultrasound breast imaging *in vivo* has been performed with the approval of the Bioethics Committee at the University of Warmia and Mazury (Resolution No. 22/2015), within the research titled: 'The evaluation of diagnostic value of breast examination using ultrasound transmission tomography and ultrasound reflection tomography'.

The test results allow a prediction that the deployed ultrasound tomography scanner offering a fusion of reconstructed images may contribute to achieving a new standard for breast cancer diagnostics through fast and inexpensive screening tests, which will provide information about the presence, basic type, location, and potential malignancy of breast tumors.

2   Ultrasound Tomography Images

Ultrasound breast tomography (USBT) is a very promising hybrid diagnostic method, as it offers multi-modal ultrasound imaging. Using both a pulse ultrasound wave transmitted through each of the breast coronal sections and a wave scattered on the structure heterogeneities of these sections in numerous directions around enables the tomographic *in vivo* reconstruction of at least three complementary ultrasound images. Each of the images shows the distribution of a separate acoustic parameter which differentiates the tissue and its lesions in a specific way. The combination of these images allows a comprehensive, both qualitative and quantitative characterization of breast tissue. A set of such images is obtained for each coronal section, thus also enabling the visualization of the complete breast volume in any breast section, with the use of the MPR (Multi-Planar Reconstruction) technique.

Ultrasound transmission and reflection tomography images constitute a new type of visualization for the structure of breast tissue. They represent the structure differently than standard images created with the currently used diagnostic devices: conventional ultrasound scanners, X-ray mammography scanners or magnetic resonance tomography scanners. The clinical significance of ultrasound tomography scanning in women breast imaging has not been yet well researched and documented. No databases exist that would contain ultrasound breast tomograms, no atlases or books describe the diagnostic approach. Only a limited number of publications describe the cases of clinical *in vivo* examinations of women's breast with the use of unique single ultrasound tomography scanners. These cases are mainly the examinations performed in the recent years in a small number of research centers involved in developing prototypes of ultrasound tomography devices capable of *in vivo* scanning [1,8,14,22,23,28].

The Polish ultrasound tomography scanner – developed by the private investor in cooperation with the authors of this paper – allows performing test on the patient lying face down on the scanner bed with her breast inserted (through an opening) into a tank containing water of temperature similar to body temperature. Breast imaging is performed automatically by scanning coronal sections at 1 or 2 mm slice intervals, using an ultrasonic ring array that moves vertically. The ultrasonic array comprises 1024 miniature piezoelectric ultrasound transducers arranged regularly on the inside of a ring having diameter $D_o = 260$ mm and surrounding the breast on all sides [21]. The elementary transducers have an active surface of 0.5×18 mm and operate in the frequency of ca. 2 MHz. Depending on breast length, the scan covers between 100 and 200 coronal sections from breast root to the nipple. On completion of the scan, two ultrasound tomographic transmission images are reconstructed for each of the coronal sections: $UTTc$ – absolute distribution of local ultrasound speeds (quantitative image) and $UTT\alpha$ – absolute distribution of local ultrasound attenuation coefficients (quantitative-qualitative image). These images are reconstructed on the basis of, respectively: average runtimes for ultrasonic pulses and average amplitudes of those pulses after they pass through the scanned breast coronal section, from all the directions around it. Moreover, during the scanning procedure, ultrasound signals are also collected, which are backscattered on heterogeneous tissue structures in breast sections, also from all the directions around it. Based on these data, each coronal section is provided with one ultrasound tomography reflection image (URT), which presents the distribution of local ultrasound backscatter coefficients (qualitative image). Transmission images are reconstructed with an FBP (Filtered Back Projection) algorithm [18] with a stochastic filter (SF) [17], and reflection images were reconstructed with a SAF (Synthetic Aperture Focusing) algorithm for transducer system arranged on the inner ring [5].

Figure 1 shows ultrasound tomography images ($UTTc$, $UTT\alpha$, URT and URT-$Edge$ – the URT image processed in order to obtain optimally sharp edges [17] of ultrasound scattering structures) for a coronal section of the right breast of a 64-year old woman with diagnosed DCIS – ductal carcinoma *in situ* (image diameter $D = 133.5$ mm); the enlarged cancer area is shown in Fig. 2. The images were obtained *in vivo*, with the use of the prototype of the ultrasound tomography scanner [21, 22]. The images of breast coronal sections (Fig. 1) are shown in views along the patient's axis in sagittal sections from the front: legs – the bottom of the image, head – the top of the image. This enables the comparison with the results obtained in conventional ultrasound scanning.

Transmission tomography images of the distribution of local ultrasound speed values in the breast tissue ($UTTc$) enable the quantitative evaluation of the tissue's elastic properties in relation to density [6, 7, 12, 25]. It is an important feature, as the cancer lumps are harder and more elastic than the surrounding tissue (Figs. 1(a) and 2). In $UTTc$ images, in the case of very small, quasi-homogeneous structures, the maximum possible contrast resolution for ultrasound speeds is below 2% (i.e. approx. 30 m/s), while in the case of sufficiently large structures it may be even below 0.1% (approx. 1 m/s) [21].

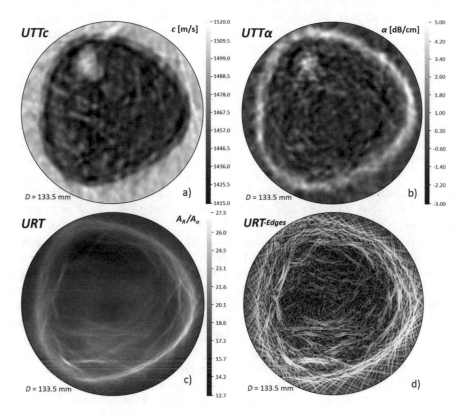

Fig. 1. Ultrasound tomography images of the coronal section of the right breast of a 64-year old woman with diagnosed DCIS, obtained *in vivo* with the use of the developed ultrasound tomography scanner: (a) *UTTc* – absolute distribution of ultrasound speed, (b) *UTTα* – absolute distribution of ultrasound attenuation, (c) *URT* – relative distribution of ultrasound scattering coefficient, (d) *URT-Edges* – the *URT* image processed to obtain sharp borders of visualized structures

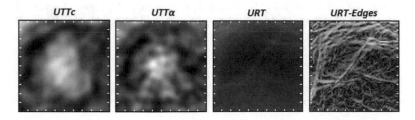

Fig. 2. The enlarged DCIS area of Fig. 1 (ROI: 36 × 36 mm)

A more precise and potentially more accurate diagnosis is possible additionally with the transmission tomogram representing the distribution of local ultrasound attenuation values ($UTT\alpha$), which only approximates actual values of this parameter in the breast structure, but provides a better contrast for the borders of heterogeneous areas (Figs. 1(b) and 2), which are blurred in the $UTTc$ images. Significant changes and negative ultrasound attenuation values on the borders of such areas in the $UTT\alpha$ images are the result of measurement errors, as the weakening of the measured amplitude of ultrasonic pulses, after they pass through the scanned tissue's structures. This amplitude is influenced not only by attenuation, but also by refraction, diffraction, anisotropy, reflection, and scattering on the borders of heterogeneous areas, as well as by beam divergence. Therefore, this image may be rather treated as a quantitative-qualitative one. The diagnosis of lesions is also significantly enhanced by the third, qualitative URT reflection tomographic image, which allows the visualization of all structures in breast tissue that effectively scatter ultrasonic waves, i.e. fibrous stroma, Cooper ligaments, breast lobe borders, blood and lymphatic vessels, milk ducts and sinuses (Figs. 1(c), (d) and 2). These structures are shown in an URT image with high spatial resolution (fractions of millimetres), allowing lesions (such as fibrosis or excessive vascularity) to be identified by sharpening their borders. URT images often show the tumor's vascularity and texture, which cause it to have a characteristic spicule shape. Malignant breast tumors provide poor contour representation in reflection images, which is due to the contrast of echo reduced from irregular contours caused by peripheral invasion or tissue interaction. Therefore, the ability of reflection images to visualize architectural deformations in fibrous strands and in connective tissue as compared to smooth contours in benign lesions provides only potential data in predicting malignancy. Notably, as breast density increases, the visibility of breast architecture in the form of strands of fibers and Cooper ligaments decreases due to increasing density of breast parenchyma.

The same breast was also examined with the use of standard US imaging, which detected a 3 cm lump of irregular shape, with calcifications, located on 12:00 o'clock, approximately 7 mm below skin. The patient was also subjected to MRT tests, which detected (in the same breast, on 12:00 o'clock) a $15 \times 10 \times 13$ mm tumor having blurred, irregular contours, showing symptoms of diffusion restriction and strong heterogeneous signal amplification upon the intravenous application of a contrast agent; the patient's breast was described as a fat-tissue breast. The examined histopathological oligobiopsy material taken from the tumor revealed the presence of a noninvasive ductal carcinoma *in situ* (DCIS).

3   The Multi-parameter Visualization of Breast Structure

In order to provide screening tests with an option of performing a multi-parameter ultrasound visualization of breast structure and of automatically discriminating tumors from healthy tissue as well as benign tumors from malignant tumors, a fusion algorithm was developed. The algorithm enables a certain combination of the $UTTc$ and $UTT\alpha$ images (Figs. 1(a), (b)), as well as the incorporation of the so-called URT-$Edge$ image, which is a specially processed URT image serving as the background. Such a multi-parameter visualization allows perfect correlation between all the three modalities of ultrasound tomography imaging, which show some common features but also provide complementary quantitative-qualitative diagnostic information [23]. The construction of the algorithm is based on the results of research, which show that increased values of ultrasound attenuation within glandular tissue and in the area with simultaneously increasing ultrasound speed values indicate high probability of malignant lesion [7,9,25]. On the other hand, independent increase in ultrasound speed indicates benign lesion [4,9,25]. By making an additional use of the specially processed URT reflection image in the form of URT-$Edge$ image (Figs. 1(d) and 2) as the background, it is possible to generate a visualization showing breast tissue structures with high spatial resolution, as these structures scatter ultrasonic waves effectively (fibrous stroma, Cooper ligaments, breast lobe borders, blood and lymphatic vessels, milk ducts and sinuses). These structures facilitate the detection of lesions, as they are characterized by sharpened borders (cysts, isolated regularly-shaped lumps) as well as by fibrosis or excessive vascularity. The developed algorithm of the USBT multi-parameter image fusion is a special arithmetic logic combination of the following three types of ultrasound tomography images:

$$I_{FR} = \underbrace{(I_{UTT_{c>c_1}})}_{\text{gray}} + \underbrace{(I_{UTT_{c>c_2}} \cap I_{UTT_{\alpha \leq \alpha_1}})}_{\text{yellow}} + \underbrace{(I_{UTT_{c>c_2}} \cap I_{UTT_{\alpha > \alpha_1}})}_{\text{red}} + \underbrace{(I_{URT_E})}_{\text{B/W}}, \quad (1)$$

where I_{FR} – the resultant multi-parameter fused image; $I_{UTT_{c>c_1}}$ – the transmission $UTTc$ image of local ultrasound speed distribution (Fig. 1(a)) with zeroed pixels having values $\leq c_1$, where c_1 is the limit value of ultrasound speed between the fat tissue and the glandular tissue for a particular breast; $I_{UTT_{c>c_2}}$ – the transmission $UTTc$ image of local ultrasound speed distribution (Fig. 1(a)) with zeroed pixels having values $\leq c_2$, where c_2 is the limit value of ultrasound speed between the healthy glandular tissue and the potentially tumorous (both benign and malignant) glandular tissue for a particular breast; $I_{UTT_{\alpha > \alpha_1}}$ – the transmission $UTT\alpha$ image of local ultrasound attenuation distribution (Fig. 1(b)) with zeroed pixels having values $\leq \alpha_1$, where α_1 is the limit value of ultrasound attenuation between the healthy glandular tissue and the glandular tissue with a potentially malignant tumor, for a particular breast; I_{URT_E} – a specially processed reflection URT image (URT-$Edge$) of relative ultrasound scattering coefficient (Fig. 1(d)); $\cap$ – the conjunction operator. Thus, the final fused image I_{FR} simultaneously shows the breast's complete architecture with oval cyst contours and regular borders of potential concentrated tumor masses (through I_{URT_E}), healthy glandular tissue represented as areas in shades of light gray (through $I_{UTT_{c>c_1}}$), benign tumor lumps represented as areas in shades of light yellow (through $I_{UTT_{c>c_2}} \cap I_{UTT_{\alpha \leq \alpha_1}}$) and lumps of potentially malignant tumors represented in shades of red (through $I_{UTT_{c>c_2}} \cap I_{UTT_{\alpha > \alpha_1}}$). The fusion algorithm of equation (1) requires the use of appropriate pixel cut-off thresholds: c_1, c_2, α_1, which are unique for a particular patient as their values increase together with the increase in the breast tissue density. Breast tissue density decreases with patient age, but also depends on other factors, such as e.g. received hormone therapy. For instance, ultrasound speeds are high for breast-feeding women, when the breast contains significant amount of milk and overgrown glandular tissue. In order to enable automatic estimation of thresholds for the examined breast, mean maximum values of ultrasound speed and attenuation can be determined for the areas of healthy glandular tissue. It is also possible to represent the thresholds in the form of tables and calculate functions for the changes in those values, using a large number of patients as the basis and correlating the results with age and additional factors, such as hormone therapies, pregnancy and breast feeding periods, or menopause. A certain preliminary, approximate, age-related decrease of ultrasound speed and attenuation in breast tissue may also be assumed [12].

Figure 3 shows images of Fig. 1, specially processed to meet the requirements of fusion algorithm (Eq. (1)): with cut-off threshold for fat tissue $c_1 = 1446\,\mathrm{m/s}$ (Fig. 3(a)), with cut-off threshold for healthy tissue $c_2 = 1487\,\mathrm{m/s}$ (Fig. 3(b)), with cut-off threshold for healthy tissue $\alpha_1 = 1.74\,\mathrm{dB/cm}$ (Fig. 3(c)) and the resultant image, fused in accordance with equation (1) (Fig. 3(d)).

The threshold values were determined in relation to patient age, using empirical linear functions prepared on the basis of tests presented in [22]:

$$c_1 = -y_p + 1510 \quad [\mathrm{m/s}], \tag{2}$$

$$c_2 = -1.3 \cdot y_p + 1570 \quad [\mathrm{m/s}], \tag{3}$$

$$\alpha_1 = -0.04 \cdot y_p + 4.3 \quad [\mathrm{dB/m}], \tag{4}$$

where y_p – patient age in years. Based on the developed algorithm (Eq. (1)), the multi-parameter ultrasound image of the breast in coronal section (Fig. 3(d)) – with appropriate scaling of the threshold ultrasound speed and attenuation values on the UTT images (Fig. 3(a), (b), (c)), with the background in the form of a specially processed URT image (URT-Edges of Fig. 1(d)) and with color patterns for fat tissue areas (black), glandular tissue (gray), benign tumors (yellow – if only the defined ultrasound speed threshold is exceeded) and malignant tumors (red – if defined thresholds of ultrasound speed and attenuation are exceeded simultaneously) – enabled automatic detection of the DCIS cancer, as confirmed in histopathological tests. The cancer area of Fig. 3(a)–(d) is shown enlarged in Fig. 4, together with an additional multi-parameter fused image with darker background in the form of the less intensive URT-Edge image (Fusion dark background). The intensity of the URT-Edge image can be modified to meet the requirements.

The tests of the fusion algorithm performed on the ultrasound tomography images of breasts obtained from initial screening of 50 patients allowed a conclusion that false positive results in the multi-parameter fused images (indicating lesions) are always explainable, never random, and are always caused by easily identifiable reasons (Fig. 3(d)). Errors, which show as small yellow or red dots (suggesting benign or malignant tumors, respectively) often occur on the

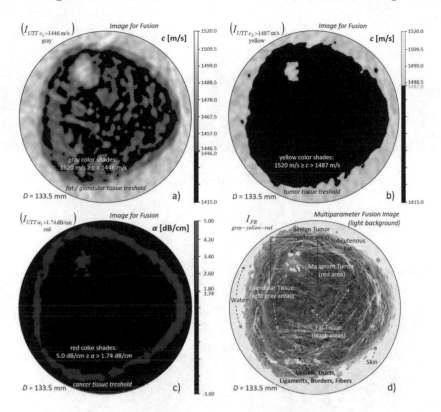

Fig. 3. Images of Fig. 1, specially processed to meet the requirements of the multi-parameter fusion algorithm (Eq. (1)): (a) with cut-off threshold for fat tissue $c_1 = 1446$ m/s, (b) with cut-off threshold for healthy tissue $c_2 - 1487$ m/s, (c) with cut off threshold for healthy tissue $\alpha_1 = 1.74$ dB/cm, (d) the resultant image of fusion with *URT-Edge* image as the background

water/skin border and occasionally in the area of the water surrounding the breast (in the case of older women), as the ultrasound speeds in such areas are higher than in the breast tissue (Fig. 3).

Yellow dots may also occur in coronal sections, in the vicinity of the nipple (especially in tests performed on dense breasts with young women) due to the concentration of milk ducts and sinuses [22]. Thus, the false positive detections of lesions may be easily eliminated by specialized diagnosticians. This task is further facilitated by the possibility to produce images of breast volumes in transverse sections (with the help of Multi-Planar Reconstructions) and in three-dimensional views (Maximum Intensity Projections). The MPR and MIP techniques are used in every tomography imaging method (CT, MRT, PET, SPECT).

Initial *in vivo* breast screening tests on a group of 50 patients confirmed the very high accuracy of the developed multi-parameter fusion algorithm (Eq. (1))

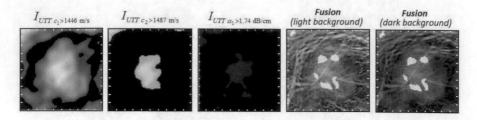

Fig. 4. The enlarged DCIS area of Fig. 3 (ROI: 36 × 36 mm)

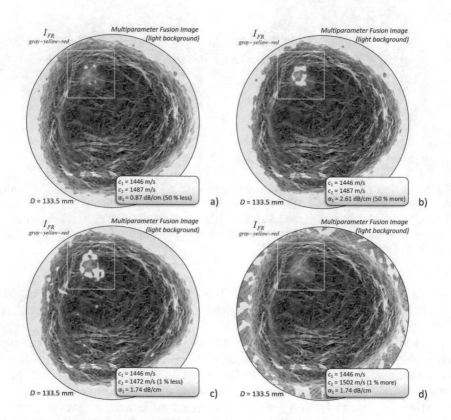

Fig. 5. Multi-parameter fused images of the coronal section of a 64-year-old woman's breast with the DCIS cancer, scanned *in vivo* with the use of the developed ultrasound tomography scanner; cut-off thresholds in the algorithm (Eq. (1)) were offset from the values calculated with equations (2) – (4) by: (a) –50% for α_1, (b) +50% for α_1, (c) –1% for c_2, (d) +1% for c_2

in automatically detecting lesions and in predicting their malignancy – all tumors present in the area analyzed with the ultrasound tomography scanner were correctly detected and qualified as benign/malignant. Moreover, multi-parameter fused images have been observed to have high (on the order of several tens of percent) tolerance to the changing values of thresholds α_1 and approximately $\pm 1\%$ tolerance to the changing values of thresholds c_1 and c_2 (Fig. 5).

These changes cause only a slight increase or decrease of the color-coded tumor areas, when the thresholds are understated or overstated, respectively. In order to increase the chances for a proper diagnosis, it is possible to perform first a preliminary, automatic configuration of thresholds c_1 and c_2 most of all, and to regulate the device within the accepted tolerances. For instance, if a hormone therapy must be allowed for, the patient's age may be lowered when defining the threshold values (Eqs. (2) – (4)) in the measurements.

The functioning and the accuracy of the designed algorithm, as well as the calibration of threshold values, are planned be tested by subjecting a group of at least 150 patients to *in vivo* screening tests.

4 Conclusions

The developed algorithm for the fusion of ultrasound tomography images allows an automatic and multi-parameter visualization of the structures of breast tissue in such a manner that one image represents simultaneously a number of characteristics. Therefore, the characteristics of breast tissue may be provided with a complex description, i.e. more effectively and with greater accuracy. The concentrated masses are clearly visible as the fused image represents both local phenomena and the immediate vicinity of the tumor, including breast parenchyma and the architecture of breast tissue. In particular, such a multi-parameter ultrasound image of any breast section allows an automatic detection of a lesion and an evaluation of its character by providing a visual representation of blood vessels or fibers in the area which has increased ultrasound speed and/or attenuation values. The obtained results allow a prediction that the ultrasound tomography scanner which uses the here-presented algorithm to fuse the reconstructed images and which is currently deployed by the private investor in cooperation with the authors of this paper will provide a new standard in breast cancer diagnostics through fast and inexpensive screening tests.

References

1. André, M., et al.: Quantitative volumetric breast imaging with 3D inverse scatter computed tomography. In: Conference Proceedings of IEEE Engineering in Medicine and Biology Society, vol. 34, San Diego (2012)
2. Birk, M., Kretzek, E., et al.: High-speed medical imaging in 3D ultrasound computer tomography. IEEE Trans. Parallel Distrib. Syst. **27**(2), 455–467 (2016)
3. Boston, W.: Siemens Tees Up Health-Care IPO in One of Biggest European Deals in Years. The Wall Street Journal, Business (2017)

4. Chang, C.-H., Huang, S.-W., et al.: Reconstruction of ultrasonic sound velocity and attenuation coefficient using linear arrays: clinical assessment. Ultrasound Med. Biol. **33**(11), 1681–1687 (2007)
5. Cobbold, R.S.C.: Foundations of Biomedical Ultrasound. Oxford University Press, New York (2007)
6. Doyley, M.M., Parker, K.J.: Elastography: general principles and clinical applications. Ultrasound Clin. **9**(1), 1–11 (2014)
7. Duck, F.A.: Physical Properties of Tissue. Academic Press, London (1990)
8. Duric, N., Littrup, P., et al.: Breast imaging with the SoftVue imaging system: first results. In: Bosch, J.G., Doyley, M.M. (eds.) Proceedings of SPIE 2013. Medical Imaging 2013: Ultrasonic Imaging, Tomography, and Therapy, vol. 8675. SPIE (2013)
9. Edmonds, P.D., Mortensen, C.L., et al.: Ultrasound tissue characterization of breast biopsy specimens. Ultrason. Imaging **13**(2), 162–185 (1991)
10. Forbes, Nauka i Społeczeństwo. Polska rodzinna firma zmienia oblicze medycyny. Przełom w diagnostyce nowotworów, 24 April 2017. https://www.forbes.pl/innogy/nauka-i-spoleczenstwo/rak.../k0et0qj. (in Polish)
11. Gordon, P.B., Goldenberg, S.L.: Malignant breast masses detected only by ultrasound: a retrospective review. Cancer **76**(4), 626–630 (1995)
12. Greenleaf, J.F., Johnson, S.A., et al.: Quantitative cross-sectional imaging of ultrasound parameters. In: Proceedings of IEEE Ultrasonics Symposium, Phoenix, USA (1977)
13. Hooley, R.J., Scoutt, L.M., Philpotts, L.E.: Breast ultrasonography: state of the art. Radiology **268**(3), 612–659 (2013)
14. Hopp, T., Zapf, M., et al.: 3D ultrasound computer tomography: update from a clinical study 2016. In: Duric, N., Heyde, B. (eds.) Proceedings of SPIE 2016. Medical Imaging 2016: Ultrasonic Imaging and Tomography, vol. 9790, pp. 97900A-1–9. SPIE (2016)
15. Hortobagyi, G.N., de la Salazar, J.G., et al.: The global breast cancer burden: variations in epidemiology and survival. Clin. Breast Cancer **6**(5), 391–401 (2005)
16. Jaeger, M., Held, G., et al.: Computed ultrasound tomography in echo mode for imaging speed of sound using pulse-echo sonography: proof of principle. Ultrasound Med. Biol. **41**(1), 235–250 (2015)
17. Jain, A.K.: Fundamentals of Digital Image Processing. Prentice Hall, USA (1989)
18. Kak, A.C., Slaney, M.: Principles of Computerized Tomographic Imaging. IEEE Press, New York (1988)
19. Klimonda, Z., Postema, M., et al.: Tissue attenuation estimation by mean frequency downshift and bandwidth limitation. IEEE Trans. Ultrason. Ferroelec. Freq. Contr. **63**(8), 1107–1115 (2016)
20. Marmarelis, V.Z., Jeong, J., et al.: High-resolution 3-D imaging and tissue differentiation with transmission tomography. Acoust. Image **28**, 195–206 (2007)
21. Opieliński, K.J., Pruchnicki, P., et al.: Imaging results of multi-modal ultrasound computerized tomography system designed for breast diagnosis. Comput. Med. Imaging Graph. **46**, 83–94 (2015)
22. Opieliński, K.J., Pruchnicki, P., et al.: Multimodal ultrasound computer-assisted tomography: an approach to the recognition of breast lesion. Comput. Med. Imaging Graph. **65**, 102–114 (2018)
23. Ranger, B., Littrup, P.J., et al.: Breast ultrasound tomography versus MRI for clinical display of anatomy and tumor rendering: preliminary results. Am. J. Roentgenol. **198**, 233–239 (2012)

24. Ricci, P., Maggini, E., et al.: Clinical application of breast elastography: state of the art. Eur. J. Radiol. **83**(3), 429–437 (2014)
25. Weiwad, W., Heinig, A., et al.: Direct measurement of sound velocity in various specimens of breast tissue. Invest. Radiol. **35**(12), 721–726 (2000)
26. Wiskin, J., Borup, D., et al.: Threedimensional nonlinear inverse scattering: quantitative transmission algorithms, refraction corrected reflection, scanner design and clinical results. POMA **19**, 075001 (2013)
27. Ying, X., Lin, Y., et al.: A comparison of mammography and ultrasound in women with breast disease: a receiver operating characteristic analysis. Breast J. **18**(2), 130–138 (2012)
28. Zografos, G., Koulocheri, D., et al.: Novel technology of multimodal ultrasound tomography detects breast lesions. Eur. Radiol. **23**(3), 673–683 (2013)

Development of a Multimodal Image Registration and Fusion Technique for Visualising and Monitoring Chronic Skin Wounds

Andre Woloshuk[1]($\boxtimes$), Michał Kręcichwost[2], Jan Juszczyk[2],
Bartłomiej Pyciński[2], Marcin Rudzki[2], Beata Choroba[2], Daniel Ledwon[2],
Dominik Spinczyk[2], and Ewa Pietka[2]

[1] Weldon School of Biomedical Engineering, Purdue University,
206 S Martin Jischke Dr, West Lafayette, IN 47907, USA
acwolosh@purdue.edu

[2] Faculty of Biomedical Engineering, Silesian University of Technology,
Zabrze, Poland

Abstract. Chronic skin wounds from diabetes, atherosclerosis, and cancer form a large source of morbidity and medical complications. While individual imaging modalities (e.g. visual images, thermograms, ultrasound) can be useful for monitoring the healing process, their use is limited because of the difficulty acquiring and registering multiple images from different modalities. This paper presents a methodology for image registration using an alignment phantom for grayscale images and thermograms. The registration system achieves a Fiducial Registration Error of 0.61 mm and Mutual Information value of 0.774. Future studies will seek to add additional imaging modalities and improve registration for other areas of the body.

Keywords: Image fusion · Thermography · Image registration
Alignment phantom

1 Introduction

Chronic wounds result mostly from three main pathologies, commonly called lifestyle diseases or diseases of civilization: diabetes mellitus, atherosclerosis, and cancer. The pathogenesis of the wounds differ in these diseases (peripheral neuropathy and microangiopathy with consequent ischaemia in diabetes, ulceration caused by critical arterial ischaemia in atherosclerosis, and bedsores as a result of prolonged bed rest, in people with cancer). The prognoses show that occurrence of chronic wounds in the coming years is going to increase, mainly because of the upward trend of mentioned diseases' morbidity. In Poland each year, 150,000 people are diagnosed with cancer and the number may increase 17% annually until 2025 [1]. Diabetes mellitus affects approximately 3 million

© Springer International Publishing AG, part of Springer Nature 2019
E. Pietka et al. (Eds.): ITIB 2018, AISC 762, pp. 138–149, 2019.
https://doi.org/10.1007/978-3-319-91211-0_12

people in Poland [2] and the number is going to increase in the future. Critical arterial ischaemia is the main cause of lower limb amputation [3]. In the year 2012, there were over 13,000 of these operations in Poland [4]. Therefore, there is a strong need for the development of new procedures which may monitor the progression and treatment of chronic skin wounds.

Current wound evaluation techniques include the *Wagner Ulcer Grade Classification Scale* or *European Pressure Ulcer Advisory Panel* [5], both of which may require the use of a ruler or, rarely, a camera for documentation. Novel methods, through the use of non-invasive devices, include consideration of the anatomical, mechanical and physiological characteristics of wound healing process [6]. The most important factors for predicting patient outcomes are wound size, depth, and duration [7]. These parameters, as well as blood flow, skin barrier function, or skin thickness, can be reproducibly evaluated by quantitative modalities such as ultrasonography (US), grayscale photography (VIS), or thermography (IR).

Color and grayscale photography has been used to assess the size of chronic wounds [8], and more recent studies have used segmentation to classify different wound types based on those images [9,10]. The use of thermographic images has been shown to provide clinically useful information about wound healing for pressure ulcers [11], diabetic ulcers [12], and vascular insufficiency in peripheral artery disease [13]. Additionally, it has been shown that applying a texture from thermographic images onto color photographs of a burn wound improves diagnostic possibilities [14]. However, the combined use of these techniques is limited by image registration error and camera positioning [15]. The use of an alignment phantom may help address these issues and a similar approach has been used for liver surface reconstruction of stereoscopic images [16,17].

The main contribution described in this article is a multimodal image acquisition setup for thermographic and grayscale images of back wounds as well as a methodology for automatic image registration and fusion using an alignment phantom.

The paper is organized in the following manner. The image acquisition setup and alignment aids are described in the Materials section. The alignment process and image registration methodology are presented in the Methods section. The registration error and other findings are presented in the Experiments and Results section, while the next steps regarding wound healing observation are described in the Discussion.

2 Materials

2.1 Measuring Station

The proposed multimodal station includes a stereo-camera, a thermal imaging camera, and a specialized, secure attachment device for individual elements of the station above the wound surface. The FLIR A300 thermal camera was used. The sensor resolution for this model is 320×240 px and the detector pitch is 25 microns. The Field of View is $25° \times 18.8°$ with a minimum focus distance of 0.4 meters. The f-number is 1.3. The Claron Bumblebee2 Hx40 stereo camera was used. The sensor resolution for this model is 1024 × 768 px. The Field of Measurement (FOM) is (radius × width × height) 120 × 120 × 90 cm. The physical case dimensions (W × H × D, approx.) are 164 × 43 × 54 mm.

The stereo-vision camera is used to determine the location of the phantom during registration. In addition, the phantom is equipped with markers that are used to locate characteristic points in both modalities. A stereo camera, Claron Hx40, from ClaroNav was calibrated by the manufacturer and supplied to the user with a dedicated calibration file. Lens distortion problem is taken into account by calibration corrective polynomials and was included in manufacturer calibration process. The image obtained from the calibrated camera is subject to rectification in accordance with the calculated correction coefficients. Dedicated software for detecting black and white markers ensures an accuracy of 0.1 mm ± 0.25 mm. The accuracy standard requires stable temperature and visual conditions in the analyzed scene.

A halogen lamp has also been included in the described station to heat the alignment phantom. The cameras included in the station have a parallel optical axis. The concept of the measuring station can be seen in Fig. 1.

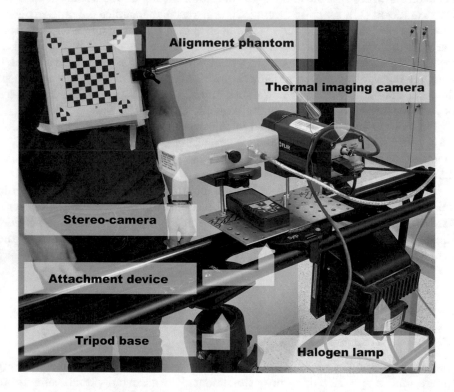

Fig. 1. Measuring station and components

2.2   Alignment Phantoms

The proposed phantom consists of two parts. Its central part is filled with alternating bright and dark fields, forming a chessboard with sides 132 mm in length. On the edges, there are markers used to determine the distance between the phantom and the camera set. Bright (white paper $\varepsilon = 0.70$) and dark (black paper $\varepsilon = 0.90$) fields have different infrared radiation emissivity, ε, which can be distinguished in the infrared image [18]. A checkerboard pattern is used because algorithms for detecting characteristic points are widely used in the literature [19–21]. These methods are used when aligning the images from both cameras. In order to develop IR contrast, the phantom must be heated, for example with a halogen lamp, before imaging. Due to the high emissivity coefficient of the material (paper $\varepsilon = 0.70, \ldots, 0.90$), approximately 10 s is enough for the phantom to develop visible contrast in the IR image.

The printed marks at the edges of the phantom track the location of the phantom over the test area. They are used by a stereo-camera built into the measurement stand. The stereo-camera software automatically detects and tracks the markers. In addition, the markers can be used to determine the distance of markers from the measurement stand.

3   Methodology

In Fig. 2, a general scheme of image acquisition and processing has been presented. The acquisition of the wound area was divided into two stages (Fig. 3). First, an image was simultaneously recorded in visible and infrared light (thermograms) with a phantom held above the wound (this phantom allows the detection of characteristic points in both modalities). Subsequently, in the second stage of acquisition, the phantom was removed and the wound image is acquired again. During acquisition, it was important to record the distance between the object and the stereo-camera.

Due to the low resolution of the infrared camera (240×320 pixels) and the location of the area of interest during the acquisition (the center of the image), image distortion reduction resulting from the camera optical systems was omitted.

For each pair of images (phantom + object, object) recorded in visible and infrared spectra (thermograms), the image registration and fusion operations were preceded by pre-processing. The preprocessing of the images consisted of several stages. Due to the different resolutions of the analyzed images (IR, VIS), each stage was carried out independently for both types of images obtained.

The purpose of the first pre-processing step was to increase the contrast of the obtained thermographic images. This step consisted of dividing the IR image into smaller sections. Each section was subjected to histogram alignment, median filtration, and sharpening to decrease the effect of uneven intensity distribution from the phantom heating process.

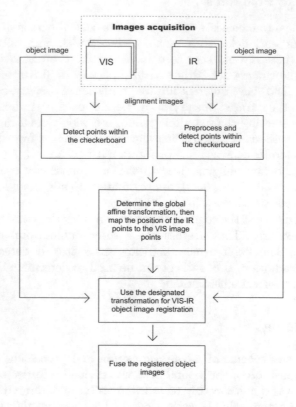

Fig. 2. General scheme of image acquisition and processing for phantom and object images

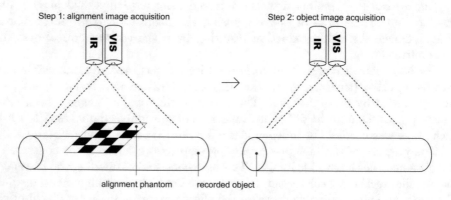

Fig. 3. Image acquisition is divided into two stages, with and without the phantom

The next stage was to determine characteristic points for pairs of images with a phantom (VIS, IR). The following steps have been used to designate these points:

- chessboard nodes were determined using corner prototypes,
- the location of nodes was improved with sub-pixel accuracy using gradients,
- regular chessboard structures were obtained by minimizing energy functions.

A detailed description of the algorithm for determining the corner points has been described in [22].

The previously described step provided characteristic points for pairs of images with a phantom (VIS, IR). However, the detection of characteristic points in the IR image was imprecise due to the low image resolution and blurred checkerboard edges. Therefore, an adjustment algorithm was used to improve the position of these points. On the basis of the detected points, the first order polynomial curves were interpolated for the horizontal, vertical and diagonal direction (Fig. 4). Then, the points were shifted to the intersection of the these lines. These lines built a grid in which the intersections of the lines constituted the target location of the characteristic point on the phantom.

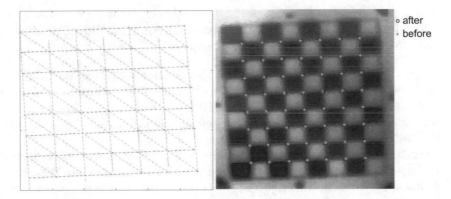

Fig. 4. Left: first order polynomial curves for the horizantal, vertical and diagonal directions, right: the characteristic points were improved using the curves

The localized points can be used to define a common region of interest for both modalities. This region was determined by first using an affine transformation from the checkerboard corner locations to align the grayscale image of the alignment phantom with the coordinate system of the thermogram. The characteristic points were used to crop the region of interest in the grayscale image. Finally, the grayscale image and thermogram were fused by the average fusion method [23].

4   Experiments and Results

In order to verify the functionality of the described methodology, a database of synthetic chronic back wound image pairs (VIS, IR) was built. These images were registered using a two-stage acquisition process using the previously described phantom. Due to the difficulty accessing patients and the pilot nature of the research, synthetic wounds with a specific geometry and different temperature than the human body were used. The database includes 24 sets of images, which include grayscale images and thermograms of the phantom and object, as seen in Fig. 3. An area of the back has been registered. As a synthetic wound, paper soaked with cold water of a specific geometry was applied to the exposed skin of the back of the subjects. The subjects were 70 cm from the measurement station. The subjects were positioned such that the wounds were in one of three positions:

- straight: the back was parallel to the phantom and in the center of the image,
- oblique: the back was angled away from the phantom and wounds were located in the center of the image,
- offset: the back was parallel to the phantom and located near the edge of the image.

Based on the image database, an experiment was carried out to determine the effectiveness of image matching and fusion of both modalities. The following quantitative measures were used for this purpose:

- Mutual Information (MI) – describes the alignment of images of different modalities and signals and is a measure of ability of one image to predict the values in another image. Mutual information can be calculated by subtracting the joint entropy of two images from the sum of the Shannon entropy from the two individual images [24],
- Normalized Mutual Information (NMI) – is the mutual information normalized by the joint entropy and is robust to significant image misalignment.
- Fiducial Registration Error (FRE) – the root-mean-square of the Euclidean distance between the fiducial markers in the IR and grayscale photo after registration. The fiducial markers are the checkerboard corners [25].

4.1   Results

Figure 5 shows examples of matching and fusion results. Mean FRE, MI, and NMI for 24 image pairs of the back using a phantom are presented in Table 1 The median FRE, MI, and NMI values prior to registration are presented in Table 2.

Figure 6 shows the median FRE distribution of the straight, oblique, and offset alignment images. The median FRE values for straight, oblique, and offset positions are 0.631, 0.819, and 0.585 mm, respectively. The phantom was placed in similar position for each alignment.

Table 1. Mean FRE, MI, and NMI for 24 image pairs of the back using a phantom, after registration

	FRE (mm)	MI	NMI
Straight	0.597	0.752	1.067
Oblique	0.638	0.729	1.063
Offset	0.580	0.918	1.081

Table 2. Mean FRE, MI, and NMI for 24 image pairs of the back using a phantom, before registration

	FRE (mm)	MI	NMI
Straight	7.824	0.699	1.061
Oblique	7.677	0.654	1.058
Offset	8.041	0.714	1.062

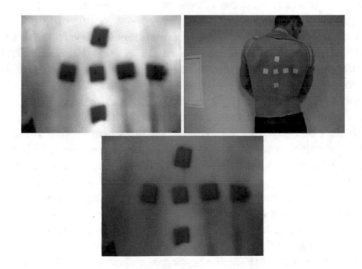

Fig. 5. Example of IR and VIS images and corresponding fusion result

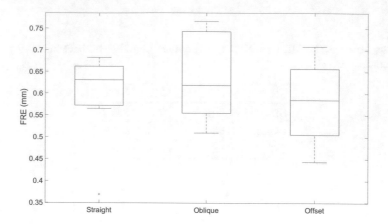

Fig. 6. FRE distribution of the straight, oblique, and offset alignment images after registration

5   Discussion

Due to the nature of the analyzed images (images of chronic wounds of the back) the acquisition time during the examination must be as short as possible. In addition, the type of analyzed area does not allow the application of markers visible in both modalities on the skin (directly, near the wound). The wound image also has no characteristic anatomical points visible in both modalities, which would facilitate image fitting and fusion. The use of an alignment phantom and simultaneous image capture allows the measurement station to be used quickly without direct contact with the patient.

Across all of the alignment images, a median FRE value of 0.61 mm was obtained. FRE has been used instead of Target Registration Error (TRE) because wounds are often amorphous and irregular, thus making it difficult to define consistent target points. For image-guided otologic surgery systems, FRE values of 0.66 mm were achieved [26].

Mutual Information is a frequently used metric for image registration, especially in medical imaging [27–30]. Using Particle Swarm Optimization and Powell's search algorithm to register IR and VIS images, an average MI of 1.17 was reached [31]. However, these images only required translational and rotational transformation. Similarly, a novel registration method achieved an MI of 0.936 based on images from an active and passive sensors [28]. The median MI of all images of was 0.774 after registration. The registration process reduced FRE by an average of 7.24 mm across all images. The difference between MI and NMI before and after registration was much less pronounced.

A limitation of using MI for evaluating registration and fusion accuracy is that it is mainly used for rigid transformation applications, such as in satellite or medical images [29]. Novel image registration metrics exist for non-rigid applications [32,33]. In this experiment, registration seems to be affected by the distance between the wound and alignment phantom, as seen in the oblique and offset images. Future experimentation should determine which metrics correspond with improved registration, then utilize a fine-tuning registration step after phantom alignment.

The acquisition setup uses markers on the alignment phantom to ensure that the phantom position is repeatable. The grayscale stereo-camera computes the three dimensional location of the makers with respect to the camera. Thus, the alignment phantom can be placed in a similar position for each measurement.

6 Conclusion

In Polish health facilities, monitoring the vast majority of chronic wound cases is carried out without the use of measuring equipment that provides an objective description of the extent of the wound. Most often, the severity of the ulcer is expressed in accordance to the five-point Torrance or Wagner scale. The only measurement method is to determine the diameter of the wound and possible photographic documentation. The proposed method for stereographic and thermographic image registration will enable the objective evaluation of chronic wounds. Future development could include ultrasound and color images in the multimodal acquisition setup.

Acknowledgement. This research is supported by the Polish National Science Centre (NCBR) grant No.: UMO-2016/21/B/ST7/02236. The funders had no role in study design, data collection and analysis, decision to publish, or preparation of the manuscript.

References

1. Didkowska, J., Zatonski, W., Wojciechowska, U., Didkowska.: Prediction of cancer incidence and mortality in Poland up to the year 2025. Centrum Onkologii. Instytut im. Marii Skłodowskiej-Curie (2009)
2. Greenwade, G.D.: Type 2 diabetes. part i. a modern epidemic. Przemysl Spozywczy **57**(6), 38–40 (2013)
3. Beard, J.D.: Chronic lower limb ischemia. West. J. Med. **173**(1), 60–63 (2000)
4. Czeleko, T., Sliwczynski, A., Nawrot, I., Karnafel, W.: The incidence of major, nontraumatic lower amputations in patients without diabetes mellitus in poland during 2009–2012, based on polish national health found data. Acta Angiologica **20**(3), 124–131 (2014)
5. Defloor, T., Schoonhoven, L., Fletcher, J., Furtado, K., Heyman, H., Lubbers, M., Witherow, A., Bale, S., Bellingeri, A., Cherry, G., Clark, M., Colin, D., Dassen, T., Dealey, C., Gulacsi, L., Haalboom, J., Halfens, R., Hietanen, H., Lindholm, C., Moore, Z., Romanelli, M., Soriano, J.V.: Statement of the european pressure ulcer advisory panel-pressure ulcer classification: differentiation between pressure ulcers and moisture lesions. J. Wound Ostomy Continence Nurs. **32**(5), 302–306 (2005)
6. Ud-Din, S., Bayat, A.: Non-invasive objective devices for monitoring the inflammatory, proliferative and remodelling phases of cutaneous wound healing and skin scarring. Exp. Dermatol. **25**(8), 579–585 (2016)

7. Emilia, M., Chaves, A., da Silva, F.S., Pinheiro, V., Soares, C., Augusto, R., Ferreira, M., Sampaio, F., Gomes, L., de Andrade, R.M., Pinotti, M.: Evaluation of healing of pressure ulcers through thermography: a preliminary study. Res. Biomed. Eng. **31**(1), 3–9 (2015)
8. Ozturk, C., Nissannov, J., Dubin, S., Wy, S., Nichols, J., Mark, R.: Measurement of wound healing by image analysis. Biomed. Sci. Instrum. **31**, 189–193 (1995)
9. Wild, T., Prinz, M., Fortner, N., Krois, W., Sahora, K., Stremitzer, S., Hoelzenbein, T.: Digital measurement and analysis of wounds based on colour segmentation. Eur. Surg. **40**(1), 5–10 (2008)
10. Mukherjee, R., Manohar, D.D., DAS, D.K., Achar, A., Mitra, A., Chakraborty, C.: Automated tissue classification framework for reproducible chronic wound assessment. Biomed. Res. Int. **2014**, 1–9 (2014)
11. Nakagami, G., Sanada, H., Iizaka, S., Kadono, T., Higashino, T., Koyanagi, H., Haga, N.: Predicting delayed pressure ulcer healing using thermography: a prospective cohort study. J. Wound Care **19**(11), 465–6, 468, 470 (2010)
12. Nagase, T., Sanada, H., Takehara, K., Oe, M., Iizaka, S., Ohashi, Y., Oba, M., Kadowaki, T., Nakagami, G.: Variations of plantar thermographic patterns in normal controls and non-ulcer diabetic patients: Novel classification using angiosome concept. J. Plast. Reconstr. Aesthetic Surg. **64**(7), 860–866 (2011)
13. Huang, C.L., Wu, Y.W., Hwang, C.L., Jong, Y.S., Chao, C.L., Chen, W.J., Wu, Y.T., Yang, W.S.: The application of infrared thermography in evaluation of patients at high risk for lower extremity peripheral arterial disease. J. Vasc. Surg. **54**(4), 1074–1080 (2011)
14. Thatcher, J.E., Squiers, J.J., Kanick, S.C., King, D.R., Lu, Y., Wang, Y., Mohan, R., Sellke, E.W., DiMaio1, J.M.: Imaging techniques for clinical burn assessment with a focus on multispectral imaging. Adv. Wound Care (New Rochelle) **5**(8), 360–378 (2016)
15. Paul, D., Ghassemi, P., Ramella-Roman, J., Prindeze, N., Moffatt, L., Alkhalil, A., Shupp, J.: Noninvasive imaging technologies for cutaneous wound assessment: a review. Wound Repair Regen. **23**(2), 149–162 (2015)
16. Spinczyk, D., Karwan, A., Rudnicki, J., WrÄsblewski, T.: Stereoscopic liver surface reconstruction. Videosurgery and Other Miniinvasive Techniques **3**, 181–187 (2012)
17. Spinczyk, D., Karwan, A., Zylkowski, J., WrÄsblewski, T.: Experimental study in-vitro evaluation of stereoscopic liver surface reconstruction. Videosurgery and Other Miniinvasive Techniques **1**, 80–85 (2013)
18. Brewster, M.Q.: Thermal Radiative Transfer and Properties. Wiley, New Jersey (1992)
19. Heikkila, J., Silven, O.: A four-step camera calibration procedure with implicit image correction. In: Proceedings of IEEE Computer Society Conference on Computer Vision and Pattern Recognition, pp. 1106–1112, June 1997
20. Zhang, Z.: A flexible new technique for camera calibration. IEEE Trans. Pattern Anal. Mach. Intell. **22**(11), 1330–1334 (2000)
21. Fuersattel, P., Dotenco, S., Placht, S., Balda, M., Maier, A., Riess, C.: Ocpad 8212: occluded checkerboard pattern detector. In: Proceedings of 2016 IEEE Winter Conference on Applications of Computer Vision (WACV), pp. 1–9, March 2016
22. Geiger, A., Moosmann, F., Car, Ã., Schuster, B.: Automatic camera and range sensor calibration using a single shot. In: Proceedings of 2012 IEEE International Conference on Robotics and Automation, pp. 3936–3943, May 2012
23. Bhujle, H.: Weighted-average fusion method for multiband images. In: Proceedings of 2016 International Conference on Signal Processing and Communications (SPCOM), pp. 1–5, June 2016

24. Pluim, J.P.W., Maintz, J.B.A., Viergever, M.A.: Mutual-information-based registration of medical images: a survey. IEEE Trans. Med. Imaging **22**(8), 986–1004 (2003)
25. West, J., Fitzpatrick, J., Wang, M., Dawant, B., Maurer, C.J., Kessler, R., Maciunas, R., Barillot, C., Lemoine, D., Collignon, A., Maes, F., Suetens, P., Vandermeulen, D., van den Elsen, P., Napel, S., Sumanaweera, T., Harkness, B., Hemler, P., Hill, D., Hawkes, D., Studholme, C., Maintz, J., Viergever, M., Malandain, G., Woods, R.: Comparison and evaluation of retrospective intermodality brain image registration techniques. J. Comput. Assist. Tomogr. **21**(4), 554–566 (1997)
26. Labadie, R., Shah, R., Harris, S., Cetinkaya, E., Haynes, D., Fenlon, M., Juscyzk, A., Galloway, R., Fitzpatrick, J.: Submillimetric target-registration error using a novel, non-invasive fiducial system for imageguided otologic surgery. Comput. Aided Surg. **9**(4), 145–153 (2004)
27. Maes, F., Collignon, A., Vandermeulen, D., Marchal, G., Suetens, P.: Multimodality image registration by maximization of mutual information. IEEE Trans. Med. Imaging **16**(2), 187–198 (1997)
28. Gong, M., Zhao, S., Jiao, L., Tian, D., Wang, S.: A novel coarse-to-fine scheme for automatic image registration based on sift and mutual information. IEEE Trans. Geosci. Remote Sens. **52**(7), 4328–4338 (2014)
29. Rivaz, H., Karimaghaloo, Z., Collins, D.L.: Self-similarity weighted mutual information: a new nonrigid image registration metric. Med. Image Anal. **18**(2), 343–358 (2014)
30. Karimi, A., Rahmati, S.M., Razaghi, R.: A combination of experimental measurement, constitutive damage model, and diffusion tensor imaging to characterize the mechanical properties of the human brain. Comput. Methods Biomech. Biomed. Eng. **20**(12), 1350–1363 (2017)
31. Zhuang, Y., Gao, K., Miu, X., Han, L., Gong, X.: Infrared and visual image registration based on mutual information with a combined particle swarm optimizationpowell search algorithm. Optik-Int. J. Light Electron Opt. **127**(1), 188–191 (2016)
32. Darkner, S., Sporring, J.: Locally ordorless registration. IEEE Trans. Pattern Anal. Mach. Intell. **35**(6), 1437–1450 (2013)
33. Rivaz, H., Karimaghaloo, Z., Fonov, V., Collins, D.: Nonrigid registration of ultrasound and MRI using contextual conditioned mutual information. IEEE Trans. Med. Imaging **33**(3), 708–25 (2014)

Rigid and Non-rigid Registration Algorithm Evaluation in MRI for Breast Cancer Therapy Monitoring

Paweł Bzowski[1(✉)], Marta Danch-Wierzchowska[1,2],
Krzysztof Psiuk-Maksymowicz[1,2], Rafał Panek[3], and Damian Borys[1,2]

[1] Institute of Automatic Control, Silesian University of Technology,
Akademicka 16, 44–100 Gliwice, Poland
`pawel.bzowski@polsl.pl`
[2] Biotechnology Centre, Silesian University of Technology,
Krzywoustego 8, 44-100 Gliwice, Poland
[3] Nottingham University Hospitals,
Darby Road, Nottingham NG7 2UH, UK

Abstract. One of the most common methods in breast cancer radio-therapy planning is Magnetic Resonance Imaging (MRI). It is also used for patient evaluation during treatment because of its sensitivity and lack of ionizing radiation. During each imaging session a patient position can be different and inaccuracies can occur. In this case it is very difficult to compare two image sets originating from different patient examination. The main goals of this work were to implement an algorithm, based on affine transformation with Mutual Information as the quality factor of images match and the method based on the Navier-Lame equation for elastic image co-registration. The rigid transformation is used for the preliminary processing, and the non-rigid transformation allows for successful co-registration of both image sets. Our results were evaluated visually, and the MI indices were calculated. These algorithms allowed for image co-registration in different imaging sessions during the course of treatment.

Keywords: MRI · Image processing · Image registration
Breast imagining

1 Introduction

Breast cancer is one of the most common types of cancer in women population. According to statistics from 2016 [1] 29% (245 660 cases) of all cancers in the USA female population were breast cancer. In 2017 this value was increased to 30% (252 710 cases) [2]. Breast cancer screening and diagnosis is based on the use of mammography and medical ultrasonography (USG). In many cases, therapy starts with the surgical removal of changed tissue, followed by the chemotherapy and/or radio-therapy. The affected tissue needs to be precisely localised, which is essential for the radiotherapy planning. Usually, MRI and CT are used for that purpose.

© Springer International Publishing AG, part of Springer Nature 2019
E. Pietka et al. (Eds.): ITIB 2018, AISC 762, pp. 150–159, 2019.
https://doi.org/10.1007/978-3-319-91211-0_13

The magnetic resonance imaging (MRI) has a higher sensitivity than computed tomography (CT) and does not introduce any additional patient exposure to ionizing radiation. This type of imaging is also used in patient monitoring during the treatment. Repeated imaging can inform on treatment effects, which can be achieved comparing two or more images. However, a patient position can be slightly different in both examinations. Internal structures can also differ in the images, as a result of medical procedure (or therapy), which makes them difficult to compare. Additionally, MRI images may not be geometrically accurate in the case of the large field of view and the presence of metallic implants. As a result of medical procedure (or therapy), the obtained fused image can be deformed and displaced. This is an unfavourable effect, especially for radiotherapy planning where tumor position location must be precise. Breast is a tissue consisting mainly of fat. This is particularly important for larger breasts where position changes during the scanning session are significant. During the treatment, the internal structure of the region of interest is changing and therefore the affine (rigid) transformation based co-registration results can be unsatisfactory, which can be addressed using non-rigid algorithms. Recently the image co-registration has become increasingly used in the clinical practise. Medical image co-registration can be performed using hybrid devices, for multi-modal image fusion, or as an 'offline' processing step, for example in case of SPECT or PET with CT and MRI fusion [3]. Here, we investigate co-registered images from the same modality acquired in different time of patient therapy.

The main goal of our work was to implement an algorithm based on rigid and non-rigid transformation.

The rigid registration was evaluated first to determine if it is sufficient to compare longitudinal MRI breast studies in time. For this purpose, we chose minimalization of the Mutual Information index [4,5] using affine transformations and the solution based on the Navier-Lame equation proposed by Modersitzki [6]. Finally, the rigid method is used for the initial registration of both images, followed by the non-rigid method using elastic image deformation.

2   Materials and Methods

2.1   Patients

The algorithm was tested in a group of women with breast cancer. Each patient was scanned at least twice. The first image was acquired during diagnosis (before treatment) the remaining images were acquired after or during the treatment. All patients undergo one of the breast cancer-related treatment procedures (chemo or radiotherapy, or both). The data was acquired at the Maria Sklodowska-Curie Memorial Cancer and Institute of Oncology, Gliwice Branch.

2.2   MRI Scanning

All of the images were in DICOM format and were acquired using Siemens Aera, 1.5 T and Siemens Avanto, 1.5 T systems, with dedicated breast coils. Each study included T1 subscript and T2 subscript weighted sequences and the whole area of breast was acquired. The image matrix was 512×512 and the number of slices were between 5–50.

2.3   Software

The algorithm based on the rigid method (minimise the mutual information index by transform image using affine transformation) and the non-rigid method (elastic image co-registration based on the Navier-Lame equation) were implemented in MATLAB 2015a on Intel Core i7-6700HQ, NVIDIA GeForce GTX 1060 6 GB, 16 GB RAM and SSD disk. The first step of the presented algorithm was to load all the images and interpolate the template image (the moving image) set to the original study image (the reference image). Here, rescaling both datasets into a joint space occurs. Next, the rigid transformation was performed. In this step, the algorithm calculates the entropy of each image set (1) and the joint entropy of both sets (2).

$$H(A) = - \sum_{i}^{n} p(a_i) \cdot \log(p(a_i)) \tag{1}$$

$$H(A, B) = - \sum_{i}^{n} p(a_i, b_i) \cdot \log(p(a_i, b_i)) \tag{2}$$

where:

– a_i, b_i – pixel value in each matrix element (for dataset A and B),
– $p(a_i)$, $p(b_i)$ – marginal distribution of elements a_i and b_i.

The mutual information (MI) index equals common entropy minus entropy of images set A and images set B [4] which was calculated according to (3).

$$MI = H(A, B) - H(A) - H(B). \tag{3}$$

The obtained index is a similarity measure. It informs on how much each dataset is similar to the other. For the same two image sets, the MI index is at the lowest level. The goal is to minimise the described index by performing an affine transformation (i.e. displacement, rotation). The method uses only changes in the pixel positions, but does not change their value. Rotation and displacement for a 2D image are presented in the Eq. (4).

$$\begin{bmatrix} x_2 \\ y_2 \\ 0 \end{bmatrix} = \begin{bmatrix} 1 & 0 & d_x \\ 0 & 1 & d_y \\ 0 & 0 & 1 \end{bmatrix} \begin{bmatrix} \cos(\alpha) & -\sin(\alpha) & 0 \\ \sin(\alpha) & \cos(\alpha) & 0 \\ 0 & 0 & 1 \end{bmatrix} \begin{bmatrix} x_1 \\ y_1 \\ 0 \end{bmatrix}, \tag{4}$$

where:

– x_1 and y_1 – coordinates of image before transformation,
– x_2 and y_2 – coordinates of image after transformation,

– d_x and d_y – translation in x and y direction,
– α – rotation (angle).

In each step, the algorithm calculates the MI index and change d_x, d_y and α (translation in the x-axis, translation in the y-axis and rotation), until the function minimum is found. Next, the non-rigid transformation is performed. We used the solution proposed by Jan Modersitzki [6], based on the Navier-Lame equation (5).

$$\mu\nabla^2 + (\mu + \lambda)\nabla(\nabla \cdot u) = F, \tag{5}$$

where the parameters are as follows:

– λ – Lame's first parameter,
– μ – Lame's second parameter,
– u – displacement,
– F – force.

This law describes the motion of viscous fluid substances. A finite difference approximation can be used to present the discrete form of the equation, where A is a matrix representing specific material (see Eq. (6)):

$$Au = F. \tag{6}$$

Each material is represented by two Lame's constants, which describe material deformation. To find the pixel displacements, a discretization of the Navier-Lame equation is required and the forces are calculated. The solution proposed by Jan Modersitzki is based on the finite difference approximation to solve the equation. As a result, the values of the forces value and of the discrete Navier-Lame equations are obtained. Next, an inversion of the Navier-Lame equation is calculated. In this work the Moore-Penrose pseudo-inverse was used. The displacement was calculated according to Eq. (7):

$$\begin{pmatrix} u^1_{k,j} \\ u^2_{k,j} \end{pmatrix} = \begin{pmatrix} D^{1,1}_{k,j} & D^{1,2}_{k,j} \\ D^{2,1}_{k,j} & D^{2,2}_{k,j} \end{pmatrix}^{\dagger} \begin{pmatrix} F^1_{k,j} \\ F^2_{k,j} \end{pmatrix}, \tag{7}$$

where:

– u – displacement each pixel in each dimension,
– D – discrete form of the Navier-Lame equation,
– F – force.

To calculate forces we used the simplest similarity method. This is the difference between study and template image sets multiplied by a gradient of template image set (see Eq. (8)).

$$F(x, u(x)) = (S(x) - T(x))\nabla T(x), \tag{8}$$

where the parameters and variables are:

- F – force,
- S – study image,
- T – template image.

This approach performs well for the monomodality registration process, such as registration of two CT or MRI datasets, which were used in this work.

3   Results

Figure 1 presents the result of registration of MRI images for the first patient. The template image set was successfully transformed into the Result image set. For these image sets the MI indexes were calculated and presented in Table 1.

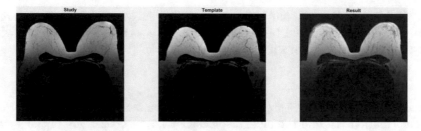

Fig. 1. Example of axial MRI breast images: study, template and result images (patient no. 1)

Table 1. MI values for pairs of images sets (patient no. 1, $\lambda = 0$, $\mu = 30$, 2000 iterations)

	MI value
Study-Study	$-3.5164 \cdot 10^4$
Study-Template	$-2.2234 \cdot 10^4$
Study-Result	$-2.9530 \cdot 10^4$

This computation was performed for $\lambda = 0$, $\mu = 30$ and the number of iterations 2000. The MI value for study-template pairs before and after registration has changed (Table 1), confirming that the image set after the registration process is more similar to study images than before registration. In Fig. 2 the checkerboard was used to present the differences between pairs of images before and after image registration. The result is satisfying, but some dissimilarities occurred in the center of the image, near the pectoralis major muscle.

Figure 3 presents results of transformation for the second patient. In this case the MI value is also lower then before transformation (Table 2).

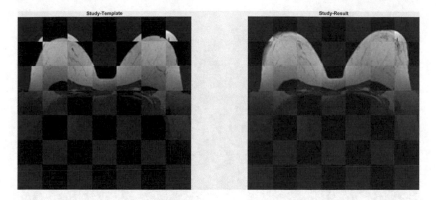

Fig. 2. Checkerboard display of study-template images and study-result images (patient no. 1)

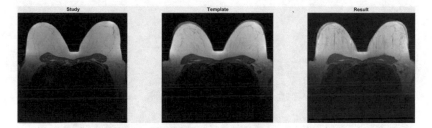

Fig. 3. Example of axial MRI breast images: study, template and result images (patient no. 2)

Table 2. MI values for pairs of image sets (patient no. 2, $\lambda = 0$, $\mu = 30$, 2000 iterations)

	MI value
Study-Study	$-3.2592 \cdot 10^4$
Study-Template	$-2.1554 \cdot 10^4$
Study-Result	$-2.4211 \cdot 10^4$

Figure 4 presents checkerboards of study-template and study-result images for that patient. The outside part of the breast was correctly matched. Some misregistrations were obtained near the pectoralis major muscle. This situation is similar to the patient no. 1 registration process.

Corresponding images for patient no. 3 are present in Figs. 5 and 6. Before the co-registration the breast boundary in the template image was more towards the image centre, than in the study image. After the co-registration the breast in the result image is in the same position as the breast in the study image. The mutual information index was also calculated and values presented in Table 3.

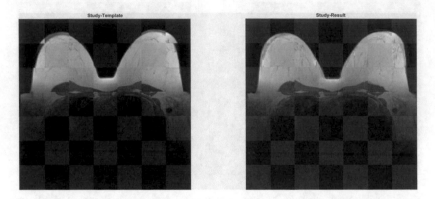

Fig. 4. Checkerboard display of study-template images and study-result images (patient no. 2)

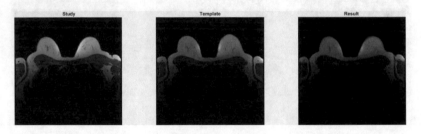

Fig. 5. Example of axial MRI breast images: study, template and result images (patient no. 3)

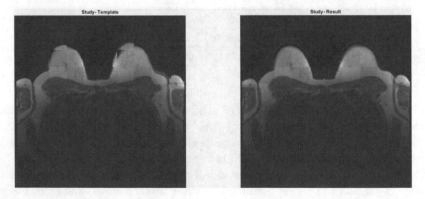

Fig. 6. Checkerboard display of study-template images and study-result images (patient no. 3)

Table 3. MI values for pairs of images sets (patient no. 3, $\lambda = 0$, $\mu = 30$, 2000 iterations)

	MI value
Study-Study	$-8.9794 \cdot 10^3$
Study-Template	$-6.2901 \cdot 10^3$
Study-Result	$-2.4211 \cdot 10^4$

We also checked the MI factor for the patient in four different MRI T2 studies (patient no. 4). This index was calculated using MI method. The first set of images is a reference (study) and the second is a moving set (template). In the first step, the rigid transformation was performed. In this step, we compared two images sets before the rigid method and prepared images size for the non-rigid method. In Tables 4, 5 and 6 mutual information values are presented for each pair in each step. Lower values indicate that the images are more similar. In our case the rigid method not always give acceptable results. In Tables 5 and 6 the mutual information indexes before and after non-rigid registration are presented. All of the results are lower than before registration.

Table 4. MI values for pairs of images sets (patient no. 4), before rigid image registration

Template		MRI T2 1	MRI T2 2	MRI T2 3	MRI T2 4
Study	MRI T2 1	$-1.2356 \cdot 10^4$	$-4.9784 \cdot 10^3$	$-6.4678 \cdot 10^3$	$-3.4091 \cdot 10^3$
	MRI T2 2	$-4.5297 \cdot 10^3$	$-1.4038 \cdot 10^4$	$-4.7678 \cdot 10^3$	$-5.9531 \cdot 10^3$
	MRI T2 3	$-5.8813 \cdot 10^3$	$-4.8005 \cdot 10^3$	$-1.3739 \cdot 10^4$	$-3.7917 \cdot 10^3$
	MRI T2 4	$-5.4271 \cdot 10^3$	$-5.9281 \cdot 10^3$	$-3.6972 \cdot 10^3$	$-1.3217 \cdot 10^4$

Table 5. MI values for pairs of images sets (patient no. 4), after rigid image registration and before non-rigid registration

Result		MRI T2 1	MRI T2 2	MRI T2 3	MRI T2 4
Study	MRI T2 1	–	$-5.4422 \cdot 10^3$	$-5.3503 \cdot 10^3$	$-3.4091 \cdot 10^3$
	MRI T2 2	$-2.4964 \cdot 10^3$	–	$-4.2160 \cdot 10^3$	$-5.7277 \cdot 10^3$
	MRI T2 3	$-4.2165 \cdot 10^3$	$-4.7949 \cdot 10^3$	–	$-3.9528 \cdot 10^3$
	MRI T2 4	$-2.0006 \cdot 10^3$	$-5.5802 \cdot 10^3$	$-3.6831 \cdot 10^3$	–

Table 6. MI values for pairs of images sets (patient no. 4, $\mu = 30$, $\lambda = 0$, 500 iterations), after non-rigid image registration

Final result		MRI T2 1	MRI T2 2	MRI T2 3	MRI T2 4
Study	MRI T2 1	–	$-7.2189 \cdot 10^3$	$-6.7218 \cdot 10^3$	$-5.7511 \cdot 10^3$
	MRI T2 2	$-3.1957 \cdot 10^3$	–	$-5.6147 \cdot 10^3$	$-7.5530 \cdot 10^3$
	MRI T2 3	$-5.7819 \cdot 10^3$	$-6.9555 \cdot 10^3$	–	$-5.4271 \cdot 10^3$
	MRI T2 4	$-2.3494 \cdot 10^3$	$-6.1581 \cdot 10^3$	$-4.2753 \cdot 10^3$	–

4   Discussion and Conclusion

The presented algorithm is capable to successfully co-register two MRI breast image sets. Obtained results were visually analysed (Figs. 1, 2, 3, 4, 5 and 6) and for each pair of image sets the mutual information index was calculated (Tables 1, 2, 3, 4, 5 and 6). The lower MI value indicated that the images were more similar. This confirms that the algorithm can be useful in breast cancer therapy monitoring and can be used in the region of interest tracking during the therapy. The combination of rigid and non-rigid methods improves results at the expense of the computation time. The processing time for two image data sets ($512 \times 512 \times 30$) was about 120 min for 2000 iterations. The long computation time sets a demand for further algorithm optimization. Sometimes the algorithm stuck in a local minimum, what causes an increase of mutual information value during the registration.

Many different methods, including B-Spline [7] or Maxwell Demons [8] for images co-registration, were presented in recent years. Usually, these algorithms were tested for brain MRI images. Breast tissue has a different structure and is more flexible than brain tissue, which causes difficulties in image co-registration. The encouraging results of this preliminary pilot study allow the possibility of further future investigation.

Acknowledgement. This work was supported by the Polish National Center of Research and Development grant no. STRATEGMED2/267398/4/NCBR/2015 (MILESTONE – Molecular diagnostics and imaging in individualized therapy for breast, thyroid and prostate cancer) (KPM, DB) and the Institute of Automatic Control, Silesian University of Technology under Grant No. BKM-508/RAU1/2017 t.1 (MDW) and BK-204/RAU1/2017 t.3 (PB). Calculations were performed on the Ziemowit computer cluster in the Laboratory of Bioinformatics and Computational Biology, created in the EU Innovative Economy Programme POIG.02.01.00-00-166/08 and expanded in the POIG.02.03.01-00-040/13 project.

References

1. Siegel, R.L., Miller, K.D., Jemal, A.: Cancer statistics, 2016. CA Cancer J. Clin. **66**, 7–30 (2016)
2. Siegel, R.L., Miller, K.D., Jemal, A.: Cancer statistics, 2017. CA Cancer J. Clin. **67**, 7–30 (2017)
3. D'Amico, A., Szczucka, K., Borys, D., Gorczewski, K., Steinhof, K.: SPECT-CT fusion: a new diagnostic tool for endocrinology. Endokrynologia Polska **57**(Suppl A), 71–4 (2006)
4. Viola, P.A.: Alignment by maximization of mutual information, A.I. Technical Report No. 1548 June (1995)
5. D'Agostino, E., Maes, F., Vandermeulen, D., Suetens, P.: A viscous fluid model for multimodal non-rigid image registration using mutual information. Med. Image Anal. **7**, 565–575 (2003)
6. Modersitzki, J.: Numerical Methods for Image Registration. Oxford University Press, New York (2004)
7. Rohr, K., Fornefett, M., Stiehl, H.S.: Spline-based elastic image registration: integration of landmark errors and orientation attributes. Comput. Vis. Image Underst. **90**, 153–168 (2003)
8. Thirion, J.: Image matching as a diffusion process: an analogy with Maxwell's demons. Med. Image Anal. **2**(3), 243–260 (1998)

Image Guided Core Needle Biopsy of the Breast

Bartłomiej Pyciński[✉], Jan Juszczyk, Agata Wijata, Marta Galinska, Joanna Czajkowska, and Ewa Pietka

Faculty of Biomedical Engineering, Silesian University of Technology, Roosevelta 40, 41-800 Zabrze, Poland
bartlomiej.pycinski@polsl.pl

Abstract. This study presents the development of a multimodal data acquisition system dedicated to assist a core needle biopsy of the breast. The system consists of the following elements: optical and electromagnetic tracking devices, Time-of-Flight camera, thermovision camera and video camera. The system has been prepared for cooperating with any ultrasound machine. The aim of proposed system is to record locations of the tissue samples. The accuracy of calibration as well as patient registration is reported.

Keywords: Breast biopsy · Image-guided procedure
Medical imaging · Image registration

1 Introduction

Breast cancer is the most common malignancy and invasive cancer in women and the second main cause of cancer death after lung cancer. However, the survival rate has increased dramatically thanks to fast development and advances in screening and treatment. Therefore, on-going research activities still focus on efficient and robust analysis of image data. Our work is a part of a research project targeting in analysing heterogeneity of the breast tumour. As a result of the whole project, therapy aggressiveness shall be reduced and social and economic burden decreases without compromising the treatment's efficacy.

Core needle biopsy performed under ultrasonographic control is currently one of the diagnostic techniques in breast cancer. The breast tissue removed during the biopsy is then examined in a laboratory. To determine the heterogeneity of the tumour, 3–5 samples of tissue are taken from its different places. Further therapy is then determined based on the obtained histological results. However, due to the movement of patient body between screening and treatment, the complete histological information can not be used. Therefore, the proposed system aims to record the locations of the samples relative to a fixed structure like the breast or patient's torso. To complete obtaining the samples, several types of image's and surface data are recorded simultaneously.

© Springer International Publishing AG, part of Springer Nature 2019
E. Pietka et al. (Eds.): ITIB 2018, AISC 762, pp. 160–171, 2019.
https://doi.org/10.1007/978-3-319-91211-0_14

Since navigation technology became a part of medical systems, medical procedures have become more accurate, precise, and repeatable. Simultaneously, fast development of imaging techniques enables including new medical procedures [12]. Existing commercial approaches, such as BrainLAB, make it possible to guide the ablation needle placement based on the preoperative 3D data. However, it is sensitive to patient anatomy changes between studies. The problem of system calibration is considered in [1]. The authors present a calibration algorithm, which computes the transformation from the ultrasound (US) image plane to the coordinate system of the sensor attached to the US transducer. The world coordinate system is therefore defined by an optical tracking system with four ARTtrack2 cameras.

Bilkova et al. [2] discuss the problem of US scanning of the breast targeting in reconstruction of US probe's trajectory. The algorithm of local 3D reconstruction is based on image data recorded by tracking the position and orientation of a free-hand US transducer. Sensors placed on the patient's body create the reference coordinate system to which all the recorded points are transformed. The choice of the sensor attached to a patient eliminates respiratory or other body motion. However, such a solution assumes the existence of nipples, which could have been removed by previous surgery, and does not take into consideration the breast deformation cause by the US probe pressure. The solutions for 3D ultrasound reconstruction are also given in [3,13].

Our multimodal acquisition system consists of: optical and electromagnetic tracking devices, a Time-of-Flight (ToF) camera, a thermovision camera, and a video camera. Due to its small size, the electromagnetic marker can be attached directly to the US probe without disturbing the physicians. Tracking the US probe makes it possible to determine the position of the US image. Because of its ferromagnetic features disrupting the function of electromagnetic marker, the biopsy gun is tracked using the optical tracking system. The position of the needle is determined by the position of biopsy gun and needle detection on the US image, if it is visible on the US image. The ToF camera is used for skin surface reconstruction and the reference point is associated with it. Video and thermovision cameras were used for collecting texture images, completing the surface reconstruction. The developed methodology brings the collected data into a common coordinate system. The software enables an automated recording at the moment of the needle shot. The use of the tracking system and 3D breast model is used to determine the biopsy sites and visualise the procedure, which increases the effectiveness of the biopsy. The system is prepared to cooperate with any ultrasound machine.

The main goal of the study is to present a multimodal data acquisition system for breast core biopsy, and to assess the accuracy of calibration and patient registration. The paper is organised as follows: Sect. 2 presents the system, the calibration procedure, data registration, and visualisation system. In Sect. 3 the results are presented. The discussion is given in Sect. 4. Section 5 concludes this phase of the study.

2   Materials and Methods

2.1   Multimodal Data Acquisition System

The scheme of the measurement station is shown in Fig. 1. It consists of a few elements:

Optical tracking system Polaris – a marker is fixed on the Magnum biopsy gun using an 3D printed overlay (Fig. 2). The marker is protected by a latex coating. The camera should be directed to the operating field and the biopsy gun should be provided within the line of sight of the camera.

Electromagnetic tracking system Aurora – main 6DOF (6 Degree of Freedom) marker is fixed on the US transducer (Fig. 2). The second marker is fixed under the medical couch. The electromagnetic field generator should be placed as close as possible to the patient's chest. There must be no ferromagnetic materials in its vicinity.

Time of Flight Camera – the patient body is in the field of view. The recorded data includes the three-dimensional surface of the patient's body. After postprocessing, this surface is the basis for the visualization of the final model [6].

VIS Camera (Visual Inspection Camera) – patient body and surroundings are in the field of view. The recorded data include the registration of the biopsy procedure and can be used as a texture for the ToF surface.

Microphone – sound recording. It is possible to automatically detect the moment of discharge of the biopsy gun which can be treated as the moment of sample collection. It is possible to exclude the microphone from the measuring station, however it requires manual indication of the moment of tissue collection.

US machine – a standard apparatus with currently used transducers to perform a biopsy procedure under ultrasound guidance.

Framegrabber – connected to the output from the ultrasound device, transmits video signal to the control unit. The quality of the resulting model depends on the quality of the captured image, which is why the appropriate resolution and the frequency of capture are important.

Computer – required the PLUS library, it processes information from tracking systems, framegrabber, ToF and VIS cameras and ensures time-space synchronization of the recorded data.

Acquired data modalities are presented in Fig. 3.

Although electromagnetic and optical tracking systems in multiple situations may be used interchangeably, we have found that during the breast biopsy it is necessary to use both of these systems. The optical tracker has a much larger measuring range and accuracy. It can also be used in the proximity of ferromagnetic materials, e.g. it can be attached to a biopsy gun. In addition, optical markers are wireless, which facilitates manipulation of the gun. On the other hand, electromagnetic system markers are smaller and more convenient to use. In addition, they do not require a line of sight between the generator and the

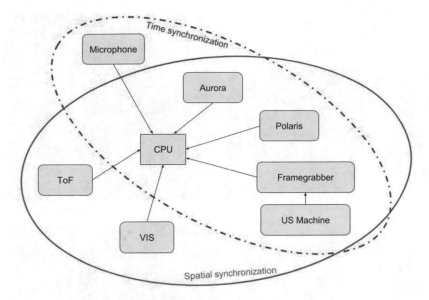

Fig. 1. The scheme of the measurement station. Red circle indicates time synchronized data, green circle indicates spatial synchronization

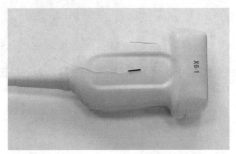

(a) Wired Aurora electromagnetic marker sticked to the probe

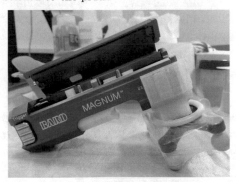

(b) Polaris optical marker

Fig. 2. Comparison of electromagnetic and optical markers

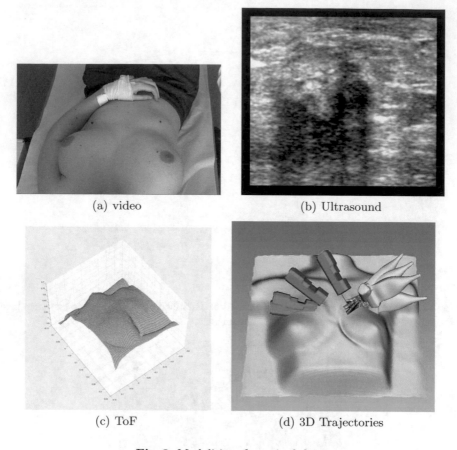

(a) video   (b) Ultrasound

(c) ToF   (d) 3D Trajectories

Fig. 3. Modalities of acquired data

sensor, which is especially important when tracking the ultrasound probe. During the procedure, the radiologist often inverts the probe or covers the markers by his hand, which interrupts optical tracking. Visibility of the optical marker attached to the US probe during the exemplary procedure is shown in Fig. 4.

2.2   ToF – Tracker Registration

The surface of the patient's body acquired by a ToF camera is registered to the tracker coordinate system. Similar approach to the method presented by Bilkova *et al.* [2] have been developed. During US examination, four distinct positions of the probe are captured. The positions are chosen separately for each patient, depending on her anatomy. They are located at the following landmarks: the nipple, the xyphoid process of the sternum, the midpoint of a line segment between the nipples, upper extremity of the sternum, and the point on the mid-clavicular line directly under the breast.

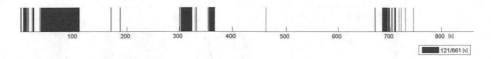

Fig. 4. Visibility of the optical marker attached to the probe during a biopsy. The blue coloured frames indicate time when the marker was in the tracker's field of view

Point positions are captured when the central point of the transducer's face touches them. Since the transducer has been calibrated, the position of each point P in the tracker's (i.e. global) coordinate frame is computed:

$$P^G = \left(M_P^G\right)_i M_I^P \begin{bmatrix} \frac{w}{2} \\ 0 \\ 0 \\ 1 \end{bmatrix}, \tag{1}$$

where i is an index of frame, M_P^G is position of the marker attached to the probe, M_I^P is a calibration matrix of the probe, and $\frac{w}{2}$ stands for the half of the image width.

Corresponding points are indicated on the ToF surface. The two sets of points are registered by minimising the distance between the pairs of the points after applying a rigid-body transformation [5].

2.3 VIS – ToF Registration

Registration between ToF camera surface data and video image is registered with the ToF amplitude image (AI). It is a gray scale image similar to the camera image. The amplitude image is in the same coordinate system as the ToF 3D data. In the first step, the camera image (VIS) is registered to the AI by using landmarks. In the second step the registered VIS is used to provide texture for the ToF 3D mesh (Fig. 5).

2.4 Calibration of the Biopsy Needle and the Ultrasound Probe

The radiologists perform a procedure using the Bard Magnum Core Biopsy System, which is intended for use in obtaining biopsies from soft tissues such as liver, kidney, breast, spleen, lymph nodes, and various soft tissue tumours. The biopsy system is equipped with a standard 14G needle (2 mm of external diameter, 13 cm of length). The whole biopsy system can not be treated as a rigid tool, because the needle is not very still attached to the base of the biopsy gun. Moreover, the needle may also deform sideways. As a result, a calibration procedure which depends on pivoting the tool around a spherical trajectory would be burdened by too much error.

Instead, in this study, the calibration of the biopsy needle was performed in a modified way. The needle was placed still. The tip of a rigid stylus tool was

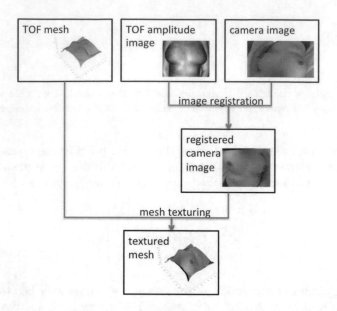

Fig. 5. ToF image and camera image registration workflow

applied to the tip of the needle and the stylus performed pivoting movement (Fig. 6). The set of transformation matrices $M_{S_i}^B, i \in \{1, \ldots, n\}$ from alternating marker on the stylus S_i to still marker on the biopsy needle B allows to determine the translation vector between marker B and the tip of the needle.

Calibration of the ultrasound probe was performed on a N-wire calibration phantom using the method provided by the PlusToolkit library [8].

2.5 Visualisation System

Data recorded during the procedure were not presented online, but an application for visualization of the acquired trajectories was created. In particular, the position of the tools is remembered at the moment of the ejecting the needle. The moment of the ejection is recognized automatically by detecting the characteristic sound which is generated by the Magnum Biopsy Instrument.

3DSlicer software has been used for visualization [9]. 3DSlicer is an open source software platform for medical computing, image processing, and three-dimensional visualization, prototyping, development, and evaluation of image analysis tools for clinical trial applications [4]. 3DSlicer is designed for doctors, researchers and the general public. 3DSlicer software is equipped with the OpenIGTLink communication module. Visualization of the navigated medical procedure is possible using this communication between 3DSlicer and Plus-Toolkit library [8], with which the tools participating in the procedure are tracked [14]. 3DSlicer software allows the users to implement their own plug-ins, which may communicate with other platform tools.

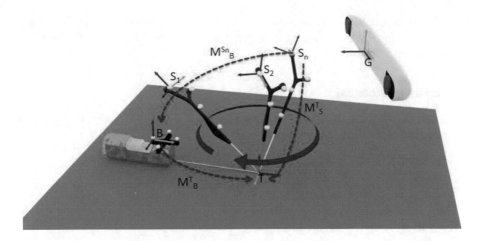

Fig. 6. Scheme of core needle calibration

In the project a scripted plug-in has been developed, which allows capturing the moment of acquiring the tissue sample during the biopsy procedure. The proposed plug-in presents positions of the probe and the needle in real time based on the transformation matrices of the tracked tools, imported tool models, and the texture of the 2D ultrasound image. Acquisition of the biopsy moment is possible by automatic detection of the sound of the biopsy gun's shot ass well as by manual indication of the selected moment.

Due to the elasticity and deformation of tissues during the examination, it is necessary to modify the solution of 3D reconstruction available in PlusToolkit, because this method assumes that there is the correspondence of the registered pixels. The proposed method is used to visualise the volume based on the acquisition time. The input data for volume reconstruction comes from congenial frames, and the factor of displacement and deformation of the examined tissue has been minimized. During each needle injection, another volume is created based only on the latest image information, which prevents the output volume from being dependent on outdated data. Reconstruction of the current volume at the time of biopsy is performed as postprocessing and, when combined with the visualization of the biopsy needle, serves to determine biopsy material location relative to the tumour. There is no need to visualize the volume online, because the procedure is carried out under 2D ultrasound control.

3 Results

Acquisition of the biopsy procedure was performed on 44 patients. In total, 270 GB of data were recorded. The average duration of the procedure and data recording was 11.09 min whilst 5323 tracked frames (each consisting of an ultrasound image and transformation matrices of probe image and biopsy gun) and 9703 images of the patient's body surface were captured. Sound recording started automatically with the registration of medical data. On average, the VIS video recorded for 12 min. During a biopsy procedure, 6–7 samples of tissue were obtained from a lesion.

3.1 System Accuracy

As the whole data acquisition system consists of multiple parts, evaluation of the following components was performed:

- accuracy of marker localisation,
- accuracy of tool calibration,
- ToF and USG data resolution,
- ToF – tracker registration accuracy,
- the patient's breast movement during the procedure.

Accuracy of tracking the optical markers is provided by the manufacturer and does not depend on the environment. Regarding electromagnetic system marker, the localisation accuracy is worse than the former, but does not exceed 1 mm unless there are external elements which interfere EM field: e.g. ferromagnetic tools, wires, or other EM emitters. Eventually, markers signal might vanish completely if disturbances are too strong.

The calibration accuracy of the biopsy needle depends on the variation of the tip position during the process of calibration. Root-mean-square error is the metric used for evaluation [10].

US probe calibration is performed either before or after the biopsy procedure. A single calibration is sufficient if more than one procedure is carried out during a day. The accuracy of the calibration is evaluated using a method implemented in PlusToolkit software.

Resolution of ToF camera is not isotropic, and previous research has stated that the highest error is along Z-axis [7,11].

Registration error of the ToF surface and the tracker coordinate frame (see Sect. 2.2) was evaluated as mean-root-square-error of the fiducial.

Obtained results have been presented in Table 1.

Table 1. Accuracies of elements of the presented system

No.	Element	Accuracy
1	Optical markers tracking	0.2 mm
2	EM markers tracking	0.6 mm
3	Needle tip calibration error	0.7 mm
4	US probe calibration	2.1 mm
5	ToF accuracy	18.3 mm
6	Tracker and ToF registration	44.1 mm

The greatest impact on total accuracy comes from the tracker and the ToF camera image registration. It depends on shape deformation as well as the ToF camera resolution.

4 Discussion

The system development and subsequent clinical tests have led to the following remarks concerning the utility, limitations, and further research associated with the system. According to the doctors opinion, the system does not interfere with the biopsy procedure and more importantly, there is no direct contact between the system and the patient. The presented combination of optical and electromagnetic tracking systems outperforms the optical one alone. Although there is high accuracy, the optical markers are often obscured by the operator and the registered signal is 'leaky' (Fig. 4). Moreover, both a sterile latex casing put on the markers and the use of a disinfectant further decrease the visibility of the markers. Unfortunately, the drawback of using the electromagnetic tracking systems is its influence on the US image – after launching the system, additional noise stripes appeared on the image at a depth greater than approx. 4 cm (Fig. 7). However, these complications do not hinder diagnosis. Moreover, it has been observed, that the biopsy needle calibration need to be performed in an unusual way. Due to the flexibility and mobility of the Magnum needle, the process of acquiring the trajectory used to determine the needle tip has been made with an additional rigid stylus tool. Finally, there has been noticed that during the procedure, the operator has occasionally changed the image resolution (depth of

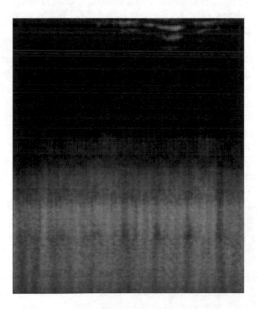

Fig. 7. Noise on US image caused by influence of an electromagnetic tracker

the image). In this situation, the position of the image is no longer tracked and the US probe calibration fails. In such case, it is necessary to manually update the value of the probe calibration matrix. Therefore, the probe calibration must be performed several times, for every resolution.

5 Conclusion

The paper presents a multimodal data acquisition system, which records locations of breast samples relative to a fixed structure of the body. It is part of bigger project aiming at the decision support of local treatment of breast cancer. The system was tested in a clinical unit on 44 patients. The underlined important feature of the system is that there is no interference in biopsy procedure between the system and the patient. The combination of optical and electromagnetic markers enables the system to be used clinically. Overall, the system is not sensitive to occlusions caused by an operator or sterilizing procedure.

Acknowledgement. This research was supported by the Polish National Centre for Research and Development (Narodowe Centrum Badań i Rozwoju) grant No. STRATEGMED2/267398/4/NCBR/2015. The funders had no role in study design, data collection and analysis, decision to publish, or preparation of the manuscript. The research was approved by the ethics committee of The Maria Skłodowska Curie Memorial Cancer Centre and Institute of Oncology in Warsaw (Poland).

References

1. Alcérreca, C., Vogel, J., Feuerstein, M., Navab, N.: A new approach to ultrasound guided radio-frequency needle placement, pp. 26–30. Springer, Heidelberg (2007). https://doi.org/10.1007/978-3-540-71091-2_6
2. Bílková, Z., Bartoš, M., Schier, J., Šroubek, F., Zitová, B., Vydra, J., Daneš, J.: Evaluating spatial coverage of breast examination with free-hand ultrasound transducer. In: Proceedings of the 10th International Joint Conference on Biomedical Engineering Systems and Technologies, pp. 128–133 (2017). https://doi.org/10.5220/0006249101280133
3. Dyer, E., Ijaz, U.Z., Housden, R., Prager, R., Gee, A., Treece, G.: A clinical system for three dimensional extended-field-of-view ultrasound. Br. J. Radiol. (2014). https://doi.org/10.1259/bjr/46007369
4. Fedorov, A., Beichel, R., Kalpathy-Cramer, J., Finet, J., Christophe Fillion-Robin, J., Pujol, S., Bauer, C., Jennings, D., Essy, F.F., Sonka, M., Buatti, J., Aylward, S., Miller, J.V., Pieper, S., Kikinis, R.: 3D slicer as an image computing platform for the quantitative imaging network. Magnet. Reson. Imaging **30**(9), 1323–1341 (2012). https://doi.org/10.1016/j.mri.2012.05.001
5. Horn, B.K.P.: Closed-form solution of absolute orientation using unit quaternions. J. Opt. Soc. Am. A **4**(4), 629–642 (1987). https://doi.org/10.1364/JOSAA.4.000629
6. Juszczyk, J., Czajkowska, J., Pyciński, B., Piętka, E.: ToF-data-based modelling of skin surface deformation. In: Advances in Intelligent Systems and Computing, vol. 472, pp. 235–244. Springer Nature (2016). https://doi.org/10.1007/978-3-319-39904-1_21

7. Kolb, A., Barth, E., Koch, R., Larsen, R.: Time-of-flight cameras in computer graphics. Comput. Graph. Forum **29**(1), 141–159 (2010). https://doi.org/10.1111/j.1467-8659.2009.01583.x

8. Lasso, A., Heffter, T., Rankin, A., Pinter, C., Ungi, T., Fichtinger, G.: Plus: open-source toolkit for ultrasound-guided intervention systems. IEEE Trans. Biomed. Eng. **61**(10), 2527–2537 (2014). https://doi.org/10.1109/TBME.2014.2322864

9. Pieper, S., Halle, M., Kikinis, R.: 3D slicer. In: IEEE International Symposium on Biomedical Imaging: Nano to Macro (2004). https://doi.org/10.1109/ISBI.2004.1398617

10. Pyciński, B.: Estimation of pointer calibration error in optical tracking system, pp. 228–239. Lecture Notes in Computer Science. Springer International Publishing (2017). https://doi.org/10.1007/978-3-319-47154-9_27

11. Pyciński, B., Czajkowska, J., Badura, P., Juszczyk, J., Pietka, E.: Time-of-flight camera, optical tracker and computed tomography in pairwise data registration. PLoS ONE **11**(7), e0159,493 (2016). https://doi.org/10.1371/journal.pone.0159493

12. Pycinski, B., Juszczyk, J., Bozek, P., Ciekalski, J., Dzielicki, J., Pietka, E.: Image navigation in minimally invasive surgery. In: Piętka, E., Kawa, J., Więcławek, W. (eds.) Information Technologies in Biomedicine, Volume 4. Advances in Intelligent Systems and Computing, vol. 284, pp. 25–34. Springer International Publishing (2014). https://doi.org/10.1007/978-3-319-06596-0_3

13. Solberg, O.V., Lindseth, F., Torp, H., Blake, R.E., Hernes, T.A.N.: Freehand 3D ultrasound reconstruction algorithms - a review. Ultrasound Med. Biol. **33**(7), 991–1009 (2007). https://doi.org/10.1016/j.ultrasmedbio.2007.02.015

14. Ungi, T., Lasso, A., Fichtinger, G.: Open-source platforms for navigated image-guided interventions. Med. Image Anal. **33**, 181–186 (2016). https://doi.org/10.1016/j.media.2016.06.011

Preliminary Study of Modeling Sagging Breasts for Support Navigation in Ultrasound Guided Biopsy

Aleksandra Juraszczyk and Dominik Spinczyk[✉]

Faculty of Biomedical Engineering, Silesian University of Technology,
Roosevelta 40, 41-800 Zabrze, Poland
dominik.spinczyk@polsl.pl

Abstract. The main challenge in the biopsy procedure is to guarantee reproducibility of the needle's tip position between biopsies. The general solution addressed to overcome this challenge is an image-based navigation system. While these are widely used for rigid tissue, applications for soft tissues are in the preliminary implementation stage. The paper presents the stages of a method for rigid registration of uncut sections and ultrasound implantation of the breast surface and the possibility of their visualization in a common coordinate system. Measurement of the quality of surface fit is based on the distance between the registered markers indicated on the breast surface by the user. The proposed methodology obtains the median Fiducial Registration Error to fit the fragile, flat, mutual surface areas and match markers in the Time of Flight image to the positions indicated in the tracker coordinate system of 12, 6.9, 5.8 and 15 mm respectively. A current challenge in breast biopsy is the changing position of the needle tip between biopsies.

Keywords: Breast deformation · Breast surface models
Computerized support of breast cancer
Ultrasound guided breast biopsy · Time of flight surface

1 Introduction

In minimally invasive surgery, one important procedure is ultrasound guided breast biopsy. The main challenge in the biopsy procedure is to guarantee reproducibility of the needle's tip position between biopsies. This is a major factor in determining the effectiveness of this intervention. The solution addressed to overcome this challenge is an image-based navigation system. While these are widely used for rigid tissue, applications for soft tissues are in the preliminary implementation stage [1–4].

Biomechanical properties of breast tissue were the subject of research. Ramiao [5] studied the relationship between the six regions of the breast for different biomechanical properties of the skin. These regions were evaluated based on how parts of the breast, for example, were related the points on the upper part of the

© Springer International Publishing AG, part of Springer Nature 2019
E. Pietka et al. (Eds.): ITIB 2018, AISC 762, pp. 172–181, 2019.
https://doi.org/10.1007/978-3-319-91211-0_15

breast, the lower part and the midline, with the purpose of verifying the existence of a relationship. According to the results obtained for the mean values of all regions of the breast, there is a similarity between the biomechanical parameters of firmness and elasticity of the breast.

Juszczyk [6] prepared the Skin Surface Deformation Model using Time of Flight (ToF) data and surface model build by implementing the Poisson equation solution. They obtained a median Hausdorff distance between input data and surface model that did not exceed 3.0 mm.

Spinczyk [7] presented the methodology of creating a model of 3D anatomical organ, which was represented by a B-spline surface, generated by the global surface interpolation algorithm.

Baroni [10] described a clinical application of an opto-electronic system for real-time three-dimensional (3D) control of patient position in breast cancer radiotherapy. The clinical application of the system revealed median 3D localization errors for directly controlled anatomical landmarks of around 4.5 mm. When the positional inaccuracies introduced by patients' respiration were also considered, the extent of the resulting 3D mis-positioning of the control points increased to median values of up to 8 mm. Spinczyk [11] found a matched bent surface with the use of non-rigid Iterative Closest Point (ICP). They obtained a mean marker alignment error as measured by the position shift error to the nearest point in the cloud of 5.63 mm. Spinczyk [12] modeled the deflection of the abdominal area using the elastic body spline based elastic field. By setting up Particle Swarm optimization algorithms, they selected the parameters of the glued curves. They achieved a median Target Registration Error (TRE) of 9.8 mm for the entire respiratory period.

From the medical point of view, the 3D visualization and the 3D models of the anatomical structures of the human body are extremely important in computer assisted surgery especially for treatment planning [8,9]. While the ultrasound-guided breast biopsy is a reference diagnostic method and must be repeated many times the main challenge is to guarantee reproducibility of the needle's tip position between biopsies. Currently, the breast surface reconstruction, which is a novelty in the presented approach, is not routinely used during biopsy, but in the presented application, the registration of the reconstructed surfaces between the treatments allows to solve the raised main challenge.

The aim of the study is to present a methodology to model sagging breasts for support navigation in ultrasound guided biopsy. It allows the registration between undeformed and deformed breast surfaces.

The paper is organized as follows: the Materials and Methods section presents the assumptions and proposed approach, including breast surface reconstruction and rigid registrations, fitting the 3D model of the ultrasound probe, and approximation of the edges of the deformed area. The Results section presents the outcomes, which are analyzed in reference to other works in the Discussion section.

2   Materials and Methods

The paper describes the proposed measurement station and methodology for the reconstruction of the surface of the breast in these two situations and their submission. The surface is observed in two situations (Figs. 1 and 2):

1. Breast free – with no touchdowns and no pressure from the ultrasound head,
2. Breast impingement – by applying pressure from the ultrasound head.

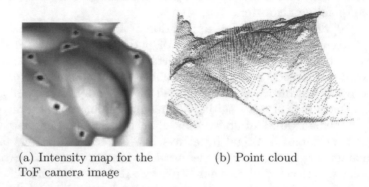

(a) Intensity map for the   (b) Point cloud
ToF camera image

Fig. 1. Figure (a) shows the breast free intensity map for the ToF camera image. Figure (b) shows the point cloud of this map

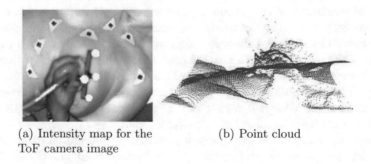

(a) Intensity map for the   (b) Point cloud
ToF camera image

Fig. 2. Figure (a) shows the breast impingement intensity map for the ToF camera image. Figure (b) shows the point cloud of this map

The proposed methodology consists of the following steps:

1. Reconstruction of the breast surface.
2. Rigid registration of undeformed and deformed surfaces.
3. Fitting of the ultrasound image to the deformed surface of the breast.
4. Visualization of the breast surface and its abrasion.

2.1   Reconstruction of the Surface of the Breast

ToF camera Swiss Range 4000 was used to capture the surface. The absolute accuracy for this ToF camera is ± 1 cm or $\pm 1\%$ [13]. The distance to the object is computed as:

$$d = \frac{c}{2f} \cdot \frac{\phi}{2\pi}, \tag{1}$$

where ϕ is shift between emitted and reflected light signal and f is frequency of the infrared (780 nm) cosine-shaped light signal. Objects within a 5 m area can be measured at a frequency of 30 MHz with an accuracy of 1 cm, which is enough to track respiratory motion. The previous works [14] shows the influence of a warm up time on distance measurement stability. The minimum relative variations of the mean value and standard deviation of average range images were performed with 3 m distance of 3 m and an integration time of 100 ms.

To evaluate the accuracy of reconstructed surface, the reference method was used. A calibrated tooltip was used to grab the point from the surface. The Fuducial Registration Error (FRE) is used to measure the distance between reference and ToF surfaces.

$$FRE = \frac{\sum_{i=1}^{n} \sqrt{(x_i - x_i')^2 + (y_i - y_i')^2 + (z_i - z_i')^2}}{n}, \tag{2}$$

2.2   Rigid Registration of Undeformed and Deformed Surfaces

To find rigid mapping between two Cartesian coordinate systems, the data must include three or more sets of corresponding non-collinear points. Horn [15], proposed a closed form solution based on a least-squares formulation. Optimal rotation Rot and translation $Trans$ was found by a singular value decomposition (SVD) of coordinal points' matrices, founded by:

$$SVD(C) = U diag(\sigma_i) V, \tag{3}$$

where $C = \sum_{i=1}^{n} S_i^T T_i$ is a correlation matrix, S_i are points in the first Cartesian coordinate system, T_i are points in the second Cartesian coordinate system, σ_i are non-negative singular values of the correlation matrix and U, V are orthonormal matrices,

$$Rot = U \begin{vmatrix} 1 & 0 & 0 \\ 0 & 1 & 0 \\ 0 & 0 & det(UV^T) \end{vmatrix} V^T, \tag{4}$$

and

$$Trans = \overline{T} - Rot(\overline{S}) \tag{5}$$

where $\overline{S}, \overline{T}$ are average values of the points' coordinates in the first and second coordinate systems, respectively. This rigid registration approach was used for the initial registration of point clouds before starting normal shooting retrieving correspondence in the proposed non-rigid iterative closest point algorithm.

2.3   Fitting of the Ultrasound Image to the Deformed Surface of the Breast

Fitting of the ultrasound image involves selecting points on the image (Fig. 3) and typing them into the breast model (Fig. 4). First, a pattern was used to calculate the points in the Polaris camera layout:

$$[XYZ1]' = Trans_{ProbeToTracker} \cdot Trans_{ImageToProbe} \cdot [xy01]' \qquad (6)$$

where $[XYZ1], [xy01]$ are selecting points on the tracker coordinate system and ultrasound image, $Trans_{ProbeToTracker}, Trans_{ImageToProbe}$ are matrices of ultrasound probe position in the tracker coordinate system and calibration transformation, respectively.

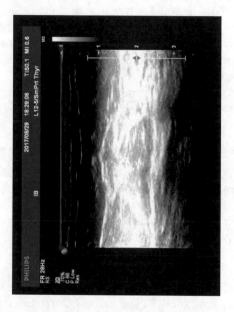

Fig. 3. Selecting points on the ultrasound image (red color)

The Public software Library for Ultra Sound imaging research (PLUS) was selected to track images during the ultrasound session. PLUS is a software package containing library functions and applications for tracked ultrasound image acquisition, calibration, and processing [16]. Development of the PLUS library is supported by Cancer Care Ontario by funding an Applied Cancer Research Unit at the Laboratory for Percutaneous Surgery at Queen's University. The main idea of PLUS is presented in Fig. 5. The position of the ultrasound head is tracked by the position tracking system. The use of a calibrated stylus and a phantom of known geometry along with a designed calibration product allows finding the calibration of the ultrasound head transformed between the marker

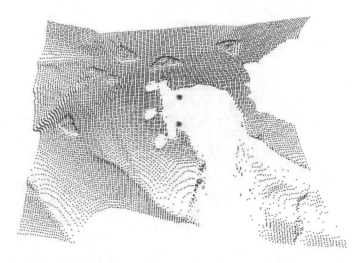

Fig. 4. Typing points into the breast model (selected points on the image – red color)

attached to the head and the beginning of the ultrasound image produced by the head. After finding the desired transform $Trans_{ImageToProbe}$ the position of any element of the ultrasound image with the coordinates x, y can be determined in the coordinate system of the tracking system using the Eq. (6).

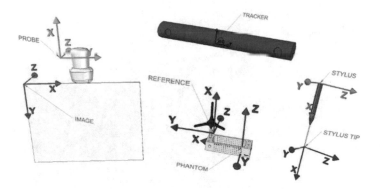

Fig. 5. Main idea of the PLUS library: presentation of a defined coordinate systems taken into account during ultrasound probe calibration process [16]

2.4 Visualization of the Breast Surface and Its Abrasion

The subsections used and described in the preceding steps enable visualization of the surface of the ring with and without a joint in the joint. Data after rigid registration are clustered in one cloud of points and presented in one color. On the background, the surface of the abdomen is presented.

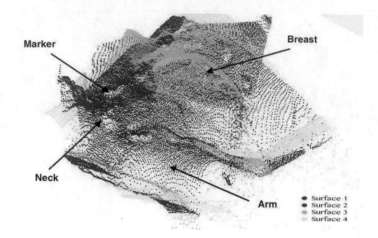

Fig. 6. Matching 4 segments (Segment 1 – Segment 4) of non-deformed surfaces

3   Results

Figures 6, 7 and 8 present examples of registered segments of non-deformed, deformed surfaces and registered deformed and non-deformed surfaces

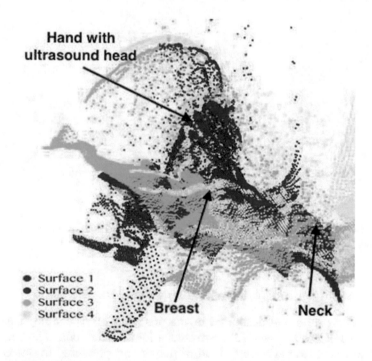

Fig. 7. Matching 4 segments (Segment 1 – Segment 4) of deformed surfaces

respectively. Segments of deformed and non-deformed surfaces (Figs. 6 and 7) do not represent corresponding anatomical segments, but result from the position of the ToF camera during the acquisition sessions. However, it is important, that areas that are not deformed in both whole surfaces after the registration (Fig. 8) are as close as possible.

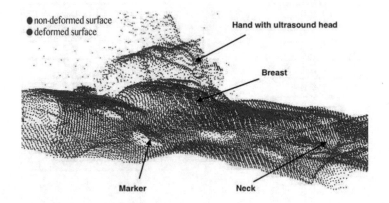

Fig. 8. Matching deformed (blue color) to non-deformed surfaces (red color)

Tables 1, 2, 3 and 4 show FRE results for: non-deformed surfaces, deformed surfaces, deformed surfaces to non-deformed surfaces, and registered ToF to tracker data respectively.

Table 1. FRE results for matching segments of non-deformed surfaces

Patient	FRE [mm]
1	16.7
2	5.9
3	13.5
4	11.4
5	12.6
6	12.7
7	8.3
8	6.9
9	15.0
10	10.9

Table 2. FRE results for matching segments of deformed surfaces

Patient	FRE [mm]
1	6.0
2	5.6
3	11.4
4	2.6
5	12.7
6	5.2
7	7.8
8	8.7
9	13.0
10	3.0

180   A. Juraszczyk and D. Spinczyk

Table 3. FRE results for matching of deformed to non-deformed surfaces

Patient	FRE [mm]
1	4.1
2	10.0
3	6.0
4	2.9
5	4.2
6	5.1
7	5.6
8	7.6
9	7.0
10	9.0

Table 4. FRE results for matching ToF surface to tracker coordinate system

Patient	FRE [mm]
1	11.2
2	10.3
3	16.5
4	19.2
5	14.2
6	16.2
7	13.0
8	15.8
9	17.0
10	10.0

4 Discussion

The proposed methodology obtains the median of FRE to fit the fragile, flat, mutual surface areas and match markers in the ToF image to the positions indicated in the tracker coordinate system of 12, 6.9, 5.8, 15 mm (Tables 1, 2, 3 and 4), respectively. Measurement the surface fit quality is based on the measure of the distance between the registered markers indicated on the breast surface by the user. As the numerical values show, the worst results were obtained when comparing the position of the ToF marker and the position tracking system (Table 4). The second worst value is the matching of non-deformed segments (Table 1). It should be noted here that similar results for the distorted surface are much better (Table 2). Here, the resolution of the ToF image can also be indicated as the main reason for the difference in the FRE error values.

Figures 6, 7 and 8 present examples of registered segments of non-deformed, deformed surfaces and registered deformed and non-deformed surfaces respectively. From the clinical point of view, the most important is the possibility of applying the breast area between treatments, as this in turn leads to the solution of the main challenge of repeatability of the biopsy position between treatments (Fig. 8).

The paper presents the stages of the method for rigid registration of uncut sections and ultrasound implantation of the breast surface and their visualization in a common coordinate system. Further research is necessary to automate the measurement of marker positions and the labeling of breast areas. This will allow for testing on a greater number of patients and the integration of the proposed methodology into the clinical workflow.

Acknowledgement. This research was supported by the Polish National Centre for Research and Development (Narodowe Centrum Badan i Rozwoju) grant No. STRATEGMED2/ 267398/4/NCBR/2015. The authors would also like to thank Andre Woloshuk for his English language corrections.

References

1. Phee, S.J., Yang, K.: Interventional navigation systems for treatment of unresectable liver tumor. Med. Biol. Eng. Comput. **48**, 103–111 (2010)
2. Neshat, H., Cool, D.W., Barker, K., Gardi, L., Kakani, N., Fenster, A.: A 3D ultrasound scanning system for image guided liver interventions. Med. Phys. **40**, 112903 (2013)
3. Kenngott, H.G., Wagner, M., Gondan, M., Nickel, F., Nolden, M., Fetzer, A., et al.: Real-time image guidance in laparoscopic liver surgery: first clinical experience with a guidance system based on intraoperative CT imaging. Surg. Endosc. **28**, 933–940 (2014)
4. Spinczyk, D.: Towards the clinical integration of an image-guided navigation system for percutaneous liver tumor ablation using freehand 2D ultrasound images. Comput. Aided Surg. **20**, 61–72 (2015)
5. Ramiao N., Martins P., Fernandes A.A: Biomechanical properties of breast tissue. In: ENBENG 2013, pp. 1–6 (2013)
6. Juszczyk, J., Czajkowska, J., Pycinski, B., Piętka, E.: ToF-data-based modelling of skin surface deformation. In: Piętka, E., et al. (eds.) Information Technologies in Medicine, pp. 235–244. Springer International Publishing, Kamien Slaski (2016)
7. Spinczyk, D., Piętka, E.: Automatic generation of 3D lung model. In: Computer Recognition Systems 2. Advances in Intelligent and Soft Computing, vol. 45, pp. 671–678 (2007)
8. Zarychta, P., Konik, H., Zarychta-Bargiela, A.: Computer assisted location of the lower limb mechanical axis. In: Pietka, E., Kawa, J. (eds.) Information Technologies in Biomedicine. Lecture Notes in Bioinformatics, vol. 7339, pp. 93–100. Springer (2012)
9. Zarychta, P.: A new approach to knee joint arthroplasty. Comput. Med. Imaging Graph. **65**, 32–45 (2017). https://doi.org/10.1016/j.compmedimag.2017.07.002
10. Baroni, G., Ferrigno, G., Orecchia, R., Pedotti, A.: Real-time opto-electronic verification of patient position in breast cancer radiotherapy. Comput. Aided Surg. **5**(4), 296–306 (2000)
11. Spinczyk, D., Karwan, A., Copik, M.: Methods for abdominal respiratory motion tracking. Comput. Aided Surg. **19**(1–3), 34–47 (2014)
12. Spinczyk, D., Fabian, S.: Target Registration Error minimization involving deformable organs using elastic body splines and Particle Swarm Optimization approach. Surg. Oncol. **26**, 489–497 (2017)
13. Mesa-Imaging – manufactor website: SR4000 Data Sheet. http://www.mesa-imaging.ch/swissranger4000.php. Accessed 16 Nov 2018
14. Chiabrando, F., Chiabrando, R., Piatti, D., Rinaudo, F.: Sensors for 3D imaging: metric evaluation and calibration of a CCD/CMOS time-of-flight camera. J. Sensors **9**(12), 10080–10096 (2009)
15. Horn, B.K.P., Hilden, H.M., Negahdaripour, S.: Closed-form solution of absolute orientation using orthonormal matrices. J. Opt. Soc. Am. A **5**, 1127–1135 (1988)
16. Lasso, A., Heffter, T., Rankin, A., Pinter, C., Ungi, T., Fichtinger, G.: PLUS: open-source toolkit for ultrasound-guided intervention systems. IEEE Trans. Biomed. Eng. **61**(10), 2527–2537 (2014)

Novel Geometric Technique of Ultrasound Probe Calibration

Beata Choroba[✉], Bartłomiej Pyciński, Michał Kręcichwost,
Dominik Spinczyk, and Ewa Pietka

Faculty of Biomedical Engineering, Silesian University of Technology,
Roosevelta 40, 41-800 Zabrze, Poland
beata.choroba@polsl.pl

Abstract. In the study a novel, simple and robust calibration technique
of ultrasound probe for image-guided navigation systems has been proposed. The method employs a LEGO phantom with known geometry
and is much simpler than other commonly used methods. Additionally,
it requires only a single US image. The method was compared to the
state-of-the-art method, which is based on a N-wire phantom. Obtained
results show an improvement in accuracy and reproducibility between
the *state-of-the-art* and the proposed method.

Keywords: Ultrasound imaging · Ultrasound probe calibration
Phantom study · Comparative study

1 Introduction

Ultrasound (US) is one of the most commonly used and easily available techniques of human body imaging. It is widely used in medical diagnostics and
during therapy as a low-cost, flexible, and real-time imaging technique. It is safe
and noninvasive, therefore it has many clinical applications. There are many
varieties of this technique that use different probes and can be used in various
branches of medicine. To enhance its capabilities, US is often integrated with
tracking systems. This approach is relatively new and is used to map the 2D
ultrasound images into the 3D space of the tracking device and then to reconstruct a 3D volume of the patient's organ.

This technique enables volume measurements as well as geometry and texture
analysis [5]. The tracked US can be also used in surgery planning and as an
intraoperative imaging modality. It allows the surgeon to monitor the procedure
with the aid of real time 2D imaging and precise localization of the organs
and tools without other tissues damage. US navigation can also be combined
with preoperative MRI or CT images that improves navigation precision and
intraoperative accuracy [4,15].

Ultrasound navigation has many advantages and is currently used in many
fields including neurosurgery, orthopedic surgery and radiation therapy. However, this technique requires a calibration procedure to find the spatial relationship between the ultrasound image frame and the position of the marker attached

© Springer International Publishing AG, part of Springer Nature 2019
E. Pietka et al. (Eds.): ITIB 2018, AISC 762, pp. 182–193, 2019.
https://doi.org/10.1007/978-3-319-91211-0_16

to the probe. Over the last two decades, ultrasound spatial calibration methods have been widely investigated in the literature. The most common approach is to scan an object with known geometry (a phantom). Some of the phantoms are very simple, *e.g.* made of bricks [19,21], others are more complicated, even mechanical [7]. Phantoms used in different investigations can be divided into few main groups: single point phantoms, wall phantoms, 2D alignment phantoms, and multiple wires phantoms [8,12].

Point-based phantoms are the simplest. They are usually constructed as a bead [1,18], crossed wires [6,9] or a center of the sphere [2]. This calibration method is based on scanning the point from different probe positions and then matching corresponding points from different coordinate frames.

In plane-based methods, the phantom can be a single-wall [14,16] or it can contain multiple planes [13]. Each plane appears as a straight line on the image and can be easily segmented. Therefore, the calibration is more precise than in methods based on a point target.

Methods which are based on 2D alignment use phantoms with known geometry and fiducial point positions (*e.g.* vertices) [11,17,20]. On each scan, these points are localized on the image and aligned with corresponding points on the phantom.

The most popular calibration methods are based on multiple wires phantoms, especially with N- or Z-shaped patterns. This type of calibration is similar to the method based on 2D alignment – fiducial points segmented on the images are matching to the points in the 3D space. One of the most known methods of this type was described in [3]. The authors used a phantom with two parallel N-wire configurations which is continuously scanned during calibration. The wires segmentation algorithm is real time and fully automatic. The calibration parameters are calculated using a closed-form formula based on segmented fiducials and corresponding coordinates in the phantom space. This method is used in the open-source Plus Toolkit ultrasound library [10] and is considered to be one of the most reliable methods of probe calibration, therefore in this study it is used as a reference method.

In this study we propose a novel, simple and robust US probe calibration method which is based on a phantom with known geometry. This geometric method can be used to calibrate probes with different depth and resolution. It requires only to capture a single image which is used to determine the relationship between the phantom and the US image coordinate systems. The final calibration result can be calculated easily just before an examination without capturing next ultrasound images. The main goal of this study is to assess the accuracy of the proposed geometric method by comparing it to the well-known N-wires method implemented in Plus Toolkit library.

2   Materials and Methods

The ultrasound probe calibration is performed to determine the spatial relationship between two coordinates frames: the first one is the coordinate frame of

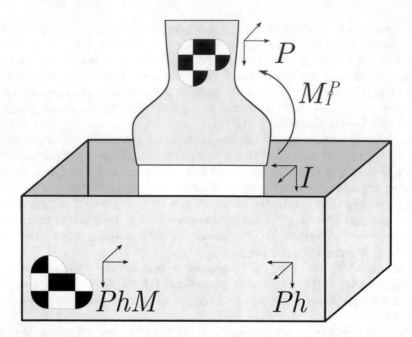

Fig. 1. Ultrasound probe calibration. Coordinates frames: I – Image; P – Marker attached to the probe; Ph – Phantom; PhM – Marker attached to the phantom. M_I^P – transformation matrix from I to P coordinate frame

ultrasound image (I), and the second one is related to a marker attached to the probe (P). Such relationship is presented as 4×4 transformation matrix M_I^P. The scheme is presented in Fig. 1.

The calibration method proposed in this study can be divided into two main steps. In the first step US images of the phantom are captured. Based on them, the correct probe position in the phantom is found. Then the geometry of the phantom is locked and the relationship between the phantom and the image plane coordinate systems is determined. In this step the markers attached to the probe and to the phantom are not needed.

In the second phase of the calibration, the final M_I^P transform is calculated based on the previously found relationship and the position of the tracked markers. It is important that in this step the US images are not captured. If the phantom geometry does not changed after the first phase of the calibration, the final transform can be determined in a quick and easy way just before an image-guided procedure. One needs only to attach the markers, place the probe on the cradle and calculate the required matrix. It is not necessary to repeat the first step of the calibration.

Both steps of the proposed calibration method are described in detail in the next section.

2.1   Geometric Phantom

To calculate the M_I^P transform between the image coordinate system and the probe coordinate system, a calibrating phantom of known geometry was used (Fig. 2). The proposed phantom is a box made of Lego bricks with a swinging cradle attached internally to the two opposite walls. This element can be rotated around one axis using a handle outside the box. It is used to find the correct angular position of the probe during calibration and acts as a stand for the probe. Moreover, there are two pairs of wires in the phantom intersecting each other in known geometrical locations and a few additional wires guided perpendicularly to the phantom walls. A tracking marker is mounted on one side of the phantom.

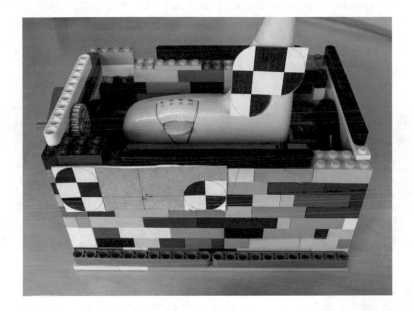

Fig. 2. Calibrating phantom

The proposed calibration method is based on geometric measurements that the determine required transforms. First, pixel dimension (s_x, s_y) in millimeters is calculated for the specific depth and resolution of the US image. This information is obtained from the rulers presented on the screen. This determines the scaling matrix M_I^{Imm} that relates points in the digital image coordinate system (in pixels) with points in the real US image coordinate system (in millimeters):

$$M_I^{Imm} = \begin{bmatrix} s_x & 0 & 0 & 0 \\ 0 & s_y & 0 & 0 \\ 0 & 0 & \frac{s_x+s_y}{2} & 0 \\ 0 & 0 & 0 & 1 \end{bmatrix}, \tag{1}$$

where s_x and s_y denote the pixel size in millimeters, in X and Y axes respectively.

The next matrix that can be calculated based on the measurements is M_{Ph}^{PhM} – a transform between coordinate system of the marker attached to the phantom and the phantom coordinate system. If these systems are not rotated relative to each other, the transform contains only a translation between the origins. Otherwise, there is a need to apply an appropriate, known rotation (in our study 180° around the Y axis). The last transform needed for the calibration is M_{Ph}^{Imm}. It relates the phantom coordinate system to the real US image coordinate system. This matrix can be calculated by finding the transformation between the points on the US image corresponding to the wires and the known real position of these points in 3D space.

Correct placement of the US probe is necessary to prepare the calibration. The probe should be put on the swinging cradle in the phantom which is then rotated using the handle to achieve the position, when the image plane is directed perpendicular to the bottom. If the phantom is filled with water, each point of crossing of the wires is visible on the image as a single point only (Fig. 3). The wires pattern is presented in Fig. 4.

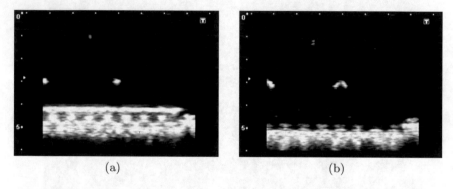

(a)   (b)

Fig. 3. Ultrasound images of the phantom with different positions of the probe: (a) correct probe placement – the image plane is perpendicular to the bottom; (b) incorrect probe placement – the image plane is tilted

When the probe is correctly placed, it is possible to calculate the M_{Ph}^{Imm} transform, and more precisely, the translation between the coordinate systems' origins. It is based on the positions of the wires on the image and in the phantom coordinate system. If the point in the US image has coordinates (x_I, y_I) and the corresponding point in the phantom coordinate system (x_{Ph}, y_{Ph}, z_{Ph}), then the following equation can be used to calculate the M_{Ph}^{Imm} transform:

$$M_{Ph}^{Imm} \cdot [x_{Ph}, y_{Ph}, z_{Ph}, 1]^T = M_I^{Imm} \cdot [x_I, y_I, 0, 1]^T . \tag{2}$$

Relative orientation of the phantom coordinate system and the US image coordinate system should be identity, therefore the M_{Ph}^{Imm} transform contains only translation and the equation is possible to be solved. The final transform matrix is the mean of the matrices obtained for each point corresponding to the wires.

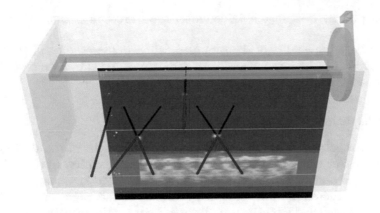

Fig. 4. The wires pattern used in the phantom with its ultrasound image

The M_I^P transform is calculated using matrices determined in the previous steps and positions of the markers attached to the probe (M_P^T) and the phantom (M_{PhM}^T) in the tracker coordinate system. The US image is not needed in this part of the calibration. The resulting matrix is obtained by multiplying the known transforms in the following order:

$$M_I^P = M_T^P \cdot M_{PhM}^T \cdot M_{Ph}^{PhM} \cdot M_{I_{mm}}^{Ph} \cdot M_I^{I_{mm}}. \tag{3}$$

3   Experiments and Results

In this work, two methods of probe calibration were compared. First was the method implemented in Plus Toolkit library [10], where the N-wire phantom is used. Second method, proposed by the authors, was described in the previous section.

The hardware setup used to acquire the data during the calibration process consisted of a US device Toshiba Nemio XG with 3–5 MHz linear probe PLF-308, Claron Micron Tracker Hx40 six degrees of freedom optical tracking device, and a framegrabber Imaging Source DFG/USB2pro.

Experiments were conducted three times independently, for three different image resolutions of the ultrasound probe. They corresponded to image depths 30 mm, 40 mm and 60 mm, respectively. The other parameters of the image acquisition were adjusted each time.

The first method of calibration was completely repeated 10 times for each image resolution. The second method was carried out in two ways. In the first way, the $M_{Ph}^{I_{mm}}$ transform (see Sect. 2.1) was calculated only once and then the cradle was locked. The calibration results were repeated and calculated 10 times, each time after shifting the phantom and re-positioning the probe in the cradle.

In the second way, the whole calibration process using the proposed method was performed 10 times. For each calibration, the $M_{Ph}^{I_{mm}}$ transform was calculated using a new US image obtained after the correct placement of the cradle and the probe.

To evaluate the quality of the proposed calibration method and to compare it with baseline method, the following metrics are used: calibration reproducibility (CR) and point reconstruction accuracy (PRA).

3.1   Calibration Reproducibility

Calibration reproducibility (CR) [8] measures the spread of the position of a single point after being transformed with multiple calibration results. If N calibrations were performed, and A^I denotes a point A in the image coordinate frame I, then there are N transformed positions of this point into the tracker coordinate system, and CR is a mean distance between the transformed positions and their centroid,

$$CR = \frac{1}{N} \sum_{i=1}^{N} \left| M_P^T \cdot \left(M_I^P \right)_i \cdot A^I - \overline{A^T} \right|, \tag{4}$$

where $\overline{A^T}$ is the centroid of transformed position of A into the tracker coordinate frame:

$$\overline{A^T} = \frac{1}{N} \sum_{i=1}^{N} M_P^T \cdot \left(M_I^P \right)_i \cdot A^I. \tag{5}$$

CR was computed for five points in the US image: for all corners and the central point. Summary values are presented in Table 1. A Kruskall test revealed that there were no significant differences between mean CR values of different points (values from 1.20 to 1.75 mm, p = 0.77).

Comparison of CR between different methods using a Wilcoxon test showed that both ways of the proposed method did not differ (p = 0.86). They both yielded significantly lower CR values than the calibration with N-wire phantom (p < 0.001).

The distribution of direction of CR has been also computed by performing the same calculations for each component X, Y, Z of the centroid $\overline{A^T}$ separately. X axis spreaded from left to right part of the image, Y from the probe alongside acoustic waves, and Z was perpendicular to image plane. The greatest impact on CR came from Z direction, especially for N-wire phantom. This is because the ultrasound image does not come from perfect plane, but rather from a thin pyramid, so position of the wires are distorted. Wilcoxon tests showed that the values of Z direction of CR (2.39, 0.65 and 0.68 mm for the consecutive calibration methods) are higher than X (0.36, 0.29, 0.22 mm) and Y (0.44, 0.27, 0.32 mm). Complete results are presented in Table 2.

Since we proved that CR of both ways of the proposed method did not differ, therefore, to calculate PRA, only transforms from the former way were taken into account.

Table 1. CR values of 5 image points for various image depths and phantoms. C – central point, LL – lower left corner, UL – upper left corner, LR – lower right corner, UR – upper right corner. All values in [mm]

	C	LL	UL	LR	UR	Mean	Std
Calibration with N-wire phantom							
30 mm	2.13	2.71	2.90	3.17	2.95	2.77	0.40
40 mm	2.59	2.50	2.83	2.55	2.77	2.65	0.14
60 mm	1.98	1.57	1.92	2.97	2.30	2.15	0.53
Geometric calibration ver. 1							
30 mm	0.39	0.77	0.42	0.92	0.51	0.60	0.23
40 mm	0.45	1.13	0.47	1.38	0.65	0.81	0.42
60 mm	0.92	1.81	0.76	1.87	0.84	1.24	0.55
Geometric calibration ver. 2							
30 mm	0.66	0.67	0.64	0.58	0.64	0.64	0.04
40 mm	0.74	1.17	0.74	0.99	0.70	0.87	0.20
60 mm	0.91	1.57	0.87	1.30	0.93	1.12	0.31
Mean	1.20	1.55	1.28	1.75	1.37		
Std	0.81	0.71	1.00	0.94	1.00		

Table 2. Distribution of CR into the directions X, Y and Z for various calibration methods phantoms. All values in [mm]

	Mean	Std	Min	25%	50%	75%	Max
Calibration with N-wire phantom							
X	0.36	0.15	0.19	0.27	0.32	0.40	0.72
Y	0.44	0.15	0.23	0.33	0.42	0.51	0.76
Z	2.39	0.43	1.46	2.06	2.50	2.72	2.93
Geometric calibration ver. 1							
X	0.29	0.13	0.17	0.19	0.23	0.42	0.50
Y	0.27	0.08	0.15	0.19	0.30	0.34	0.36
Z	0.65	0.48	0.22	0.25	0.49	0.90	1.59
Geometric calibration ver. 2							
X	0.22	0.11	0.11	0.13	0.15	0.35	0.39
Y	0.32	0.09	0.19	0.25	0.38	0.39	0.43
Z	0.68	0.29	0.39	0.50	0.54	0.77	1.39

3.2   Point Reconstruction Accuracy

Given two coordinate systems X and Y, point A in the former coordinate system, A^X, and its correspoding point in the latter, A^Y, and the transformation matrix M_X^Y (calibration result) from X to Y, then point reconstruction accuracy

(PRA) is a metric that measures the Euclidean distance between A^Y and A^X transformed into the X coordinate frame:

$$PRA = \left| A^Y - M_X^Y \cdot A^X \right|. \tag{6}$$

In the experiment there were three different coordinates system, hence for each point three values of PRA were computed. Namely, P was the phantom's coordinates frame, T was the frame connected to the tracked stylus and I was an ultrasound image coordinate frame. Therefore the pairs $I - T$, $I - P$ and $P - T$ denotes PRA values between the above pairs of coordinates frames.

In the experiment, the corner point on the N-wire phantom was indicated by the calibrated and tracked stylus tip (T coordinate frame), and its position on the US image was acquired using tracked probe (I coordinate frame). Geometry of the phantom was known, so the P coordinates were also known.

For each of 10 probe calibration results for both phantom and each probe depth, 10 points were obtained and three PRA values were computed. A Saphiro test indicated that the distribution of the results were not normal, so non parametric statistical tests were used.

PRA values of $I - P$ were significantly higher than $I - T$ (p = 0.048 and p < 1e–6 for N-wire and geometrical phantom, respectively). PRA of $I - T$ were also significantly higher for $P - T$ (p = 0.03 and p < 1e–3 for N-wire and geometrical, respectively).

There were no significant differences between PRA values of N-wire and geometric phantom, except for $I-T$, where the geometrical phantom had smaller value (5.45 mm vs 6.18 mm, p = 0.002).

A Wilcoxon test proved that overall, PRA results were the smallest for depth 60 mm and the highest for 40 mm. There were some differences if three PRA values were compared separately.

Complete numerical results are presented in Tables 3 and 4.

Table 3. PRA distances of N–wire phantom. Row definitions are described in the text. All values in [mm]

	Mean	Std	Min	25%	50%	75%	Max
30 mm							
$I - T$	7.33	3.76	0.99	3.72	8.03	10.47	15.00
$I - P$	5.95	3.26	0.58	3.38	5.24	8.05	14.95
$P - T$	4.10	1.91	1.06	2.89	3.83	4.94	10.39
40 mm							
$I - T$	5.57	2.10	1.74	3.77	5.55	6.87	12.99
$I - P$	8.83	4.43	1.97	5.01	8.79	11.80	19.27
$P - T$	8.26	2.97	3.12	6.08	8.03	10.17	15.42
60 mm							
$I - T$	5.80	1.59	2.43	4.73	5.81	6.69	10.23
$I - P$	5.83	2.75	0.89	3.73	5.31	7.57	13.21
$P - T$	3.45	2.24	0.62	1.90	2.88	4.40	13.11

Table 4. PRA distances of geometric phantom. Row definitions are described in the text. All values in [mm]

	Mean	Std	Min	25%	50%	75%	Max
30 mm							
$I - T$	5.12	3.06	1.48	2.76	3.79	8.27	12.06
$I - P$	7.26	3.85	2.90	4.42	5.75	9.03	18.81
$P - T$	4.74	3.00	1.25	2.46	4.10	5.88	15.83
40 mm							
$I - T$	5.82	2.97	2.54	3.73	4.42	8.06	15.37
$I - P$	6.35	2.97	2.31	3.99	5.67	7.59	17.77
$P - T$	6.36	3.02	2.21	3.92	5.82	8.06	18.88
60 mm							
$I - T$	5.44	1.79	2.00	4.10	5.43	6.70	10.34
$I - P$	7.18	3.15	2.38	4.73	6.15	9.02	15.37
$P - T$	4.21	2.59	0.36	2.17	3.77	5.45	12.83

4   Summary

In this study a novel US probe calibration method based on the known geometry of the phantom was described. This way of calibration is simpler than most of the known methods. It can be divided into two steps which can be performed independently. Acquiring an US image is needed only in the first step. After locking the cradle and determining the required matrices dependent on the image, the probe and the marker attached to it can be moved. The final calibration can be performed without capturing US images of the phantom.

The results obtained in the study show that the accuracy of the proposed calibration method is not worse than in the N-wires method. The low calibration reproducibility values (mean CR less than 1.3 mm) indicate that the method is repeatable. The Z component of the CR is significantly lower than in the N-wires method. The cradle in the phantom enables precise placement of the probe during calibration, which reduces the impact of the US beam thickness. There were no significant differences between point reconstruction accuracy values of the N-wire and the geometric phantom. The proposed method can be successfully used to calibrate US probes with different image depth and resolution.

Acknowledgement. This research is supported by the Polish National Science Centre (Narodowe Centrum Nauki) grant No.: UMO-2016/21/B/ST7/02236. The funders had no role in study design, data collection and analysis, decision to publish, or preparation of the manuscript.

The authors would like to thank Mr. Andre Woloshuk B.Sc. for his valuable English language corrections.

References

1. Amin, D., Kanade, T., Jaramaz, B., Digioia, A.M., Nikou, C., LaBarca, R., Moody, J.E.: Calibration method for determining the physical location of the ultrasound image plane. In: Proceedings of the 4th International Conference on Medical Image Computing and Computer-Assisted Intervention (MICCAI 2001), Pittsburgh, PA (2001)
2. Brendel, B., Winter, S., Ermert, H.: A simple and accurate calibration method for 3D freehand ultra-sound. Biomed. Tech. **49**, 872–873 (2004)
3. Chen, T.K., Thurston, A.D., Ellis, R.E., Abolmaesumi, P.: A real-time free-hand ultrasound calibration system with automatic accuracy feedback and control. Ultrasound Med. Biol. **35**(1), 79–93 (2009). https://doi.org/10.1016/j.ultrasmedbio.2008.07.004
4. Chen, X., Bao, N., Li, J., Kang, Y.: A review of surgery navigation system based on ultrasound guidance. In: 2012 IEEE International Conference on Information and Automation, pp. 882–886 (2012). https://doi.org/10.1109/ICInfA.2012.6246906
5. Czajkowska, J., Pyciński, B., Piętka, E.: HoG feature based detection of tissue deformations in ultrasound data. In: 2015 37th Annual International Conference of the IEEE Engineering in Medicine and Biology Society (EMBC), pp. 6326–6329. Institute of Electrical & Electronics Engineers (IEEE) (2015). https://doi.org/10.1109/embc.2015.7319839
6. Detmer, P.R., Bashein, G., Hodges, T., Beach, K.W., Filer, E.P., Burns, D.H., Strandness, D.: 3D ultrasonic image feature localization based on magnetic scan-head tracking: in vitro calibration and validation. Ultrasound Med. Biol. **20**(9), 923–936 (1994). https://doi.org/10.1016/0301-5629(94)90052-3
7. Gee, A.H., Houghton, N.E., Treece, G.M., Prager, R.W.: A mechanical instrument for 3D ultrasound probe calibration. Ultrasound Med. Biol. **31**(4), 505–518 (2005). https://doi.org/10.1016/j.ultrasmedbio.2004.12.022
8. Hsu, P.W., Prager, R.W., Gee, A.H., Treece, G.M.: Freehand 3D ultrasound calibration: a review. In: Sensen, C.W., Hallgrímsson, B. (eds.) Advanced Imaging in Biology and Medicine, pp. 47–84. Springer, Heidelberg (2009). https://doi.org/10.1007/978-3-540-68993-5_3
9. Huang, Q., Zheng, Y., Lu, M., Chi, Z.: Development of a portable 3D ultrasound imaging system for musculoskeletal tissues. Ultrasonics **43**(3), 153–163 (2005). https://doi.org/10.1016/j.ultras.2004.05.003
10. Lasso, A., Heffter, T., Rankin, A., Pinter, C., Ungi, T., Fichtinger, G.: Plus: open-source toolkit for ultrasound-guided intervention systems. IEEE Trans. Biomed. Eng. **61**(10), 2527–2537 (2014). https://doi.org/10.1109/TBME.2014.2322864
11. Lindseth, F., Tangen, G.A., Langø, T., Bang, J.: Probe calibration for freehand 3-D ultrasound. Ultrasound Med. Biol. **29**(11), 1607–1623 (2003). https://doi.org/10.1016/S0301-5629(03)01012-3
12. Mercier, L., Langø, T., Lindseth, F., Collins, L.D.: A review of calibration techniques for freehand 3-D ultrasound systems. Ultrasound Med. Biol. **31**(4), 449–471 (2005). https://doi.org/10.1016/j.ultrasmedbio.2004.11.015
13. Najafi, M., Afsham, N., Abolmaesumi, P., Rohling, R.: A closed-form differential formulation for ultrasound spatial calibration: multi-wedge phantom. Ultrasound Med. Biol. **40**(9), 2231–2243 (2014). https://doi.org/10.1016/j.ultrasmedbio.2014.03.006
14. Prager, R., Rohling, R., Gee, A., Berman, L.: Rapid calibration for 3-D freehand ultrasound. Ultrasound Med. Biol. **24**(6), 855–869 (1998). https://doi.org/10.1016/S0301-5629(98)00044-1

15. Pyciński, B., Juszczyk, J., Bożek, P., Ciekalski, J., Dzielicki, J., Pietka, E.: Image navigation in minimally invasive surgery. In: Piętka, E., Kawa, J., Więcławek, W. (eds.) Information Technologies in Biomedicine Volume 4. Advances in Intelligent Systems and Computing, vol. 284, pp. 25–34. Springer International Publishing (2014). https://doi.org/10.1007/978-3-319-06596-0_3
16. Rousseau, F., Hellier, P., Barillot, C.: Confhusius: a robust and fully automatic calibration method for 3D freehand ultrasound. Med. Image Anal. 9(1), 25–38 (2005). https://doi.org/10.1016/j.media.2004.06.021
17. Sato, Y., Nakamoto, M., Tamaki, Y., Sasama, T., Sakita, I., Nakajima, Y., Monden, M., Tamura, S.: Image guidance of breast cancer surgery using 3-D ultrasound images and augmented reality visualization. IEEE Trans. Med. Imaging 17(5), 681–693 (1998). https://doi.org/10.1109/42.736019
18. State, A., Chen, D., Tector, C., Brandt, A., Chen, H., Ohbuchi, R., Bajura, M., Fuchs, H.: Case study: observing a volume rendered fetus within a pregnant patient. In: Proceedings Visualization, pp. 364–368 (1994)
19. Walsh, R., Soehl, M., Rankin, A., Lasso, A., Fichtinger, G.: Design of a tracked ultrasound calibration phantom made of LEGO bricks. In: Medical Imaging 2014: Image-Guided Procedures, Robotic Interventions, and Modeling (2014). https://doi.org/10.1117/12.2043533
20. Welch, J.N., Johnson, J.A., Bax, M.R., Badr, R., Shahidi, R.: A real-time freehand 3D ultrasound system for image-guided surgery. In: 2000 IEEE Ultrasonics Symposium, Proceedings, An International Symposium (Cat. No. 00CH37121), vol. 2, pp. 1601–1604 (2000). https://doi.org/10.1109/ULTSYM.2000.921630
21. Xiao, Y., Yan, C.X.B., Drouin, S., De Nigris, D., Kochanowska, A., Collins, D.L.: User-friendly freehand ultrasound calibration using lego bricks and automatic registration. Int. J. Comput. Assist. Radiol. Surg. 11(9), 1703–1711 (2016). https://doi.org/10.1007/s11548-016-1368-5

An Application of a Haptic Device in a Computer Aided Surgery

Magdalena Żuk(✉), Jakub Mazur, Matylda Żmudzińska, Marcin Majak,
Michał Popek, and Ewelina Świątek-Najwer

Wroclaw University of Science and Technology, Wrocław, Poland
magdalena.zuk@pwr.edu.pl

Abstract. The purpose of this work was to asses the application of
haptic device for preoperative virtual planning and intraoperative aiding oncological treatment in maxillofacial area, as well as to preliminarily evaluate an accuracy of intraoperative model registration using
Geomagic Touch device. The skull anatomical phantom with mounted
titanium screws, previously scanned using CBCT, was used for validation. Preoperative planning, including indication of 6 fiducial registration
points and 5 target registration points, was performed for 4 different
data sets and repeated 10 times by single user. An average fiducial registration error was 2.46 ± 0.25 mm, while an average target registration
error was 2.88 ± 0.44 mm. Although, obtained accuracy is lower than in
the case of optical and electromagnetic navigation system, it still can
improve surgery procedure in less demanding applications being a low
cost alternative. Geomagic Touch haptic device can be used for preoperative virtual planning of maxillofacial surgery, as well as for intraoperative
navigation.

Keywords: Haptic device · Computer aided surgery

1 Introduction

In the last few years haptic technology has gained huge popularity among
researchers, educators, medical specialists and many others. In general, haptics is a technology which allows a user to create, feel or manipulate virtual
objects, as well as to communicate with other devices or users by sense of touch
[18]. There are a few distinctions of haptic systems, but in general there are two
groups. The former are active systems where the user can generate and manipulate objects, while the latter are passive systems, where the user can feel e.g.
forces or shapes of objects. It is possible for one device to act as active and
passive device simultaneously.

With the growing popularity of haptic devices, the number of their applications in both industry and medicine is also growing. Art, entertainment and
education applications also should not be overlooked [22]. In all of those fields,
great importance lies in the possibility of creating and manipulating objects

© Springer International Publishing AG, part of Springer Nature 2019
E. Pietka et al. (Eds.): ITIB 2018, AISC 762, pp. 194–204, 2019.
https://doi.org/10.1007/978-3-319-91211-0_17

(e.g. 3D modelling for engineering, and manipulating virtual objects for education and medicine). Beside these, especially in medicine and medical training, haptic technology has some characteristic applications like in minimally invasive surgeries (MIS) and laparoscopy training (Fig. 2), in telemedicine and medical robots (e.g. the da Vinci Surgical System – Fig. 1). Haptic technology is also used in rehabilitation robotics (e.g. HapticWalker – haptic foot device for gait rehabilitation) and in surgery planning, what is described below. Other interesting applications cover automotive field, where new systems for car control are being expanded of haptics [5], and fashion, where system for haptic sensing of virtual textiles has been developed [12].

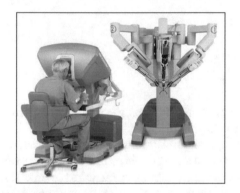

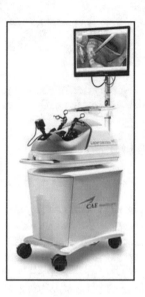

Fig. 1. The da Vinci surgical system by intuitive surgical [2]

Fig. 2. LapVR haptic laparoscopic surgical simulator by CAE healthcare [3]

In recent years, great advancement has been done in the field of computer-aided surgery and related medical interventions. Several different fields can be distinguished: preoperative virtual planning [10], preoperative planning using personalized 3D printed models [8], surgical simulation [4], guided surgery [11,19], and autonomous and semi-autonomous surgery [6,7,14].

Current study is a part of a wide project which aims to develop new computer and fluorescence-guided system for planning and aiding oncological treatment. General idea of the developed system was presented in paper [24]. The purpose of the current work was to asses the application of haptic device in MentorEye system for preoperative planning and intraoperative aiding oncological treatment in maxillofacial area, as well as to preliminarily evaluate an accuracy of intraoperative model registration using Geomagic Touch device (Fig. 3).

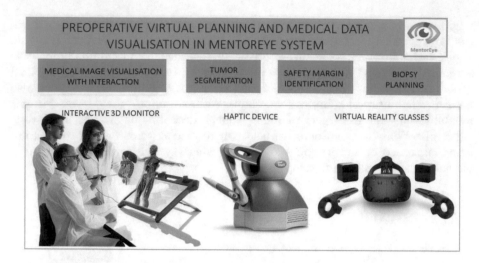

Fig. 3. Application of virtual reality tools for preoperative planning and medical image visualization in MentorEye system

2 Method

2.1 Geomagic Haptic Device

The Touch haptic device, used in described work, is a commercial product from 3D Systems. The robot allows users to touch, manipulate, create or mark points on different virtual models. Device's range of motion covers hand movement pivoting at wrist, with nominal position resolution at 0.055 mm. Position sensing along X,Y and Z is realized by digital encoders, mounted on joints, while the rotations about roll, pitch and yaw axis are measured using potentiometers. Force feedback realized by holding torque and the resistance of the motors is executed with 3 degrees of freedom, covering the workspace of 160 mm × 120 mm × 70 mm. Other 3, non-actuated degrees of freedom correspond to wrist joints.

The stylus of the device (Fig. 4) is removable, which allows the user to customize the robot and its application. Another feature of the device, which facilitates customization, is software support with Open Haptics Software toolkit and QuickHaptics micro API. Toolkit delivers the ability to integrate The Touch into an application with tools such as device control, sensor readings or 3D navigation.

As the device is delivered with the software of Geomagic Freeform and Geomagic Sculpt, so after installation, it is almost instantly ready to work. Applications mentioned by the manufacturer are possible to be executed with the device and software are e.g. 3D modeling, medical surgery and rehabilitation simulations, artwork and sculpting, training, entertainment and virtual reality, teleoperation and robotic control, virtual assembly and collision detection [1].

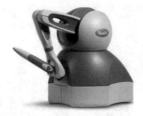

Fig. 4. The touch haptic device by 3D systems [1]

2.2   Application of a Haptic Device in Virtual Planning and Computer Aided Surgery

The software tool for a preoperative virtual planning and an intraoperative assistance using Geomagic Touch haptic device has been developed. Software was implemented in C++ programming language in Visual Studio 2017. VTK (Visualisation Toolkit, Kitware) and ITK (Insight Segmentation and Registration Toolkit, Kitware) libraries were used for model visualisation and rendering, as well as model transformations. Open Haptic library was applied for data acquisition from Geomagic Touch haptic device. Developed tool includes two phases: preoperative phase and intraoperative phase (presented in Fig. 5). In the preoperative phase, user can load a 3D patient anatomical model in STL format which is interactively visualised. Conversion from DICOM medical imaging data into 3D model was done using precise marching cubes algorithm with further two smoothing iterations. Finally, the haptic device workspace can be adjusted to the model coordinate system. The matching procedure is necessary to calculate transformation matrix between virtual and real objects. The point-based registration method was applied. Alternative solution would be surface matching or hybrid approach were point-based and surface methods are used [25].

During preoperative, virtual planning step user has to indicate on a virtual model 6 fiducial registration points used for matching procedure. Furthermore, user can select target registration points which are useful for validation during intraoperative phase. Target registration points have many potential application in intraoperative phase: resection line indication, planning position of fixating plate or indication of anatomical structures, which have to be preserved during surgery.

The intraoperative phase begins with matching procedure, where fiducial registration points are marked on a real object (anatomical phantom or human face) according to preoperatively prepared virtual plan. Then, virtual anatomical model is transformed using calculated matrix. The accuracy of matching procedure can be quantitatively evaluated using fiducial registration error (FRE) and target registration error (TRE). Fiducial registration error (FRE) is the root-square distance between corresponding fiducial points after registration. While target registration error (TRE) is the root-square distance between corresponding target points (any other than fiducial points) [9]. In clinical practice, if fiducial registration error is relatively high, registration procedure should be repeated. After successful matching procedure, the tip of a haptic device is visualized in the reference of virtual model and preoperative plan.

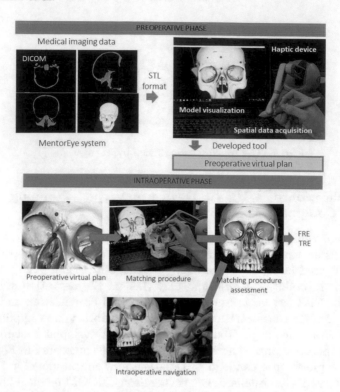

Fig. 5. Application of a haptic device for computer aided surgery including the preoperative planning and intraoperative navigation

2.3   Software Validation Phase

The skull anatomical phantom with mounted titanium screws was used for validation (Fig. 6). In advance, the phantom was scanned in Cone Beam CT scanner (Iluma CT, Imtec) with spatial resolution 0.3 mm. Standard DICOM data was converted into 3D model in STL format using MentorEye software previously developed by authors [24]. Then, 3D phantom model was loaded into software developed within current work. Eleven points were indicated by stylus on the virtual skull model during preoperative phase: six points intended for matching procedure and five target points. In intraoperative phase: first six fiducial registration points corresponding to preoperative plan were indicated on phantom, then matching procedure was applied, finally five target registration points were indicated on phantom according to software assistance. Four different data sets (various fiducial registration points and target registration points) were designed, what is presented in Fig. 8. Described procedure was repeated for each data set ten times by one user (a total of 40 procedures, 240 fiducial registration points and 200 target registration points). Mean FRE and TRE errors were calculated for each procedure.

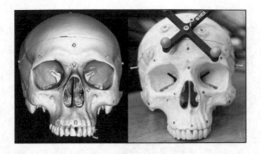

Fig. 6. Phantom evaluation

Moreover, the measurement repeatability of stylus tip position was carried out due to the fact that its accuracy and repeatability is not provided by the producer. Eight different points were indicated using haptic device stylus in different areas of the haptic device's workspace. Specially prepared stand with conical recess was used to ensure high repeatability (Fig. 7). Measurement was repeated twelve times for each point for various stylus and arm orientations.

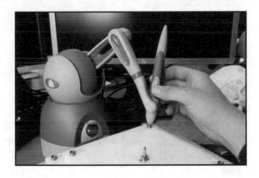

Fig. 7. Position measurement repeatability test using a stand with conical recess

3   Results

Qualitative assessment of the matching procedure accuracy and the target registration accuracy for selected trials are shown in Fig. 8. Results of quantitative assessment, represented as fiducial registration error (FRE) and target registration error (TRE), averaged over different data points and all repetitions for four data sets are presented in Fig. 9. Fiducial registration error averaged over four collected data sets is $2.46 \pm 0.25\,\text{mm}$, while target registration error averaged over four collected data sets is $2.88 \pm 0.44\,\text{mm}$.

Results of repeatability test of stylus position measurement are presented in Fig. 10. RMS error averaged over all points is $0.63 \pm 0.12\,\text{mm}$.

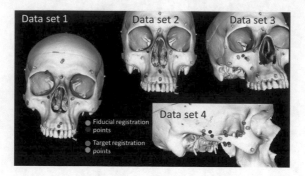

Fig. 8. Qualitative visualization of matching procedure accuracy and target registration accuracy for one selected trial. Red and green circles represent points indicated on a virtual model and a real phantom, which have been applied in matching procedure for a transformation matrix calculation, while grey and purple circles represent the other indicated points

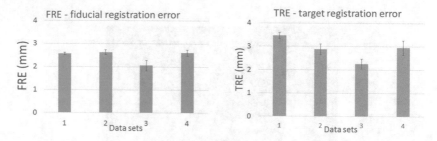

Fig. 9. Fiducial registration error (FRE) and target registration error (TRE) averaged over all points (6 points for FRE and 5 points for TRE) collected during ten repetitions for four different data sets

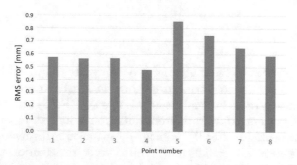

Fig. 10. Results of repeatability test of stylus position measurement. RMS error for various point in haptic device workspace

4 Discussion

In current work, Geomagic Touch haptic device was applied as 3D navigation tool for computer aided surgery using a custom made software. Application of haptic device is a low cost alternative for expensive tracking devices. The cost of such haptic device is about 3 000 \$, while the cost of an accurate navigation system with very limited workspace is about 13 000 \$. Developed tool enables preoperative planning, as well as intraoperative navigation preceded by the registration procedure. The potential applications of the haptic device together with a proposed software are: preoperative planning of a biopsy procedure, an osteotomy line, a position of fixating plates, and intraoperative navigation of the stylus in regard to the anatomical model and the preoperative plan and finally, as a simulator tool. However, the utility of proposed tools in a clinical practice would depend on their accuracy, availability, an ergonomy of use, and of course benefits. Advantages of the navigation during maxillofacial surgery preceded by virtual planning have been extensively discussed in previous papers [11].

Proposed procedures were validated using the skull anatomical phantom. Obtained accuracy of registration procedures (fiducial registration errors 2.46 ± 0.25 mm and target registration errors 2.88 ± 0.44 mm) can be compared to another studies [13, 15–17, 21, 23]. In paper [23], authors compared accuracy of three commercially available optical navigation systems for computer aided maxillofacial surgery. Mean target registration errors measured for four cadaveric heads were: 1.00 ± 0.04 mm (StealthStation), 1.13 ± 0.05 mm (VectorVision), and 1.34 ± 0.04 mm (Voxim). In papers [16, 17], an objective assessment of the accuracy of craniomaxillofacial resection simulation using optical navigation system and custom made software was performed on anatomical phantoms. Obtained mean TRE was 0.95 ± 0.19 mm, while mean FRE was respectively 0.70 ± 0.16 mm and 0.80 ± 0.11 mm. In paper [15], commercially available optical navigation system was applied in orthognathic surgery of mandible, mean target registration was 1.51 mm obtained for skull modes and 1.51 mm for six patients. An electromagnetic tracking device in maxillofacial surgery on a skull phantom was evaluated in paper [21]. The average target registration error for 6 points registration was 1.03 ± 0.53 mm under operating room conditions, but increased to 1.76 ± 0.81 mm in presence of metallic tool.

An accuracy, obtained in current study using the haptic device is lower than those obtained by other authors using optical and electromagnetic navigation systems. Fiducial and target registration errors depend on the accuracy of tracking device, applied algorithm for data processing and registration procedures, number and choice of points, as well as user's experience. It should be emphasized, that adopted haptic device is not a typical coordinate-measuring device with a declared high accuracy of stylus position, but it is quite cheap counterpart. In current study, preliminary prepared software was validated. Further software optimization, including improved point indication or point position averaging could increase accuracy.

What is a substantial limitation in the haptic device application in intraoperative navigation is position measurement of merely stylus. There is no possibility to measure a position of surgical instruments as a sagittal saw, a drill or a biopsy needle in contrast to optical or electromagnetic navigation systems. Moreover, patient or model position should be preserved relative to the haptic device coordinate system due to inability to measure stylus coordinated with the respect to patient coordinate system. In the case of an optical or an electromagnetic navigation systems, reference frames can be mounted to the selected segments of human body and tracked during the surgical procedure. Therefore, in clinical practice, if the patient is not immobilized during surgery, the stylus of haptic device can be used as a pointer for indicating points or curves immediately after matching procedure, what would limit clinical application of such solutions. Geomagic Touch is a mid-range haptic device and tracking workspace is limited.

However, on the other hand, there are advantages arising from this device application. First of all we do not need to preserve direct visibility, as it is required in case of optical navigation. It may also be very useful to apply haptic device to indicate osteotomy line for example in case of autografts from fibula bone. An important advantage of haptic device is low price, lower than any tracking system and many application possibility, both in planning or surgery simulation. The device may be helpful for educating medicine students and young physicians. Another important advantage is that haptic device provides force feedback and it would be possible in the future to model tissue response to exerted pressure.

Further development of system is planning of surgery on projections, currently we provided the planning on 3D models. We will also focus on optimizing software in order to increase accuracy.

5 Conclusions

Geomagic Touch haptic device can be used for preoperative virtual planning of maxillofacial surgery, as well as for intraoperative navigation. The registration accuracy obtained using custom made software (TRE 2.88 ± 0.44 mm, FRE 2.46 ± 0.25 mm) is lower than in the case of optical and electromagnetic navigation system. However, it still can improve surgery procedure in less demanding applications being a low cost alternative. Furthermore, haptic devices have many other application possibility in computer aided surgery and medical education.

Acknowledgement. The work is supported by National Centre of Research and Development in Poland, in frames of the project: 'Development of Polish complementary system of molecular surgical navigation for tumor treatment', STRATEGMED1/233624/4/NCBR/2014.

References

1. 3Dsystem. https://www.3dsystems.com/haptics-devices/touch. Accessed 31 Dec 2017
2. The da Vinci Surgical System by Intuitive Surgical. https://www.intuitivesurgical. com/company/media/images/singlesite/SingleSite_PC_SC_Surgeon_head_in_conso le.jpg. Accessed 31 Dec 2017
3. LapVR haptic laparoscopic surgical simulator by CAE Healthcare. https://www. intechopen.com/source/html/39043/media/image2.jpeg. Accessed 31 Dec 2017
4. Badash, I., Burtt, K., Solorzano, C.A., Carey, J.N.: Innovations in surgery simulation: a review of past, current and future techniques. Ann. Transl. Med. **4**(23), 453 (2016)
5. Bernstein, A., Bader, B., Bengler, K., Künzner, H.: Visual-Haptic Interfaces in Car Design at BMW, pp. 445–451. Birkhäuser Basel, Basel (2008). https://doi.org/10. 1007/978-3-7643-7612-3_36
6. Ciszkiewicz, A., Lorkowski, J., Milewski, G.: A novel planning solution for semi-autonomous aspiration of baker's cysts. Int. J. Med. Robot. Comput. Assist. Surg. e1882–n/a. https://doi.org/10.1002/rcs.1882. E1882 RCS-16-0207.R3
7. Ciszkiewicz, A., Milewski, G.: Path planning for minimally-invasive knee surgery using a hybrid optimization procedure. Comput. Methods Biomech. Biomed. Eng. **21**(1), 47–54 (2018). https://doi.org/10.1080/10255842.2017.1423289. PMID: 29318898
8. Farooqi, K.M., Mahmood, F.: Innovations in preoperative planning: Insights into another dimension using 3d printing for cardiac disease. J. Cardiothorac. Vasc. Anesth. (2017, in Press). https://doi.org/10.1053/j.jvca.2017.11.037
9. Fitzpatrick, J.M.: Fiducial registration error and target registration error are uncorrelated. In: Proceedings Volume 7261, Medical Imaging 2009: Visualization, Image-Guided Procedures, and Modeling, vol. 726102, pp. 7261:1–7261:12 (2009). https://doi.org/10.1117/12.813601
10 Joskowicz, L.: Computer-aided surgery meets predictive, preventive, and personalized medicine. EPMA J. **8**(1), 1–4 (2017). https://doi.org/10.1007/s13167-017-0084-8
11. Lubbers, H.T., Jacobsen, C., Matthews, F., Gratz, K.W., Kruse, A., Obwegeser, J.A.: Surgical navigation in craniomaxillofacial surgery: expensive toy or useful tool? A classification of different indications. J. Oral Maxillofac. Surg. **69**(1), 300–308 (2011). https://doi.org/10.1016/j.joms.2010.07.016
12. Magnenat-Thalmann, N., Bonanni, U.: Haptic Sensing of Virtual Textiles, pp. 513–523. Birkhäuser Basel, Basel (2008). https://doi.org/10.1007/978-3-7643-7612-3_43
13. Majak, M., Żuk, M., Świątek-Najwer, E., Popek, M., Pietruski, P.: Biopsy procedure applied in Mentoreye Molecular Surgical Navigation System. In: Proceedings of the VI ECCOMAS Thematic Conference on Computational Vision and Medical Image Processing, VipIMAGE 2017, Porto, Portugal, 18–20 October 2017, pp. 338–344. Springer International Publishing, Cham (2018). https://doi.org/10. 1007/978-3-319-68195-5_37
14. Moustris, G.P., Hiridis, S.C., Deliparaschos, K.M., Konstantinidis, K.M.: Evolution of autonomous and semi-autonomous robotic surgical systems: a review of the literature. Int. J. Med. Robot. Comput. Assist. Surg. **7**(4), 375–392 (2011). https:// doi.org/10.1002/rcs.408

15. Naujokat, H., Rohnen, M., Lichtenstein, J., Birkenfeld, F., Gerle, M., Florke, C., Wiltfang, J.: Computer-assisted orthognathic surgery: evaluation of mandible registration accuracy and report of the first clinical cases of navigated sagittal split ramus osteotomy. Int. J. Oral Maxillofac. Surg. **46**(10), 1291–1297 (2017). https://doi.org/10.1016/j.ijom.2017.05.003

16. Pietruski, P., Majak, M., Świątek-Najwer, E., Popek, M., Jaworowski, J., Żuk, M., Nowakowski, F.: Image-guided bone resection as a prospective alternative to cutting templates-a preliminary study. J. Cranomaxillofac. Surg. **43**(7), 1021–1027 (2015). https://doi.org/10.1016/j.jcms.2015.06.012

17. Pietruski, P., Majak, M., Świątek-Najwer, E., Popek, M., Szram, D., Żuk, M., Jaworowski, J.: Accuracy of experimental mandibular osteotomy using the image-guided sagittal saw. Int. J. Oral Maxillofac. Surg. **45**(6), 793–800 (2016). https://doi.org/10.1016/j.ijom.2015.12.018

18. Robles-De-La-Torre, G.: Virtual reality: touch/haptics. In: Encyclopedia of Perception, vol. 2. Sage Publications (2009)

19. Rosenthal, E.L., Warram, J.M., Bland, K.I., Zinn, K.R.: The status of contemporary image-guided modalities in oncologic surgery. Ann. Surg. **261**(1), 46 (2015). https://doi.org/10.1053/j.jvca.2017.11.037

20. Schneider, O., MacLean, K., Swindells, C., Booth, K.: Haptic experience design: what hapticians do and where they need help. Int. J. Hum. Comput. Stud. **107**(Supplement C), 5–21 (2017). https://doi.org/10.1016/j.ijhcs.2017.04.004. Multisensory Human-Computer Interaction

21. Seeberger, R., Kane, G., Hoffmann, J., Eggers, G.: Accuracy assessment for navigated maxillo-facial surgery using an electromagnetic tracking device. J. Craniomaxillofac. Surg. **40**(2), 156–161 (2012). https://doi.org/10.1016/j.jcms.2011.03.003

22. Sreelakshmi, M., Subash, T.: Haptic technology: a comprehensive review on its applications and future prospects. In: Materials Today: Proceedings of the International Conference on Computing, Communication, Nanophotonics, Nanoscience, Nanomaterials and Nanotechnology, vol. 4, no. 2, Part B, pp. 4182–4187 (2017). https://doi.org/10.1016/j.matpr.2017.02.120

23. Strong, E., Rafii, A., Holhweg-Majert, B., Fuller, S., Metzger, M.: Comparison of 3 optical navigation systems for computer-aided maxillofacial surgery. Arch. Otolaryngol. Head Neck Surg. **134**(10), 1080–1084 (2008). https://doi.org/10.1001/archotol.134.10.1080

24. Świątek-Najwer, E., Majak, M., Żuk, M., Popek, M., Kulas, Z., Jaworowski, J., Pietruski, P.: The new computer and fluorescence-guided system for planning and aiding oncological treatment. In: CARS 2017–Computer Assisted Radiology and Surgery–Proceedings of the 31th International Congress and Exhibition, vol. 2, pp. S1–S286 (2017)

25. Świątek-Najwer, E., Żuk, M., Majak, M., Popek, M.: The rigid registration of CT and scanner dataset for computer aided surgery. In: Proceedings of the VI ECCOMAS Thematic Conference on Computational Vision and Medical Image Processing, VipIMAGE 2017, Porto, Portugal, 18–20 October 2017, pp. 345–353. Springer International Publishing, Cham (2018). https://doi.org/10.1007/978-3-319-68195-5_38

Time Regarded Method of 3D Ultrasound Reconstruction

Jan Juszczyk[(⊠)], Marta Galinska, and Ewa Pietka

Faculty of Biomedical Engineering,
Silesian University of Technology, Roosevelta 40, Zabrze, Poland
jan.juszczyk@polsl.pl

Abstract. Ultrasound (US) examination is the most commonly used method for visualizing internal organs, and is usually used as a 2D visualisation method. Despite the fact that many ultrasound machines have '3D free hand' protocols or they are equipped with a volumetric US probe, 3D volumetric reconstruction is popular mainly in obstetrics. 3D reconstruction and visualization of abdominal organs is difficult for two reasons. First – abdominal organs are large and the entire organ cannot be shown at once, and second – organs are moving. In this paper, a new approach to freehand 3D ultrasound reconstruction and visualisation is presented. The main idea of this approach is to not use all recorded data in the same time, but dynamically change the reconstruction model. Besides, typical order of the algorithm steps was changed. In the first step the segmentation is performed and in the second step the volume reconstruction is done. Usefulness of this approach was tested on Z-shaped phantom images. The median of error (RMSE) for obtained models is less than 0.41 mm with respect to the reference models. For the same data set the median RMSE for the standard reconstruction method (excluded the impact of registration time) is about 0.71 mm.

Keywords: Ultrasound volume reconstruction · 3D visualization
Ultrasound image segmentation

1 Introduction

Ultrasound examination is a widely used non-invasive diagnostic procedure because of its efficiency, safety and low costs. The main disadvantages of this technique are high noise and lack of the visibility of surrounding tissues in other directions. A 3D US probe may be useful for observing large and complicated shapes but because of the low image quality, radiologists commonly uses 2D image presentations. It is impossible to avoid lack of the visibility of surrounding tissues using 2D US probe without a tracking system. Currently, electromagnetic and optical tracking systems are widely used during neurosurgery procedures. A study performed on 50 surgeons proved that an augmented reality positively affects the time and precision of the performed procedures [1]. An intra-operative

© Springer International Publishing AG, part of Springer Nature 2019
E. Pietka et al. (Eds.): ITIB 2018, AISC 762, pp. 205–216, 2019.
https://doi.org/10.1007/978-3-319-91211-0_18

ultrasound-based navigation system has been successfully used for craniotomy planning [2] and brain shift correction [3,4].

However, the difference between neuro and soft tissue surgery lies in the rigidity of the surrounding tissues. Assumptions underlying navigation system requires stabilization of the observed object. In the case of soft tissue, this assumption cannot be met. For this type of chirurgical intervention (e.g. a breast surgery), a new method of the 3D visualization is needed.

The PLUS (Public software Library for Ultrasound) open source toolkit is widely used for image-guided interventions [5] and procedures (e.g. needle tracking [6]). The toolkit enables the calibration, data acquisition, preprocessing, real-time visualization of scanned areas in 3D space, reconstruction the path of the tracked probe, and volume reconstruction of image data. The tool for 3D volume reconstruction requires a set of 2D images and corresponding transform matrices. The basis of this method is the iterative insertion of the values of the pixels into the reconstructed volume. This process enables the transition between local 2D image space with its 3D global position and 3D global space. Calculation of the voxel values may be based on different types of interpolation (nearest neighbor or linear interpolation) and compounding overlapping pixels may be computed based on mean, maximum or latest values. A hole-filling algorithm has been implemented also for quality improvement when recorded data are insufficient to fill all voxels (output spacing is too low). The foregoing article arose based on study published by Gobbi in 2002 [7], where authors described a real-time method for 3D volume reconstruction of the phantom imitated cranium.

In 1999 Rohling proposed a new Radial Basis Function (RBF) reconstruction technique [8]. It is an interpolation method based on a 3D kernel. The RBF based method were compared to the other techniques - Pixel Nearest Neighbor (PNN), Voxel Nearest Neighbor (VNN) and Distance-Weighted (DW) interpolation. According to the results, the RBF method performed at least as well as the other methods and in some cases improved results. One disadvantage of RBF is the processing speed. Recently published papers show an adaptive kernel regression method which reduces speckles in homogeneous regions and preserves edges in inhomogeneous areas [9]. The main disadvantage of this method - time consumption - is minimized by the parallel computing [10].

Another approach to improve the reconstruction is to use filters [11]. Median and Weighted-Median Filters produced smaller interpolation errors, preserved tissue boundaries, and reduced speckles.

In a review of freehand 3D US reconstruction algorithms, the autors divided the methods into three groups: Voxel-Based Methods (VBM), Pixel-Based Methods (PBM) and Function-Based Method (FBM) [12]. According to this comparison, PNN methods are more accurate than VNN ones. Using a 3D kernel may improve results but it requires disproportionate computational costs.

All of the above 3D volume reconstruction methods are efficient for observing rigid objects. According to our best knowledge, there are no methods for visualization deformable or moving volumes which take into account the time dependency.

We decided to describe an issue and find a solution by making the data adequacy and reliability dependent on the acquisition moment. The data subset collected in shorter time period should be more reliable than larger data subset collected in longer one.

The main purpose of this study is to propose a new method for 3D data visualization taking into account a confidence map depending on the time of the recorded frames. It enables the visualization of a reliable image of the tissues under radiological observation at the specific time of the examination. Simultaneous reinforcing voxels lying near the target in the specified moment and weakening unreliable areas (due to the tissue shift) may improve visualization of the lesion area. The method is especially useful for tissues undergoing large displacement and deformations.

2 Materials and Methods

The proposed solution is to create a new, time dependent visualization method for dynamic 3D US image data, where the data sets consists of 2D US image series and corresponding affine transformations.

Datasets are collecting during a freehand scan of the phantom. The object can be fixed or moving up and down. In the moving case, the rate of collected frames should be suitable for the movement speed. Quality of a volume reconstruction might be poor when frame-rate is too low.

The obtained model is fully correct only when the imaged object is fixed. Otherwise, when the object is moving, there is no possibility to obtain a whole model simultaneously without information about the object trajectory. It is necessary to assume the width of the time window when the object can be treated as static. Value of the width parameter depends on the movement speed of the object. The idea of the method is to divide the dataset into several time windows and reconstruct each of them separately. Partial models can be used for full model reconstruction in post-processing if needed.

The method can be divided into several steps (Fig. 1).

First, images are pre-segmented in preprocessing step to simplify the model. During acquisition, images are manually preprocessed to decrease the size of the volumes and to cut out unnecessary layout elements. The size of each frame is limited to useful image information only.

Next, the object elements are segmented on 2D images. In general, the 2D segmentation method should be fast and simple because it is time consuming. The method is assumed to be a real time method, e.g. for the Z-shaped phantom (Fig. 2), 2D segmentation algorithm consists of a thresholding step and morphological dilation using circular structural element.

For different types of objects, any other segmentation method can be used. For example, if doppler images are recorded and the blood vessels are segmented, the Red-channel or the Blue-channel separation (from RGB images) should be the one of the steps in 2D segmentation. However, the quality of obtained results of 2D segmentation directly affects the quality of the whole 3D reconstruction.

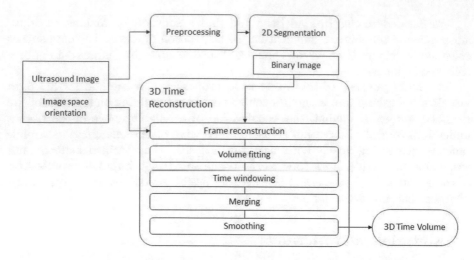

Fig. 1. Workflow, all steps have beend descibed in text

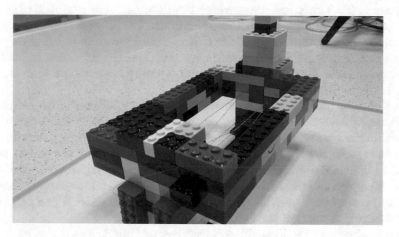

Fig. 2. Constructed Z-shaped Lego bricks phantom

The first recorded frame is a point of reference for each subsequent frames. Each raster 2D image is converted into a 3D raster volume according to the corresponding affine transformation matrix. This frame reconstruction is performed using linear interpolation. Each volume may have a different size depending on the angle between the first and current frame. Based on extreme points of singular volumes, the size of the output volume is estimated. Each frame is inserted into an empty volume of known dimensions.

In the next step, the frames of interest are selected from the dataset. The number of frames in the time window must be adjusted to the frame rate and the object speed. The narrower the time window, the more accurate the reconstruction is, but a smaller part of the imaged object is visible at the same time and more partial models are needed.

In the merging step, selected frames are accumulated in an output volume. A common coordinate system allows a logical disjunction. Each voxel which is marked as belonging to the object in at least one frame belongs to the output mask.

The next step is the smoothing model. Based on the output mask obtained from logical operations on frames, a partial model is formed. It is subjected to morphological dilation using spherical structuring element due to the lack of information about voxels omitted during a freehand scan. The size of the sphere is determined by the resolution of input images, framerate, and speed of the probe during scanning.

For visualization purposes and the quality tests, the obtained volume-raster model is converted to a surface by using the Marching Cubes algorithm. Finally, the obtained vector model can be visualized in many 3D graphic environments, for example Slicer.

3   Experiment

The Z-shaped phantom used to perform the experiment consists of Lego bricks and seven fishing lines (Fig. 2). The phantom was submerged in water at room temperature.

The layout of the lines is designed to easily assess the accuracy of 3D reconstruction and determine the position of the 2D image. The thickness of the lines was constant at 0.3 mm. Four lines were placed in parallel connecting the opposite corners of the frame and the other three lines were angled to determine the distance from the corners. The full dimensions have been presented in Fig. 3.

US data were recorded using the Philips iU22 ultrasound machine with linear transducer Philips L12-5 and Small Parts Breast Advanced proBot. NDI Polaris Vicra camera and 2 markers attached to the US transducer and phantom base surface were used as a tracking system. The tracking system was calibrated using the PLUS toolkit [5]. Full probe calibration is needed to register a proper dataset. Epiphan DVI2USB3.0 Video Grabber with frame rate 10 Hz was used to capture the image data from the ultrasound machine. PLUS library version 2.4 was used for probe calibration and reference reconstruction. Reference 3D volumes (US) were obtained using the same ultrasound machine with matrix convex transducer Philips X6-1. The virtual model (VM) was created based on dimensional measurements of the constructed phantom. The diameter of the fishing lines was set as the size of the ultrasound echo from the wire on the US image. The virtual model was subjected to the same processing steps as other data sets.

The experiment can be divided into two stages (Fig. 4). First, the tracking system calibration was performed and the fixed phantom was scanned along the long axis. Next, the same phantom was moved up and down with straight linear movement in both directions with an average speed of the phantom of 1 mm/s, however US scanning was performed in-line and independently also. Images and their position data were computed and 3D static (FM) and 3D dynamic (WT)

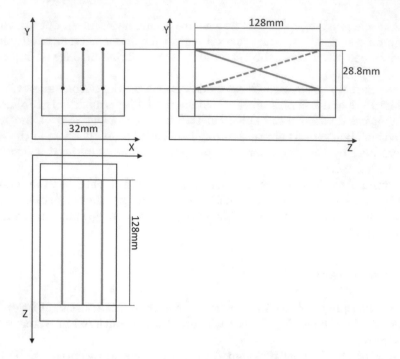

Fig. 3. Dimmensions of the phantom used in three ortogonal plane

models were reconstructed using all recorded frames. Dynamic data has been divided into several time windows and reconstruction has been performed for each window separately (TR). The results have been compared with the static model, virtual metric model, and model obtained from the volumetric US probe.

4   Results and Discussion

The dataset, acquired for Time Regarded Reconstruction, was divided into 10 subsets of 30 frames, except the last subset was 23 frames only. The remaining four data sets (Virtual Metric Model, Fixed Model, Whole Time Reconstruction Model and 3D Ultrasound Model) were divided into 10 subsets corresponding to the volume and position of the TR sets. The subsets from each type of model, have been brought to a common coordinate system. Because in the experiment the global position of each set was not important, the registration was performed for each subset separately. The registration was performed by using the Iterative Closest Point (ICP) algorithm [15] after manual pre-registration. The ICP algorithm can be useful for the registration of point clouds or surfaces obtained from many various types of 3D data [16].

Root Mean Squared Error (RMSE) was used for verifying of the efficiency of the proposed reconstruction method. RMSE was calculated according to the formula:

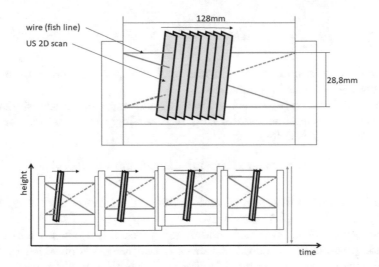

Fig. 4. Static and dynamic stage of the experiment; during whole experiment the phantom was scanned along the long axis; in the static stage the phantom was fixed and in the dynamic stage it was moved up and down during scanning

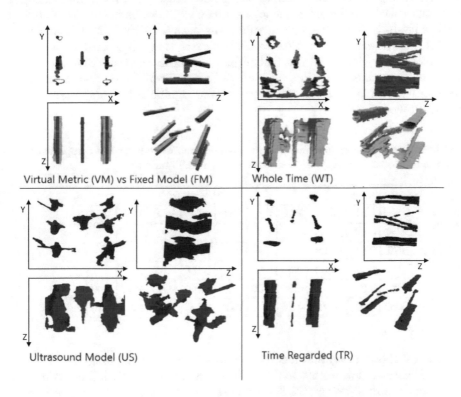

Fig. 5. Visualisation of obtained models for first subset contains 30 frames, Virtual Metric Model (cyan) and Fixed Model (yellow) are treated as refrence model

$$RMSE = \sqrt{\frac{1}{n}\sum_{t=1}^{n} e_t^2} \tag{1}$$

where n denotes a number of verticles and e is a fitness error between two corresponding verticles in milimeters.

Hausdorff distance (d_H) has been used as a measure of the sets similarity for evaluation of the obtained results [13]. It is a widely used method for surface comparison [14]. It is defined as:

$$d_H(X,Y) = \max\{\sup_{x \in X} \inf_{y \in Y} d(x,y), \sup_{y \in Y} \inf_{x \in X} d(x,y)\} \tag{2}$$

where d is Euclidean distance, X and Y denotes two non-empty sets, x and y are samples in X and Y, respectively.

Visualization of all obtained models are presented in Figs. 5 and 6. Mean and median values of Hausdorff distances between models obtained by the five different techniques are presented in Table 1. The abbreviations used in tables below signifies various methods.

The highest values of the Hausdorff distances was observed for the model obtained using 3D US probe. This data has been recorded using a matrix convex transducer with a different frequency range and will not be taken into account in further analysis. The lowest mean value was between Virtual Metric and Fixed Models and it was 3.4 mm. This result indicates that 3D reconstruction of the Fixed Model is similar to the real object. Proposed method achieved similar or even better median values to Virtual Metric and Fixed Models (2.9 mm). Results for Whole Time Reconstruction were significantly worse than for proposed method.

Table 1. The juxtaposition of various reconstruction methods; paired comparison analysis for Hausdorff distances between methods (in millimeters)

	Mean					Median				
	VM	WT	FM	US	TR	VM	WT	FM	US	TR
VM	0.00					0.00				
WT	9.01	0.00				5.43	0.00			
FM	3.41	9.02	0.00			3.09	5.03	0.00		
US	9.55	10.32	8.04	0.00		8.03	9.06	7.87	0.00	
TR	4.04	5.12	4.70	8.01	0.00	2.90	3.59	2.95	7.10	0.00

Table 2 shows mean and median values of RMSE after using the ICP algorithm. Relatively low results confirmed efficiency of the ICP method. Almost all of obtained values, except US 3D Volume, were lower than 0.7 mm. As before, the best results were obtained using the for proposed method and Fixed Model compared to Virtual Model.

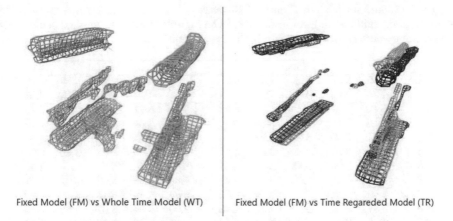

Fixed Model (FM) vs Whole Time Model (WT)   Fixed Model (FM) vs Time Regareded Model (TR)

Fig. 6. Wireframe visualisations shows differences between Fixed Model (yellow, as a reference model) and Whole Time Model (green) and Time Regarded Model (red) respectively, the quality of the model has been artificially reduced

Table 2. The juxtaposition of various reconstruction methods; paired comparison analysis for Root Mean Squared Error after ICP between methods (in millimeters)

	Mean					Median				
	VM	WT	FM	US	TR	VM	WT	FM	US	TR
VM	0.00					0.00				
WT	0.54	0.00				0.54	0.00			
FM	0.66	0.75	0.00			0.35	0.71	0.00		
US	1.37	1.44	**2.38**	0.00		1.05	1.45	2.23	0.00	
TR	0.68	1.79	0.75	2.19	0.00	0.46	1.44	0.41	**2.37**	0.00

In Tables 3 and 4, d_H and $RMSE$ values of each time window reconstruction are presented. The first column denotes the quality of fit for the Virtual Metric and Fixed models. Second refers to Virtual Metric vs. Whole Time Reconstruction Model. The next column describes the fit of the Fixed and Whole Time Models. In last two columns there are comparisons of the Time Regarded with the Virtual Metric Model and the Fixed Model. In consecutive rows, corresponding time windows are presented. Mean results for different time intervals are heterogeneous for all compared methods because the object was scanned freehand with uneven speed. Comparing the median value is more suitable because of this inconsistency. Median d_H values for Time Regarded Reconstruction are significantly lower than Whole Time Reconstruction Method. Median $RMSE$ values of both methods compared to the Virtual Metric Model are similar but matching is better for the proposed method and Fixed Model.

Table 3. Mean and median Hausdorff distances obtained using various methods for all subsets (in millimeters); for each subset the highest values are marked red and the lowest are green; yellow background indicates reference value

ID	Mean					Median				
	VM--FM	VM--WT	FM--WT	VM--TR	FM--TR	VM--FM	VM--WT	FM--WT	VM--TR	FM--TR
1	5.02	11.09	13.25	2.88	6.22	3.63	5.71	6.02	2.36	2.12
2	2.23	8.22	7.92	3.59	3.27	1.67	5.69	5.98	3.19	2.89
3	3.55	9.20	8.03	5.23	4.88	3.02	5.41	4.72	3.76	3.06
4	2.74	3.62	2.86	3.57	3.41	2.74	3.45	2.81	3.30	2.95
5	3.52	10.38	9.95	3.99	4.21	3.06	5.68	5.54	1.94	2.44
6	2.19	7.27	7.50	3.34	3.47	1.69	5.53	6.32	1.92	1.81
7	4.49	11.39	12.66	5.37	7.52	3.84	5.49	6.15	4.29	7.02
8	2.87	6.54	5.01	4.22	4.28	2.90	5.04	4.07	2.80	2.73
9	3.76	11.02	11.32	4.01	4.64	3.35	5.45	5.11	2.90	4.49
10	3.69	11.38	11.11	4.26	5.05	3.45	5.97	5.20	4.50	3.50

Table 4. Mean and median $RMSE$ values obtained using various methods for all subsets (in millimeters); for each subset the highest values are marked red and the lowest are green; yellow background indicates reference value

ID	Mean					Median				
	VM--FM	VM--WT	FM--WT	VM--TR	FM--TR	VM--FM	VM--WT	FM--WT	VM--TR	FM--TR
1	1.32	0.57	0.83	0.47	0.65	0.35	0.48	0.71	0.40	0.36
2	0.48	0.46	0.60	0.49	0.43	0.34	0.45	0.65	0.46	0.40
3	0.36	0.70	0.92	1.42	1.59	0.35	0.71	0.81	0.45	0.49
4	0.52	0.71	0.75	0.72	0.66	0.43	0.70	0.65	0.64	0.70
5	0.40	0.53	0.88	0.45	0.74	0.35	0.53	0.72	0.42	0.38
6	0.53	0.44	0.57	0.45	0.40	0.32	0.41	0.57	0.46	0.37
7	1.08	0.48	0.79	0.86	0.84	0.33	0.53	0.73	0.56	0.44
8	0.38	0.57	0.76	0.54	0.59	0.36	0.58	0.72	0.49	0.48
9	0.77	0.49	0.73	0.52	0.66	0.33	0.54	0.73	0.50	0.42
10	0.64	0.45	0.74	0.89	1.02	0.32	0.50	0.68	0.49	0.40

5   Conclusion

The results (shown in tables and figures) confirm that it is possible to improve the quality of the 3D ultrasound reconstruction by using a time regrading method. Further improvement is necessary especially for moving objects. The proposed method does not give better results for stationary models because of using only partial data but might accelerate reconstruction and facilitate visualization of interesting parts of the object, especially when the visualised object is moving.

Numerical results clearly show that the object displacement during scanning makes it impossible to create a reliable model using static methods.

Using the 3D volumteric US probe for 3D reconstruction does not give the best results, however the frequency of the ultrasound should be taking into account. Even the models obtained using this type of acquisition should not be use as a reference model.

Switching the typical order of image processing (using segmentation, rather than reconstruction, as the first step) accelerates image processing, which could enable on-line visualization.

The proposed solution might be implemented into clinical practice as an on-line visualization of a scanned moving and deformed object, for example breast tissue. For clinical use it is necessary to develop an automatic or semi-automatic algorithm to adjust time window width according to movement speed and to adapt the segmentation method based on the dataset.

Acknowledgement. This research was supported by the Polish National Centre for Research and Development (NCBR) grant No.: STRATEGMED2/267398/4/NCBR/ 2015. The funders had no role in study design, data collection and analysis, decision to publish, or preparation of the abstract.

References

1. Marcus, H.J., Pratt, P., Hughes-Hallett, A., Cundy, T.P., Marcus, A., Yang, G.Z., Darzi, A., Nandi, D.: Comparative effectiveness and safety of image guidance systems in neurosurgery: a preclinical randomized study. J. Neurosurg. **123**(2), 307–313 (2015). https://doi.org/10.3171/2014.10.JNS141662
2. Prada, F., Del Bene, M., Mattei, L., Casali, C., Filippini, A., Legnani, F., Mangraviti, A., Saladino, A., Perin, A., Richetta, C., Vetrano, I., Moiraghi, A., Saini, M., DiMeco, F.: Fusion imaging for intra-operative ultrasound-based navigation in neurosurgery. J. Ultrasound **17**(3), 243–251 (2014). https://doi.org/10.1007/ s40477-014-0111-8
3. Letteboer, M.M.J., Willems, P.W.A., Viergever, M.A., Niessen, W.J.: Brain shift estimation in image-guided neurosurgery using 3-D ultrasound. IEEE Trans. Biomed. Eng. **52**(2), 268–276 (2005). https://doi.org/10.1109/TBME.2004.840186
4. Comeau, R.M., Sadikot, A.F., Fenster, A., Peters, T.M.: Intraoperative ultrasound for guidance and tissue shift correction in image-guided neurosurgery. Med. Phys. **27**(4), 787–800 (2000). https://doi.org/10.1118/1.598942
5. Lasso, A., Heffter, T., Rankin, A., Pinter, C., Ungi, T., Fichtinger, G.: PLUS: opensource toolkit for ultrasound-guided intervention systems. IEEE Trans. Biomed. Eng. **61**(10), 2527–2537 (2014). https://doi.org/10.1109/TBME.2014.2322864
6. Czajkowska, J., Pyciński, B., Juszczyk, J., Pietka, E.: Biopsy needle tracking technique in US images. Comput. Med. Imaging Graph. **65**, 93–101 (2017). https:// doi.org/10.1016/j.compmedimag.2017.07.001
7. Gobbi, D.G., Peters, T.M.: Interactive intra-operative 3D ultrasound reconstruction and visualization. In: International Conference on Medical Image Computing and Computer-Assisted Intervention, vol. 2489, pp. 156–163 (2002). https://doi. org/10.1007/3-540-45787-9_20
8. Rohling, R., Gee, A., Berman, L.: A comparison of freehand three-dimensional ultrasound reconstruction techniques. Med. Image Anal. **3**(4), 339–359 (1999). https://doi.org/10.1016/S1361-8415(99)80028-0

9. Wen, T., Yang, F., Gu, J., Chen, S., Wang, L., Xie, Y.: An adaptive kernel regression method for 3D ultrasound reconstruction using speckle prior and parallel GPU implementation. Neurocomputing **275**, 208–223 (2017). https://doi.org/10.1016/j.neucom.2017.06.014

10. Daoud, M.I., Alshalalfah, A.L., Al-Najar, M.: GPU accelerated implementation of kernel regression for freehand 3D ultrasound volume reconstruction. In: Biomedical Engineering and Sciences (IECBES), pp. 586–589 (2016). https://doi.org/10.1109/IECBES.2016.7843517

11. Huang, Q.H., Zheng, Y.P.: Volume reconstruction of freehand three-dimensional ultrasound using median filters. Ultrasonics **48**(3), 182–192 (2008). https://doi.org/10.1016/j.ultras.2007.11.005

12. Solberg, O.V., Lindseth, F., Torp, H., Blake, R.E., Hernes, T.A.N.: Freehand 3D ultrasound reconstruction algorithms–a review. Ultrasound Med. Biol. **33**(7), 991–1009 (2007). https://doi.org/10.1016/j.ultrasmedbio.2007.02.015

13. Huttenlocher, D.P., Klanderman, G.A., Rucklidge, W.J.: Comparing images using the Hausdorff distance. IEEE Trans. Pattern Anal. Mach. Intell. **15**(9), 850–863 (1993). https://doi.org/10.1109/34.232073

14. Aspert, N., Santa-Cruz, D., Ebrahimi, T.: Mesh: measuring errors between surfaces using the Hausdorff distance. In: Proceedings of the 2002 IEEE International Conference on Multimedia and Expo, ICME 2002, vol. 1, pp. 705–708 (2002). https://doi.org/10.1109/ICME.2002.1035879

15. Besl, P.J., McKay, N.D.: A method for registration of 3-D shapes. IEEE Trans. Pattern Anal. Mach. Intell. **14**(2), 239–256 (1992). https://doi.org/10.1109/34.121791

16. Pycinski, B., Czajkowska, J., Badura, P., Juszczyk, J., Pietka, E.: Time-of-flight camera, optical tracker and computed tomography in pairwise data registration. PloS One **11**(7), e0159493 (2016). https://doi.org/10.1371/journal.pone.0159493

Statistical Analysis of Radiographic Textures Illustrating Healing Process After the Guided Bone Regeneration Surgery

Gabriela Girejko[1(✉)], Marta Borowska[2], and Janusz Szarmach[3]

[1] Institute of Mechatronics, Warsaw University of Technology,
św. Andrzeja Boboli 8, 02-525 Warsaw, Poland
girejkogabriela@gmail.com
[2] Faculty of Mechanical Engineering, Białystok University of Technology,
Wiejska 45C, 15-351 Białystok, Poland
[3] Department of Oral Surgery, Medical University of Białystok,
M. Curie-Skłodowskiej 24A, 15-276 Białystok, Poland

Abstract. Radiographic images of post-gastrectomy and after the cyst removal in dental bone loss registered within 1 year period. Images of 28 patients (8 images directly after the procedure and 20 images after 12 months) who underwent the Guided Bone Regeneration surgery. The X-rays were obtained using Kodak RVG 6100 set with a resolution higher than 14 pl/mm. Textural analysis of these areas included: cropping rectangular ROIs (Regions of Interest) from both types of images (right after and '1 year after' the procedure), computing following features: 3 basic (minimum, maximum, average value of pixels), GLRL matrix and GLCM. The final step was the assessment of the features and analysis of those which are statistically significant.

Keywords: Texture analysis · Radiographic images
Guided Bone Regeneration · Grey Level Run Length Matrix
Grey Level Co-occurrence Matrix

1 Introduction

Various techniques which are implemented in order to activate the process of bone regeneration are called the Guided Bone Regeneration (GBR technique). What is vital to perform such a regeneration is the use of barrier membranes. These membranes are divided into nonresorbable and resorbable membranes [1]. This technique was not clinically recognised and implemented until the early 1980s when Karring and Nyman's team performed an examination of barrier membranes in different experiments and studies for periodontal regeneration. First clinical testing of membranes was initialised among implant patients in the late 1980s. GBR is a surgical procedure with a wide biologic and biomaterial background [4].

© Springer International Publishing AG, part of Springer Nature 2019
E. Pietka et al. (Eds.): ITIB 2018, AISC 762, pp. 217–226, 2019.
https://doi.org/10.1007/978-3-319-91211-0_19

Widely studied is also the ability of bone regeneration in the neighbourhood of physical barrier such as nonporous or porous membranes, what is more the resorbable membranes are divided into natural or synthetic. Many features of the membrane such as: biocompatibility, cell occlusiveness, proper clinical manageability or the process of integration by the host tissue have an impact on the bone regeneration process [1,8]. GBR may be introduced in two cases/approaches in implant therapy: before implant placement or at a simultaneous approach during implant placement [9].

Radiographs in dentistry are commonly used, especially when it comes to analyses of a particular dental process in time. In this study parts after resection and cyst removal were taken into consideration. The wounds after such procedure are tough to heal as in these parts there is an inadequate bone volume and undesired cells may determine the type of tissue that will occupy this space. Thus, Guided Bone Regeneration technique which using barrier membranes enables the allowed cells to populate a wound area, was performed [1]. This study is based on the analysis of radiographic images of teeth. In particular, the Guided Bone Regeneration after resection and cyst removal was observed. Each image of X-ray through the analysed area was registered using Kodak RVG 6100 system. The experiment involved X-rays on the day of surgical procedure and 12 months later. The wounded areas were treated using xenogeneic bones inserted into them which are osteoconductive. What is more, barrier membranes were also implemented.

The gathered X-rays images are difficult to be analysed in detail, thus new computer-aided texture analysis methods can show the integration of the bone and proper or improper regeneration. Therefore, it is important to develop methods for radiographic interpretation of the treatment. In this analysis following textural parameters are proposed: basic features of an image (e.g. min., max, average value of pixels, entropy), Grey Level Co-Occurrence Matrix (GLCM) and Grey Level Run Length Matrix (GLRLM).

2   Materials and Methods

2.1   Patients and Surgical Procedure

In this study X-rays of 25 patients (17 women, 8 men) with diagnosis of root cysts, from Department of Oral Surgery Medical University of Białystok, were gathered. Patients were generally healthy, their medical condition did not affect the process of bone regeneration. Their average age was 35.6 years (aging from 18 to 53). The analysed areas include: 25 intraosseous cavities of IInd Dietrich's class situated in the frontal surface of maxilla (22) and mandible (3) near 34 teeth. There were no other conditions before the procedure for the patients to be qualified, so that the group could be randomised. All the surgical procedures were performed by the same authorised person. Beforehand, the group of patients underwent: endodontic treatment of teeth qualified to the GBR procedure, cleansing the oral cavity and a professional instruction related to the hygiene of oral cavity. Clinical assessment was conducted just before the surgical procedure, 2 weeks and 12 months after. Inner RTG photos were taken right after the procedure and 12 months later using Kodak RVG 6100 set with a resolution higher than 14 pl/mm. In order to gather these X-rays a narrowing beam collimator which is based on the right-angle technique with a constant time of exposure: 0.08 s was introduced. The photos were saved as MPG files, archived and later converted to bitmaps (.bmp) and analysed [3].

All the mentioned procedures were performed in a typical way due to the protocol and under a local anaesthesia. Bone deficits were filled with a BioOss$^{®}$ xenogeneic material and covered with a resorbable membrane: BioGide$^{®}$. Bone substitute, BioOss$^{®}$, in small granules (0.25–1 mm), is a natural formulation received from deproteinised beef bone. Its topographic and chemical structure, morphology and hydrophilic properties show its high resemblance to biological bone. The porosity of this material is also very similar to biological properties as it reaches 60%. Each wound after surgical procedure was stabilised with single stitches using synthetic thread (5–0 thick). Postoperative care included antibiotics, pain relievers and oral rinse with a 0.12% chlorhexidine gluconate. After performing GBR procedure using Geistlich BioOss$^{®}$ osteoconductive material and Geistlich BioGide$^{®}$ collagen membranes in order to fill bone loss parts no postoperative complications were observed and all the cases reached a good (stable) clinical result [2].

2.2   Image Analysis

Textural analysis methods implemented in this study include: basic image parameters such as: maximum, minimum and average pixel value, entropy, standard deviation, GLRL (Grey Level Run Length Matrix) and GLCM (Grey Level Co-occurrence Matrix. Grey Level Co-Occurrence matrix is a mathematical tool based on the analysis of grey tone spatial dependence in texture [7]. If we consider $I : Z^2 \ni D \to G = \{1, \ldots, N_g\}$ as a two-dimensional discrete image, the co-occurrence matrix for this image is defined as:

$$P_o(k, l|d, \delta) = \# \{m, n \in D : I(m) = k, l(n) = l, |m - n| = d, \angle(m - n) = \delta\} \qquad (1)$$

where k, l are grey levels of points m and n, $\angle(m - n)$ represents the angle between vector $\mathbf{mn}$ and axis $\mathbf{OX}$, d respectively is the distance between m and n, δ is the direction of co-occurrence, the power of set X is represented by $\#X$. In the particular code which was implemented following features are computed: autocorrelation, contrast, correlation, cluster prominence, cluster shade, dissimilarity, energy (Matlab), entropy, homogeneity (Matlab), homogeneity, maximum probability, sum of squares: variance, sum average, sum variance, sum entropy, difference variance, difference entropy, information measure of correlation 1, information measure of correlation 2, inverse difference, diagonal moment. The process used to create the GLCM is shown in Fig. 1. The point (1, 1) in GLCM has a value of 1 as there is only one case in the input image where two horizontally adjoining pixels have the values 1 and 1. Cognately, point (2, 1) in GLCM has a value of 2.

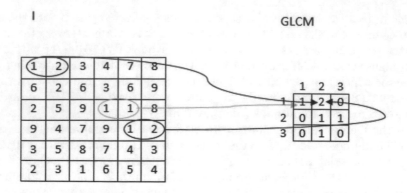

Fig. 1. Illustration of GLCM method, I: input image, GLCM: GLCM values

The coefficients are defined in the paper by Śmietanski [11]. The potential of GLCM matrix is high as it is a universal method [11]. If run-length matrix is considered, it is a method which enables searching an image across a particular direction. The aim of the run-length matrix is to find runs of consecutive pixels with the same grey level value in the given direction [4]. Most often, four matrices are computed: vertical, horizontal and two diagonal directions. The code derived from Mathworks: File Exchange offers computing 7 features: short run emphasis (SRE), long run emphasis (LRE), grey level non-uniformity (GLN), run percentage (RP), run length nonuniformity (RLN), low grey level run emphasis (LGRE), high grey level run emphasis (HGRE). For instance, short run emphasis is defined as: a value of proportion of runs which occur in the image and have short length [5]. Let $I(i, j)$ be the number of runs of pixels with a run length j and grey level i, n_r – total runs in GRLR matrix. Four basic parameters of run length matrix are defined in Table 1.

Table 1. Basic coefficients of GLRL matrix [6]

Texture features	Formulae
Short run emphasis	$f_1 = \frac{1}{n_r} \sum_i \sum_j I(i, j)/j^2$
Long run emphasis	$f_2 = \frac{1}{n_r} \sum_i \sum_j I(i, j) \times j^2$
Gray level nonuniformity	$f_3 = \frac{1}{n_r} \sum_i (\sum_j I(i, j))^2$
Run-length nonuniformity	$f_4 = \frac{1}{n_r} \sum_j (\sum_i I(i, j))^2$

3   Results

In total, there were 28 registered images, 8 right after the surgical procedure and 20 of them twelve months after. The preparation process of images included: cropping a rectangular ROI (Region of Interest), and converting each image into a bitmap. The separation of the 28 areas of interest of a size of 128 × 128 pixels (Figs. 2 and 3) was performed in CorelDRAW software. The next step was textural analysis based on computing: minimum, maximum, average value of pixels, entropy, standard deviation as well as GLRL (Gray Level Run Length) matrix and GLCM (Grey-Level Co-Occurrence Matrix) for each region [10]. The mentioned features were computed using a self-designed Graphical User's Interface in Matlab, version: 9.3.0.713579 (R2017b). In order to calculate basic image features, built-in functions were used. Considering GLRL matrix and GLCM, the codes were derived from a free-source website: https://www.mathworks.com/matlabcentral/fileexchange/. Afterwards, each of the 56 computed features was tested using Mann–Whitney U–test in Matlab software. A hypothesis that features right after the procedure and 12 months later come from continuous distribution with equal medians, assuming that samples are independent and their length might differ was proposed. The results of this test prove the statistical significance for 11 out of 56 features. In all 11 cases, the p value of the Mann–Whitney test is smaller than 0.05. Following parameters are statistically significant: 3 basic – average, maximum and minimum value of pixels and 8 derived from GLCM matrix: autocorrelation 1 and 2, sum squares variance 1 and 2, sum average 1 and 2, sum variance 1 and 2. None parameters computed by GLRL matrix show statistically significant differences. First order statistics (value $\pm SD$) for the features shows Table 2 considering basic image parameters, whereas Tables 3 and 4: GLCM statistically significant features.

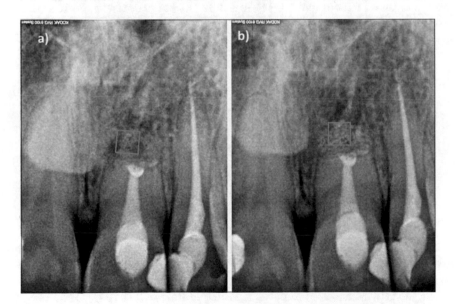

Fig. 2. Two X-ray images of the bone loss regions: (a) image right after the procedure, (b) image after 12 months, both rectangles represent regions of interest

a)    b)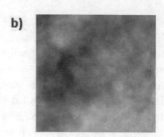

Fig. 3. Rectangular ROIs: (a) X-ray right after the procedure, (b) X-ray 12 months after

Table 2. Statistical significance and first order statistics for basic image features

	Average pixels value	Maximum pixels value	Minimum pixels value
After procedure	102.74 ± 5.31	143.00 ± 10.49	62.00 ± 7.93
After 12 months	126.99 ± 12.71	176.50 ± 20.69	78.60 ± 12.38
p value	<0.001	<0.001	<0.001

Table 3. Statistical significance and first order statistics for GLCM features

	Autocorrelation 1	Autocorrelation 2	Sum squares: variance 1	Sum squares: variance 2
After procedure	14.17 ± 1.27	14.18 ± 1.27	14.12 ± 1.27	14.12 ± 1.28
After 12 months	20.51 ± 3.71	20.45 ± 3.72	20.43 ± 3.70	20.43 ± 3.70
p value	<0.001	<0.001	<0.001	<0.001

Table 4. Statistical significance and first order statistics for GLCM features (2)

	Sum			
	Average 1	Average 2	Variance 1	Variance 2
After procedure	7.47 ± 0.35	7.47 ± 0.35	142.87 ± 5.24	42.94 ± 5.18
After 12 months	8.97 ± 0.80	8.97 ± 0.80	62.64 ± 11.57	62.64 ± 11.57
p value	<0.001	<0.001	<0.001	<0.001

In this study, all the features which characterize images after the procedures have lower values than the features in '1 year after' images. This is shown on the box plots in the Figs. 4, 5, 6 and 7.

For the GLCM features in pairs, a Multiple Range Test (95%, LSD test) was obtained using Statgraphics 18® centurion software. The results are presented in Table 5.

Table 4 represents multiple comparison method which determines which means are significantly different from which others. The method used to discriminate among the means is Fisher's least significant difference (LSD). There is a significant difference between features computed for images right after the surgery and parameters calculated for images registered '1 year after' Table 5.

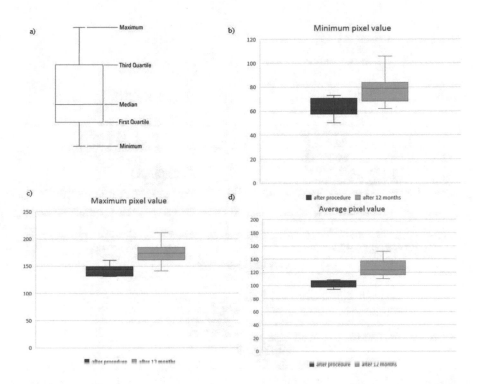

Fig. 4. Results of box plots of: (a) scheme of whisker plot, (b) minimum pixel value, (c) maximum pixel value, (d) average pixel value, computed on the basis of radiographic ROIs registered directly after the surgery (dark gray) and '1 year after' (light gray)

Table 5. Multiple Range Test performed for GLCM features of images directly after surgery and 12 months after (names with_1 ending), * – denotes a statistically significant difference (significance level was set to 5%, SoS: sum of squares)

	Significant difference	Difference	± Limits
Autocorrelation 1 – Autocorrelation 1_1	*	−6.34	2.72
Autocorrelation 2 – Autocorrelation 2_1	*	−6.33	2.72
SoS: Variance 1 – Sos: Variance 1_1	*	−6.33	2.71
SoS: Variance 2 – Sos: Variance 2_1	*	−6.32	2.71
Sum average 1 – Sum average 1_1	*	−1.49	0.59
Sum average 2 – Sum average 2_1	*	−1.49	0.59
Sum variance 1 – Sum variance 1_1	*	−19.76	8.60
Sum variance 2 – Sum variance 2_1	*	−19.69	8.60

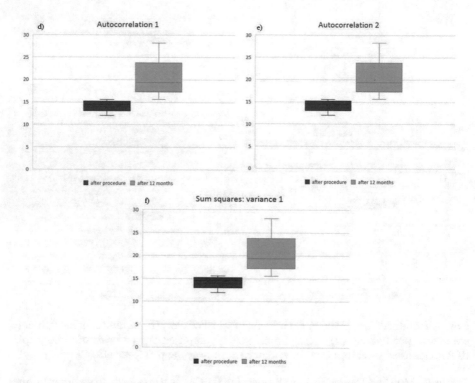

Fig. 5. Results of box plots of: (d) autocorrelation 1, (e) autocorrelation 2, (f) sum squares: variance 1, computed on the basis of radiographic ROIs registered directly after the surgery (dark gray) and '1 year after' (light gray)

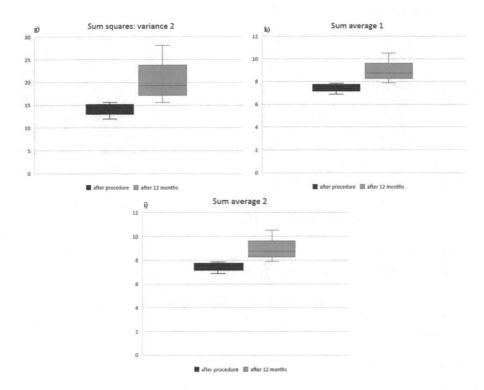

Fig. 6. Results of box plots of: (g) sum squares: variance 2, (h) sum average 1, (i) sum average 2, computed on the basis of radiographic ROIs registered directly after the surgery (dark gray) and '1 year after' (light gray)

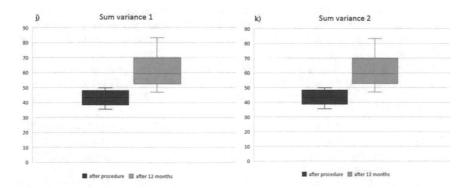

Fig. 7. Results of box plots of: (j) sum variance 1, (k) sum variance 2, computed on the basis of radiographic ROIs registered directly after the surgery (dark gray) and '1 year after' (light gray)

4   Conclusion

Textural analysis, including basic image parameters as well as GLCM or GLRL matrix are very useful considering quantitative assessment of radiological images. In this study, 11 out of 56 features describing relations between grey tone pixels have an impact on the result. All the computed factors reached much higher values in the images registered '1 year after' than the ones in the images right after the procedure. A higher homogeneity of the '1 year after' images may be assumed and also the process of healing may be observed. On the grounds of statistical results and clinical opinion, combining radiology and textural analysis of an image, the process of healing after performing the Guided Bone Regeneration procedure can be evaluated in detail.

Compliance with Ethical Standards

Conflicts of Interest

The authors declare that they have no conflict of interest.

Acknowledgement. The research was performed as a part of the projects S/WM/1/ 2017 and was financed with the founds for science from the Polish Ministry of Science and Higher Education.

References

1. Benic, I.G., Hämmerle, F.H.C.: Horizontal bone augmentation by means of guided bone regeneration. Periodontology **2000**(66), 13–40 (2014)
2. Borowska, M., et al.: Fractal dimension in textures analysis of xeno transplants, SIViP (2017). https://doi.org/10.1007/s11760-017-1108-5
3. Borowska, M., et al.: Fractal texture analysis of the healing process after bone loss. Comput. Med. Imaging Graph. **46**, 191–196 (2015)
4. Buser, D.: 20 Years of Guided Bone Regeneration in Implant Dentistry, 2nd edn. Quintessence Publishing Co, Inc., Chicago (2009). ISBN 978-0-86715-401-6
5. Castellano, G., et al.: Texture analysis of medical images. Clin. Radiol. **59**, 1061–1069 (2004)
6. Gunduz–Demir C., Burak Tosun A.: Graph run-length matrices for histopathological image segmentation. IEEE Trans. Med. Imaging **30**(3), 721–732 (2011)
7. Haralick, M.R.: Statistical and structural approaches to texture. Proc. IEEE **67**(5), 786–804 (1979)
8. Hardwick, R., Scantlebury, T., Sanchez, R., Whitley, N., Ambruster, J.: Membrane design criteria for guided bone regeneration of the alveolar ridge. In: Buser, D., Dahlin, C., Schenk, R. (eds.) Guided Bone Regeneration in Implant Dentistry, pp. 101–136. Quintessence, Chicago (1994)
9. Liu, J., Kerns, G.D.: Mechanisms of guided bone regeneration: a review. Open Dent. J. **8**(Suppl 1-M3) 56–65 (2014)
10. MathWorks—Makers of MATLAB and Simulink. https://www.mathworks.com/ help/images/ref/graycomatrix.html
11. Śmietański, J., et al.: Texture analysis in perfusion images of prostate cancer - a case study. Int. J. Appl. Math. Comput. Sci. **20**(1), 149–156 (2010)

Computer-Aided Diagnosis

Determination of the Cognitive Model: Compressively Sensed Ground Truth of Cerebral Ischemia to Care

Artur Przelaskowski[1]([✉]), Ewa Sobieszczuk[2], and Izabela Domitrz[3]

[1] Faculty of Mathematics and Information Science,
Warsaw University of Technology, 75 Koszykowa st., 00-662 Warsaw, Poland
arturp@mini.pw.edu.pl
[2] Department of Neurology, 1st Faculty of Medicine,
Medical University of Warsaw, 1a Banacha st., 02-097 Warsaw, Poland
[3] Department of Neurology, 2nd Faculty of Medicine,
Medical University of Warsaw, 80 Ceglowska st., 01-809 Warsaw, Poland

Abstract. Reported research concerns optimized methods of computerized clinical decision support on the example of stroke care management. New paradigm of compressive cognition is presented and discussed including implementation of the proposed empirical model designed to improve ischemia description and aid reperfusion therapy. The concept of semantic compressed sensing was developed to analyze clinically conditioned consensus of ground truth formulated basing on semantic descriptors of objectified expert ratings, interview data analysis, monitoring of vital signs, lab measurements, the results of physical examinations and imaging studies. The designated sparse model allows determining the interrelationship between subjective interpretations of physicians completing comprehensive picture of pathology in emergency conditions. According to the experiments carried out, the obtained effectiveness of stroke diagnosis and prediction of the effects of applied therapy is very high. The potential benefit is not only important for the patient and the physician, but also for the whole society, by significantly reducing the socio-economic costs of caring for a stroke patient.

Keywords: Compressed sensing · Cognitive models
Semantic patterns · Computer-aided diagnosis
Clinical decision support · Stroke care

1 Introduction

Computerized support of medical diagnosis and, in the wide range, clinical decision support (CDS) systems are the application context of the reported research. The keynote is the development of compressive cognition paradigm based on reliably recovered sparse model of domain knowledge and skills invariant to clinical conditioning of decision making. The cognitive model is designed and then

© Springer International Publishing AG, part of Springer Nature 2019
E. Pietka et al. (Eds.): ITIB 2018, AISC 762, pp. 229–242, 2019.
https://doi.org/10.1007/978-3-319-91211-0_20

adaptively optimized in a given clinical area for constituting clinical decisions. These concepts refer to the traditional model-based cognition based on the experimental knowledge (sensing of the real signals and phenomenons, data analysis, verification and inference), resulting in model design and implementation, next cognitive model verification and optimization rooted in experienced effectiveness and suitability with feedback according to improved cognitive criteria. Semantic descriptors are used to sparsify and consequently to simplify the problem defining kernel understanding its specificity instead of data-dependent uncontrolled assumptions. Development and implementation of the proposed paradigm is possible through use new concepts of signal measurement, representation and processing called compressed sensing (CS) [1]. Sparse signal representations were used to control sensing and signal recovery procedures while structured representations and semantic models can be used in direct signal analysis and information reconstruction according to predefined user-model [2]. This concept of the cognitive model is innovative, different from the ones used so far, e.g using linguistic description of the image content and artificial intelligence methodology [3].

This paper outlines the theoretical assumptions of the paradigm of the compressive cognition model (CCogModel) and clarifies the implementation details of the cognitive model as applied to clinical decision support for diagnosis and therapy of early stroke. An important complement is the description of the experiments performed together with a discussion of results and conclusions. The philosophy of the research undertaken is as follows: (a) initial experimental verification of the lasso selector applied for ischemia numerical descriptors of clinical cases (defined in [4]) with confirmed high efficiency in stroke recognition and treatment outcome prediction on large dataset; the statistical selector was used to significantly reduce the number of case descriptors resulting in increased efficiency, (b) extending reference to the concept of empirical model that puts forward the search for an effective method of building the clinical CCogModel based on representative measurements; (c) adaptation and using the growing potential of model-dependent CS methods based on a reduced number of measurements and a sparse problem descriptors; (d) developing the model construction method based on experimentally adjusted pattern of ground truth and semantic descriptors of pathology embodiments; experimentally verified pattern was based on common expert opinion on reference cases; (e) presented attempt to implement the proposed model for stroke care problem with its experimental verification.

2   Cognitive Model Concept

Proposed model of compressive cognition is empirical one designed and optimized in iterative retrospective-to-prospective procedure based on integrated, possibly complete and reliable, sensed clinical picture of the pathology. Thus, the model is determined on the bases of accumulated knowledge and experience of the team of experts expressed in the retrospective evaluation of representative or reference cases. The learned model of numerical descriptors defining patient clinical picture is recovered basing on CS procedures, especially model-based, as sparse as possible to be effectively and possibly clearly interpreted, used to suggest clinical decisions (diagnosis, therapy).

Initially, retrospectively established Sensed Pattern of Ground Truth (Sen-PatGT) is constituted basing on gathered results of clinical sensing, rating and decision making procedures (IntResults) completed by the establishment of a joint, consistent opinion of experts with regard to a representative group of full medical histories including follow-up of treatment effects.

Next, the CCogModel is the solution of ill-posed inverse problem recovered basing on theory and algorithms of compressed sensing, including structural models and semantics. Such model could be understood as formalized description of representative expert interpretations and decision priorities. In general, it can constitute the numerical equivalence of expert experience. Moreover, using the CCogModel may balance the subjective and incomplete clinical experience of individual doctors working in emergency conditions, constituting a significant added value to their own experience, current knowledge and skills. More clarified idea of cognitive model extraction and use is presented in Fig. 1.

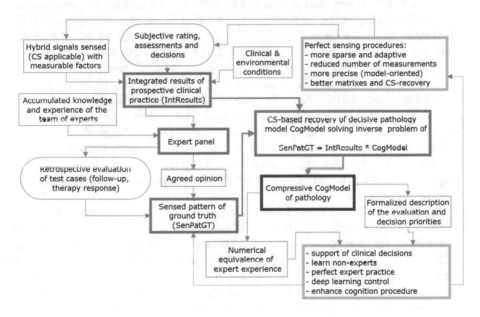

Fig. 1. The cognitive model estimation and use for clinically defined acute stroke care

More precisely, the CCogModel is compactly characterized as follows:

– integrated hybrid sensing of signals, images and vital signs, lab measurements, subjective ratings and scaled opinions (rooted in expert knowledge and skills), results of physical examinations and interview data arising from the prospective clinical practice are used to discover the meaning of the clinical reality being examined, interpret it, and then determine the right decision;

– objectified consensus of expert opinions (ground truth) is done in retrospective perspective having regard to applied diagnostic and therapeutic procedures (thrombolysis), signal sensing equipment and consequences of made decisions for credible, representative cases;
– formalized cognitive model for specific, difficult and demanding application (example of stroke care) to support key decisions is recovered basing on CS paradigm with reduced number of measurements because of assumed sparsity of reconstructed reality; sparsity of the CCogModel, regarding the dimensionality of the clinical description data space, is assumed mostly because of: (a) known and expected dependencies of the clinical observations influencing data interpretation, (b) specificity of measured signals and collected data sets, used information models, semantic descriptions, domain knowledge representatives etc., (c) repeatable monitoring and data sensing etc.; thus, the CCogModel is solution of inverse problem defined as follows

$$\mathbf{y} = \mathbf{A}\mathbf{x} + \varepsilon \tag{1}$$

where $\mathbf{x} \in \mathrm{I\!R}^N$ is searched K-sparse CCogModel in redundant space describing the clinical picture numerically while often $K \ll N$ – the sparsity ratio is defined as $\beta = K/N$; $\mathbf{y} \in \mathrm{I\!R}^M$ is resulting vector of agreed arrangements, i.e. retrospectively verified and established ground truth of made decisions and observed effects (SenPatGT); generally assuming that $K < M < N$ we express difficulty and often extremal complexity of reliable ground truth obtaining – adopted optimization method refers rather to the determination of credibly interpreted, possibly representative and complete cases of pathology description than to automatic methods of analyzing countless data sets (big data); $\mathbf{A} \in \mathrm{I\!R}^{M \times N}$ is sensing matrix consisting N descriptors/measurants for each of the M reference cases; standard random sensing errors ε can also represent random imperfectness of SenPatGT estimation to be minimized in the experimental stage.
– recovered numerical model of the studied pathology is the essence of a measurable pathology pattern, which is the established composition of key characteristics useful in application and interpretation; it enables: (a) enhanced cognition of lesion expressions causing more effective pathology recognition and interpreting descriptions which results in perfected follow-up care activities and therapeutic decisions; (b) perfecting procedures of information sensing and description in establishment of optimized clinical picture of stroke cases, (c) use as numerical equivalence of expert experience to learn non-experts or to control deep learning algorithms.
– computerized balancing the unavailable unique experience of reference experts with the clinical practice-based cognitive model of hybrid indicators (or descriptors) of pathology allows for the emergence of an important measurable pattern facilitating interpretation – objectified, adaptively perfected, susceptible to continuously improved learning procedures.

Cognitive model of stroke care $\tilde{\mathbf{x}}$ was extracted basing on CS formula (1) with clinically determined numerical measurements of reference cases $\mathbf{A}$ constituting the IntResults and the vector **y** of common expert ground truth determinants of the SenPatGT.

2.1   Integrated Results of Clinical Stroke Assessment

The implemented criterion of selecting complete pathology description (i.e. IntResults) included all the relevant clinical data of stroke care (neurological, radiological, acquired in the pre-hospital phase) including a series of image descriptors based on CT as the method of choice. Such numerical description of a representative set of reference cases is the result of the analysis of the reference stroke database, including about 200 cases collected over a period of 10 years in 3 centers using the evolving equipment and the imaging method in emergency. The applied measure of effectiveness was the usefulness of the respective descriptors in estimation of reliable SenPatGT.

Prehospital Descriptors of Risk of Ischemic Stroke. The set of descriptors was created based on: (a) sensed real data of vital signs measurements, i.e. blood pressure, heart rate, oxygen saturation, blood glucose level, and the assessment of consciousness on the Glasgow Coma Scale, (b) medical history data and data of physical examination, i.e. age, aggregate time of symptom onset and presence of diabetes mellitus, (c) measurable sudden signs of neurological deficit: -numbness, weakness or the inability to move one limb/side of the body, reduced, in relation to contralateral, muscular strength or fatigue which can affect arms, hands, legs and facial muscles, -trouble speaking, slurred speech or other speech disturbances, abnormal articulation or language content, -trouble seeing in one or both eyes, loss of vision, visual impairment or balance disorder, hemisensory deficit/loss, -severe headache with no known cause, dizziness or nystagmus, -confusion, trouble understanding, or consciousness disorders.

Neurological Descriptors of Stroke. The measures taken into account are primarily the assessments carried out by a neurologists in a form of: (a) NIH Stroke Scale (NIHSS) [5] used to objectively quantify the impairment to assess stroke severity basing on clinical findings such as symptom intensity and duration, (b) Stroke Bricks (StBr) [6] scale used to identify and describe the dysfunctional areas of the brain responsible for the observed symptoms, (c) the results of laboratory CITISSIMO and observational tests including primarily morphology, coagulogram, blood sodium and potassium level, cardiac enzymes and markers of inflammation, and updated vital signs measurements confirming stabilization of vital conditions.

Radiological Descriptors of Ischemia. The respective descriptors are as follows: (a) subjective radiological study resulting in ischemic stroke confirmation (Y/N type) and subjectively established subtlety of ischemic signs, expressed on a scale of 1 to 5 (higher score means increased evidence), representing certainty of decision taken; (b) a standardized, systematic radiological assessment of CT scans according to a 10-point quantitative topographic CT scan score used in patients with middle cerebral artery (MCA) stroke, called ASPECTS (The Alberta Stroke Program Early CT Score) [7], (c) NCCT[1]-based extended set of numerical ischemia measures designed to identify tissue impairment, predict tissue fate during the acute phase and estimate final tissue outcome (infarct vs recovery) affecting stroke confirmation and influencing the treatment applicability [4,8].

2.2   Sensed Pattern of Ground Truth

The SenPatGT $\in [0,1]$ is understood as the most reliable exponent of clinical assessment of representative cases (IntResults), obtained on the basis of retrospective analyzes and interpretations of collected data, made by experts according to current knowledge and experience. Realized implementation of ground truth is subjective common opinion of two supervising clinicians-experts participating emergency procedures. It concludes approximately optimum thrombolysis outcome being formulated as the expected results of the normalized outcome prediction. Such opinion was based on clinical evidence gathered in two hospital centers used in the retrospective study, agreed by the supervisors of constituted clinical evidence. Follow-up clinical data of representative cases were used to confirm (or not) the stroke occurrence and evaluate the treatment outcome (beneficial or not) confirming (or not) usefulness of applied therapy. Improved prognosis was constituted in follow-up assessment to recommend (or not, with more or less conviction) therapy for test cases of stroke untreated with thrombolysis in analyzed dataset. Such suggestions were predicted or proved basing on clinical analysis of stroke progression monitored in the context of all documented conditions and assessments. In particular, NIHSS -in and -out, stroke severity, subjective assessment of treatment outcome (SATO), occurrence of symptomatic intracranial haemorrhage (SICH), HAT score (risk of SICH and risk of fatal ICH after rtPA) [9], DRAGON score (likelihood of good outcome, likelihood of miserable outcome after rtPa, probability of good clinical outcome) [10], iSCORE (risk of SICH, risk of 30 day mortality, risk of 30 day disability) [11] were taken into account above all.

2.3   Compressed Sensing of the Cognitive Model

Standard CS framework relies on: (a) limited, possibly minimal number of fixed in advance measurements related to K-sparsity of recovered $\mathbf{x}$, (b) the sparsity or approximate sparsity of the signal of interests while required sparsity could be modeled with additional sparsifying basis $\mathbf{\Psi} \in \mathbb{R}^{N \times N}$, (c) RIP[2]-conditioning of the random measurement matrix with high probability or computationally tractable mutual coherence of $\mathbf{A}$ low enough; in case of additional basis used to sparsify the model, measurement matrix is $\mathbf{A} = \mathbf{\Phi}\mathbf{\Psi}$ while $\mathbf{\Phi} \in \mathbb{R}^{M \times N}$ defines

---

[1] NonContrast Computerized Tomography.

[2] Restricted Isometry Property.

real conditions of the target sensing; (d) nonlinear recovery process with a variety of algorithms including computationally tractable convex-optimization based methods or greedy iterative relaxations [12]. Thus, nonadaptive process of standard CS measurements is modeled with random projections incoherent with any fixed sparsifying basis with high probability. However, adaptive measurements can lead to significant performance increase.

Construction of measurement matrix is aimed to acquire, represent and enable recovery of all important information contained in the sensed reality. Structured sparsity models of Ψ exists to fit recovery algorithms more precisely to signal specificity, including predefined semantic model [2]. Reduced degree of freedom to represent information, the structured models enable better differentiate signal semantics from recovery irrelevances or artifacts to get more robust and accurate recovery. Moreover, leveraging the structure present among the sensed signals leads to better recovery.

Commonly used $\mathbf{A}$ are random dense matrices generated by an independent identically distributed Gaussian or Bernoulli process. Computably easier matrices are sparse random or binary sparse random satisfying, structured (e.g. Toeplitz, block diagonal, permuted) or even deterministic (e.g. chirp, binary block diagonal, graph-based, Reed-Miller) all satisfying the RIP and low coherence criteria [13,14]. Because RIP condition is difficult to verify for a given $\mathbf{A}$, mutual coherence of $\mu(\mathbf{A}) = \max \frac{|\langle \mathbf{a}_i, \mathbf{a}_j \rangle|}{\|\mathbf{a}_i\|_2 \|\mathbf{a}_j\|_2} \leq 1, \ i,j = 1,\ldots,N$ is used to measure efficiency of considered measurement matrix. In case of additional sparsifying basis, coherence of $\Phi\Psi$ was beneficially verified.

The second clue problem is accurate information recovery from $\mathbf{y}$ is extremely important for cognitive model estimation based on the adopted CS framework. In standard CS we have recovered $\tilde{\mathbf{x}} = \arg\min_{\mathbf{x}} \mathcal{S}(\mathbf{x})$ subject to $\mathcal{C}(\mathbf{Ax}, \mathbf{y})$ to find the sparsest solution consistent with sensed $\mathbf{y}$. More useful equivalent unconstrained formula is

$$\tilde{\mathbf{x}} = \arg\min_{\mathbf{x}} \mathcal{S}(\mathbf{x}) + \lambda\mathcal{C}(\mathbf{Ax}, \mathbf{y}) \qquad (2)$$

The sparsity prior is number of nonzeros in $\mathbf{x}$, i.e. $\mathcal{S}(\mathbf{x}) = \|\mathbf{x}\|_0 = |\text{supp}(\mathbf{x})|$ while the consistency prior is often defined as $\mathcal{C}(\mathbf{Ax}, \mathbf{y}) = \|\mathbf{y} - \mathbf{Ax}\|_2 < \varepsilon$ for imperfect measurements for noisy conditions. Because $\|\cdot\|_0$ is nonconvex, zero pseudonorm is replaced with its convex approximation $\|\cdot\|_1$ more computationally tractable. Moreover, other forms or combinations of priors representing sparsity and consistency of the recovery are applied, e.g. $TV(\mathbf{x}) = |\nabla\mathbf{x}|$ or $\frac{1}{2}\|\mathbf{x}\|_2^2$, respectively. An opposed to convex optimization is sparse approximation used to find the sparsest solution by greedily selecting columns of $\mathbf{A}$ and iteratively forming better approximations to $\mathbf{y}$.

The procedure of ground truth sensing refers to adaptively redefined human-oriented sensing to extract iteratively recovered information-based model: expert evidence-based assessment procedure is 'sensing system'. The SenPatGT is used to develop the CCogModel basing on CS paradigm. Consequently we applied: (a) enhanced measurement matrix based on perfected numerical description of clinical cases, (b) model-oriented recovery of such measurements. Use of the

CCogModel the use of the model boils down to (a) recognition of informative objects or features in sparse reconstructed domain, (b) synergistic improvement of human sensing, numerical representation of expert decisions and recovery priors through adoption of perfected usability criteria.

Formulation of Measurement Matrix. In details, the measurement matrix of the proposed SenPatGT consists of N-dimensional numerical descriptors of M subsequent clinical reference cases. The descriptors of IntResults represent complete case description in sense of measured signal, effects of signal processing, clinical rating scores and any useful data explaining the reality of clinical picture. Thus, $\mathbf{A}$ consists of clinically determined numerical measurements representative for experimentally selected reference cases according to common opinion of experts.

Optimized sensing procedure was based on adjusting effective measurement matrix, i.e. conditioning of processed clinical $\mathbf{\Phi}$ and selection of the sparsifying $\mathbf{\Psi}$. Criterion used is relation between monitored level of mutual coherence of $\mathbf{A}$ and the efficiency of recovered implementation of stroke CCogModel. According to Welch theorem, for an $M \times N$ sensing matrix $\mathbf{A}$, the mutual coherence bound is given by $\sqrt{\frac{N-M}{M(N-1)}} \leq \mu(\mathbf{A}) \leq 1$ [14]. It means that for used $M = 32$ and $N = 115$ (radiological descriptors) or $N = 132$ (integrated clinical descriptors) we have $0.151 \leq \mu(\mathbf{A})$ or $0.155 \leq \mu(\mathbf{A})$, respectively. Mutual coherency of clinical sensing $\mathbf{\Phi}$ used in the experiments was equal to 1.

Model Recovery. The method of CCogModel recovery was initially perfected by selection of respective quality and regularization priors, including verification of different sparsifying bases $\mathbf{\Psi}$. Among tested matrices we have: (a) Perturbed Jordan block, (b) diagonally dominant, ill-conditioned, tridiagonal, (c) with eigenvalues lying on a vertical line in the complex plane, (d) symmetric sine basis, (e) symmetric Hankel, (f) tridiagonal sparse, (g) cosine basis and their random variations. Resulting mutual coherence was $.619 \leq \mu(\mathbf{\Phi\Psi}) \leq .967$ while cosine bases occurred the most effective.

Next, the optimization of procedure (2) concerned relaxed sparsity prior $\mathcal{S} = ||\mathbf{\Psi x}||_p$ while $p = 1$ for lasso or $0 < p < 1$ with elastic net. In addition, we have gradient-based regularizers $|\nabla \mathbf{x}||_p$, $p = 1$ (TV prior) or $p = 2$ (Sobolev). Then, the consistency for lasso is $\mathcal{C} = \frac{1}{2}||\mathbf{y} - \mathbf{Ax}||_2^2$ (least squares) or more generally $\mathcal{C} = ||\mathbf{y} - \mathbf{Ax}||_p^s$ where $p, s \geq 1$ (e.g. $p = 2, s = 1$ for mean squares or $p = \infty, s = 1$ for Dantzig selector).

Different algorithms of recovery were verified including implemented convex optimization of norms p_1 or p_2 in constrained or unconstrained formula. In particular, $p = 1$-based regularizer with constrained limit of $s = 2$ for imperfect measurements $- l_1\text{eq\_pd}^3$ was tested. Moreover, we considered greedy procedures related to nonconvex problem of zero pseudonorm minimization including OMP

---

[3] In implementation written by: Justin Romberg, Caltech.

[15]. But other methods tries to joint convex problem with optimization of non-smooth, possibly nonconvex regularizer implemented as Sparse Reconstruction by Separable Approximation (spaRSA) [16]. Also multiple linear regression (ML regression) was tested as reference optimizer of least squares consistency without sparsity prior.

2.4   Use of Clinical Model

Verification of the usefulness of the designated compressive cognitive model concerns the effectiveness of prediction of the thrombolytic therapy effects, i.i. probability of the favorable outcome. Formula of anticipated success of the therapy based on sparse $\tilde{\mathbf{x}}$ of (2) – i.e. recovered implementation of the CCogModel – was simply calculated as Hadamard product[4] of the CCogModel and clinical case description numerically interpreted according to the model

$$TOP(\mathbf{a}) = \mathbf{a}(\tilde{\mathbf{x}}) \circ \tilde{\mathbf{x}} \tag{3}$$

where $\mathbf{a}$ is the vector of integrated clinical descriptor for the selected test case. The Thrombolysis Outcome Predictor (TOP) is sparse exponent of susceptibility to such thrombolysis which can be classified as suggestive of therapy or warning against (Y/N). For classification, Discriminant Analysis (DA) model was applied with linear discrimination type fitted to the calculated values of TOP for test cases benchmarked according to the binarized SenPatGT.

In addition, scalar score of Thrombolysis Outcome Predictor (TOR) was proposed in a form corresponding to the subjective exponent of clinical assessment (SenPatGT) to explain in a more understandable way the model's indications. Thus, $TOR(\mathbf{A}) = \mathbf{A}\tilde{\mathbf{x}}$ was calculated for sensed set of cases $\mathbf{A}$ while $TOR(\mathbf{A}) \in [0, 1]$. To verify the efficiency of TOR, the level of linear correlation (PCorr) with SenPatGT was calculated. The numerical similarity of the numerical suggestion to the joint opinion of experts could be acceptable in clinical practice.

3   Experiments and Discussion

The research involved on the one hand verification of the sparsifying methods of the effective feature selection for classic stroke recognition and prediction of thrombolysis outcome, and on the other hand optimization of the proposed CCogModel using criteria of possibly sparse representation and accuracy of the computed model and high effectiveness of its implementation for supporting stroke treatment decisions.

---

[4] Each element i, j of resulting matrix is the product of elements i, j of the source two matrices.

3.1   Data and Test Procedures

Three datasets were formed to develop, verify and confirm the CCogModel. The first two sets were carefully selected with their clinical value confirmed to test variational sparse representations of test cases. The homogeneous one consists of the clinical data of test cases including CT scans collected in only one hospital center (two scanners), according to its own protocols and clinical paths. The clinical data were collected from 71 patients, including 36 cases of stroke group and 35 cases of control group. Mean age of patients classified to stroke group was 67 years (29–83) while 50% of this group was male patients. Mean age of the controls was 64 years (26–97) with 54% of male ones. Median time onset-first CT for the stroke group patients was approximately 2 h 10 min (45 min–6 h). The control group consisted of cases with misdiagnosis of stroke or stroke mimics. For that group we have had approximately 3 h 20 min (45 min–168 h) of time onset-first CT.

The second test set extends the first one with another clinical cases collected in another hospital center with different specificity of stroke procedures and documentation standards. In total such heterogeneous set includes 71 patients of the stroke group and 74 ones of the control group. Mean age of patients classified to the stroke group was 71 years (29–92) while 58% of this group was male ones. Mean age of 74 controls was 58 years (20–97) with 50% of male ones. Median time onset-first CT for stroke patients was approximately 3 h (45 min–8 h). The control group consisted of patients with non-confirmed stroke and with other neurological or general non-neurological diseases. For that group we have had approximately 3 h 30 min (45 min–336 h) of time onset-first CT.

Retrospective verification of the sparse case representation was applied in patient-oriented procedures of stroke recognition and prediction of treatment outcome in clinical practice. A leave-one-patient-out crossvalidation was used where numerical description of one patient case, determined according to the proposed model, was cross-validated against the modeled descriptors of other patients. In such procedure, two measures of efficiency were used: the Area Under the Curve (AUC) computed from the estimated ROC curve and Correct Rate (CR) with detailing Sensitivity (Se) and Specificity (Sp). The ROC curve was determined basing on posterior probabilities estimated for each test patients in procedure one against the others. In our experiments, AUC is interpreted as mean prediction ability of ischemia (i.e. tissue fate from onset specificity to follow-up findings) or treatment outcome, respectively, for all crossvalidated test cases. Set of estimated posterior probabilities is considered as a measure of stroke probability or severity according to computerized support of complete clinical evidence, assisting clinical decision making process separately in each test case. Analogically in prediction of treatment outcome, posterior probabilities are interpreted as each-case probability of beneficial treatment. Correct Rate directly determines the effectiveness of automatic suggestions that relate to a decision-making processes in confirming the stroke or execution of thrombolytic therapy.

Thereafter, we retrospectively analyzed 32 patients from which 7 underwent thrombolytic treatment to define carefully the pattern of ground truth and verified calculated cognition model in a context of stroke treatment conditions. Patients were selected from DDIS II database[5]. Baseline clinical characteristics of selected test group included general patient info, vital signs measurements, laboratory test results, patient neurological description and results of NCCT imaging.

3.2 Results and Discussion

The selected results of realized experiments verifying the effectiveness of the optimized method in question are presented in Tables 1 and 2.

Table 1. Efficiency of stroke recognition and prediction for thrombolytic successful outcome applied for more extensive test sets. Descriptors of image data and clinical data were verified using classical feature selection/recognition procedure (RCS – Rank key features by Class Separability criteria) and the lasso Selector (lassoS); ts1 and ts2 are data test sets of 145 heterogeneous and 71 more homogeneous test cases; OFS means the dimension of optimal feature space experimentally adjusted

Methodology	Effectiveness				
(method, features: data)	Size of OFS	AUC	CR	Sn	Sp
Stroke recognition					
RCS, image: ts1/ts2	21/57	.86/.94	.81/.90	.82/.91	.79/.89
RCS, clinical: ts1/ts2	45/27	.96/.98	.90/.92	.95/.86	.86/.97
LassoS, image: ts1/ts2	35/25	.98/1	.96/1	.97/1	.94/1
lassoS, clinical: ts1/ts2	45/31	**.99/1**	**.99/1**	**1/1**	**.97/1**
Treatment outcome prediction (binary decisions)					
RCS, image: ts1/ts2	27/15	.81/.94	.77/.90	.80/.91	.64/.87
RCS, clinical: ts1/ts2	11/13	.91/.94	.86/.92	.88/.91	.79/.93
lassoS, image: ts1/ts2	43/31	.91/1	.88/.97	.89/.98	.86/.93
lassoS, clinical: ts1/ts2	45/33	**.95/1**	**.92/1**	**.94/1**	**.86/1**

The implemented cognitive model allowed to obtain significantly higher effectiveness of stroke recognition and prediction of therapy effects, comparing to traditional paradigm of feature selection and classification (RCS) – Table 1. This efficiency is very high – in several variants of the CCogModel implementations practically unmistakable on the presented reference datasets. The CCogModel made it possible to set a more stable and representative set of ischemia descriptors in relation to different test data sets, indicating the possibility of obtaining a more reliable cognitive model. In case of the RCS, the selection of the type

---

[5] Digital Database of Ischemic Stroke Cases (DDIS II) – http://aidmed.pl/.

Table 2. Selected effects of prediction for thrombolytic successful outcome – optimization of cognitive model implementation. Radiologic and integrated clinical descriptors are used. The 32 representative cases of sensed pattern of ground truth were used

Implementation of the CCogModel		Effectiveness					
Test data	Method	β ratio	AUC	CR	Sn	Sp	PCorr
Radiological	lasso	.17	1	1	1	1	.969
	elastic net	.21	1	.97	1	.95	.981
	ML regression	.24	1	.78	.92	.8	1
	OMP	.17	.93	.78	.92	.85	.943
	spaRSA	.15	.93	.69	.83	.75	.751
Integrated	lasso/sparseΨ	.13/.09	1/1	1/1	1/1	1/1	.981/.982
	elastic net/sparseΨ	.17/.09	1/1	1/1	1/1	1/1	.985/.981
	ML regression/ sparseΨ	.19/.15	1/1	.97/1	1/1	.95/1	1/1
	OMP/sparseΨ	.16/.15	1/1	1/1	1/1	1/1	1/1
	spaRSA/ sparseΨ	.02/.02	1/1	.81/.81	.92/.92	.75/.75	.85/.89
	$l_1$eq_pd/sparseΨ	.08/.06	1/1	.87/.91	.84/.92	.9/.9	.934/.945

of features and their number was much more accidental. The use of full clinical information is more advantageous than the numerical description of only image features.

The selected procedures of cognitive model implementation used for prognosis of favorable thrombolysis of stroke cases gave comparably high effectiveness – Table 2. Especially, PCorr equal to 1 or almost 1 means ability of perfect repetition of experts opinions by the implemented model-based cognition of complex clinical picture in emergency. Going into details, the selection of the matrix Ψ allowed an increase of the model sparisty sometimes even close to half with the same or higher prediction efficiency. Deterministic matrices were more stable and effective comparing randomized ones while cosine bases gave the most stable improvement in the effectiveness of the model. Among the methods of reconstruction, above all, convex optimization-based methods (lasso, elastic net) that achieved sparse models with relatively high efficiency were distinguished.

Thus, the proposed concept of compressive cognitive model implemented to support clinical decisions of stroke care seems to positively verified. However, further methods of its optimization and prospective verification are required.

4   Conclusions

Essential contribution of this research is the concept of compressive cognitive model determined on the basis of empirical procedures including clinical protocols and objectified assessments followed by numerical analysis and description of complete pathology picture including signal processing and image analysis. Sparsity of the model was achieved using modeled CS paradigm with recovery of decisive clinical parameters important for description of pathology core possibly invariant to the clinical and technical conditions of stroke care.

These studies will be continued in the direction of prospective verification of the designated model in clinical conditions and further optimization of the CCogModel by: improving the methods of determining ground truth pattern, implementing better determinants of the measurement matrix and introducing structural adaptation to the model reconstruction algorithms in ill-posed inverse problem of the CS paradigm.

Not only from a clinical point of view (general practitioner, emergency, neurologist) but also from the point of view of the patient, it is very important to diagnose the disease as soon as possible and start further steps of proper and deliberate therapeutic process. Shortening the time of diagnosis and thus the decision to undertake thrombolytic treatment, and in the future and the consequences of therapeutic decisions, throbectomy, significantly increases the patient's chances not only for survival but also for reducing the neurological deficit (e.g. speech problems, limb paralysis/paresis, visual problems). The benefit of the proposed cognitive model is therefore not only important for the patient and the physician, but also for the whole society, by significantly reducing the socio-economic costs of caring for a stroke patient.

Acknowledgement. This publication was funded by the National Science Centre (Poland) based on the decision DEC-2011/03/B/ST7/03649.

References

1. Donoho, D.L.: Compressed sensing. IEEE Trans. Inf. Theory **52**(4), 1289–1306 (2006)
2. Baraniuk, R.G., Cevher, V., Duarte, M.F., Hegde, C.: Model-based compressive sensing. IEEE Trans. Inf. Theory **56**(4), 1982–2001 (2010)
3. Ogiela, M.R., Tadeusiewicz, R.: Cognitive vision systems in medical applications. In: Zhong, N., Ras, Z.W., Tsumoto, S., Suzuki, E. (eds.) Foundations of Intelligent Systems. Lectures Notes on Artificial Intelligence, vol. 2871, pp. 116–123. Springer, Heidelberg (2003)
4. Przelaskowski, A., Sobieszczuk, E., Sklinda, K, Domitrz, I.: CT-based morphological ischemia measure. Preprint submitted to Neuroimage: Clinical
5. Brott, T., Adams, H.P., Olinger, C.P., Marler, J.R., Barsan, W.G., et al.: Measurements of acute cerebral infarction: a clinical examination scale. Stroke **20**, 864–870 (1989)
6. Ciszek, B., Jozwiak, R., Sobieszczuk, E., Przelaskowski, A., Skadorwa, T.: Stroke bricks - spatial brain regions to assess ischemic stroke location. Folia Morphol. **76**(4), 568–573 (2017)
7. Barber, P.A., Demchuk, A.M., Zhang, J., Buchan, A.M.: Validity and reliability of a quantitative computed tomography score in predicting outcome of hyperacute stroke before thrombolytic therapy. ASPECTS Study Group. Alberta Stroke programme early CT score. Lancet **355**(9216), 1670–1674 (2000)

8. Przelaskowski, A.: Recovery of CT stroke hypodensity - an adaptive variational approach. Comp. Med. Im. Graph. **46**, 131–141 (2015)
9. Lou, M., Safdar, A., Selim, M., et al.: The HAT score: a simple grading scale for predicting hemorrhage after thrombolysis. Neurology **71**(18), 1417–1423 (2008)
10. Strbian, D., Meretoja, A., Ahlhelm, F.J., Pitkäniemi, J., Lyrer, P., Kaste, M., Engelter, S., Tatlisumak, T.: Predicting outcome of IV thrombolysis-treated ischemic stroke patients: the DRAGON score. Neurology **78**(6), 427–32 (2012)
11. Saposnik, G., Fang, J., Kapral, M., Tu, J., Mamdani, M., Austin, P., Johnston, S.: On behalf of the investigators of the registry of the Canadian Stroke Network (RCSN) and the Stroke Outcomes Research Canada (SORCan) working group: the iScore predicts effectiveness of thrombolytic therapy for acute ischemic stroke. Stroke **3**(5), 1315–1322 (2012)
12. Baraniuk, R., Davenport, M.A., Duarte, M.F., Hegde, C.: An introduction to compressive sensing. In: Connexions. Rice University, Houston (2010)
13. Ravelomanantsoa, A., Rabah, H., Rouane, A.: Compressed sensing: a simple deterministic measurement matrix and a fast recovery algorithm. IEEE Trans. Inst. Meas. **64**(12), 3405–3413 (2015)
14. Nguyen T.L.N., Shin, Y.: Deterministic sensing matrices in compressive sensing: a survey. Sci. World J. 6 p. (2013) ID 192795
15. Davis, G., Mallat, S., Zhang, Z.: Adaptive time-frequency decompositions with matching pursuits. Opt. Eng. **33**, 2183–2191 (1994)
16. Wright, S.J., Nowak, R.D., Figueiredo, M.A.T: Sparse reconstruction by separable approximation. Trans. Sig. Process. **57**(7), 2479–2493 (2009)

Evaluation of Puberty in Girls by Spectral Analysis of Voice

Marcin D. Bugdol[1]([✉]), Maria J. Bieńkowska[1], Monika N. Bugdol[1],
Anna M. Lipowicz[2], Andrzej W. Mitas[1], and Agata Wijata[1]

[1] Faculty of Biomedical Engineering, Silesian University of Technology,
Roosevelta 40, 41-800 Zabrze, Poland
marcin.bugdol@polsl.pl
[2] Department of Anthropology,
Wroclaw University of Environmental and Life Sciences, Wrocław, Poland

Abstract. In this paper, a method for girls' pubertal status evaluation is presented. The proposed algorithm uses voice features. Spectral analysis, Support Vector Machine and Random Forest Trees were employed. The obtained results are promising. Sensitivity reached 89.38%, when all features were included in the calculations (SVM). The highest specificity was achieved when only standard deviations were used (80.14% for the RF). Accuracy was greater than 80% for both classifiers when all features were used.

Keywords: Voice analysis · Spectral analysis · Puberty evaluation

1 Introduction

The age and tempo of maturation is a very important factor for assessing the living conditions of children and adolescents. Even small changes in the environment of human development results in different time of the first menstruation (menarche) and thus this information can be used to evaluate social inequalities [19]. In surveys researchers usually use one of three methods for menarcheal age estimation [15]:

- the status quo method – asking girls whether they menstruate or not,
- the recall or retrospective method – asking menstruating women about their age of menarche,
- the prospective method – a longitudinal survey in which each girl is asked regularly, whether or not she has already begun to menstruate.

All the above mentioned methods are based on somebody's answers and there are some situations (i.e. criminology), where other more reliable tests are needed. The proposed idea is to employ voice for pubertal status evaluation.

The production of sounds by a human being, as in other animals, is used for inter-individual communication and is associated with functioning in a group.

© Springer International Publishing AG, part of Springer Nature 2019
E. Pietka et al. (Eds.): ITIB 2018, AISC 762, pp. 243–250, 2019.
https://doi.org/10.1007/978-3-319-91211-0_21

Units inform each other about their condition (including sex, age, body structure), as well as emotions and motivation of action (aggression, interest, fear, boredom, etc.). Sounds help determine the place of an individual in society, create group membership, establish a hierarchy, show interest in a potential partner or detour an intruder or rival.

The speech apparatus, which consists of vocal folds (producing vibrations), lower (trachea, bronchi, lungs, diaphragm) and upper voice resonators (paranasal sinuses, nasal cavity, pharynx, oral cavity), is responsible for producing sounds with specific parameters [20].

During adolescence the girls' (and boys') body structure changes rapidly and so does their voice. Before maturation, male and female voices do not differ significantly (voice pitches are similar, however formants are somewhat closer in boys) [21], then after puberty, the fundamental frequency of young women is higher than the fundamental frequency of young men by about 100 Hz [7,8].

An approach to evaluating menarcheal status of girls has been presented in [3], where voice and anthropometric features were employed and 85% average accuracy was achieved. The only similar works were focused on evaluation of boys' pubertal age but mainly using mathematical modelling rather than machine learning techniques [9,11,12]. One of the ideas to evaluate the stage of the boys' voice development, which is correlated with pubertal status, was presented by Cooksey [5]. He analysed spectrograms and found that they had a different shape according boys' actual pubertal state. However, no further analysis was proposed. Recently, image processing methods were employed for feature extraction from raw spectrogram of voice signal [4,13,14].

The aim of the presented work was to create a method for classifying pre- and post-menarche girls using voices features extracted on the basis of spectrogram analysis.

The paper is organized as follows. In Sect. 2 information about the collected voices samples, extracted features and employed classifier are presented. The results of the experiment are provided in Sects. 3 and 4 summarizes the paper.

2   Materials and Methods

The voice samples were collected from girls who were pupils of elementary, secondary and high school. The age range of registered girls was from 9 to 18. The mean age was 13.41 and standard deviation was 2.74. The information about girls' menarcheal status was obtained using a questionnaire. During five measurement session, which took place between September 2015 and September 2017, 98 girls were registered of which 39 were before first menstruation and 49 were after menarche.

The samples have been recorded in 16 bit quality with 44100 Hz sampling rate and saved in WAVE audio format. They have been gathered using a system which consisted of a microphone, Sontronic STC-80 a microphone pre-amplifier, IMG Stageline MPA-202, and a computer.

The voice samples were gathered according to the following protocol: the first task was to introduce herself aloud. Next, the examined girl articulated the vowels a, e, i, o, u, which were viewed on the computer screen for 3 s, in extended phonation (this stage was repeated three times). The vowels appeared in a random order. There was a 2 s break between the vowels for taking a breath. The whole procedure lasted about 2 min. All of the acquired signals made one voice sample.

2.1 Voice Features Extraction

The pre-processing step of speech analysis consisted of extracting a stable part of the signal of approximately 200 ms on which the analysis was carried out. The next steps included signal normalization, windowing with the Hanning function and half-frame overlapping (Fig. 1). Each frame was 30 ms long.

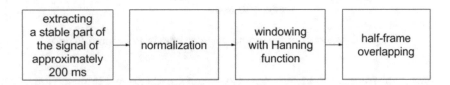

Fig. 1. Voice preprocessing algorithm

All of the proposed methods are based on searching for signal changes in time. Because only single vowel is used, detected changes refer to a voice break, which is characteristic for pubertal period.

A spectrogram is a representation of the magnitude spectrum of a speech signal as a time vs. frequency chart. It is calculated as Short Time Fourier Transform (STFT) in particular frames of the signal [1, 16]. A spectrogram was subdivided into ranges of 33.36 Hz, what was the result of the applied sampling frequency (44100 Hz) and length of the frame (30 ms). In this paper, means and standard deviations of magnitude were computed for each frequency range for the analysis of potential signal changes in time (Fig. 2). Two (mean and standard deviation) 331-elements vectors were obtained for each of analyzed vowel.

When the speech signal is divided into smaller frames, it can be assumed that the signal is quasi-stationary. Nevertheless, there may be some changes in the energy of particular frames, which can be informative feature. Spectral flux (SF) measures the quantity of variation in the spectrum across time [17] and can be calculated according to Eq. (1). For each vowel, an 8-element vector containing spectral-flux of every frame were obtained.

$$SF(n) = \sum \left(|X|(n) - |X|(n-1) \right)^2 \tag{1}$$

where: $|X|(n)$ – the magnitude spectrum of n-th frame.

To complete the information given by the spectral flux, the energy (E) of each frame was added to the feature vector. In spectral flux, differences between

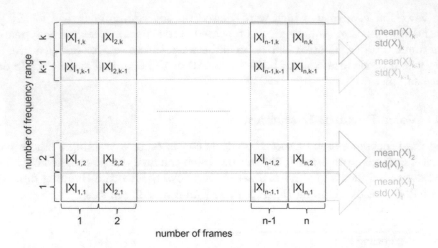

Fig. 2. Extraction of mean and standard deviation of amplitude

the energy of frames are always positive numbers; therefore, information about its direction is lost. Including the energy vector of each frame retains the full information of the signal variability. The energy of single frame can be computed according to Eq. (2). For each each vowel 8-elements vector containing energies of consecutive frames were obtained.

$$E(n) = \sum |X|(n)^2 \qquad (2)$$

where: $|X|(n)$ – the magnitude spectrum of n-th frame.

For each vowel a vector of length 678 was obtained using MATLAB. Due to the fact that every vowel was recorded three times, there was a need to choose a representative feature vector for a single vowel. It was performed according to the following procedure. First, individually for each feature, the median was found. Next, the feature vector including the highest number of medians was the input vector for further analysis. The representatives of each five vowels are combined into one vector of 3390 elements. More details about this algorithm can be found in [3].

In order to provide insight into the data, boxplots of exemplary obtained coefficients were included in Fig. 3. Since the majority of the computed features did not follow a Gaussian distribution, nonparametric statistics such as medians, quartiles and outliers range were presented. Exploratory data analysis revealed that pre-pubertal girls exhibited the tendency to achieve much higher values of feature and to have a large range, compared to post-menarche examined subjects.

2.2   Classification

For classification, a Support Vector Machine (SVM) [6,18] and Random Forest (RF) [2,10] were used. They are well established and the most popular

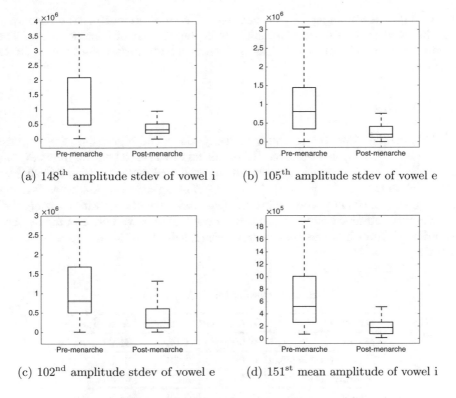

(a) 148th amplitude stdev of vowel i

(b) 105th amplitude stdev of vowel e

(c) 102nd amplitude stdev of vowel e

(d) 151st mean amplitude of vowel i

Fig. 3. Boxplots of exemplary features

approaches in two-class classification problems. All experiments have been carried out using toolboxes available in MATLAB environment. The number of trees for RF classifier was set to 200 and the values of other parameters were default. For the SVM classifier the linear kernel with default parameters has been employed.

The database used to train and test the classifier consisted of 98 measurements and 678 features each. Tests were carried out using individual types of features and also for the set consisting all parameters. Ten-fold cross validation was performed 1000 times and the obtained results were averaged.

The effectiveness of the proposed method has been evaluated using following parameters: sensitivity (Eq. (3)), specificity (Eq. (4)) and accuracy (Eq. (5)):

$$sen = \frac{TP}{TP + FN}, \tag{3}$$

$$spec = \frac{TN}{FP + TN}, \tag{4}$$

$$acc = \frac{TP + TN}{TP + FP + TN + FN}, \tag{5}$$

where TP is the number of true positives, TN the number of true negatives, FP the number of false positives and FN is the number of false negatives. The girls after menarche are treated as positives and the girls before menarche as negatives.

3   Results

Table 1 includes the results obtained using the SVM algorithm. The highest sensitivity (89.38%) was achieved, when all features served as the input for the SVM. Performing calculations on means or standard deviations implied slightly lower values of sensitivity (87.90% and 87.98% respectively). Means as features gave highest specificity and accuracy. The worst results for all the computed metrics were obtained when energies were used. Flux gave better outcome than energies, but much worse than means, standards deviations, and all features together.

Table 1. Results for SVM classifier

Features	Sensitivity	Specificity	Accuracy
Means	87.90	76.02	81.90
Standard deviations	87.98	73.48	81.26
Spectral flux	68.86	60.37	64.59
Energies	57.55	51.82	54.92
All	89.38	71.97	81.51

The classification results from the RF method were presented in Table 2. The best results were obtained for means, standard deviations, and all features. The differences between the values of sensitivity, specificity and accuracy were for those coefficients insignificant. The lowest values of all the computed parameters occurred when the labelling was performed using energies. Employing flux gave better results, but still performed worse than means, standard deviations and the whole feature set.

Table 2. Results for RF classifier

Features	Sensitivity	Specificity	Accuracy
Means	88.78	79.06	83.72
Standard deviations	87.48	80.14	83.67
Spectral flux	67.73	65.21	65.94
Energies	64.25	54.45	58.97
All	87.72	79.28	83.40

For each feature set specificity and accuracy was higher for the RF than for the SVM. Sensitivity did not exhibit such dependency, but the differences between the respective values were small. Therefore, it can be concluded, that the RF classifier better suits the problem of assessing girls' pubertal status on the basis of their voice samples. On the other hand, the training and test process is more time-consuming for RF classifier than for SVM.

4   Conclusions

In the paper, a method for assessing girls' pubertal status based on the voice spectral features has been presented. The obtained results are satisfying and proves that the proposed approach can be employed in surveys in which there are no possibilities to ask girls about their menarcheal status or when their answers are unreliable.

Further research will be focus on creating a similar method for evaluating boys' maturation status, which do not have a measure similar to the menarche for girls.

Acknowledgement. We would like to thank Andre Woloshuk for his English language corrections.

References

1. Allen, J.: Short term spectral analysis, synthesis, and modification by discrete fourier transform. IEEE Trans. Acoust. Speech Signal Process. **25**(3), 235–238 (1977). https://doi.org/10.1109/TASSP.1977.1162950
2. Breiman, L.: Random forests. Mach. Learn. **45**(1), 5–32 (2001). https://doi.org/10.1023/A:1010933404324
3. Bugdol, M.D., Bugdol, M.N., Lipowicz, A.M., Mitas, A.W., Bienkowska, M.J., Wijata, A.M.: Prediction of menarcheal status of girls using voice features. Computers in Biology and Medicine (2017). https://doi.org/10.1016/j.comp biomed.2017.11.005, http://www.sciencedirect.com/science/article/pii/S00104825 17303657
4. Carbonneau, M.A., Granger, E., Attabi, Y., Gagnon, G.: Feature learning from spectrograms for assessment of personality traits. IEEE Trans. Affect. Comput. (2017)
5. Cooksey, J.: Voice transformation in male adolescents, pp. 731–733 (2000)
6. Cortes, C., Vapnik, V.: Support-vector networks. Mach. Learn. **20**(3), 273–297 (1995)
7. Feinberg, D.R., Jones, B.C., Little, A.C., Burt, D.M., Perrett, D.I.: Manipulations of fundamental and formant frequencies influence the attractiveness of human male voices. Anim. Behav. **69**(3), 561–568 (2005)
8. Fouquet, M., Pisanski, K., Mathevon, N., Reby, D.: Seven and up: individual differences in male voice fundamental frequency emerge before puberty and remain stable throughout adulthood. Open Sci. **3**(10) (2016). https://doi.org/10.1098/rsos.160395

9. Harries, M.L.L., Walker, J.M., Williams, D.M., Hawkins, S., Hughes, I.A.: Changes in the male voice at puberty. Arch. Dis. Child. **77**(5), 445–447 (1997)
10. Ho, T.K.: A data complexity analysis of comparative advantages of decision forest constructors. Pattern Anal. Appl. **5**(2), 102–112 (2002). https://doi.org/10.1007/s100440200009
11. Hodges-Simeon, R., Gurven, M., Cardenas, R.A., Gaulin, S.J.C.: Voice change as a new measure of male pubertal timing: a study among bolivian adolescents. Ann. Hum. Biol. **40**(3), 209–219 (2013)
12. Hughes, I.A., Kumanan, M.: A wider perspective on puberty. Mol. Cell. Endocrinol. **254–255**(Suppl. C), 1–7 (2006). https://doi.org/10.1016/j.mce.2006.04.014. Puberty: A Sensor of Genetic and Environmental Interactions, http://www.sciencedirect.com/science/article/pii/
13. Ishikawa, K., MacAuslan, J., Boyce, S.: Toward clinical application of landmark-based speech analysis: landmark expression in normal adult speech. J. Acoust. Soc. Am. **142**(5), EL441–EL447 (2017)
14. Jeffery, T., Cunningham, S., Whiteside, S.P.: Analyses of sustained vowels in down syndrome (DS): a case study using spectrograms and perturbation data to investigate voice quality in four adults with DS. Journal of Voice (2017)
15. Karapanou, O., Papadimitriou, A.: Determinants of menarche. Reprod. Biol. Endocrinol. **8**(1), 115 (2010)
16. Prasad, K.S., Ramaiah, G.K., Manjunatha, M.: Speech features extraction techniques for robust emotional speech analysis/recognition. Indian J. Sci. Technol. **8**(1) (2017)
17. Sadjadi, S.O., Hansen, J.H.: Unsupervised speech activity detection using voicing measures and perceptual spectral flux. IEEE Signal Process. Lett. **20**(3), 197–200 (2013)
18. Scholkopf, B., Smola, A.J.: Learning with Kernels: Support Vector Machines, Regularization, Optimization, and Beyond. MIT Press, Cambridge (2001)
19. Strickland, S.S., Shetty, P.S.: Human Biology and Social Inequality, vol. 39. Cambridge University Press, Cambridge (1998)
20. Titze, I.R.: Principles of Voice Production. Prentice Hall (1994). https://books.google.pl/books?id=m48JAQAAMAAJ
21. Vuorenkoski, V., Lenko, H.L., Tjernlund, P., Vuorenkoski, L., Perheentupa, J.: Fundamental voice frequence during normal and abnormal growth, and after androgen treatment. Arch. Dis. Child. **53**(3), 201–209 (1978)

Boys' Age Modeling Using Voice Features

Monika N. Bugdol[1]([✉]), Andrzej W. Mitas[1], Anna M. Lipowicz[2],
Marcin D. Bugdol[1], and Maria J. Bieńkowska[1]

[1] Faculty of Biomedical Engineering, Silesian University of Technology,
Roosevelta 40, 41-800 Zabrze, Poland
monika.bugdol@polsl.pl
[2] Department of Anthropology,
Wroclaw University of Environmental and Life Sciences, Wrocław, Poland

Abstract. The paper presents the results of boys' age modeling on the basis of the features of their voice. The research group has been divided according to age and the threshold been 14 years. 98 boys have been examined (57 aged less than 14 years, 41 aged 14 years or more). Voice data has been acquired and processed. The obtained coefficients have been subjected to Principal Component Analysis and then linear models have been built, estimeting the boys' age. The obtained results are promising and are especially good in case of the group of younger boys, where the median absolute error has been less than 6 months and the median relative error has been equal to 2.1%.

Keywords: Voice · Age estimation · Boys' puberty

1 Introduction

In non-verbal interpersonal communication two main acoustic attributes play an important role – fundamental frequency (F_0) and formant structure (formant dispersion and formant position [4,18]). The fundamental frequency, also called the laryngeal tone, is produced by the vibration of vocal folds in the larynx under the influence of the air stream flowing out of the lungs and depends on the length and thickness of the vocal folds – it is responsible for the pitch of the voice. Formants, i.e. the spectral maxima resulting from the resonances of the oral cavities, depend on the length and shape of the vocal tract.

Voice is a distinctive dimorphic trait, its changes occur with age differently in boys and girls. Since in childhood the vocal tract does not anatomically show sexual differences, the voice of children of both sexes does not differ much. Distinct changes appear at puberty when the size of the chest and the lung capacity increase. The entire voice track extends, including nasopharyngeal cavity and tongue. Significant changes occur within the larynx, the place of phonation. The vocal cords lengthen, the cartilages, that build the larynx, increase their size and the larynx itself moves in the lower direction [8]. Development in the speech apparatus involve changes in the quality of the voice and the process lasts usually from one to three years [6]. The most abrupt changes occur between Tanner

© Springer International Publishing AG, part of Springer Nature 2019
E. Pietka et al. (Eds.): ITIB 2018, AISC 762, pp. 251–259, 2019.
https://doi.org/10.1007/978-3-319-91211-0_22

stage G3 and G4 [9]. As a result of these transformations, the voice lowers, much more in boys than in girls, which leads to the development of differences in the dimorphic and interpersonal maturity differences.

From the biological point of view, the pitch of the voice measured by the fundamental frequency (F_0) gives information about the sex of the individual, his/her age and maturational status [15, 16, 19]. It has been proven, that voice quality and speaking rate are perceptually relevant cues of age in male voices [7]. In case of speakers aged 2–34 years, most respondents misestimated their age by less than 5 years [12].

Therefore, we assume that voice can be used as one of the traits for assessing age, both chronological and biological, wherever there is no possibility of conducting a direct interview (questionnaire), or it is not possible to obtain a reliable answer. This method brought the expected results in the case of girls in the peri-pubertal age, where the analysis of the voice parameters allowed to assess the girl's maturing status with 86% accuracy [1]. This work is the first step towards the development of a new method for assessing the biological age of boys based on their voice and includes estimating the chronological age based on their acoustic parameters.

2   Materials and Methods

Voice data has been acquired in the years 2015–2017 in the Lutheran Primary School, Lutheran Junior High School and Lutheran High School in Cieszyn, Poland. This has been a part of a longitudinal study (Longitudinal Voice Study LoVoiS) and so far, 5 measurements have taken place, each every 6 months. For the purposes of the research presented in this article only the first measurement of each subject has been considered, which was due to avoid data overfitting.

Voice samples have been recorded for 98 boys aged 8 to 19. The task of the participants was to loudly pronounce vowels a, e, i, o and u. The samples have been recorded in 16 bits quality with 44100 Hz sampling rate and saved in WAVE audio format. They have been gathered using a system consisting of a microphone Sontronic STC-80, a microphone pre-amplifier IMG Stageline MPA-202 and a computer. Audio data have been obtained in stable acoustic conditions, in an isolated room, and the individual is subjected to functionally stabilizing relaxation activities, without informing about the purpose of such stabilization. Breath alignment, pulse compensation, obtained by taking a relaxed sitting position, reading a text fragment and saying simple sequences also allows to achieve stable and natural conditions for the emission of periodic sounds, subjected to final analysis. The unhurried formula of the study in the conditions of psychological comfort is dictated by the need to ensure a repeatable condition of the subject. The natural exclusion is a throat disease, eliminating the tested person by her absence from school, where research is carried out nominally. The order of the person conducting the research, so that the examined person would naturally pronounce a vowel, does not have to be supplemented with a command to position the sound at a given pitch, because the measurement task is to analyze the dominant, most convenient, anatomical frequency associated with the energy minimization necessary to generate an audible and distinctive sound.

The following voice features have been computed: tristimulus, total harmonic distortion (THD), mean autocorrelation, period, fundamental frequency (F_0), formants, jitter, shimmer, noise to harmonic ration (NHR), linear prediction coefficients (LPC) and mel frequency cepstral coefficients (MFCC). Tristimulus and THD have not been used in age assessment issues before, nevertheless they are based on the voice timbre. Other proposed features are commonly used in studies concerning voice maturity [1].

Tristimulus (T_1, T_2, T_3) is a measure of sound timbre, which is based on the spectral energy of the signal. During puberty the voice timbre is changing. Energy is divided into 3 bands, which corresponds to three primary colors in image analysis. Tristimulus assesses the energy in the fundamental, the next three partials, and the higher partials in relation to the whole energy of the signal, it can be presented as [3]:

$$T_1 = \frac{a_1}{\sum_{k=1}^{N} a_k}, \tag{1}$$

$$T_2 = \frac{a_2 + a_3 + a_4}{\sum_{k=1}^{N} a_k}, \tag{2}$$

$$T_3 = \frac{\sum_{k=5}^{N} a_k}{\sum_{k=1}^{N} a_k}, \tag{3}$$

where a_k are the amplitudes of particular harmonics.

Total Harmonic Disortion (THD) is used to quantify the level of harmonics of a waveform. In this paper it is defined as the harmonic content of a waveform divided by its fundamental and can be described as [20]:

$$THD = \frac{\sqrt{\sum_{k=2}^{n} a_k^2}}{a_1}. \tag{4}$$

Mean autocorrelation value depends on periodicity of the signal. For periodic signal it reaches high values, which decrease for an unstable voice (noticed during puberty).

Period determines a duration of a repeatable fragment of speech signal. Women's voices have shorter periods than men, additionally during puberty the voice period elongates in both genders. In this paper mean value of calculated period and its standard deviation were used.

Fundamental frequency (F_0) is the inverse of the period. It refers to the pitch of the voice, which changes during ontogeny.

Formants are characteristic frequencies, which refer to resonances in the vocal tract during speech signal production. They depend on the spoken phone and the size of the vocal tract, which changes during puberty.

Jitter corresponds to the absolute difference between following periods of the signal divided by the average period. Shimmer is equivalent of jitter parameter computed for amplitudes. Both of them refer to voice stability.

Noise to Harmonic Ration (NHR) assesses the ration of energy in the noise part of the signal to its periodic part.

Linear Prediction Coefficients (LPC) permit estimating the fundamental speech parameters. They represent normally spectral envelope, which is strongly correlated with the vocal tract properties. The idea of LPC is based on the assumption, that any speech sample can be approximated as a linear combination of past data [17].

Mel Frequency Cepstral Coefficients (MFCC) are coefficients obtained in Mel frequency Cepstrum (inverse Fourier transform of the logarithm of the estimated spectrum of a signal) representation [17]. They represent a compressed version of the spectral envelope. Both LPC and MFCC are the complex set of voice features commonly used in literature.

The examined boys have been considered as the whole group and as 2 separate groups (57 boys aged up to 14 and 41 boys aged 14 or more). The value of 14 years has been indicated as the contractual threshold between pre-pubertal and post-pubertal boys, accordingly to the age at peak height velocity fitted for Polish boys with the Preece-Baines Model 1 [14].

Principal Component Analysis [11] has been employed on the evaluated voice features. Following the Kaiser Criterion [13], further analysis has been performed on those components, for which the eigenvalue was higher than 1. The PCA has been used independently on all the gathered data and on the two groups divided with respect to the boys' age, which has implied the emergence of three sets of components.

For each set the extracted components have served as independent variables in a multiple linear regression model [5] with age as the exogenous variable. Due to considering 3 groups of subjects, 3 linear models have been computed.

3   Results

The goodness of fit results have been presented in Table 1. The standard errors of estimates are in all cases smaller than 2 years. Best results have been obtained in the group of pre-pubertal boys, where the standard error was lower than 10 months. The largest standard error has been noted for boys at 14 years and more, which might caused by the fact, that at the age range 14–15 years in boys, many biological traits are characterised by increased variability influenced by differences in tempo of growth. The values of adjusted R^2 coefficient are high for boys under 14 and for the whole examined group, whereas the elder group has a much lower value of that coefficient, which implies the need to gather more data, especially from that particular age group.

Table 1. Results of multiple linear regression of age on voice features (R—multiple correlation coefficient, R^2—coefficient of determination)

	Multiple R	Multiple R^2	Adjusted R^2	Standard error of estimation [years]
Boys under 14	0.930	0.866	0.604	0.813
Boys at 14 and more	0.846	0.715	0.266	1.854
All boys	0.912	0.831	0.727	1.475

The mean absolute errors have not exceeded 1 year, regardless of the age group (Table 2). The best result (error lower than 4 months) has been obtained for younger subjects, and the worst for the combined group (almost 9 months). The median absolute errors have been lower than 6 months for each of the analyzed groups. Moreover, for each group 75% of the estimated age values have been computed accurate to less than one year and in case of the younger group less than 5 months.

Table 2. Absolute errors of age estimation [years]

	Mean	Std dev	Median	Q_1	Q_3	Min	Max
Boys under 14	0.32	0.34	0.23	0.10	0.40	0.001	1.70
Boys at 14 and more	0.58	0.49	0.40	0.17	0.90	0.04	1.85
All boys	0.66	0.62	0.44	0.23	0.86	0.003	2.95

Figure 1 presents histograms of the absolute error. The distribution of each of those random variables is exponential, which has been confirmed by the outcomes of the chi-square goodness-of-fit test [2]. All the obtained p-values have been higher than 0.6 and for the examined individuals under the age of 14, the computed p-value has been equal to 0.91. All the estimations have been accurate up to 3 years. In the group of the older boys the absolute errors has exceeded 1 year 5 months only twice. Best accuracy has been achieved for the pre-pubertal group, where only one boy's age has been misestimated by more than 15 months.

The relative errors values, presented in Table 3, confirm that the goodness of fit is satisfying. The average relative error did not exceed 6% and was even smaller, when boys have been considered separately, according to their age. In case of boys under the age of 14 the relative error has been lower than 3% and the relative error obtained for the older examined has been equal to 3.69%. In all cases the distribution has been right-skewed, which implies that the median has been noticeably lower than the mean. The age of 50% younger boys has been estimated with a relative error smaller than 2.11%.

The distributions of the relative errors have been presented in Fig. 2. In all cases relative errors follow the exponential distribution, which has been tested

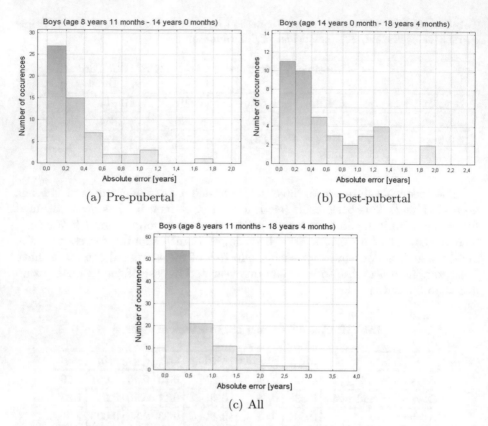

(a) Pre-pubertal   (b) Post-pubertal

(c) All

Fig. 1. Absolute error, exponential distribution confirmed with chi-squared test with the p-value respectively (a) p = 0.91 (b) p = 0.64 (c) p = 0.63

Table 3. Relative errors of age estimation [%]

	Mean	Std dev	Median	Q_1	Q_3	Min	Max
Boys under 14	2.93	3.01	2.11	0.82	3.65	0.01	12.39
Boys at 14 and more	3.69	3.20	2.52	1.07	5.86	0.27	12.92
All boys	5.42	5.23	3.58	1.68	7.11	0.02	24.42

with the chi-square goodness-of-fit test. When all examined boys' results have been analyzed, the p-value of the test has been equal to 0.69, yet in some cases the relative error has exceeded 20%. Using the threshold of 14 years has improved the results considerably, since the relative error has very rarely exceeded 9%. The p-value for the goodness-of-fit test has confirmed the exponential distribution (p = 0.76 and p = 0.31 for the younger and older boys respectively). The characteristics of the relative error distribution confirms, that the proposed algorithm is accurate and effective, especially in case of boys in pre-pubertal age.

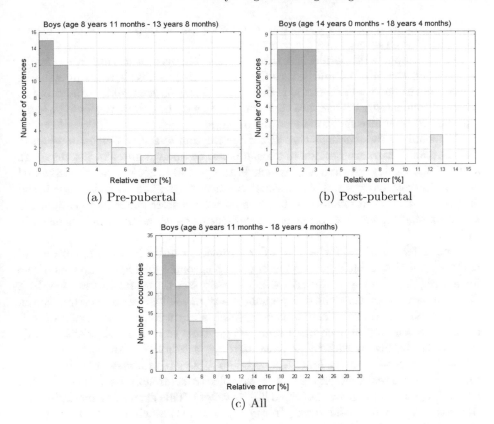

Fig. 2. Relative error, exponential distribution confirmed with chi-squared test with the p-value respectively (a) p = 0.76 (b) p = 0.31 (c) p = 0.69

4   Discussion

The results of this study indicate the high usefulness of the voice, as one of the biological features, to assess the chronological age of boys in the peri-pubertal age. It has been shown that the age of the speaking boy can be estimated in a large approximation on the basis of his voice. This estimate is more accurate for boys under the age of 14. The error in this age group was 0.6 years which gives about 7 months of overestimation or underestimation of the correct chronological age. In the case of boys aged 14 or more, the error was larger—1.5 years. Hodges-Simeon et al. [10], based on the data of Bolivian adolescents, modeled the dependencies between the youths' age and their voice parameters (the fundamental frequency, the frequency range of the voice and the analysis of formants) for both sexes. However, after implementing the model and applying it to the voice data collected for the purpose of this study, the accuracy error had achieved even 40% in case of children aged 12–14 years. This inconsistency confirms the large difference in the rate of biological development between those two ethnic groups and indicates, that it is probably not possible to apply the evaluated algorithms to all populations, without taking into account their ethnic or social diversity.

The Periopubertal period is a time of rapid changes occurring in the body, both within the internal and external organs. This process depends on genetic, gender, environmental and cultural factors. Maturation is an individual process, which is connected with the fact that the changes do not start at all of the same age, nor do they last the same amount of time.

It should be remembered that the direction and speed of these changes are not constant, there are periods of acceleration, no change and slowing down. In spite of this biological diversity, which is the probable reason for the assumed error in the relative method of assessing the chronological age of older boys based on their voice, it is worth noting that this method is more accurate in estimating the chronological age than other biological features such as body height or body weight.

The differentiation of the rate of maturation results in the appearance of children of different biological age in the same chronological age. In terms of the formal requirements of social life, this diversity can be useful in practice. In a direct contact with an identified person, many physiological biometrics remain for use (behavioral are of course very helpful, and perhaps even in certain circumstances leading, but require a much longer time to acquire diversified data). It is worse, if this contact takes place through a sound transmission medium. Consumer devices, usually functionally compatible with phones in their various forms, meet the requirements of telephone voice transmission, i.e. a three-decibel natural telephony band (in the 300–3400 Hz range). This extremely modest (from the point of view of music lovers) frequency range is sufficient to transfer up to the tenth harmonic of the human voice signal (in relation to the above-mentioned averaged, comfortable frequency of emission). What is more, three-decibel rigors impose a stable quality of telephone transmission for the analysis of the characteristics of the voice. Thanks to this, it is possible to use the presented method, especially where the voice is available only on the phone (also in computer messengers). The use of the proposed concept of voice characteristics analysis can therefore be useful in verifying the declaration of an unseen interviewee.

The key conclusion is the positively verified usefulness of the method in multicriteria analysis of dynamic parameters of the maturation curve over time. The specification of such characteristics is a great contribution to the personalization of not only the teaching-learning process, but above all of undertaking activities defined by the developmental psychology of children and youth.

Acknowledgement. We would like to thank Andre Woloshuk for his English language corrections.

References

1. Bugdol, M.D., Bugdol, M.N., Lipowicz, A.M., Mitas, A.W., Bieńkowska, M.J., Wijata, A.M.: Prediction of menarchal status of girls using voice. Comput. Biol. Med. (2017, in press)
2. Cochran, W.G.: The chi-square goodness-of-fit test. Ann. Math. Stat. **23**, 315–345 (1952)
3. Datta, A.K., Solanki, S.S., Sengupta, R., Chakraborty, S., Mahto, K., Patranabis, A.: Signal Analysis of Hindustani Classical Music. Springer, Singapore (2017)
4. Fitch, W.T.: Vocal tract length and formant frequency dispersion correlate with body size in rhesus macaques. J. Acoust. Soc. Am. **102**, 1213–1222 (1997)
5. Freedman, D.A.: Statistical Models: Theory and Practice, vol. 23. Cambridge University Press, New York (2009)
6. Hagg, U., Taranger, J.: Menarche and voice change as indicators of the pubertal growth spurt. Acta Odontol. Scand. **38**(3), 179–186 (1980)
7. Harnsberger, J.D., Brown Jr., W.S., Shrivastav, R., Rothman, H.: Noise and tremor in the perception of vocal aging in males. J. Voice **24**(5), 523–530 (2010)
8. Harries, M.L.L., Hawkins, S., Hacking, J., Hughes, I.A.: Changes in the male voice at puberty: vocal fold length and its relationship to the fundamental frequency of the voice. J. Laryngol. Otol. **112**(5), 451–454 (1998)
9. Harries, M.L.L., Walker, J.M., Williams, D.M., Hawkins, S., Hughes, I.A.: Changes in the male voice at puberty. Arch. Dis. Child. **77**(5), 445–447 (1997)
10. Hodges-Simeon, C.R., Gurven, M., Cardenas, R., Gaulin, S.J.C.: Voice change as a new measure of male pubertal timing: a study among Bolivian adolescents. Ann. Hum. Biol. **40**(3), 209–219 (2013)
11. Hotelling, H.: Analysis of a complex of statistical variables into principal components. J. Educ. Psychol. **24**, 417–441, 498–520 (1933)
12. Hughes, S.M., Rhodes, B.C.: Making age assessments based on vioce: the impact of the reproductive viability of the speaker. J. Soc. Evol. Cult. Psychol. **4**(4), 290–304 (2010)
13. Kaiser, H.F.: The varimax criterionfor analytic rotation in factor analysis. Psychometrika **23**, 187–200 (1958)
14. Kozieł, S.M., Malina, R.M.: Modified maturity offset prediction equations: validation in independent longitudinal samples of boys and girls. Sports Med. **48**(1), 221–236 (2018)
15. Linders, B., Massa, G.G., Boersma, B., Dejonckere, P.H.: Fundamental voice frequency and jitter in girls and boys measured with electroglottography: influence of age and height. Int. J. Pediatr. Otorhinolaryngol. **33**, 61–65 (1995)
16. Nicollas, R., Garrel, R., Ouaknine, M., Giovanni, A., Nazarian, B., Triglia, J.-M.: Normal voice in children between 6 and 12 years of age: database and nonlinear analysis. J. Voice **22**(6), 671–675 (2008)
17. Prasad, K.M.S., Ramaiah, G.N.K., Manjunatha, M.B.: Speech features extraction techniques for robust emotional speech analysis/recognition. Indian J. Sci. Technol. **8**, 1 (2017)
18. Puts, D.A., Apicella, C.L., Cardenas, R.A.: Masculine voices signal men's threat potential in forager and industrial societies. Proc. Biol. Sci. **279**(1728), 601–609 (2012)
19. Ringel, R.L., Chodzko-Zajko, W.J.: Vocal indices of biological age. J. Voice **1**(1), 31–37 (1987)
20. Shmilovitz, D.: On the definition of total harmonic disortion and its effect on measurement interpretation. IEEE Trans. Power Delivery **20**(1), 526–528 (2005)

CAD of Sigmatism Using Neural Networks

Andre Woloshuk[1]($^{\boxtimes}$), Michał Kręcichwost[2], Zuzanna Miodońska[3],
Pawel Badura[2], Joanna Trzaskalik[4], and Ewa Pietka[2]

[1] Weldon School of Biomedical Engineering, Purdue University,
206 S Martin Jischke Dr, West Lafayette, IN 47907, USA
acwolosh@purdue.edu
[2] Faculty of Biomedical Engineering, Silesian University of Technology,
Roosevelta 40, 41-800 Zabrze, Poland
[3] Faculty of Automatic Control, Electronics and Computer Science,
Silesian University of Technology, Akademicka 16, 44-100 Gliwice, Poland
[4] Non-Resident Faculty of Jesuit University Ignatianum in Cracow, Cracow, Poland

Abstract. Sigmatism, or lisp, is a common speech pathology defined by the misarticulation of sibilants and commonly appears in preschool-age children. Automated diagnosis from speech data has been used for other disorders, and the use of acoustic features could objectify the diagnosis procedure. 1593 multichannel recordings from 85 young children were subjected to feature extraction and classification using a neural network. The classification performance was evaluated for single and multichannel input as well as multiple feature sets and articulation phases. Multichannel recordings increased the classifier accuracy from 78.75% to 87.27% when using cepstral and spectral features. The introduction of a multichannel acoustic features was shown to increase sigmatism detection accuracy.

Keywords: ANNs · Multichannel signal processing
Computer-aided pronunciation evaluation · Sibilants
Sigmatism diagnosis

1 Introduction

Computer-aided diagnosis is becoming a more utilized technology in speech pathology and speech mispronunciation to improve therapy as well as give fast feedback to patients and clinicians [1]. Using automated classifiers of voice recordings presents a uniform method to quickly identify these errors and potentially create an at-home therapy for speech pathologies.

Sigmatism, or lisp, is the misarticulation of ($/s, z, ts, dz/, sibilants$ $/S, Z, tS, dZ/, /C, , tC, d/$) and commonly appears in children at the pre-school age [2,3]. Due to the fact that most lisps are caused by functional rather than physical inaccuracies, different positions of the tongue during articulation can

© Springer International Publishing AG, part of Springer Nature 2019
E. Pietka et al. (Eds.): ITIB 2018, AISC 762, pp. 260–271, 2019.
https://doi.org/10.1007/978-3-319-91211-0_23

produce different sounds, which are identified by a speech therapist. Treatment usually begins at the phoneme level, where children can pronounce only a single phoneme with or without the aid of tactile indicators placed in the mouth.

There have been a wide number of signal features used for voice pathology detection, including wavelet packet decomposition (WVD) [4], Linear Prediction Cepstrum Coefficients (LPCC) [5], and most commonly Mel-frequency Cepstral Coefficients (MFCC) [6]. MFCCs work well because they are based on the critical frequencies perceived by the human ear, with linearly spaced filters below 1000 Hz and logarithmically spaced filters over 1000 Hz [7]. Additionally, spectral moments (power (M0), mean (M1), variance (M2), skewness (M3), and kurtosis (M4)) have been shown to be robust features for identifying fricative sounds [8].

A number of different classifiers have been used in the literature for speech pathology detection. Traditionally, Hidden Markov Models (HMM) [9,10] and Support Vector Machines (SVM) [11] have been combined with feature reduction techniques such as Linear Discrimination Analysis (LDA) [12,13] to achieve pathology discrimination accuracies of up to 90% [11,14]. More recently, neural networks present an alternative to these machine learning algorithms [4]. The ability to classify multiple pathological states as well as to use a large number of features makes neural networks a good candidate to handle voice features from multiple microphones to classify speech into three categories (normative, interdental sigmatism, or other sigmatism).

In the previously referenced experimentation, only features extracted from a single-channel have been used for classification purposes. Multichannel analysis has shown promise in the areas of distant speech recognition and spatial learning [15,16]. Adding additional information from neighboring microphones may expose more features with high pathology prediction capabilities because the air patterns around the mouth may be disturbed.

The main contribution described in this paper is the creation of a neural network classifier for multiclass speech pathology diagnosis on a novel, multichannel dataset. Additionally, the network performance was evaluated for single-channel and multichannel data for up to 15 microphones. The authors of [16] created a database with pathological and normal speech signals from children using a multichannel recording device that it is further described in data collection and database section.

The paper is organized as follows. The methods section describe the data set, processing steps, and neural network architecture. The results and discussion sections evaluate the performance of the classifier and compare it to other speech pathology classifiers, respectively.

2 Methods

2.1 Data Collection and Database

Since there is no available database for pathological children's speech, a database was created. It includes 1593 recordings. Speech samples come from 85 children aged 6-8 years prior to any speech therapy. For each child, a speech pathology description was provided by speech therapists along with the diagnosis. The diagnosis consisted of assigning a given child to one of three classes (normative, interdental sigmatism, or another type of sigmatism). The dictionary used during measurements consists of the following logatomes: ASA, ESE, ISI, OSO, USU, YSY, SAS, SES, SIS, SOS, SUS and SYS. The test sequence has been registered at least twice from each child. Table 1 contains a test sequence along with information on how many recordings are in the database. Sequences are used in speech therapy diagnosis [3] and allow phonemes /s/ in various acoustic environments. Analyzed by phoneme, there are three articulation phases: the beginning, middle, and end of a logatome.

Table 1. Count of logotomes of different types in the database

ASA (93)	ESE (92)	ISI (87)	OSO (87)	USU (89)	YSY (91)
SAS (87)	SES (88)	SIS (83)	SOS (92)	SUS (86)	SYS (91)

For the needs of this research, a measuring device for multichannel speech signal recording has been designed and manufactured. The prototype of the device is described in the paper [16]. Measurements were made using its newer version (this version has 15 audio channels and an improved mounting system to ensure accurate placement on the subject's head). Figure 1 shows the location of the microphones during the recording process. To ensure repeatability of the device's position relative to the sound source, the distance between the patient's philtrum and the central microphone was measured.

The directional microphones used are characterized by a linear transmission characteristic in the frequency range of the speech signal. The signal was recorded with a sampling rate of 44100 Hz due to the relevant information contained in the higher frequency bands.

All logatomes were manually segmented in order to mark the boundaries of the segment /s/ occurring in various articulation phases.

2.2   General Workflow

The general workflow for the proposed method is presented in Fig. 2. At first, the registered multichannel waveforms are preprocessed and segmentation. Then, the sibilant part of each utterance is manually segmented. Next, the features are extracted. Finally, the classification of segments is conducted and verified with their logopaedic evaluation.

2.3   Preprocessing and Feature Extraction

For each recorded audio channel, feature extraction was carried out independently and each channel was treated as an independent source of information.

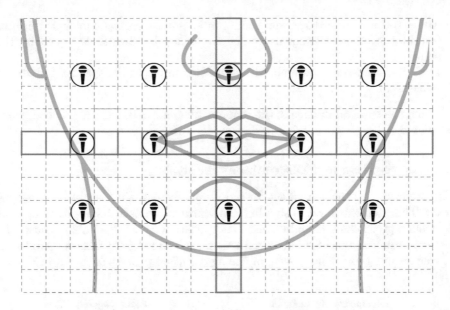

Fig. 1. Microphone configuration on a semicylindrical mask

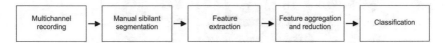

Fig. 2. The general workflow for the proposed method

The first processing step of the /s/ segment was to carry out the pre-amplification process, i.e. to scale the power so that different frequencies had a similar reference level. A framing process was carried out with overlaying and windowing of the analyzed signal fragment. The frame length was 25-ms with a 15-ms shift. The Hamming window was used for windowing.

Feature separation was carried out for individual frames included in the analyzed phoneme /s/. The first feature set determined from a single frame was 13 Mel-frequency Cepstral Coefficients. These features correspond to the vector of cepstrum coefficients in the corresponding mel-bands. They are characterized by low sensitivity to noise and are often used in the literature [17–19].

Spectral moments for particular frames of the segment /s/ have also been determined [20]. They were calculated based on the estimate of the signal's spectrum density [21, 22]. Four spectral moments have been used:

- M0 – the zero-order spectral moment was used for normalization and indicates the signal power.
- M1 – the first-order normalized spectral moment was used to determine the moments of higher orders. In addition, it carries information about the center of gravity of the spectrum.

- M2 – the second-order normalized center-point spectral moment contains information about the square of the frequency bandwidth occupied by the signal.
- M3 – the third-order normalized reference moment in the spectral imbalance (skewness).

From the spectral moments, the amount of spectral flattening (kurtosis) was calculated.

2.4   Aggregation and Discriminant Analysis

After determining the feature set for individual frames, the features were aggregated. This step was used to simplify the features representing a given segment /s/ from a given channel and increase computation speed. For this purpose, the average value was used for individual features obtained from frames included in a given segment /s/. The scheme of the aggregation process is shown in Fig. 3.

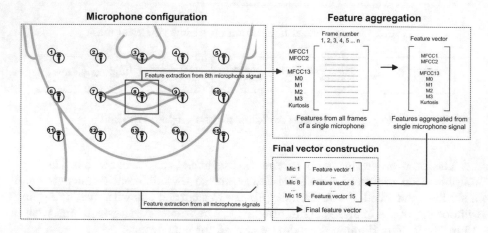

Fig. 3. Feature aggregation process. The features from each channel are extracted and then averaged across the recorded frames

From the average values of each feature, a feature vector was constructed from each channel. This vector contained 13, 18, 195, or 270 features, depending on the number of microphones and features used. The following vectors have been proposed:

- 13 features: 1 channel × 13 MFCC features,
- 18 features: 1 channel × (13 MFCC features + M0, M1, M2, M3, and Kurtosis),
- 95 features: 15 channels × 13 MFCC features,
- 270 features: 15 channels × (13 MFCC features + M0, M1, M2, M3, and Kurtosis).

In order to further reduce the dimensionality of the proposed feature vector and to find a linear combination of features that would best differentiate the analyzed groups, Fisher's linear discriminant analysis (FLDA) was used [12].

2.5 Classification

Data Preparation. A total of 1593 labeled voice samples were obtained, which were split randomly into training, validation, and testing sets. The data was split for a 10-fold cross validation training structure. 80% of the samples were used for training, 10% for validation, and 10% for testing. Ten networks were trained, each with a different subset of the data used for the testing and validation sets so that each section of the data was used for testing and validation once.

Network Design. A feed-forward neural network design was implemented to classify the speech recordings into 3 categories (normative, interdental, or other sigmatism). The design of the network consisted of two main variables that influenced the accuracy: the number of hidden nodes and regularization amount. All networks had a single hidden layer. Because the number of inputs varied from single to multichannel analysis and when using different features, it was necessary to adjust the structure to maximize the validation accuracy of each network. The highest performing structure of each network can be seen in Table 2.

Table 2. Highest performing parameters for each network after FLDA

Channels, Features	Hidden nodes	Regularization
Single, 13 MFCC features	26	0.1
Multi, 71 of 195 MFCC features	31	0.3
Single, 18 features (MFCC + Moments)	28	0.1
Multi, 91 of 270 features (MFCC + Moments)	26	0.6

Scaled conjugate gradient (SCG) backpropagation has been used successfully on MFCC features for classification [4]. Conjugate backpropagation searches for alternative gradient descents, which usually results in faster convergence compared to traditional backpropagation, which uses the largest gradient. SCG optimizes this search to reduce the number of computations in each layer, but may result in more iterations overall [23,24]. Each individual network was trained until the model validation error increased 150 times or the backpropagation error gradient was less than $1e-5$. The performance was evaluated using mean squared error (MSE).

Feature Comparison. In previous experimentation, only MFCC features have been used for classification purposes. Spectral moment and kurtosis data could improve network classification performance. To test this hypothesis, the network trained on 13 MFCC features per channel was compared to a network trained on 18 features (MFCC, spectral moments, and kurtosis) per channel.

Articulation Phase Comparison. The database contains three different articulation phases for the six logatoms. A neural network trained on a specific articulation phase may achieve higher accuracy than one trained on all phases because there is less variation in the original signal.

Analysis. After all the networks were trained and tested, the aggregate number of true positives (TP), true negatives (TN), false positives (FP), and false negatives (FN) were used to calculate the sensitivity (1), specificity (2) and accuracy (3) of the classifier. These values were calculated from a 3×3 confusion matrix as follows. All experiments were repeated 50 times and the results were averaged.

- sensitivity:
$$TPR = \frac{TP}{TP + FN} \cdot 100\%, \tag{1}$$

- specificity:
$$SPC = \frac{TN}{FP + TN} \cdot 100\%, \tag{2}$$

- accuracy:
$$ACC = \frac{TP + TN}{TP + FP + FN + TN} \cdot 100\%. \tag{3}$$

3   Experiments and Results

The network structure for each data type with the highest accuracy can be seen in Table 2, including both the number of hidden neurons and regularization. Both of these values were determined empirically, as seen in Figs. 4 and 5, and used in all resulting experimentation.

The average accuracy, sensitivity, and specificity can be seen in the Table 3. After FLDA, multichannel data using all features had the highest accuracy, sensitivity, and specificity of all feature vectors, 82.27%, 88.56%, and 91.33%, respectively.

The accuracy distribution for the networks trained on different channel and feature types is shown in Fig. 6.

Figure 7 shows the boxplot and distribution of each phase type. Phase 3 logatomes (SAⓈ SEⓈ, etc.) had a higher accuracy than Phase 1 (ⓈAS, ⓈES, etc.) and Phase 2 (AⓈA, EⓈE, etc.) logatomes, 86.36% compared to 84.89% and 82.36%, respectively. However, the network trained on all logatome phases had the highest accuracy. In all cases, feature reduction using FLDA outperformed those networks that did not use FLDA.

Table 3. Average accuracy, sensitivity, and specificity of each network

Channels, Features	Accuracy (%)	Sensitivity	Specificity
Single, MFCC	79.19 ± 0.16	77.29	84.63
Multi, MFCC	86.35 ± 0.14	86.30	90.23
Single, MFCC + Moments	78.75 ± 0.13	76.31	84.41
Multi, MFCC + Moments	87.27 ± 0.14	88.56	91.33

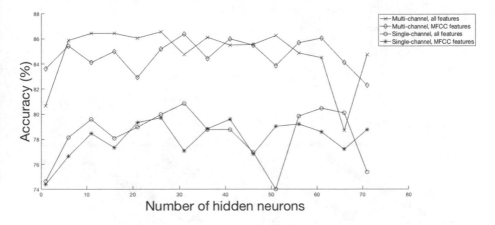

Fig. 4. The accuracy of different numbers of hidden neurons for each feature and channel type

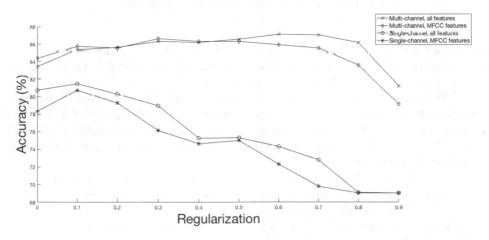

Fig. 5. The accuracy of different regularization for each feature and channel type

4   Discussion

The highest performing structure for each neural network varied in both network size and regularization. In all cases, the number of neurons with the highest

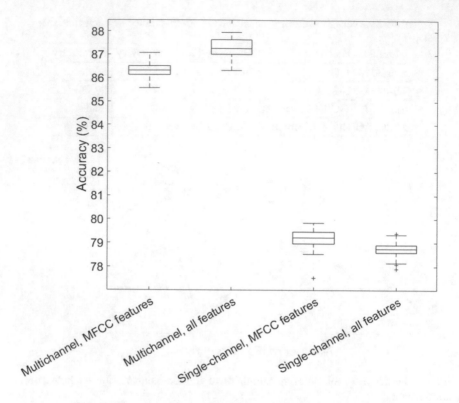

Fig. 6. Accuracy of variable feature and channel selection

accuracy was approximately 30. For single-channel data, high amounts of regularization crippled performance, while it increased performance in multichannel data. FLDA reduced the number of features in each network.

In all of the experiments, FLDA produced a statistically significant ($p = 0.01$) increase in the accuracy of the classifier and reduced the number of features by up to 66% (from 270 to 91 features). Feature reduction techniques including PCA [25] and LDA [12] have been shown to improve classifier accuracy in voice impairments and disorders.

The number of features used by each microphone did not vary by distance from the philtrum. The channels closest to the center (microphones 3, 7, 8, 9, and 13) did not provide more features than the average channel for MFCC (4.8 vs. 4.6 features, respectively) or MFCC and spectral moments (6.8 vs. 6.86, respectively). For multichannel data, it seems that the microphones closest to the philtrum do not provide more discriminating features (based on FLDA) than other microphones, and it is the aggregate features from all microphones which contribute to the observed accuracy increase between single and multichannel data.

Additionally, using a combination of MFCC features and spectral moments improved results for multichannel data, but worsened the accuracy in

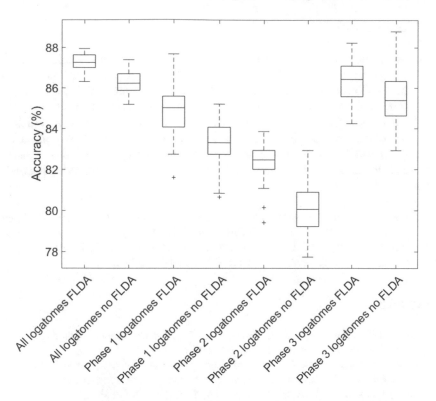

Fig. 7. Accuracy of the multichannel, all feature network for individual articulation phases with and without FLDA

single-channel data. One explanation for this result is that while static acoustic features, such as spectral moments, can aid in fricative identification [25], they could not reliably distinguish between further subclassification (interdental vs. labiodental fricatives). For multichannel data, using both MFCC and spectral moments increased the accuracy from 86.25% to 87.27% when classifying the speech samples into three classes (normative, interdental sigmatism, or another type of sigmatism).

For all feature sets, multichannel data performed better than data from a single-channel. The multichannel recording device may improve accuracy by capturing information about the spatial changes in sound associated with tongue misplacement and sigmatism. Using single-channel data, the authors of [26] were able to achieve an accuracy of 75% in identifying multiple /r/ misarticulations in Arabic using an I-vector classification system, and 92% in binary classification.

The performance of each individual articulation phase was worse than the entire dataset. Phases 1 and 2 performed much worse, while Phase 3 only slightly differed from the network trained on all phases. The number of samples to train the network seems to be more important than the specific type of samples used.

5   Conclusion

While neural networks have been used for speech pathology classification, their use in multiclass discrimination, especially regarding sigmatism, has been limited. The development of a new network to classify different types of sigmatism has the potential to standardize and aid in pathology diagnosis. Similarly, current speech pathology databases come from a single audio channel. The multichannel speech database used showed a significant performance increase compared to the single-channel equivalent. Further experimentation could seek to increase the number of classes or improve the classification accuracy from a single articulation phase.

Acknowledgement. The work has been partially financed by: Polish Ministry of Science and Silesian University of Technology statutory financial support for young researchers BKM-510/RAu-3/2017 and Faculty of Biomedical Engineering statutory financial support No. BK-209/RIB1/2018 (07/010/BK_18/0021).

References

1. Borsel, J.V., Rentergem, S.V., Verhaeghe, L.: The prevalence of lisping in young adults. J. Commun. Disord. **40**(6), 493–502 (2007)
2. Lobacz, P., Dobrzanska, K.: Acoustic description of sybilant phones in pronunciation of pre-school children, (PL) Opis akustyczny glosek sybilantnych w wymowie dzieci przedszkolnych. Audiofonologia **15**, 7–26 (1999). (in Polish)
3. Trzaskalik, J.: Sigmatismus lateralis in polish logopedics literature. theoretical considerations, (PL) Seplenienie boczne w polskiej literaturze logopedycznej. Rozważania teoretyczne. Forum Logopedyczne **24**, 33–46 (2016). (in Polish)
4. Majidnezhad, V.: A novel hybrid of genetic algorithm and ANN for developing a high efficient method for vocal fold pathology diagnosis. EURASIP J. Audio Speech Music Process. **2015**(1), 3 (2015)
5. Ai, O.C., Hariharan, M., Yaacob, S., Chee, L.S.: Classification of speech dysfluencies with MFCC and LPCC features. Expert Syst. Appl. **39**(2), 2157–2165 (2012)
6. Majidnezhad, V., Kheidorov, I.: An ANN-based method for detecting vocal fold pathology. CoRR abs/1302.1772 (2013)
7. Muda, L., Begam, M., Elamvazuthi, I.: Voice recognition algorithms using Mel Frequency Cepstral Coefficient (MFCC) and Dynamic Time Warping (DTW) techniques. CoRR abs/1003.4083 (2010)
8. Kong, Y.Y., Mullangi, A., Kokkinakis, K.: Classification of fricative consonants for speech enhancement in hearing devices. PLOS ONE **9**(4), 1–8 (2014)
9. Miodońska, Z., Kręcichwost, M., Szymańska, A.: Computer-Aided Evaluation of Sibilants in Preschool Children Sigmatism Diagnosis, pp. 367–376. Springer International Publishing, Cham (2016)
10. Hu, W., Qian, Y., Soong, F.K., Wang, Y.: Improved mispronunciation detection with deep neural network trained acoustic models and transfer learning based logistic regression classifiers. Speech Commun. **67**(Suppl. C), 154–166 (2015)
11. Ali, S.M., Karule, P.T.: MFCC, LPCC, formants and pitch proven to be best features in diagnosis of speech disorder using neural networks and SVM. Int. J. Appl. Eng. Res. **11**(2), 897–903 (2016)

12. Akbari, A., Arjmandi, M.K.: An efficient voice pathology classification scheme based on applying multi-layer linear discriminant analysis to wavelet packet-based features. Biomed. Signal Process. Control **10**, 209–223 (2014)
13. Bugdol, M.D., Bugdol, M.N., Lipowicz, A.M., Mitas, A.W., Bienkowska, M.J., Wijata, A.M.: Prediction of menarcheal status of girls using voice features. Computers in Biology and Medicine (2017)
14. El Hanine, M., Abdelmounim, E., Haddadi, R., Belaguid, A.: Electrocardiogram signal denoising using discrete wavelet transform. Comput. Technol. Appl. **5**(2) (2014)
15. Król, D., Lorenc, A., Świcęiński, R .: Detecting laterality and nasality in speech with the use of a multi-channel recorder. In: 2015 IEEE International Conference on Acoustics, Speech and Signal Processing (ICASSP), pp. 5147–5151, April 2015
16. Kręcichwost, M., Miodońska, Z., Trzaskalik, J., Pyttel, J., Spinczyk, D.: Acoustic Mask for Air Flow Distribution Analysis in Speech Therapy, pp. 377–387. Springer International Publishing, Cham (2016)
17. Miodonska, Z., Bugdol, M.D., Krecichwost, M.: Dynamic time warping in phoneme modeling for fast pronunciation error detection. Comput. Biol. Med. **69**, 277–285 (2016)
18. Srinivasan, V., Ramalingam, V., Arulmozhi, P.: Artificial neural network based pathological voice classification using MFCC features (2014)
19. Hossan, M.A., Memon, S., Gregory, M.A.: A novel approach for MFCC feature extraction. In: 2010 4th International Conference on Signal Processing and Communication Systems, pp. 1–5, December 2010
20. Korkko, P.: Spectral moments analysis of /s/ coarticulation development in Finnish-speaking children. paper 470
21. Ravan, M., Beheshti, S.: Speech recognition from adaptive windowing PSD estimation. In: 2011 24th Canadian Conference on Electrical and Computer Engineering (CCECE), pp. 000524–000527, May 2011
22. Percival, D.B., Walden, A.T.: Spectral Analysis for Physical Applications. Cambridge University Press, Cambridge (1993)
23. Hagan, M.T., Demuth, H.B., Beale, M.: Neural Network Design. PWS Publishing Co., Boston (1996)
24. Moller, M.F.: A scaled conjugate gradient algorithm for fast supervised learning. Neural Netw. **6**(4), 525–533 (1993)
25. Ali, A.M.A., der Spiegel, J.V., Mueller, P.: Acoustic-phonetic features for the automatic classification of fricatives. J. Acoust. Soc. Am. **109**(5), 2217–2235 (2001)
26. Hanani, Abualsoud, A.: Automatic identification of articulation disorders for arabic children speakers. Birzeit University Open Access Repository (2016)

Arterial Flows in Bronchopulmonary Dysplasia Prediction

Wiesław Wajs[1]([✉]), Piotr Kruczek[2], Piotr Szymański[3], Piotr Wais[4], and Marcin Ochab[1]

[1] University of Rzeszów, Rzeszów, Poland
wwa@agh.edu.pl
[2] Medical College, Jagiellonian University, Kraków, Poland
[3] Obstetric Hospital Ujastek, Kraków, Poland
[4] Krosno State College, Krosno, Poland

Abstract. The paper presents Bronchopulmonary Dysplasia, BPD, prediction for extremely premature infants after their first week of life using LR (Logit Regression). Presented models give accuracy up to 84.6% using only three independent variables and 81.7% with two of them. That novelty was possible to achieve thanks to unique use of arterial flows measurements, which are not a common clinical practice. That original data was collected thanks to the Neonatal Intensive Care Unit of The Department of Pediatrics at Jagiellonian University Medical College. The main pulmonary artery (MPA) and patent ductus arteriosus (PDA) flows were considered as predictors. Beyond classic statistic significance analysis and LR forecast paper presents some other results and discussion, which give an outlook on possible repeatability of results and its quality on some other's patients data set.

Keywords: Bronchopulmonary dysplasia · Logit regression
Prediction · Prematurity · Low-birth-weight infant · Newborn
Arterial flows · Main pulmonary artery

1 Introduction

Bronchopulmonary dysplasia (BPD) is a chronic pulmonary disease which affects premature infants [22]. It results in significant morbidity and mortality, affecting nearly a third of newborns with birth weight lower than 1000 g [25]. Apart from mentioned factor BPD is mostly diagnosed among those who received prolonged mechanical ventilation needed to treat respiratory distress syndrome [8,9]. Due to the fact that the disease is poorly understood, many projects are focused on identifying its risk factors. Although it is widely known that steroids applied before the 8th day of life can prevent BPD development, the risk of complications when applied unnecessarily is very high [6]. Unfortunately BPD can not be diagnosed before a 28th day of life [24]. That is why prediction of such a result by the end of the first week is so important. The accurate forecast could enable

© Springer International Publishing AG, part of Springer Nature 2019
E. Pietka et al. (Eds.): ITIB 2018, AISC 762, pp. 272–278, 2019.
https://doi.org/10.1007/978-3-319-91211-0_24

early intervention and an increased likelihood of preventing the disease with limited risk of side effects. Therefore so much effort has been put to find a classifier, which based on known features would be able to predict the diagnosis. For that purpose researchers mostly use static parameters gathered after birth. Some of works propose dynamic ones as well, which are collected during the first week of life. Although some prediction models of BPD have been proposed, any of them could be adopted in common clinical practice due to a variety of reasons [16]. What is more arterial flows measurements have never been used for that purpose.

2   Data

There are numerous works related to BPD prediction and its risk factors [1,5,12,13,17,18]. The most easily available are static parameters among which gestational age (*gage*) and birth weight (*bweight*) is most commonly used [3,4,10,12,17,19]. The other independent variables mentioned in the literature are admission of surfactant (*surfact*) [1,6,11,13,17], presence of patent ductus arteriosis (*pda*) [2,4–6,8,11,13,17,18,20], or respiratory support (*respimv*) [2,12]. Use of alveolar-arterial ratio (*aa*) [7,21] is a little less frequent. Doppler blood flow measurements are not a common clinical practice, so such data is very difficult to get. Only one paper [23] refers to use of a corrected acceleration time to right ventricular ejection time ratio (AT:RVET(c)) in BPD prediction, but authors mention of problems with collecting reasonable set of data. Thanks to the Neonatal Intensive Care Unit of The Department of Pediatrics at Jagiellonian University Medical College we were able to collect data of 52 patients, which contain mentioned above parameters. Moreover we were able to acquire main pulmonary artery (MPA) (*mpaflow*) and patent ductus arteriosus (PDA) (*pdaflow*) flows. Depending on the conditions we collected 4 to 16 samples on each patients during the first week of its life. Due to suspicion that prolonged increased flow may escalate risk of BPD we analyzed mean values of samples. We also defined total arterial flow (*sumflow*) as sum of *mpaflow* and *pdaflow*.

3   Statistical Analysis

In that part computations were performed with StatSoft Statistica package. As a first step of classic medical prediction procedure we calculated Pearson correlation of parameters (Table 1). It should be mentioned that *mpaflow* is highly correlated with *gage* and *bweight*. That is natural, since flow is measured in l/min, it is simply higher for every child with greater weight (dividing the flow value by *bweight* we get correlation 0.04 and such data modification does not affect prediction results in any way). Exactly the same situation occurs with *sumflow*. As might be expected parameters *gage* and *bweight* are also highly correlated – older child in most cases weights more.

Table 1. Pearson correlation of parameters

Variable	gage	bweight	bpd	aa	surfact	respimv	pda	pdaflow	mpaflow	sumflow
gage	1.00	**0.65**	−0.38	0.08	−0.28	−0.33	0.09	−0.03	0.61	0.58
bweight	**0.65**	1.00	−0.55	0.12	−0.40	−0.51	0.10	−0.04	0.74	0.70
bpd	−0.38	−0.55	1.00	−0.20	0.26	0.37	−0.02	0.06	−0.23	−0.20
aa	0.08	0.12	−0.20	1.00	−0.50	−0.19	−0.04	0.04	0.04	0.05
surfact	−0.28	−0.40	0.26	−0.50	1.00	0.38	0.19	0.38	−0.19	−0.06
respimv	−0.33	−0.51	0.37	−0.19	0.38	1.00	−0.14	−0.20	−0.23	−0.28
pda	0.09	0.10	−0.02	−0.04	0.19	−0.14	1.00	0.41	0.18	0.30
pdaflow	−0.03	−0.04	0.06	0.04	0.38	−0.20	0.41	1.00	−0.01	0.30
mpaflow	**0.61**	**0.74**	−0.23	0.04	−0.19	−0.23	0.18	0.01	1.00	0.95
sumflow	0.58	0.70	−0.20	0.05	−0.06	−0.28	0.30	0.30	0.95	1.00

Table 2. Kolmogorov-Smirnov test results; variables significant at $p < 0.05000$ are bolded

Variable	p-level	Mean		Std. Dev.		Samples	
		Positive	Negative	Positive	Negative	Positive	Negative
gage	**p < 0.005**	27.21	29.15	2.52	1.95	33	19
bweight	**p < 0.005**	968	1258	229	185	33	19
aa	p > 0.10	0.226	0.286	0.123	0.170	33	19
surfact	p > 0.10	0.818	0.579	0.392	0.507	33	19
respimv	p < 0.10	0.788	0.421	0.415	0.507	33	19
pda	p > 0.10	0.878	0.895	0.331	0.315	33	19
pdaflow	p > 0.10	0.037	0.033	0.035	0.026	33	19
mpaflow	**p < 0.05**	0.37	0.41	0.11	0.06	33	19
sumflow	p > 0.10	0.408	0.45	0.113	0.073	33	19

Table 3. Traditional approach BPD logit prediction results obtained using MPA flow, brith weight and gestational age; accuracy (ACC) of prediction was 84.62%, specifity (SPC) 73.68%, sensitivity (TPR) 90.90%, positive predictive value (PPV) 85.71%, negative predictive value (NPV) 82.35%

Real BPD diagnosis	Predicted positive diagnosis	Predicted negative diagnosis	Percent of correct diagnosis
Positive	30	3	90.90%
Negative	5	14	73.68%

By the reason of not well known distribution of parameters a Kolmogorov-Smirnov test was performed (Table 2). As a result we get three statistically significant predictors: *gage*, *bweight* and *mpaflow*. The very same independent variables were used for prediction of future diagnosis using logit regression. Results are presented in Table 3.

4   Results Repeatability

Authors are aware of small number of samples used in calculations which may cause results glitches. On the other hand Doppler measurements results are hardly available [23] and expansion of the database is not possible. That is why we decided to use method similar to Jacknife proposed in [15]. Repeating tests with removed some random data each time are deliberately lowering results, but these we get are more data independent and can be considered as more likely possible to achieve on different patients set. Due to the low computational complexity of Algorithm 1 we were able to analyze all 2^9 feature combinations using Matlab environment. Most interesting results are presented in Table 4.

```
for each feature_combination do
    for 1...30 do
        patients = delete_5_random(all_patients);
        for each test_patient of patients do
            logit_learn_patients = patients - test_patient;
            logit_predict(test_patient, learn_patients);
        end
        calculate ACC, TPR, SPC;
    end
    for ACC, TPR, SPC do
        calculate mean_value and dev;
    end
    best_results[feature_combination] = best(meanACC);
end
```

Algorithm 1. Models evaluation algorithm

Table 4. Most interesting Jacknife logit regression results

Accuracy %	Sensitivity %	Specifity %	Parameter 1	Parameter 2	Parameter 3	Parameter 4
83.03	93.80	64.43	aa	$bweight$	$mpaflow$	pda
82.41	93.31	63.48	aa	$bweight$	$pdaflow$	$sumflow$
82.32	93.24	62.90	aa	$bweight$	$mpaflow$	
82.11	93.38	62.08	aa	$bweight$	$mpaflow$	$sumflow$
82.08	93.13	62.90	aa	$bweight$	$mpaflow$	$pdaflow$
81.90	93.44	61.73	$respimv$	$bweight$	$mpaflow$	
81.70	92.92	61.92	$bweight$	$mpaflow$		

5   Conclusions

Presented results show that arterial flows give important information that can be used in bronchopulmonary dysplasia prediction. These presented in Table 3 (ACC 84.62% , SPC 73.68%, TPR 90.90%) are better even than other complex

models based on dynamic data (ACC 83.29%, SPC 79.08%, SPC 86.4%) [16].
However due to small amount of data it is unlikely that they would be repeatable.
Even looking at Table 4 can be seen that with the same data missing only 5
random samples results are worse. Despite that comparing Table 4 to results
from [14] (obtained with the same Algorithm 1) we see that considering only
2-parameter models we get 81.7% of ACC, 92.92% of SPC, 61.92% of TPR
versus respectively 81.06%, 84.39% and 78.62% – MPA flows give little higher
accuracy and about 8% increase in specifity. Looking at 3-parameter models
we get accordingly 82.32%, 93.24% and 62.9% vs obtained with dynamic data
81.29%, 88.7% and 75.9%, which is also better in favour of MPA. Comparing the
highest accuracy results we get 83.03%, 93,80% and 64,43% computed with MPA
flow and three other features vs 83.29%, 79.08% and 86.4% from [16] which is
little better, but involves much more computationally complex SVM algorithm
and as much as nine variables. Best reported logit regression result in [16] was
obtained with six predictors and gave respectively 82.79%, 84.2% and 81.73%
which is worse and also much more complex.

As proved arterial flow measurements can be successfully used to construct
simple and powerful BPD prediction models. It seems that MPA could provide
some new quality in that field. It would be very interesting to try some new
models consisting arterial flows analysis combined with other dynamic data.
Unfortunately as of today, we do not have such data.

References

1. Ambalavanan, N., Van Meurs, K.P., Perritt, R., Carlo, W.A., Ehrenkranz, R.A.,
   Stevenson, D.K., Lemons, J.A., Poole, W.K., Higgins, R.D.: Predictors of death or
   bronchopulmonary dysplasia in preterm infants with respiratory failure. J. Perina-
   tol. **28**(6), 420–426 (2008). https://doi.org/10.1038/jp.2008.18
2. Bhering, C.A., Mochdece, C.C., Moreira, M.E., Rocco, J.R., Sant'Anna, G.M.:
   Bronchopulmonary dysplasia prediction modelfor 7-day-old infants. Jornal de pediatria **83**(2), 163–170 (2007). https://doi.org/10.1590/S0021-75572007000200011
3. Bhutani, V.K., Abbasi, S.: Relative likelihood of bronchopulmonary dysplasia
   based on pulmonary mechanics measured in preterm neonates during the first
   week of life. J. Pediatr. **120**(4), 605–613 (1992). https://doi.org/10.1016/S0022-
   3476(05)82491-6
4. Corcoran, J., Patterson, C., Thomas, P., Halliday, H.: Reduction in the risk of bronchopulmonary dysplasia from 1980–1990: results of a multivariate logistic regression analysis. Eur. J. Pediatr. **152**(8), 677–681 (1993). https://doi.org/10.1007/
   BF01955247
5. Cunha, G.S., Mezzacappa-Filho, F., Ribeiro, J.D.: Risk factors for bronchopulmonary dysplasia in very low birth weight newborns treated with mechanical ventilation in the first week of life. J. Trop. Pediatr. **51**(6), 334–340 (2005). https://
   doi.org/10.1093/tropej/fmi051
6. Farstad, T., Bratlid, D., Medbø, S., Markestad, T.: Bronchopulmonary dysplasia-
   prevalence, severity and predictive factors in a national cohort of extremely premature infants. Acta Paediatr. **100**(1), 53–58 (2011). https://doi.org/10.1111/j.1651-
   2227.2010.01959.x

7. Gilbert, R., Keighley, J.: The arterial-alveolar oxygen tension ratio. an index of gas exchange applicable to varying inspired oxygen concentrations. Am. Rev. Respir. Dis. **109**(1), 142 (1974)
8. Groothuis, J.R., Makari, D.: Definition and outpatient management of the very low-birth-weight infant with bronchopulmonary dysplasia. Adv. Therapy **29**(4), 297–311 (2012). https://doi.org/10.1007/s12325-012-0015-y
9. Jobe, A.H.: The new bronchopulmonary dysplasia. Curr. Opin. Pediatr. **23**(2), 167 (2011). https://doi.org/10.1097/MOP.0b013e3283423e6b
10. Kim, Y.D., Kim, E.A.R., Kim, K.S., Pi, S.Y., Kang, W.: Scoring method for early prediction of neonatal chronic lung disease using modified respiratory parameters. J. Korean Med. Sci. **20**(3), 397–401 (2005). https://doi.org/10.3346/jkms.2005.20.3.397
11. Kim, Y.D., Kim, K.S., Kim, E.A.R., Lee, J.J., Park, S.J., Pi, S.Y.: Perinatal risk factors for the development of bronchopulmonary dysplasia in premature infants less than 32 weeks' gestation. J. Korean Soc. Neonatol. **8**(1), 78–93 (2001)
12. Laughon, M.M., Langer, J.C., Bose, C.L., Smith, P.B., Ambalavanan, N., Kennedy, K.A., Stoll, B.J., Buchter, S., Laptook, A.R., Ehrenkranz, R.A., et al.: Prediction of bronchopulmonary dysplasia by postnatal age in extremely premature infants. Am. J. Respir. Crit. Care Med. **183**(12), 1715–1722 (2011). https://doi.org/10.1164/rccm.201101-0055OC
13. Marshall, D.D., Kotelchuck, M., Young, T.E., Bose, C.L., Kruyer, L., O'Shea, T.M.: Risk factors for chronic lung disease in the surfactant era: a north carolina population-based study of very low birth weight infants. Pediatrics **104**(6), 1345–1350 (1999). https://doi.org/10.1542/peds.104.6.1345
14. Ochab, M., Wajs, W.: Bronchopulmonary dysplasia prediction using support vector machine and LIBSVM. In: Proceedings of the 2014 Federated Conference on Computer Science and Information Systems, Annals of Computer Science and Information Systems, vol. 2, pp. 201–208. IEEE (2014). https://doi.org/10.15439/2014F111
15. Ochab,M.,Wajs,W.: Bronchopulmonary dysplasia prediction using support vector machine and logit regression. Inf. Technol. Biomed. **4**, 365–374 (2014). https://doi.org/10.1007/978-3-319-06596-0_34
16. Ochab, M., Wajs, W.: Expert system supporting an early prediction of the bronchopulmonary dysplasia. Comput. Biol. Med. **69**, 236–244 (2016). https://doi.org/10.1016/j.compbiomed.2015.08.016
17. Oh, W., Poindexter, B., Perritt, R., Lemons, J., Bauer, C., Ehrenkranz, R., Stoll, B., Poole, K., Wright, L.: Neonatal research network. association between fluid intake and weight loss during the first ten days of life and risk of bronchopulmonary dysplasia in extremely low birth weight infants. J. Pediatr. **147**(6), 786–790 (2005). https://doi.org/10.1016/j.jpeds.2005.06.039
18. Rojas, M.A., Gonzalez, A., Bancalari, E., Claure, N., Poole, C., Silva-Neto, G.: Changing trends in the epidemiology and pathogenesis of neonatal chronic lung disease. J. Pediatr. **126**(4), 605–610 (1995). https://doi.org/10.1016/S0022-3476(95)70362-4
19. Sinkin, R.A., Cox, C., Phelps, D.L.: Predicting risk for bronchopulmonary dysplasia: selection criteria for clinical trials. Pediatrics **86**(5), 728–736 (1990)
20. Sosenko, I., Bancalari, E.: New developments in the pathogenesis and prevention of bronchopulmonary dysplasia. The Newborn Lung: Neonatology Questions and Controversies: Expert Consult-Online and Print, pp. 217–233 (2012)

21. Stoch, P.: Zastosowanie narzędzi statystycznych i matematycznych metod sztucznej inteligencji do predykcji wystąpienia dysplazji oskrzelowo-płucnej u noworodków. Praca doktorska , Akademia Górniczo-Hutnicza, Kraków, pp. 60–72 (2007). (in Polish)
22. Stoll, B.J., Hansen, N.I., Bell, E.F., Shankaran, S., Laptook, A.R., Walsh, M.C., Hale, E.C., Newman, N.S., Schibler, K., Carlo, W.A., et al.: Neonatal outcomes of extremely preterm infants from the nichd neonatal research network. Pediatrics **126**(3), 443–456 (2010). https://doi.org/10.1542/peds.2009-2959
23. Subhedar, N., Hamdan, A., Ryan, S., Shaw, N.: Pulmonary artery pressure: early predictor of chronic lung disease in preterm infants. Arch. Dis. Childhood-Fetal Neonatal Ed. **78**(1), F20–F24 (1998). https://doi.org/10.1136/fn.78.1.F20
24. Tapia, J.L., Agost, D., Alegria, A., Standen, J., Escobar, M., Grandi, C., Musante, G., Zegarra, J., Estay, A., Ramírez, R.: Bronchopulmonary dysplasia: incidence, risk factors and resource utilization in a population of south-american very low birth weight infants. Jornal de pediatria **82**(1), 15–20 (2006). https://doi.org/10.1590/S0021-75572006000100005
25. Walsh, M.C., Szefler, S., Davis, J., Allen, M., Van Marter, L., Abman, S., Blackmon, L., Jobe, A.: Summary proceedings from the bronchopulmonary dysplasia group. Pediatrics **117**(Supplement 1), S52–S56 (2006). https://doi.org/10.1542/peds.2005-0620I

Attribute-Based Assessment of Lung Nodules in CT Using Support Vector Machine and Random Forest

Beata Choroba[✉] and Pawel Badura

Faculty of Biomedical Engineering, Silesian University of Technology,
Roosevelta 40, 41-800 Zabrze, Poland
beata.choroba@polsl.pl

Abstract. An attempt to provide a tool for detection of certain attributes of pulmonary nodules is presented in this paper. The support vector machine and random forest are employed to determine the nodule calcification and likelihood of malignancy on the basis of ten intensity and geometric features. Training and validation relies on lung nodule cases from the public LIDC-IDRI database with over a thousand computed tomography studies. Lesion annotation provided by four radiologists in terms of delineation and quantitative assessment of selected attributes yields ca. 2500 nodules available for the analysis. In both classifications involving two classifiers the accuracy exceeding 80% was achieved.

Keywords: Computer-aided diagnosis · Lung cancer · Classification
Support vector machine · Random forest

1 Introduction

Lung cancer causes ca. 1.7 million deaths worldwide each year, which is the most of all cancers [36]. It is, however, considered the most preventable cancer, since ca. 80% deaths are thought to result from tobacco smoking [1]. Early detection of lung cancer significantly increases the curability rate. Usually, the diagnosis relies on thoracic computed tomography (CT) studies. The lesion appearance can routinely be assessed in clinical practice for lung cancer diagnosis. Although the physician remains responsible for these actions, her/his work is often supported by dedicated computer-aided diagnosis (CAD) systems, able to effectively analyse huge amount of data in an automated way and provide valuable findings or help in quantitative lesion assessment.

One of the main concerns in CAD may be identified in an access to reliable and versatile reference data. CAD training and validation requirements force a need to prepare large datasets of images, at best with expert annotations in terms of, *e.g.*, delineations of the object of interest, quantitative or text annotations [31,35,37]. In a lung nodule field of study this problem was addressed by the Lung Image Database Consortium (LIDC). The consortium

© Springer International Publishing AG, part of Springer Nature 2019
E. Pietka et al. (Eds.): ITIB 2018, AISC 762, pp. 279–289, 2019.
https://doi.org/10.1007/978-3-319-91211-0_25

constituted by multiple research units in the US prepared a database of CT studies containing various types of lesions. The LIDC first dataset [3] consisted of 23 cases subjected to a blinded and unblinded reviews performed by six radiologists. The experiment yielded a voxel probability map per each nodule reflecting an inter-observer pathology confidence level. The dataset was used by multiple researchers as a gold standard in studies on automated detection and segmentation of lung nodules [4,5,14,23,25,26,33,34]. Further database development concluded with a publication of the LIDC-IDRI (Image Database Resource Initiative) database [2,29] containing 1018 cases, each including a clinical thoracic CT along with an XML file, recording results of a two-phase annotation process involving four radiologists. Each expert described the lesion by means of a voxel-wise delineation as well as subjective assessment of nine selected characteristics, *e.g.*, subtlety, calcification, spiculation, lobulation, or likelihood of malignancy. Since the LIDC-IDRI dataset publication, its cases were employed to validate computer-aided detection algorithms [9,21,32], segmentation techniques [6,10,11,13,15,27], studies on intra- and interobserver variability [20,28], or studies on textural features of pulmonary nodules appearance in CT [24].

Visual analysis of the nodule texture enables subjective assessment of certain attributes, describable by means of some linguistic standards. However, they can also be evaluated quantitatively, using some predefined scales. Such approach was used in the LIDC-IDRI dataset, where the proposed attributes were rated in a predefined scale reflecting the level of their likelihood noticed by the expert. Numerical reference data can be employed as a gold standard by automated detection or recognition system for certain property, *e.g.* likelihood of malignancy. Such an improved support of a physician decision-making process based on mining of high-dimensional feature spaces describing the image data is called radiomics [16]. Its application in lung cancer domain became quite common recently [7,17,19,22,30].

The main goal of this study is to create and verify a tool for automated detection of certain types of lung nodules. With a large LIDC-IDRI database of various lesions, we are able to take advantage of expert annotations when training and testing the radiomic classifier. Based on proposed feature vector for each nodule object, two classifiers are used to distinguish lesions according to selected properties (calcification and malignancy): the support vector machine (SVM) [12] and the random forest (RF) [8].

The paper is organized as follows. Section 2 presents the materials and methods including specification of the lung nodule database with expert annotations, procedures for the extraction of a lung nodule object and its features, and tools used for classification. Obtained detection results are shown, assessed, and discussed in Sect. 3. Section 4 concludes the paper.

2   Materials and Methods

2.1   The LIDC-IDRI Database

As introduced in Sect. 1, the LIDC-IDRI database contains 1018 thoracic CT studies with a number of lesions [2]. During a two-step evaluation procedure, each of the four radiologists were asked to assess each lesion by assigning to one of three categories: 'nodule $\geq$ 3 mm', 'nodule $<$ 3 mm', 'non-nodule $\geq$ 3 mm'. As a result, 7371 'nodule' lesions of any type were marked by at least one expert.

In case of each 'nodule $\geq$ 3 mm', the expert was obliged to prepare a delineation covering the nodule in her/his subjective judgement. Finally, such a lesion was assessed in terms of nine attributes, all in a four-, five-, or six-point integer scale: subtlety, internal structure, calcification, shape (sphericity), margin, lobulation, spiculation, solidity (texture), and likelihood of malignancy. All the data were stored in the XML file appended to the study.

Appropriate interpretation of the XML file enables preparation of a voxel probability map M_{pr}. Each voxel is assigned a number of its individual inclusions in the nodule object divided by the number of experts (4). Thus, a five-level scale is applied (from 0% for a certainly non-nodule voxel to 100% for a voxel delineated by all four radiologists). Figure 1 shows a single slice containing a 'nodule $\geq$ 3 mm' along with corresponding probability map.

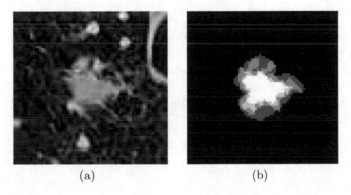

(a)   (b)

Fig. 1. Sample slice with a nodule (a) and corresponding voxel probability map (b). Gray level in (b) reflects the probability map values with 100% shown in white

2.2   Lung Nodule Extraction

The nodule extraction procedure transforms the probability map M_{pr} to a binary volume by thresholding each voxel $\mathbf{v}$ with a fixed threshold t:

$$M(\mathbf{v}) = \begin{cases} 1 \Leftrightarrow M_{pr}(\mathbf{v}) > t, \\ 0 \Leftrightarrow M_{pr}(\mathbf{v}) \leq t. \end{cases} \tag{1}$$

When $t = 0\%$, the object contains all voxels marked by at least one radiologist. On the other hand, $t = 75\%$ extracts only the nodule core – a region covered by all four expert delineations. Four different binary objects extracted from a slice from Fig. 1(b) are shown in Fig. 2. In general, each study may contain more than one lesion. Thus, the binary volume M is labelled and each connected component is investigated separately. Annotations assigned to a particular nodule are used later at the classification stage.

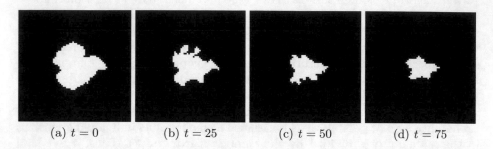

(a) $t = 0$ (b) $t = 25$ (c) $t = 50$ (d) $t = 75$

Fig. 2. Binary nodule masks extracted from a probability map from Fig. 1(b) using Eq. (1) with different t

2.3 Feature Extraction

In order to describe the 3D nodule object and provide input data for the classifier, $n_F = 10$ texture and geometric features were proposed: mean, median, minimum, and maximum intensity, standard deviation of intensity, entropy, energy, kurtosis, skewness, and the shape coefficient. The latter is calculated as the mean of the aspect ratios determined on the basis of Feret diameters in three orthogonal projections within the volume:

$$C_s = \frac{AR_x + AR_y + AR_z}{3}, \tag{2}$$

where, *e.g*:

$$AR_x = \min\left\{\frac{F_y}{F_z}, \frac{F_z}{F_y}\right\}, \tag{3}$$

with F_y, F_z denoting Feret diameters along axes y and z, respectively. Nine texture features are extracted from the volume with intensities normalized to a $[0, 1]$ range, with kurtosis and skewness calculated from the normalized intensity histogram.

2.4 Classification

Support Vector Machine: The binary SVM classifier determines a hyperplane separating training samples from two classes and thus divides the problem space into two subspaces [12]. The non-linear classification can be performed by mapping the inputs into high-dimensional feature space with a kernel function. Examples of kernel functions frequently used for classification include linear kernel, Gaussian kernel, or polynomial kernels. The classifier requires also tuning of a regularization parameter C to achieve optimal generalization performance, which controls the trade-off between the training error and the model complexity. A large value of C leads to hard-margin SVM, which does not allow errors in the trained model and fits better to the training dataset, but can perform poorly on new samples. Smaller value of C causes classification errors over the training set, but produces a more general model when applied to new datasets.

Random Forest: The RF is one of the ensemble learning methods for classification [8,18]. It is a combination of individual decision tree predictors such that each tree is created independently based on a random sample dataset and a random split selection. The trees are grown to gather observations from only one class in each leaf – they are not pruning. After a large number of trees is generated, each individual predictor votes for one class for each observation. The final forest classification is obtained by aggregating the results from individual trees. During construction of each tree a different dataset is drawn with replacement from the original data (bootstrap sample). These observations are only a fraction of all training cases – other samples, called out-of-bag (OOB), are not used for the tree growth. They are different for each individual predictor and they enable estimation of the classification error. RF classification depends on several parameters, *e.g.* a number of trees n_T and a number of features m involved in the split selection in each individual predictor.

3   Results and Discussion

3.1   Validation Protocol

Classification accuracy assessment relies on three basic measures: sensitivity, specificity, and accuracy:

$$SE = \frac{TP}{TP + FN} \cdot 100\%, \tag{4}$$

$$SP = \frac{TN}{TN + FP} \cdot 100\%, \tag{5}$$

$$ACC = \frac{TP + TN}{TP + TN + FP + FN} \cdot 100\%, \tag{6}$$

where TP, TN, FP, FN denote number of true positive, true negative, false positive, and false negative matches, respectively. In case of each of the following experiments, the available dataset was randomly divided into the training and testing groups in a 2:1 ratio. In order to secure validation reliability, each experiment was repeated 30 times with different divisions of the dataset. Only nodules acknowledged ≥ 3 mm were taken into consideration. Depending on the analysis, different thresholds t were applied during extraction of binary masks for the nodules: 0, 25, 50, 75%. Summary of the amount of considered nodules is shown in Table 1. The algorithm was implemented using Matlab® software. In the experiments, the following parameters were set: SVM was trained with $C = 12$ and two different kernels (linear and Gaussian), and RF was trained with $n_T = 20$ and $m = 3$.

Table 1. Probability map threshold t vs. the sizes of training and testing groups

t [%]	Total cases	Training cases	Testing cases
0	2471	1647	824
25	1787	1191	596
50	1327	885	442
75	868	579	289

3.2   Calcification Detection

Detection of calcified nodules was based on quantitative evaluation provided by experts in the case of each 'nodule ≥ 3 mm'. A positive (P) case of calcified nodule was identified by at least one expert assessment indicating a value from a $[1, 5]$ range. In this case note 6 denotes a non-calcified lesion, which – if confirmed by all involved experts – refers to a negative (N) case. Table 2 presents the number of positive and negative cases as well as validation accuracy measures in four experiments depending on probability map threshold t. Since there is a consistent imbalance between both groups (generally much more negative than positive samples), an additional experiment was performed for $t = 0\%$ (bottom row in Table 2) with downsampling of the N set. For each run, 500 negative samples were randomly selected from the entire group in order to train and validate the classification.

3.3   Malignancy Detection

Likelihood of malignancy was assessed in a five-point scale $[1, 5]$ without a sixth grade pointing unquestionable benignity, as in the case of calcification (Sect. 3.2). Thus, in this experiment a threshold was set to the expert assessment in order to divide each dataset into positive and negative groups. Namely, a lesion was considered malignant (P) if a mean likelihood of malignancy assigned by involved experts was greater or equal 3. Other nodules constituted the negative (N) group. Summary of the experiment is presented in Table 3. Similarly to the calcification assessment (Sect. 3.2), bottom row in Table 3 shows the results of detection validation with equated cardinalities of P and N groups, this time with 650 randomly selected N cases.

Table 2. Summary of nodule calcification detection validation

t [%]	P cases	N cases	SVM, linear			SVM, Gaussian			RF		
			SE [%]	SP [%]	ACC [%]	SE [%]	SP [%]	ACC [%]	SE [%]	SP [%]	ACC [%]
0	388	2083	59.8	99.3	93.2	55.4	98.6	91.8	63.8	97.8	93.0
25	319	1468	62.1	99.4	92.8	55.9	97.8	90.5	70.3	99.1	93.7
50	246	1081	59.4	99.0	91.7	53.2	97.6	89.6	64.2	98.8	92.1
75	186	682	58.5	99.3	90.5	52.9	96.2	87.2	58.8	97.2	88.3
0	388	500	71.3	94.9	84.4	71.0	87.1	79.9	75.4	92.8	85.2

Table 3. Summary of nodule malignancy detection validation

t [%]	P cases	N cases	SVM, linear			SVM, Gaussian			RF		
			SE [%]	SP [%]	ACC [%]	SE [%]	SP [%]	ACC [%]	SE [%]	SP [%]	ACC [%]
0	620	1851	66.9	91.8	85.5	62.7	82.6	85.1	67.5	92.6	86.3
25	570	1217	73.0	89.1	83.9	68.8	89.2	82.7	68.9	91.7	84.6
50	498	829	76.7	86.0	82.5	73.6	86.1	81.4	68.3	90.2	81.8
75	376	492	81.1	82.3	81.8	75.4	79.8	77.9	78.1	80.5	79.5
0	620	650	82.3	82.1	82.2	78.5	83.2	80.9	77.5	82.8	80.2

3.4   Discussion

The proposed radiomic system is able to assess calcification of the nodule with accuracy over 85% and estimate the likelihood of malignancy with accuracy over 82%. In both cases the system favours rather cautious diagnostic decisions reflected in classification specificity exceeding sensitivity. Such observation was generally confirmed by the experiments with equated positive and negative group cardinalities. Obtained results may be found well justified with the available reference data. Almost 2.5 K lesions annotated by multiple experts in the publicly accessible LIDC-IDRI database constitute a basis for wide and representative analysis in this matter. The reported detection accuracy metrics look particularly encouragingly with the proposed number of features and their relative simplicity and generality. Possible employment of different features of a various type (especially texture or shape-based) in the future research is supposed to improve the system performance.

Our reports can be compared only to earlier reports in automated detection of pulmonary nodule malignancy. Most of the studies use their own datasets with smaller number of cases (note Table 1 in [17]) with malignancy detection area under the receiver operating characteristic curve (AUC) between 0.79 and 0.91. The LIDC-IDRI database was employed by [17,22] with $ACC = 82.5\%$ over a complete dataset (with expert assessment of attributes used as input data) [22] and $AUC = 0.962$ over a dataset limited to 300 nodules [17]. To the best of our knowledge, automated calcification assessment was not reported thus far.

Both support vector machine and random forest prove to be repeatable and efficient tools for classification in the lung cancer radiomics area. The experiments show a relatively low sensitivity for parameter settings within their reasonable ranges except the SVM kernel and the RF number of trees n_T, being the most important factors in adjusting each classifier. The obtained results are comparable, though RF is more efficient in calcification detection and SVM with linear kernel outperforms the other approaches in malignancy assessment. In general, the linear mapping in SVM is able to provide more accurate detection than the Gaussian kernel.

Presented approach addresses a final part of the lung cancer CAD. Beneficial character of the LIDC-IDRI database annotations enables comprehensive analysis of substantial features of well and reliably defined lesion object without taking care of its proper extraction. Thus, the issues of automated detection and segmentation commonly addressed in this CAD area could be omitted. However, possible implementation of the system in clinical use requires selected procedures yielding the nodule object for advanced radiomic analysis to be incorporated in the processing workflow.

4 Conclusion

A radiomic attempt to employ the LIDC-IDRI expert annotations of pulmonary nodule attributes is described in this paper. The support vector machine and random forest classifiers with adjusted settings enable detection of lesion calcification and likelihood of malignancy with accuracies exceeding 85% and 82%, respectively. Exploration of such a CAD field has a potential to significantly support the lung cancer diagnosis.

Acknowledgement. Publication supported by the Rector's Grant in the field of research and development. Silesian University of Technology, grant number 07/010/RGJ17/0014.

References

1. American Cancer Society: Lung Cancer. https://www.cancer.org/cancer/lung-cancer.html. Accessed 02 Nov 2017
2. Armato, S.G., McLennan, G., Bidaut, L., McNitt-Gray, M.F., Meyer, C.R., Reeves, A.P., et al.: The lung image database consortium (LIDC) and image database resource initiative (IDRI): a completed reference database of lung nodules on CT scans. Med. Phys. **38**(2), 915–931 (2011)
3. Armato, S.G., McLennan, G., McNitt-Gray, M.F., Meyer, C.R., Yankelevitz, D., Aberle, D.R., et al.: Lung image database consortium: developing a resource for the medical imaging research community. Radiology **232**(3), 739–748 (2004)

4. Badura, P., Pietka, E.: Semi-automatic seed points selection in fuzzy connectedness approach to image segmentation. In: Kurzynski, M., Puchala, E., Wozniak, M., Zolnierek, A. (eds.) Advances in Intelligent and Soft Computing: Computer Recognition Systems, vol. 2(45), pp. 679–686 (2007)
5. Badura, P., Pietka, E.: Pre- and postprocessing stages in fuzzy connectedness-based lung nodule CAD. In: Pietka, E., Kawa, J. (eds.) Advances in Intelligent and Soft Computing: Information Technologies in Biomedicine, vol. 47, pp. 192–199 (2008)
6. Badura, P., Pietka, E.: Soft computing approach to 3D lung nodule segmentation in CT. Comput. Biol. Med. **53**, 230–243 (2014). https://doi.org/10.1016/j.compbiomed.2014.08.005
7. Bartholmai, B., Koo, C., Johnson, G., White, D., Raghunath, S., Rajagopalan, S., Moynagh, M., Lindell, R., Hartman, T.: Pulmonary nodule characterization, including computer analysis and quantitative features. J. Thorac. Imaging **30**(2), 139–156 (2015). https://doi.org/10.1097/RTI.0000000000000137
8. Breiman, L.: Random forests. Mach. Learn. **45**(1), 5–32 (2001). https://doi.org/10.1023/A:1010933404324
9. de Carvalho Filho, A.O., de Sampaio, W.B., Silva, A.C., de Paiva, A.C., Nunes, R.A., Gattass, M.: Automatic detection of solitary lung nodules using quality threshold clustering, genetic algorithm and diversity index. Artif. Intell. Med. **60**(3), 165–177 (2014)
10. Cavalcanti, P.G., Shirani, S., Scharcanski, J., Fong, C., Meng, J., Castelli, J., Koff, D.: Lung nodule segmentation in chest computed tomography using a novel background estimation method. Quant. Imaging Med. Surg. **6**(1), 16 (2016)
11. Chen, K., Li, B., Tian, L., Zhu, W., Bao, Y.: Vessel attachment nodule segmentation using integrated active contour model based on fuzzy speed function and shape-intensity joint Bhattacharya distance. Sig. Process. **103**(Supplement C), 273–284 (2014). https://doi.org/10.1016/j.sigpro.2013.09.009
12. Cortes, C., Vapnik, V.: Support-vector networks. Mach. Learn. **20**(3), 273–297 (1995)
13. Diciotti, S., Lombardo, S., Falchini, M., Picozzi, G., Mascalchi, M.: Automated segmentation refinement of small lung nodules in CT scans by local shape analysis. IEEE Trans. Biomed. Eng. **58**(12), 3418–3428 (2011)
14. Diciotti, S., Picozzi, G., Falchini, M., Mascalchi, M., Villari, N., Valli, G.: 3-D segmentation algorithm of small lung nodules in spiral CT images. IEEE Trans. Inf Technol. Biomed. **12**(1), 7–19 (2008)
15. Farhangi, M.M., Frigui, H., Seow, A., Amini, A.A.: 3-D active contour segmentation based on sparse linear combination of training shapes (SCoTS). IEEE Trans. Med. Imaging **36**(11), 2239–2249 (2017). https://doi.org/10.1109/TMI.2017.2720119
16. Gillies, R.J., Kinahan, P.E., Hricak, H.: Radiomics: images are more than pictures, they are data. Radiology **278**(2), 563–577 (2016). https://doi.org/10.1148/radiol.2015151169
17. Gonçalves, L., Novo, J., Cunha, A., Campilho, A.: Learning lung nodule malignancy likelihood from radiologist annotations or diagnosis data. J. Med. Biol. Eng. (2017). https://doi.org/10.1007/s40846-017-0317-2
18. Hastie, T., Tibshirani, R., Friedman, J.: The Elements of Statistical Learning: Data Mining, Inference, and Prediction. Springer Series in Statistics, 2nd edn. Springer, Heidelberg (2009)
19. Hawkins, S., Wang, H., Liu, Y., Garcia, A., Stringfield, O., Krewer, H., et al.: Predicting malignant nodules from screening CT scans. J. Thorac. Oncol. **11**(12), 2120–2128 (2016). https://doi.org/10.1016/j.jtho.2016.07.002

20. Heckel, F., Meine, H., Moltz, J.H., Kuhnigk, J.M., Heverhagen, J.T., Kiessling, A., Buerke, B., Hahn, H.K.: Segmentation-based partial volume correction for volume estimation of solid lesions in CT. IEEE Trans. Med. Imaging 33(2), 462–480 (2014)
21. Jacobs, C., van Rikxoort, E.M., Twellmann, T., Scholten, E.T., de Jong, P.A., Kuhnigk, J.M., Oudkerk, M., de Koning, H.J., Prokop, M., Schaefer-Prokop, C., van Ginneken, B.: Automatic detection of subsolid pulmonary nodules in thoracic computed tomography images. Med. Image Anal. 18(2), 374–384 (2014)
22. Kaya, A., Can, A.B.: A weighted rule based method for predicting malignancy of pulmonary nodules by nodule characteristics. J. Biomed. Inform. 56(Supplement C), 69–79 (2015). https://doi.org/10.1016/j.jbi.2015.05.011
23. Kostis, W.J., Reeves, A.P., Yankelevitz, D.F., Henschke, C.I.: Three-dimensional segmentation and growth-rate estimation of small pulmonary nodules in helical CT images. IEEE Trans. Med. Imag. 22(10), 1259–1274 (2003)
24. Krewer, H., Geiger, B., Hall, L.O., Goldgof, D.B., Yuhua, G., Tockman, M., Gillies, R.J.: Effect of texture features in computer aided diagnosis of pulmonary nodules in low-dose computed tomography. In: 2013 IEEE International Conference on Systems, Man, and Cybernetics (SMC), pp. 3887–3891 (2013)
25. Kubota, T., Jerebko, A.K., Dewan, M., Salganicoff, M., Krishnan, A.: Segmentation of pulmonary nodules of various densities with morphological approaches and convexity models. Med. Image Anal. 15(1), 133–154 (2011)
26. Kuhnigk, J.M., Dicken, V., Bornemann, L., Bakai, A., Wormanns, D., Krass, S., Peitgen, H.O.: Morphological segmentation and partial volume analysis for volumetry of solid pulmonary lesions in thoracic CT scans. IEEE Trans. Med. Imag. 25(4), 417–434 (2006)
27. Lassen, B.C., Jacobs, C., Kuhnigk, J.M., van Ginneken, B., van Rikxoort, E.M.: Robust semi-automatic segmentation of pulmonary subsolid nodules in chest computed tomography scans. Phys. Med. Biol. 60(3), 1307 (2015)
28. Li, G., Kim, H., Tan, J.K., Ishikawa, S., Hirano, Y., Kido, S., Tachibana, R.: Semantic characteristics prediction of pulmonary nodule using artificial neural networks. In: 2013 35th Annual International Conference of the IEEE Engineering in Medicine and Biology Society (EMBC), pp. 5465–5468 (2013)
29. Lung Image Database Consortium LIDC-IDRI Collection. https://wiki.cancerimagingarchive.net/display/Public/LIDC-IDRI. Accessed 02 Nov 2017
30. Ma, J., Zhou, Z., Ren, Y., Xiong, J., Fu, L., Wang, Q., Zhao, J.: Computerized detection of lung nodules through radiomics. Med. Phys. 44(8), 4148–4158 (2017). https://doi.org/10.1002/mp.12331
31. Pietka, E., Kawa, J., Badura, P., Spinczyk, D.: Open architecture computer-aided diagnosis system. Expert Syst. 27(1), 17–39 (2010). https://doi.org/10.1111/j.1468-0394.2009.00524.x
32. Tan, M., Deklerck, R., Cornelis, J., Jansen, B.: Phased searching with NEAT in a time-scaled framework: experiments on a computer-aided detection system for lung nodules. Artif. Intell. Med. 59(3), 157–167 (2013)
33. Wang, J., Engelmann, R., Li, Q.: Segmentation of pulmonary nodules in three-dimensional CT images by use of a spiral-scanning technique. Med. Phys. 34(1), 4678–4689 (2007)
34. Wang, Q., Song, E., Jin, R., Han, P., Wang, X., Zhou, Y., Zeng, J.: Segmentation of lung nodules in computed tomography images using dynamic programming and multidirection fusion techniques. Acad. Radiol. 16(6), 678–688 (2009)

35. Wieclawek, W., Pietka, E.: Fuzzy clustering in segmentation of abdominal struc-
    tures based on CT studies. In: Pietka, E., Kawa, J. (eds.) Advances in Intelligent
    and Soft Computing: Information Technologies in Biomedicine, vol. 47, pp. 93–104
    (2008)
36. World Health Organization: Cancer factsheet. http://www.who.int/mediacentre/
    factsheets/fs297/en/. Accessed 02 Nov 2017
37. Zarychta, P.: A new approach to knee joint arthroplasty. Comput. Med. Imaging
    Graph. (2017, in press). https://doi.org/10.1016/j.compmedimag.2017.07.002

Games with Resources and Their Use in Modeling Effects of Anticancer Treatment

Andrzej Swierniak[(✉)], Michal Krzeslak, and Damian Borys

Institute of Automatic Control, Silesian University of Technology,
Akademicka 16, 44-100 Gliwice, Poland
andrzej.swierniak@polsl.pl

Abstract. In this work, we study an extension to evolutionary game models with the possibility to model the change and influence of the environment fluctuations for the fitness of the players. Using spatial games, those changes can be taken into account as an additional lattice dimension. In classical spatial evolutionary games (SEGT) each position on the lattice is represented by a single player or single phenotype (strategy). The local payoff for this player arises from the interactions with the neighbouring cells. With the newer approach each cell represents heterogeneous subpopulation, so can be considered as mixed or multidimensional spatial games (MSEG). This allows performing the game on a multidimensional lattice where an additional dimension is representing the evolution of resources.

Keywords: Game theory · Spatial model · Tumour modeling

1 Introduction

Evolutionary game theory (EGT) introduced by Smith and Price [10,11] allowed us to link Darwinian fitness of the species and their evolution with game theory machinery. This created a very useful methodology for simulation and analysis of dynamics of populations of players that belong to the real and biological world. Those individuals can be characterized by some strategies or phenotypes which can cooperate or compete with others to fulfill their evolutionary objectives. Players act without any rationality, which differs this method from the standard game theory, as they follow their instincts. The reward and expected result should be an achievement of better access to some resources like food, females, living space etc. The change of this evolutionary achievement is called the payoff, and by the term fitness, we call the evolutionary adjustment. Those payoffs, represented in a matrix form, consist all costs and benefits resulting from this change in the consequence of players interactions. Due to interactions between players in time, the population composition may stabilise and achieve some equilibrium state (either mono- or polymorphic). Such state is called evolutionary stable and phenotype that when implemented by the majority of the

© Springer International Publishing AG, part of Springer Nature 2019
E. Pietka et al. (Eds.): ITIB 2018, AISC 762, pp. 290–299, 2019.
https://doi.org/10.1007/978-3-319-91211-0_26

population cannot be replaced by any other is called evolutionary stable strategy (ESS) [12]. The opposite situation may happen. EGT methodology allows us to predict in general the behaviour of the population if it tends to become homo- or heterogeneous. The former means that only one strategy will survive and will dominate the population. Additional information can give us the usage of so-called replicator dynamics [6] where one can observe the change in population composition in time starting from an initial state. However, this is only information about the entire population, and it lacks the knowledge about the local arrangements inside. Using spatial evolutionary games (SEGT), based on cellular automata, one can recover missing spatial information in the dynamics of the population. One of the first author, that used spatial tools in modeling carcinogenesis was Bach et al. [2]. This approach, similarly to EGT, is also based on iterated procedure. In SEGT to obtain a new state of the population we have to perform following steps: payoff update – calculate a payoff using local fitness information, cell mortality – remove randomly selected individuals, reproduction – define which strategy will take a free place. Bach et al. were not the first who used game theory to model the cancer development. Tomlinson and Bodmer [16] described one of the first models based on EGT, and this model will be studied later in our work. Other authors also proposed further models that include different types of cancer cell interactions, bystander effects [8], resistance to chemotherapy [3], the interaction between different tumours [5]. Some survey of those models is available in the literature [4,13]. In this work, we aimed to include information about resources in the game itself. Those resources can influence the way that players interact with each other, that is why we have modified two games – one classical Hawk and Dove problem and second angiogenic game by changing they payoff matrix. In our approach, the payoff matrix does not remain constant during the game, so we have modified the game matrix and extended them by an additional parameter representing resources. To allow taking into account this new knowledge during the spatial simulation an extension of spatial evolutionary games has to be used. In SEGT the main assumption is that each cell represents one strategy or one phenotype. Swierniak and Krzeslak [14] proposed a new type of SEGT called MSEG where each cell contains information about the composition of the phenotypes in that specific cell, representing rather a heterogenous subpopulation, that is why its name is mixed or multidimensional spatial evolutionary games (MSEG).

2   Materials and Methods

In our simulations MSEG methodology was used to include resource changes in the spatial game. For both models, games were played on the lattice forming torus, and in the case of a tie during any competition, we choose the result randomly and for MSEG is the average of phenotypic compositions. The game is iterated in three main steps: payoff update, cell mortality and reproduction. Bach et al. [2] presented three ways of mortality: synchronous (all die simultaneously), asynchronous (one cell in one step) and semi-synchronous (some amount of population die simultaneously, here 10%). In all simulations, semi-synchronous updating was used. In the original article for SEGT two reproduction possibilities were proposed: deterministic (the strongest player is the winner) or probabilistic (an adaptation for each player is divided by the total score in the neighbourhood). Using MSEG allows us to treat each cell as a composition of different phenotypes and this results in multidimensional game and lattice. The number of layers depends on the number of phenotypes and each layer corresponds each phenotype. This fact enabled [9, 14, 15] new reproduction approaches:

- weighted mean of the strongest players – weighted mean from phenotypes is computed for cells with highest scores
- weighted mean of the best interval – cells are divided into intervals by their payoffs, weighted mean is computed for players from the best interval.

Both selected models were extended with an additional parameter r which means resources, like food, territory, drugs etc. For Hawk and Dove model a mean field calculations were also performed and r was changed for the entire population. In spatial games, it can be changed spatially.

2.1 Resources in Hawk and Doves Game

In this classical game theory model we have two kinds of strategies – fight or avoid. The payoff matrix (Tables 1 and 2) contains parameters: v – possible benefit from the conflict and c – possible cost of escalation. The stable polymorphism has the form $H = v/c$ and $D = 1 - v/c$. That is why if we want to keep stable polymorphic result then $v < c$ has to be true.

Table 1. The payoff matrix for the original Hawk and Dove model

Phenotypes	Hawk	Dove
Hawk	v−c	0
Dove	2v	v

In this model a new parameter r was introduced that represents resources, as well as new rules:

- Hawks are more aggressive (better adjusted) when r is small;
- Doves obtain a better fitness when resources are greater;
- for large r Hawks bear the cost of escalation and Dove share the benefits.

When $r = 0$ the payoff matrix is the same as for original model. With increasing r more chances are gained by Doves. This parameter is limited to the [0,1] interval for this model. Both spatial and mean field game was simulated. Both situations are presented for $v = 6$, $c = 9$ and $v = 9$, $c = 6$ representing both cases where $v < c$ and $v > c$. For MSEG model additional rules for resources have been introduced:

- players that present more aggressive phenotype (more Hawks) take from less aggressive an amount of resources (equal the difference between Hawk's frequency of occurrence);
- a Dove shares its resources with other Doves that have more resources (depending on Dove's frequency of occurrence).

Table 2. The payoff matrix for modified Hawk and Dove model with resources. Parameter r is for the resources

	r = 0	r = 1
H,H	v−c	v−c
D,D	v	**2v**
D,H	0	**1/2v**
H,D	2v	2v

2.2 Tumour Modeling with Resources

This model, introduced by Tomlinson and Bodmer [16], was one of the first game theory models describing the interactions between tumour cells. Here, the paracrine production of growth factors with angiogenic promoters was described. Two strategies are to produce or not the growth factors $(A+, A-)$. Parameters of the model are related to the costs of proangiogenic factor production (i) and benefit (j) resulting from those factors. When costs are smaller than benefits, we can obtain a stable dimorphism. In the opposite case, the cells that do not produce $(A-)$ are dominating. This model was also analyzed by other authors [1,7,13]. Here, an external intervention (for example in the form of treatment) is added by the resources parameter r, which can be, for example, proangiogenic factors and r is limited here to the $[0,2]$ interval. Payoff tables are given in Tables 3 and 4.

Table 3. The payoff matrix for the original angiogenic game model

Phenotypes	A+	A−
A+	1−i+j	1+j
A−	1−i+j	1

Table 4. The payoff matrix for modified angiogenic game model with resources. Parameter r is for the resources

Phenotypes	A+	A−
A+	1−i+j+r/2	1+j+r/2
A−	1−i+j+r/2	1+r/2

3 Results

Results for Hawk and Doves model are presented in Figs. 2 and 3 for parameters $v = 6$, $c = 9$ and Figs. 4 and 5 for parameters $v = 9$, $c = 6$. Mean field dynamics, for those two parameter settings, is presented and compared in Fig. 1. According to the theory, when $v < c$ we should obtain the polymorphic stable state, and this can be observed in Fig. 1(a). When resources (red line) are equal to 0, we have obtained situation known from the original model, but for the high level of resources, Doves are dominating in the population. Also in Fig. 1(b), with the high level of resources, when we should have only one population of Hawks (because $v > c$), we have almost an opposite situation. The model with an additional dimension will lead to increased adjustment for Doves, especially for high values of resources. Therefore for $v = 6$, $c = 9$ and $r = 1$ Doves totally dominate in the population for the mean-field model (if r does not change).

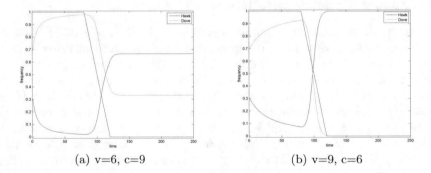

| (a) v=6, c=9 | (b) v=9, c=6 |

Fig. 1. Meanfield dynamics for Hawk and Doves model. On the left (a) for $v = 6$, $c = 9$, right (b) for $v = 9$, $c = 6$. Green line presents Dove population, blue – population of Hawks and red line shows the resources level. Time is expressed in generations

Figure 3 shows the change of particular phenotypes in the entire population for the spatial model with resources. We can observe differences in probabilistic and other reproductions (deterministic and both weighted means). The dynamics of changes within the probabilistic one oscillate more than in the primary MSEG (without resources), and Hawks are a bit better adjusted. Significant differences are seen within the deterministic reproduction where Hawks no longer dominate in the population. Surprisingly, Doves have better adjustment than in the primary MSEG model. For the set of parameters $v = 9$ and $c = 6$ only probabilistic

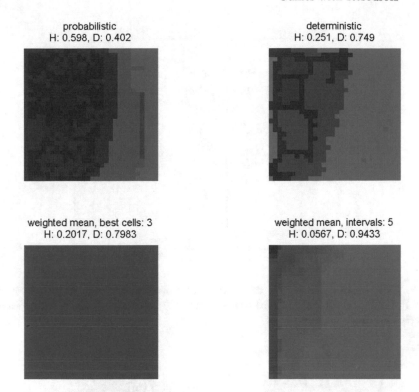

Fig. 2. Final lattices for Hawk and Doves model with resources, $v = 6$, $c = 9$. Results for reproductions: (a) probabilistic, (b) deterministic, (c) weighted mean, (d) weighted mean with intervals. Blue colour means Hawk phenotype, green – Dove phenotype, mixed colour represents mixed content of the cell

reproduction gives similar results to those for the model without resources. Other reproductions show some discrepancies in contrast to the original model, especially those with the weighted mean (with best cells and intervals). The main discrepancy is that the Hawks' frequency has been decreased, which is why in the weighted mean reproduction Doves became the dominant strategy in the population which is seen in Fig. 4.

Results for angiogenic model are presented in Figs. 6 and 7. The first image presents final results and final lattices for all types of reproductions: (a) probabilistic, (b) deterministic, (c) weighted mean, (d) weighted mean with intervals – as well as dynamics of phenotypes for all types of reproductions. Figure 7 presents changes in resources for this model. Parameters of the model for presented results were $i = 0.8$ and $j = 6$, and this should correspond to stable dimorphism situation in the model (according to the original model).

Here, again we can observe an interesting difference between reproduction methods. In the case of probabilistic reproduction, some patterns are created.

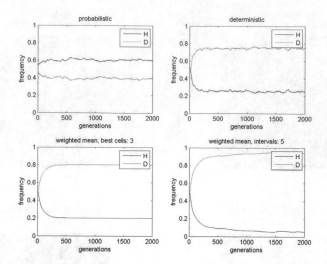

Fig. 3. Dynamics of phenotypes for Hawk and Doves model with resources, v = 6, c = 9. Results for reproductions: (a) probabilistic, (b) deterministic, (c) weighted mean, (d) weighted mean with intervals

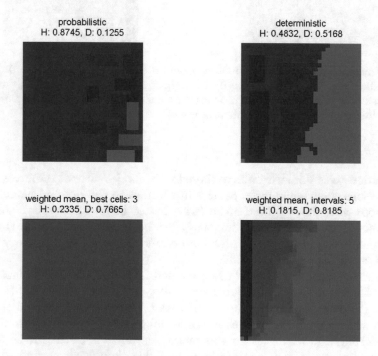

Fig. 4. Final lattices for Hawk and Doves model with resources, v = 9, c = 6. Results for reproductions: (a) probabilistic, (b) deterministic, (c) weighted mean, (d) weighted mean with intervals; blue colour means Hawk phenotype, green – Dove phenotype, mixed colour represents mixed content of the cell

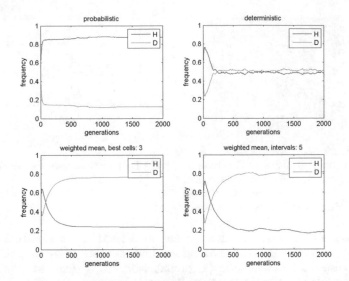

Fig. 5. Dynamics of phenotypes for Hawk and Doves model with resources, v = 9, c = 6. Results for reproductions: (a) probabilistic, (b) deterministic, (c) weighted mean, (d) weighted mean with intervals

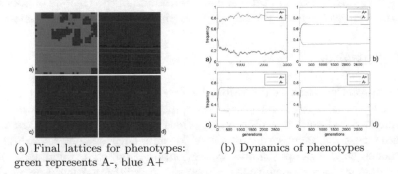

(a) Final lattices for phenotypes: (b) Dynamics of phenotypes
green represents A-, blue A+

Fig. 6. Results for the simulation of angiogenic model with resources, left: final lattices, right: dynamics of phenotypes with parameters i = 0.8, j = 6. In both parts are presented reproductions: (a) probabilistic, (b) deterministic, (c) weighted mean, (d) weighted mean with intervals

Moreover, in this case, phenotype responsible for the production of growth factors dominates in localizations where external resources have a higher level. We can observe that additional external growth factors result in changes of final distribution especially in the case of the probabilistic reproduction. Production of angiogenic factors becomes more profitable than in the case when there is no external intervention. Moreover, the spatial distribution of the use of resources by the cells depends on the distribution of phenotypes on the lattice. Another one

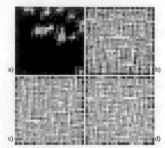
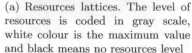
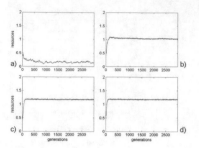

(a) Resources lattices. The level of resources is coded in gray scale, white colour is the maximum value and black means no resources level

(b) Dynamics of resources level

Fig. 7. Results for the simulation of angiogenic model with resources, left: final lattices for resources, right: dynamics of resources for different types of reproduction. In both parts are presented reproductions: (a) probabilistic, (b) deterministic, (c) weighted mean, (d) weighted mean with intervals. Resources level can change the value from 0 to 2

finding is that in the case of probabilistic reproduction the clusters of phenotypes are mostly covered by clusters in resources giving a similar spatial pattern.

4   Discussion

We have proposed some modifications for two known in the literature models to verify how the changes in resources can influence results of well-known models. Multidimensional spatial evolutionary games have been used to allow to take into account those changes in resources. Results suggest that regarding mean field model, as well as spatial one, we can obtain significant differences this will lead to prepare new models that will contain an additional layer for modelling changes in resources for the players.

Acknowledgement. This work was supported by the Polish National Science Centre Grant no. DEC-2016/21/B/ST7/02241 (AS), the Institute of Automatic Control, Silesian University of Technology under Grant No. BK-204/RAU1/2017 (MK) and the National Centre for Research and Development Grant no. STRATEGMED2/267398/4/NCBR/2015 (MILESTONE – Molecular diagnostics and imaging in individualized therapy for breast, thyroid and prostate cancer) (DB). Calculations were performed on the Ziemowit computer cluster in the Laboratory of Bioinformatics and Computational Biology, created in the EU Innovative Economy Programme POIG.02.01.00-00-166/08 and expanded in the POIG.02.03.01-00-040/13 project.

References

1. Bach, L., Bentzen, S., Alsner, J., Christiansen, F.: An evolutionary-game model of tumour-cell interactions: possible relevance to gene therapy. Eur. J. Cancer **37**(16), 2116–2120 (2001). https://doi.org/10.1016/S0959-8049(01)00246-5
2. Bach, L.A., Sumpter, D.J.T., Alsner, J., Loeschcke, V.: Spatial evolutionary games of interaction among generic cancer cells. J. Theor. Med. **5**(1), 47–58 (2003). https://doi.org/10.1080/10273660310001630443
3. Basanta, D., Gatenby, R.A., Anderson, A.R.A.: Exploiting evolution to treat drug resistance: combination therapy and the double bind. Mol. Pharm. **9**(4), 914–921 (2012). https://doi.org/10.1021/mp200458e
4. Basanta, D., Hatzikirou, H., Deutsch, A.: Studying the emergence of invasiveness in tumours using game theory. Eur. Phy. J. B **63**, 393–397 (2008). https://doi.org/10.1140/epjb/e2008-00249-y
5. Basanta, D., Scott, J.G., Fishman, M.N., Ayala, G., Hayward, S.W., Anderson, A.R.A.: Investigating prostate cancer tumour-stroma interactions: clinical and biological insights from an evolutionary game. Br. J. Cancer **106**(1), 174–181 (2012). https://doi.org/10.1038/bjc.2011.517
6. Hofbauer, J., Schuster, P., Sigmund, K.: A note on evolutionary stable strategies and game dynamics. J. Theor. Biol. **81**(3), 609–612 (1979). https://doi.org/10.1016/0022-5193(79)90058-4
7. Krześlak, M., Borys, D., Świerniak, A.: Angiogenic switch - mixed spatial evolutionary game approach. Intell. Inf. Database Syst. **9621**, 420–429 (2016). https://doi.org/10.1007/978-3-662-49381-6_40
8. Krześlak, M., Świerniak, A.: Spatial evolutionary games and radiation induced bystander effect. Arch. Control Sci. **21**(2), 135–151 (2011). https://doi.org/10.2478/v10170-010-0036-1
9. Krześlak, M., Świerniak, A.: Multidimensional extended spatial evolutionary games. Comput. Biol. Med. **69**, 315–327 (2016). https://doi.org/10.1016/j.compbiomed.2015.08.003
10. Sigmund, K., Nowak, M.A.: Evolutionary game theory. Curr. Biol. **9**(14), R503–R505 (1999). https://doi.org/10.1016/S0960-9822(99)80321-2
11. Smith, J.M.: Evolution and the Theory of Games. Cambridge University Press, Cambridge (1982). https://doi.org/10.1017/CBO9780511806292
12. Smith, J.M., Price, G.R.: The logic of animal conflict. Nature **246**, 15–18 (1973). https://doi.org/10.1038/246015a0
13. Świerniak, A., Krześlak, M.: Application of evolutionary games to modeling carcinogenesis. Math. Biosci. Eng. MBE **10**(3), 873–911 (2013). https://doi.org/10.3934/mbe.2013.10.873
14. Świerniak, A., Krześlak, M.: Cancer heterogeneity and multilayer spatial evolutionary games. Biol. Direct **11**(1), 53 (2016). https://doi.org/10.1186/s13062-016-0156-z
15. Świerniak, A., Krześlak, M., Student, S., Rzeszowska-Wolny, J.: Development of a population of cancer cells: observation and modeling by a mixed spatial evolutionary games approach. J. Theor. Biol. **405**, 94–103 (2016). https://doi.org/10.1016/j.jtbi.2016.05.027
16. Tomlinson, I., Bodmer, W.: Modelling the consequences of interactions between tumour cells. Br. J. Cancer **75**(2), 157–160 (1997). https://doi.org/10.1038/bjc.1997.26

Signal Processing and Medical Devices

The Higher-Order Spectra (HOSA) as a Tool for the Rehabilitation Progress Estimation Referred to the Patients Diagnosed with Various Cardiac Diseases

Ewaryst Tkacz[✉], Zbigniew Budzianowski, Wojciech Oleksy, and Anna Tamulewicz

Faculty of Biomedical Engineering, Department of Biosensors and Biomedical Signals Processing, Silesian University of Technology, Roosevelta 40, 41-800 Zabrze, Poland
ewaryst.tkacz@polsl.pl

Abstract. This article explores the possibility of using the higher-order spectra to identify different types of diseases. In order to assess the effectiveness of such tool the HRV (Heart Rate Variability) recordings obtained from patients suffering from three different cardiac problems are listed and compared to the results recorded for healthy subjects. Each set of HRV signals is processed with bispectral and bicoherent analysis. In both cases three statistical parameters are observed. For each type of the investigated analysis the parameters under examination differ enough to allow clear distinction of the specific cardiac disease. The obtained results show usefulness of higher-order spectra as a tool for differentiation between specific diseases. Authors believe that further work would greatly improve potential of the described tool, allowing to identify number of different diseases or even stage of the illness or progress in the rehabilitation process.

Keywords: Heart rate variability · Higher-order statistics
Signal processing

1 Introduction

The aim of this work was to answer the question whether higher-order spectral analysis, based on the records of heart rate variability, could be a valuable diagnostic tool that allows the identification of specific diseases. To achieve this the HRV registrations taken from four different groups of subjects were compared. The first group consisted of healthy individuals and served as a reference one. Three other groups consisted of people burdened with different cardiac diseases: arrhythmia, tachyarrhythmia and congestive heart failure. For each of these groups bispectral and bicoherent analyses were performed. The results are summarized below.

© Springer International Publishing AG, part of Springer Nature 2019
E. Pietka et al. (Eds.): ITIB 2018, AISC 762, pp. 303–314, 2019.
https://doi.org/10.1007/978-3-319-91211-0_27

2   Materials and Methods

2.1   Description of the Data Used

All the used data were collected from the sets of signals stored in an online database PhysioNet [1]. The main source of comparison have become records collected under the file name Normal Sinus Rhythm RR Interval Database (nsr2db) [1]. This database includes beat annotation for long-term ECG recordings of subjects in normal sinus rhythm.

For comparative purposes three other sets were also used:

- MIT-BIH Arrhythmia Database (mitdb) – HRV signals database of patients diagnosed with arrhythmia (A) [1].
- CU Ventricular Tachyarrhythmia Database (cudb) – HRV signals database of patients diagnosed with tachyarrhythmia (TA) [1].
- Congestive Heart Failure RR Interval Database (chf2db) – HRV signals database of patients diagnosed with congestive heart failure (CHF) [1].

2.2   Signal Processing

In order to eliminate artifacts simple filtering mechanism was applied. In case of each long-term recording the average length of RR interval was calculated. Next, the length of each RR interval in this recording was compared with the previously computed average. If the length of interval was shorter than 80% or longer than 120% of the average, such interval was rejected. It was assumed that all the intervals that remained after filtration were NN ones.

In case of each bispectral and bicoherent analysis authors used the first 256 registered NN intervals, dividing them into 8 equal segments (each of 32 intervals) [15]. The analysis was performed using Matlab's HOSA Toolbox [15]. Each analysis was performed using the direct method [2, 4].

2.3   Higher Order Spectra

Assuming that $\varphi(t)$ denotes characteristic function of continuous random variable defined as [5]:

$$\varphi\left(t\right) = \int_{-\infty}^{\infty} e^{-jxt} f\left(x\right) dx \tag{1}$$

where: $f(x)$ is a probability density function.

The nth derivative of the characteristic function is given by [5]:

$$\frac{d^n \varphi(t)}{dt^n} = \left(j\right)^n \int_{-\infty}^{\infty} x^n f\left(x\right) dx \tag{2}$$

The characteristic function (1) can also be obtained by the Taylors series expansion [12, 14]:

$$\varphi\left(t\right) = \int_{-\infty}^{\infty} e^{-jxt} f\left(x\right) dx = \sum_{n=0}^{\infty} \frac{1}{n!} \frac{d^n \varphi(0)}{dt^n} (jt^n) = \sum_{n=0}^{\infty} \frac{1}{n!} (jt^n) m_n \tag{3}$$

where: $m_n = \frac{1}{j^n} \frac{d^n \varphi(0)}{dt^n}$ is a nth order moment.

Using Taylors series expansion once again, n^{th} order cumulant c_n can be defined as:

$$ln \varphi(t) = \ln \left(\int_{-\infty}^{\infty} e^{-jxt} f(x)\, dx \right) = \sum_{n=0}^{\infty} \frac{1}{n!} (jt^n) c_n \qquad (4)$$

where: $c_n = (-j)^n \frac{d^n (ln\varphi(0))}{dt^n}$ is a nth order cumulant.

The n-th order moment can also be defined as:

$$m_n(t_1, t_2, \ldots, t_{n-1}) = E\left\{ x(k) \cdot x(k+t_1) \cdot x(k+t_2) \cdot \ldots \cdot x(k+t_{n-1}) \right\} \qquad (5)$$

and be dependent on differences in time $t_1, t_2, \ldots, t_{n-1}$, where $t_j = 0, \pm 1, \pm 2, \ldots$ for every j.

Thus, using a simple reasoning, one can say that the second moment $m_2(t_1)$ is the autocorrelation function of the signal $x(k)$.

By a similar procedure cumulant can be defined in a slightly different manner than above (4).

N^{th} order cumulant of non-Gaussian stationary signal $x(k)$ is given by [10, 11]:

$$c_n(t_1,\ t_2,\ \ldots, t_{n-1}) = m_n(t_1,\ t_2,\ \ldots, t_{n-1}) - m_n^G(t_1,\ t_2,\ \ldots, t_{n-1}) \qquad (6)$$

where: $m_n^G(t_1,\ t_2, \ldots, t_{n-1}) = E\{g(k) \cdot g(k+t_1) \cdot g(k+t_2) \cdot \cdots \cdot g(k+t_{n-1})\}$, $g(k)$ – is a Gaussian signal having the same second order statistic as $x(k)$.

If the analyzed signal is Gaussian one, then:

$$m_n(t_1,\ t_2,\ \ldots, t_{n-1}) = m_n^G(t_1,\ t_2,\ \ldots, t_{n-1}) \qquad (7)$$

Thus, n^{th} order cumulant $c_n(t_1,\ t_2,\ \ldots, t_{n-1}) = 0$.

The following relations can be distinguished among the nth (for $n \leq 4$) order cumulants and moments of the $x(k)$ signal:

– First cumulant:
$$c_1 = m_1 = E\left\{x(k)\right\} \quad -\ \text{mean} \qquad (8)$$

– Second cumulant:

$$c_2(t_1) = m_2(t_1) - (m_1)^2 \quad -\ \text{covariance} \qquad (9)$$

Thus, one can notice that second cumulant is a function of covariance of the $x(k)$ signal and second moment is a function of autocorrelation of the $x(k)$ signal.

If mean value of the $E\{x(k)\} = 0$, then $c_2(t_1) = m_2(t_1)$ and this is an autocorrelation function.

– Third cumulant:

$$c_3(t_1, t_2) = m_3(t_1, t_2) - m_1[m_2(t_1) + m_2(t_2) + m_2(t_1 - t_2)] + 2(m_1)^3 \quad (10)$$

If $E\{x(k)\} = 0$, then:

$$E\{x(k) \cdot x(k + t_1) \cdot x(k + t_2)\} = c_3(t_1, t_2) = m_3(t_1, t_2) \quad (11)$$

– Fourth moment assuming that $E\{x(k)\} = 0$,

$$m_4(t_1, t_2, t_3) = c_4(t_1, t_2, t_3) + c_2(t_1) c_2(t_3 - t_2) + c_2(t_2) c_2(t_3 - t_1) \\ + c_2(t_3) c_2(t_2 - t_1) \quad (12)$$

The last four equations lead to the conclusion that the moments and cumulants to the third order are equal as long as the assumption of signal's $x(k)$ zero mean is valid.

In frequency domain n^{th} order spectrum can be defined as $n - 1$ Fourier transform:

$$C_n(\omega_1, \omega_2, \ldots, \omega_{n-1})$$
$$= \sum_{t_1=-\infty}^{+\infty} \cdots \sum_{t_{n-1}=-\infty}^{+\infty} c_n(t_1, t_2, \ldots, t_{n-1}) \, exp\{-j(\omega_1 t_1 + \omega_2 t_2 + \cdots + \omega_{n-1} t_{n-1})\}$$
$$(13)$$

Assuming that $x(k)$ is a stationary, random Gaussian signal then all of its moments (for $n \geq 3$) carry no information about $x(k)$.

Hence the conclusion that it is preferable to use cumulant's spectrum, which (for $n \geq 3$) is equal to 0. Another important reason for using the cumulants is the fact that when samples of a random signal are split into two (or more) groups, which are statistically independent, then the cumulants of the nth order are equal to 0.

Thus, the spectra of the cumulants can be useful in the assessment of statistical independence of the samples.

Power spectrum, bispectrum, trispectrum are special cases of the nth order spectrum defined by the equation below:

– Power spectrum:

$$C_2(\omega) = \sum_{\tau=-\infty}^{+\infty} c_2(\tau) e^{-j\omega\tau} \quad (14)$$

where: $|\omega| \leq \pi$
– Bispectrum:

$$B(\omega_1, \omega_2) = C_3(\omega_1, \omega_2) = \sum_{\tau_1=-\infty}^{+\infty} \sum_{\tau_2=-\infty}^{+\infty} c_3(\tau_1, \tau_2) e^{-j(\omega_1\tau_1 + \omega_2\tau_2)} \quad (15)$$

where: $|\omega_1| \leq \pi$, $|\omega_2| \leq \pi$, $|\omega_1 + \omega_2| \leq \pi$

– Trispectrum:

$$C_4(\omega_1, \omega_2, \omega_3) = \sum_{\tau_1=-\infty}^{+\infty} \cdot \sum_{\tau_2=-\infty}^{+\infty} \sum_{\tau_3=-\infty}^{+\infty} c_4(\tau_1, \tau_2, \tau_3)\, e^{-j(\omega_1\tau_1 + \omega_2\tau_2 + \omega_3\tau_3)}$$ (16)

where: $|\omega_1| \le \pi$, $|\omega_2| \le \pi$, $|\omega_3| \le \pi$, $|\omega_1 + \omega_2 + \omega_3| \le \pi$

Basing on Fourier transform of $x(k)$ signal:

$$X(\omega) = \sum_{k=-\infty}^{+\infty} x(k) e^{-j\omega k}$$ (17)

Power spectrum is equal to:

$$P(\omega) = X(\omega) X^*(\omega)$$ (18)

Bispectrum:

$$B_{xxx}(\omega_1, \omega_2) = X(\omega_1) X(\omega_2) X^*(\omega_1 + \omega_2)$$ (19)

Trispectrum:

$$T_{xxxx}(\omega_1, \omega_2, \omega_3) = X(\omega_1) X(\omega_2) X(\omega_3) X^*(\omega_1 + \omega_2 + \omega_3)$$ (20)

In DFT domain all above equations can be written as:

$$P(n) = X(n) X^*(n)$$ (21)
$$B_{xxx}(n, m) = X(n) X(m) X^*(n + m)$$ (22)
$$T_{xxxx}(n, m, p) = X(n) X(m) X(p) X^*(n + m + p)$$ (23)

where: $X(n)$ – are the coefficients od DFT of $x(k)$.

For bispectrum: $n, m = 0, 1, 2, \ldots, N/4 - 1$.

By using normalization procedure one can obtain relationship between higher order spectra, or n^{th} order coherence, and power spectrum ($n = 2$). Bicoherence ($n = 3$) and tricoherence ($n = 4$) can be defined as:

$$P_3(\omega_1, \omega_2) = \frac{C_3(\omega_1, \omega_2)}{\sqrt{C_2(\omega_1) C_2(\omega_2) C_2^*(\omega_1 + \omega_2)}}$$ (24)

$$P_3(\omega_1, \omega_2, \omega_3) = \frac{C_4(\omega_1, \omega_2, \omega_3)}{\sqrt{C_2(\omega_1) C_2(\omega_2) C_2(\omega_3) C_2^*(\omega_1 + \omega_2 + \omega_3)}}$$ (25)

3   Calculation

Frequency analysis allows the separation of the individual components of the spectrum. This type of study allows to detect cyclicality in change of the NN intervals length [3, 8, 9].

The aim of the analysis in the frequency domain is to decompose the total variability of NN intervals into individual frequency components. The result is a plot of the power spectrum as a function of frequency [7].

To evaluate the total spectra power of NN intervals variability the following parameters are used [14]:

- ULF – ultra low frequency component (under 0.0033 Hz). The value expressed in ms2
- VLF – very low frequency component (between 0.0033 to 0.04 Hz). The value expressed in ms2.
- LF – low frequency component (from 0.04 to 0.15 Hz). The value expressed in ms2
- HF – high frequency components (from 0.15 to 0.4 Hz). The value expressed in ms2

During the work it was decided not to treat ULF band as a separate one. Instead, it is assumed that VLF band covers a range from 0 to 0.04 Hz.

Table 1 shows final division into six regions of analysis based on combinations of four sub-bands:

Table 1. Regions of bispectral and bicoherent analyses

Region	Range	Band f1 [Hz]	Band f2 [Hz]
1	VLF-VLF	0–0.04	0–0.04
2	LF-VLF	0.04–0.15	0–0.04
3	LF-LF	0.04–0.15	0.04–0.15
4	HF-VLF	0.15–0.4	0–0.04
5	HF-LF	0.15–0.4	0.04–0.15
6	HF-HF	0.15–0.4	0.15–0.4

Due to the symmetry of the bispectrum [6, 13], regions 1, 3 and 6 are limited by a diagonal of coordinates 0, 0, and 0.5, 0.5.

The final distribution of the analyzed regions is illustrated in Fig. 1.
In each of the six analyzed regions the maximum and average values of bispectrum are calculated along with its variance. The results are presented in tabular form.

4   Results

The charts below show the values obtained during bispectral and bicoherent analyses of HRV records. As mentioned before, there were four groups. Three of them were patients suffering from different cardiac diseases. The last one was the reference (healthy ones).

Objective of the study was to verify whether it's possible to identify specific diseases based on the data obtained from HRV signal.

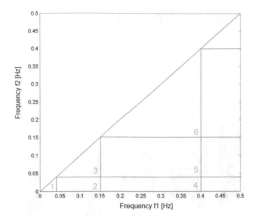

Fig. 1. Distribution of the analyzed regions

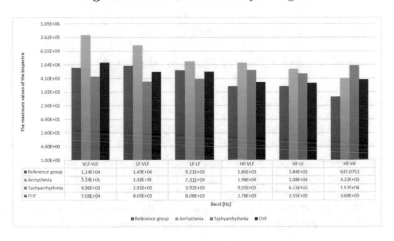

Fig. 2. Comparison of the maximum values of the bispectra

4.1 Bispectral Analyses

Comparison of the Maximum Values of the Bispectra. In order to improve the readability of the chart the logarithmic scale was used (Fig. 2).

Observations:

- Observing the maximum value of bispectrum in different frequency ranges, one can see that in each band, other than HF-HF one, results from patients suffering from arrhythmia exceed the results calculated for other groups. This difference is particularly evident in the case of the lowest frequencies (VLF-VLF and LF-VLF bands).
- In the VLF-VLF band maximum value of bispectrum calculated for the group suffering from arrhythmia is 16 times higher than the second highest result (CHF).

Comparison of the Average Values of the Bispectra. In order to improve the readability of the chart the logarithmic scale was used (Fig. 3).

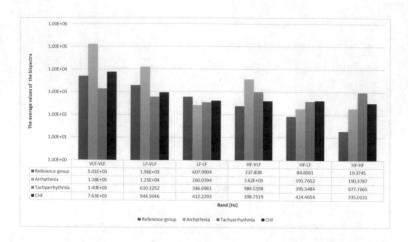

Fig. 3. Comparison of the average values of the bispectra

Observations:

- Observing the average values of bispektra in different frequency ranges, one can see that the in case of VLF-VLF, LF-VLF and HF-VLF bands results of the group suffering from arrhythmia exceed the results calculated for other groups.
- This difference is particularly evident in the case of VLF-VLF band, where average value of bispectrum calculated for the group suffering from arrhythmia is over 16 times higher than the second highest result (CHF).

Comparison of the Variance of the Bispectra. In order to improve the readability of the chart the logarithmic scale was used.
Observations:

- Comparing the variances in the different bands, once again one can observe that the results calculated for group suffering from arrhythmia stand out.
- The biggest difference can be spotted in the VLF-VLF band. However, this time it's up to 800 times higher than in the case of the second highest result (CHF) (Fig. 4).

4.2   Bicohrent Analyses

Observations:

- In each band, except the VLF-VLF one, the maximum value of bicoherence obtained for a group suffering from tachycardia significantly exceeds other registrations (Fig. 5).

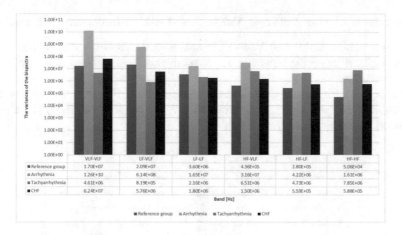

Fig. 4. Comparison of the variances of the bispectra

– The biggest difference was recorded in the LF-LF band, where the result calculated for patients with tachycardia was almost 9 times higher than the second highest (reference group) (Fig. 6).

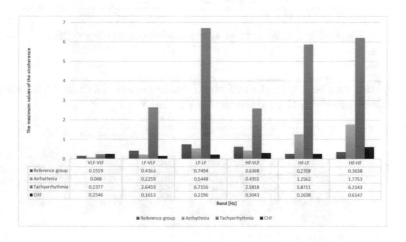

Fig. 5. Comparison of the maximum values of the bicoherence

Comparison of the Average Values of the Bicoherence. Observations:

- In each band, except the VLF-VLF one, the maximum value of bicoherence obtained for a group suffering from tachycardia significantly exceeds other registrations.
- The biggest difference was recorded in the LF-LF band, where the result calculated for patients with tachycardia was almost 9 times higher than the second highest (reference group).

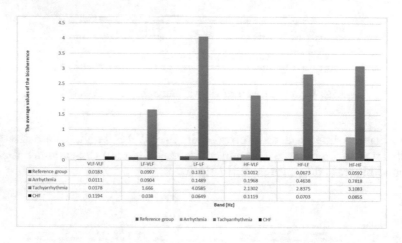

Fig. 6. Comparison of the average values of the bicoherence

Comparison of the Variances of the Bicoherence. In order to improve the readability of the chart the logarithmic scale was used (Fig. 7).

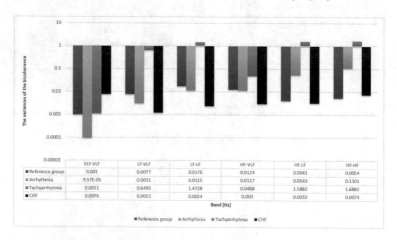

Fig. 7. Comparison of the variances of the bicoherence

Observations:

- Just like in the case of a comparison of the maximum values of bicoherence, in each band, except the VLF-VLF one, the results of the group suffering from tachycardia clearly stand up.
- The highest difference can be observed in the LF-LF band. The average value of bicoherence is more than 26 times higher than the second highest result (arrhythmia).

5   Discussion

5.1   Bispectral Analysis – Summary

Comparison of the results of the reference group and patients suffering from arrhythmia, tachycardia and CHF showed the usefulness of the bispectral analysis as a tool for differentiation between specific diseases.

For each of the analyzed parameters one can easily distinguish results registered for patients suffering from arrhythmia.

The differences between arrhythmia and other cases were so significant that high effectiveness of such identification can be assumed. Particularly in the case of comparing the variations in VLF-VLF band. The variation obtained for the patients suffering from arrhythmia was over 800 times higher than in the any other observed case.

5.2   Bicoherent Analysis – Summary

Comparison of the results of the reference group and patients suffering from arrhythmia, tachycardia and CHF showed the usefulness of the bicoherent analysis as a tool for differentiation between specific diseases. For each of the analyzed parameters a significant alternation of the results registered for patients suffering from tachycardia can be observed.

The biggest differences occurred in the LF-LF band. They were so significant that high efficiency of such identification can be assumed. Particularly in the case of comparing the variations in the above-mentioned frequency range, where the result obtained for the tachycardia was over 80 times greater than other ones.

6   Conclusions

As the result of the work the analysis of the suitability of the higher-order spectra as a tool for the identification of patients diagnosed with various cardiac diseases was presented.

To simplify, only three parameters were taken under consideration (variance, maximum and average value). Each of them can be used to identify registrations taken from healthy individuals and patients suffering from arrhythmia or tachycardia. However, in each case the most robust analysis was the one based on comparison of the variances.

Only for a third group, that is the patients diagnosed with CHF the results were not conclusive. Therefore, it seems that the key to improving the identification mechanism is to extend the list of investigated parameters.

In the present work this step was abandoned due to the fact that the efficiency of the described analysis has already been confirmed for the groups with tachycardia and arrhythmia.

References

1. Physionet. http://physionet.org/. Accessed 5 Mar 2015
2. Chua, K.C.: Analysis of cardiac and epileptic signals using higher order spectra. Ph.D. thesis, Queensland University of Technology (2010)
3. Gałąska, R.: Analiza fraktalna zmienności rytmu zatokowego u pacjentów z upośledzoną funkcją lewej komory mięśnia serwcowego. Ph.D. thesis, The Medical University of Gdańsk (2006). (in Polish)
4. Goshvarpour, A., Goshvarpour, A.: Comparison of higher order spectra in heart rate signals during two techniques of meditation: chi and kundalini meditation. Cogn. Neurodyn. **7**(1), 39–46 (2012)
5. Hellwig, Z.: Elementy rachunku prawdopodobieństwa i statystyki matematycznej. Wydaw, Naukowe PWN (1995). (in Polish)
6. Jouny, I., Moses, R.: The bispectrum of complex signals: definitions and properties. IEEE Trans. Sig. Process. **40**(11), 2833–2836 (1992)
7. Kłopocka, M., Budzyński, J., Bujak, R., Świątkowski Maciej and. Sinkiewicz, W., Ziółkowski, M.: Dobowa zmienność rytmu zatokowego serca jako wskaźnik aktywności autonomicznego układu nerwowego u mężczyzn z zespołem zależności alkoholowej w okresie abstynencji. Alkocholizm i Narkomania **13**(4), 491–501 (2000). (in Polish)
8. Krauze, T., Guzik, P., Wysocki, H.: Zmienność rytmu serca: aspekty techniczne. Nowiny Lekarskie **70**(9), 973–984 (2001). (in Polish)
9. Mazur, P., Matusik, P., Pfitzner, R.: Analiza parametrów częstotliwościowych zmienności rytmu serca po pomostowaniu aortalno-wieńcowym. Folia Cardiologica Excerpta **6**(1), 76–81 (2011). (in Polish)
10. Mendel, J.: Tutorial on higher-order statistics (spectra) in signal processing and system theory: theoretical results and some applications. Proc. IEEE **79**(3), 278–305 (1991)
11. Nikias, C., Mendel, J.: Signal processing with higher-order spectra. IEEE Sig. Process. Mag. **10**(3), 10–37 (1993)
12. Pander, T.: Zastosowanie metod częstotliwościowych do wyznaczania przesunięcia sygnałów biomedycznych w dziedzinie czasu. Ph.D. thesis, Silesian University of Technology (1999). (in Polish)
13. Saliu, S., Birand, A., Kudaiberdieva, G.: Bispectral analysis of heart rate variability signal. In: 2002 11th European Signal Processing Conference, pp. 1–4 (2002)
14. Socha, L.: Równania momentów w stochastycznych układach dynamicznych. Wydaw. Naukowe PWN (1993). (in Polish)
15. Swami, A., Mendel, J.M., Nikias, C.L.M.: Higher-order spectral analysis toolbox: For use with MATLAB (1993). (User's Guide)

Spatio-Temporal Extension
of Independent Component Analysis
for Fetal ECG Extraction

Michał Piela and Tomasz Moroń[(✉)]

Silesian University of Technology, Gliwice, Poland
Tomasz.Moron@polsl.pl

Abstract. We propose an extension of independent component analysis when applied for fetal ECG extraction. Before using the classical ICA method, we multiply the number of measured signals using the technique of delays (each signal channel delayed by a proper time interval is regarded as a new measured signal). After this duplication of the measured signal channels, the classical JADE algorithm is applied to perform blind separation of independent source signals. Then we use a simple algorithm to select the estimated source signal that contains the fetal ECG of the best quality. We compare the results obtained using the classical ICA and the approach proposed. The experiments performed on 4-channel maternal abdominal ECG signals confirm the superior performance of this approach.

Keywords: Spatio-temporal filtering
Independent component analysis · Blind source separation

1 Introduction

Analysis of fetal electrocardiogram (fECG) has been the subject of numerous researches in recent years [1,2,6,7,10,16,18]. Its attractiveness results from the non-invasiveness of the examination, which does not affect the mother and the fetus, and also from its relatively low costs. Research on this topic centre around overcoming the challenges and problems associated with fECG analysis based on maternal abdominal signals. Among the most important challenges, we can distinguish rather low energy of the fetal ECG, in comparison to noise sources like maternal ECG or bioelectric activity of muscles. Many methods and algorithms have been developed, which aim in improvement of fetal ECG signal quality and its extraction from maternal abdominal signals [4,5,8,19]. The basic approach includes methods that solve blind source separation problem. Independent component analysis implemented using JADE algorithm is one of the most significant and popular methods used for that purpose [3,15]. However, the algorithm applied on the signals with low number of channels is insufficient. It is confirmed in our experiments on maternal abdominal signals containing 4 channels. In this

© Springer International Publishing AG, part of Springer Nature 2019
E. Pietka et al. (Eds.): ITIB 2018, AISC 762, pp. 315–324, 2019.
https://doi.org/10.1007/978-3-319-91211-0_28

paper, we propose the spatio-temporal extension of the ICA method. The proposed approach will be called as the spatio-temporal ICA method (STICA). In Sect. 2, we describe both ICA and STICA methods, and latter signal processing for assessment of fECG signal quality. In Sect. 4, numerical experiments are presented and discussed. Finally, conclusions are formulated.

2 Methods

2.1 Independent Component Analysis

Independent component analysis is one of several techniques which can be used to solve the blind source separation problem (BSS). The BSS model assumes that the signal from every lead is a linear combination of the source signals, according to equation

$$\mathbf{x}(n) = \mathbf{A}\mathbf{s}(n) + \eta(n) \tag{1}$$

where $\mathbf{x}(n)$ represents the measured signal vector, $\mathbf{s}(n)$ is the vector containing source signals and $\eta(n)$ involves noise components. A is the mixing matrix.

ICA assumes statistical independence of the source signals to be separated. It is restricted to non-gaussian signals (at most one of them can have a Gaussian distribution) [4]. In our experiments we used the JADE algorithm [15], which exploits the second and the fourth moments: covariances and cumulants in order to determine both separating and mixing matrices. Having the separating matrix $\mathbf{A}_{JADE}^{-1}$ calculated, we can estimate the independent source signals using

$$\hat{\mathbf{s}}(n) = \mathbf{A}_{JADE}^{-1}\mathbf{x}(n) \tag{2}$$

2.2 Spatio-Temporal Generalization of Independent Component Analysis

The method proposed in this article extends capabilities of the classical ICA. It makes use of spatio-temporal information present in the recorded multichannel signal. We increase the dimension of the observation vector – the number of channels – by using the original signal channels, shifted in time according to the following equation

$$\mathbf{x}'(n) = [x_1(n - \tau), x_1(n), x_1(n + \tau), \ldots, x_K(n - \tau), x_K(n), x_K(n + \tau)]^T \tag{3}$$

where K denotes the number of the measured signal channels (dimension of the measured signals vector). This way we obtain the extended measured signals vector $(\mathbf{x}\prime(n))$ whose dimension is three times larger than the dimension of the original vector $\mathbf{x}(n)$. Following this operation, we apply the JADE algorithm to estimate $3K$ independent source signals.

2.3   Assessment of ECG Signal Quality

To assess the ECG signals quality, we apply the approach proposed in [12]. In this approach, we assume that ECG signals are repeatable. Assessment of their quality is based on the autocorrelation function. However, to make it immune to noise, the signals are firstly enhanced. Thus, to calculate the quality index, the following steps are performed:

1. First, we calculate a so called detection function, using linear filtering, squaring and moving window integration. As a result, we obtain a nonnegative plot conditioned for further processing (Fig. 1(B)).
2. The autocorrelation function is applied to the selected, equidistant signal parts of the same length.
3. For every selected part of the signal, we look for the largest value (h_1) obtained for the dominant period (τ_1) of repeatability, and for the smallest one (h_2) (Fig. 2(B)). Quality index Q_i is determined as the quotient of these two values: $Q_i = \frac{h_1}{h_2}$.
4. Finally, index Q, used to assess the ECG signals quality, is calculated, as the median value of the Q_i indices obtained in the previous step.

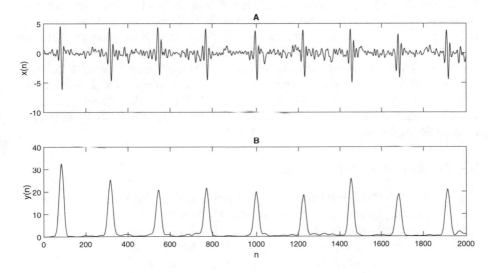

Fig. 1. A segment of an ECG signal whose quality is to be assessed ($x(n)$) and the calculated detection function ($y(n)$)

2.4   Selection of the Fetal ECG

Following application of ICA or STICA, we obtain a set of estimates of independent source signals. These estimates can contain maternal ECG, fetal ECG,

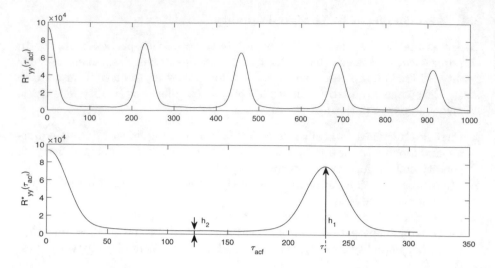

Fig. 2. (A) A plot of the autocorrelation function obtained for the detection function from Fig. 1(B), (B) its selected part

noise and all these component mixed. Our aim is to find the estimate that contains the fetal ECG of the best quality. To this end, we apply the index defined in the previous subsection. In the first step, we search for the estimate with the best maternal ECG (we assume that this estimate obtains the highest value of index Q). Then, assuming that other estimates containing maternal ECG have the same dominant period of repeatability (like the one selected), we exclude these estimates from the search for the fetal ECG. Finally, among the other ones, we select the source signal estimate with the best fetal ECG (it is the one that achieved the highest value of index Q).

3   Numerical Experiments

The proposed STICA method was tested using fECG Challenge 2013 training set A database, facilitated by Physionet [18]. The first 5 files (a01–a05) were selected. Original sampling frequency for each file was 1000 Hz, during the preprocessing step we performed decimation by a factor of 2. Every file consists of 4 channels from electrodes collecting maternal abdominal bioelectric signals. An exemplary signal is presented in Fig. 3. Results of the classical independent component analysis performed on this signal are drawn in Fig. 4. To perform its STICA decomposition, we formed the extended measured signals vector $\mathbf{x}(n)$ according to (3) using $\tau = 5$. Since the length of the formed vector equals $3K = 12$, by its ICA decomposition we obtained 12 estimates of independent source signals (presented in Fig. 5). Applying the described algorithm of fECG selection, we chose the estimate indicated in the figure by the horizontal arrow.

Quantitative results of ICA and STICA application to the selected test signals are presented in Table 1. For the classical ICA method, we presented the single

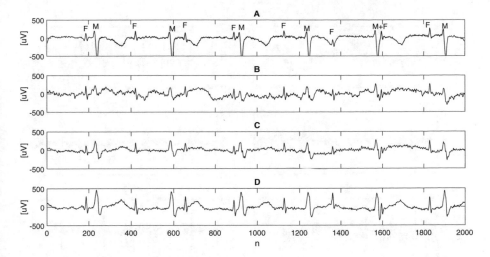

Fig. 3. An exemplary maternal abdominal 4-channel ECG signal. Letters M and F mark the maternal and the fetal QRS complexes, respectively. M+F signifies a case of the both complexes coincidence

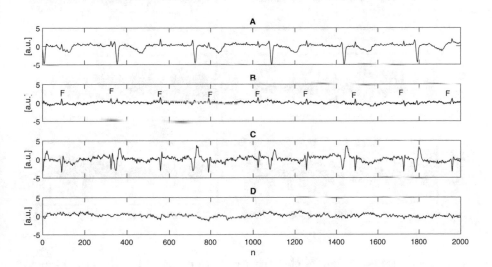

Fig. 4. Source signals estimates obtained using the classical ICA method on the basis of the signals from Fig. 3. The signals are presented in arbitrary units

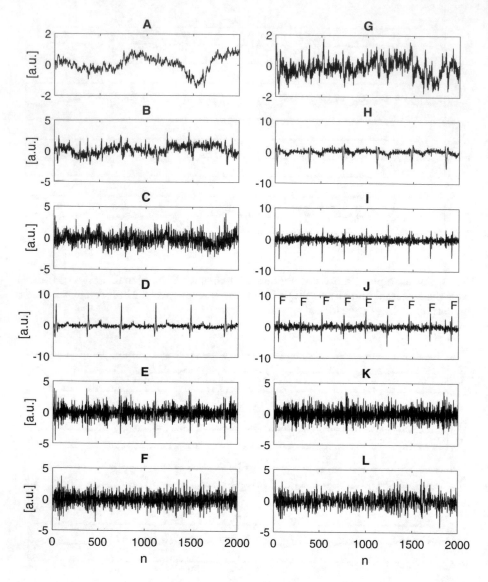

Fig. 5. Source signals estimates obtained using the proposed STICA method on the basis of the signals from Fig. 3. The arrow indicates the automatically selected fECG component of the best quality. The signals are presented in arbitrary units

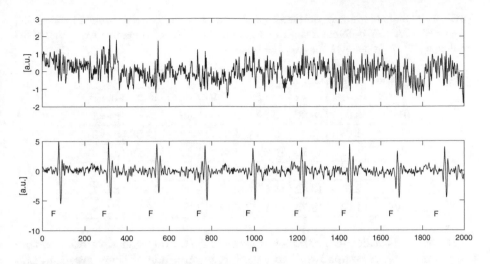

Fig. 6. Visual comparison of the results obtained by applying ICA (A) and STICA (B) to a03 record. The signals are presented in arbitrary units

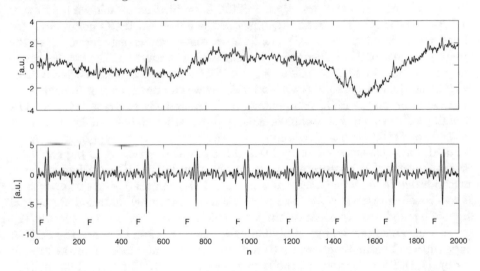

Fig. 7. Visual comparison of the results obtained by applying ICA (A) and STICA (B) to a05 record. The signals are presented in arbitrary units

Q index achieved for the best fetal ECG. The STICA method was applied with different values of parameter τ (it was varied from 1 to 15). In the table, we presented the Q index obtained for $\tau = 1$, 5, 10 and 15 and the best value achieved. As we can notice for different signals, different values of parameter tau appeared advantageous. However for signal a02 none of the values tested allowed for significant enhancement of the fECG signal. It is caused by particular properties of this signal.

Table 1. The quality indices obtained for the best fetal ECGs, determined using either ICA or STICA (for different values of tau) on the basis of 5 signals from the fECG challenge [18]. Avg denotes the average results

File no.	Q_{ICA}	Q_{STICA}				
		$\tau = 1$	$\tau = 5$	$\tau = 10$	$\tau = 15$	Best value (τ)
01	3.03	3.07	3.29	3.29	3.40	3.40 ($\tau = 15$)
02	1.07	1.37	1.08	1.04	1.10	1.83 ($\tau = 3$)
03	1.17	10.10	16.44	1.45	1.32	18.92 ($\tau = 6$)
04	1.16	40.59	37.36	27.91	5.36	40.59 ($\tau = 1$)
05	2.31	13.52	15.52	10.66	2.60	18.19 ($\tau = 7$)
AVG	1.75	13.73	14.74	8.87	2.76	16.59

It contains artificially constructed cases of A/D converter saturation within the maternal QRS complexes. The very large amplitude of these artefacts prevented the ICA method from successful separation of independent source signals irrespective of the length of the measured signals vector (4 for ICA and 12 for STICA). For other test signals STICA enabled us to achieve a substantial improvement of the results. Quality of the extracted fECG component (as measured by the index defined) was in most cases significantly higher than the quality of the signal obtained using the classical ICA method. To visualize these effects, in Figs. 6 and 7 we presented the fECGs extracted using either ICA or STICA on the basis of signals a03 and a05. As we can notice in Fig. 6, using ICA a rather poor quality fECG component was extracted. By contrast, using STICA a high quality signal was obtained. Although for other signals the improvement caused by STICA was not so imposing (see Fig. 6), nevertheless in most cases studied, the substantial increase of the Q index was observable. In papers [9, 12] it was shown that it is advantageous to combine the spatial ICA method with the methods developed to enhance single channel ECG signals. Using this approach, it was possible to extract the fetal ECG from the 3-channel maternal abdominal signals [9], and even to separate the twins fECGs using the 4-channel ones [12].

It seems also possible to apply this approach to extend further the STICA capabilities. The method can be combined with the methods of projective filtering [9, 11, 12] or various methods of time-averaging [13, 14, 17]. Like in [12], such combinations can be applied to accomplish a very demanding task of ECG signals decomposition during twin pregnancies.

4   Conclusion

Effective decomposition of multichannel biomedical signals can often be achieved using the method of independent component analysis. This method performs separation of individual source signals using the conditions of their statistical independence and exploiting the model of blind source separation. However, one of the restrictions imposed by this model concerns the number of the source signals that can be separated. This number cannot be greater than the number of the measured signals (signal channels). Our experiments showed that recording 4-channel abdominal signals does not always assure successful separation of the fetal ECG. Applying the proposed spatio-temporal representation of the recorded signals, we were able to improve the method capabilities to extract this component. For most test signals investigated, this approach led to significant improvement of the fECG quality.

Acknowledgement. This work was partially supported by the Ministry of Science and Higher Education funding for statutory activities of young researchers (BKM-BKM-510/RAu-3/2017). The work was performed using the infrastructure supported by POIG.02.03.01-24-099/13 grant: GeCONiI–Upper Silesian Center for Computational Science and Engineering.

References

1. Almeida, R., Gonçalves, H., Bernardes, J., Rocha, A.P.: Fetal QRS detection and heart rate estimation: a wavelet-based approach. Physiol. Measur. **35**(8), 1723 (2014)
2. Behar, J., Oster, J., Clifford, G.D.: Non-invasive fECG extraction from a set of abdominal sensors. In: Computing in Cardiology Conference (CinC), pp. 297–300. IEEE (2013)
3. Cardoso, J.F.: Multidimensional independent component analysis. In: 1998 Proceedings of the 1998 IEEE International Conference on Acoustics, Speech and Signal Processing, vol. 4, pp. 1941–1944. IEEE (1998)
4. De Lathauwer, L., De Moor, B., Vandewalle, J.: Fetal electrocardiogram extraction by blind source subspace separation. IEEE Trans. Biomed. Eng. **47**(5), 567–572 (2000)
5. De Lathauwer, L., De Moor, B., Vandewalle, J.: SVD-based methodologies for fetal electrocardiogram extraction. In: 2000 IEEE International Conference on Acoustics, Speech, and Signal Processing, ICASSP 2000, Proceedings, vol. 6, pp. 3771–3774. IEEE (2000)
6. Jezewski, J., Matonia, A., Kupka, T., Roj, D., Czabanski, R.: Determination of fetal heart rate from abdominal signals: evaluation of beat-to-beat accuracy in relation to the direct fetal electrocardiogram. Biomed. Tech./Biomed. Eng. **57**(5), 383–394 (2012)
7. Jezewski, J., Wrobel, J., Matonia, A., Horoba, K., Martinek, R., Kupka, T., Jezewski, M.: Is abdominal fetal electrocardiography an alternative to Doppler ultrasound for FHR variability evaluation? Front. Physiol. **8** (2017)
8. Kotas, M.: Projective filtering of time-aligned beats for foetal ECG extraction. Tech. Sci. **55**(4) (2007)
9. Kotas, M.: Combined application of independent component analysis and projective filtering to fetal ECG extraction. Biocybernetics Biomed. Eng. **28**(1), 75 (2008)
10. Kotas, M., Blaszczyk, J., Moron, T.: Spatio-temporal FIR filter for fetal ECG extraction. Int. J. Inf. Electron. Eng. **5**, 10–14 (2015)
11. Kotas, M.: Projective filtering of time warped ECG beats. Comput. Biol. Med. **38**(1), 127–137 (2008)

12. Kotas, M., Leski, J., Wrobel, J.: Sequential separation of twin pregnancy electrocardiograms. Bull. Pol. Acad. Sci. Tech. Sci. **64**(1), 91–101 (2016)
13. Kotas, M., Pander, T., Leski, J.M.: Averaging of nonlinearly aligned signal cycles for noise suppression. Biomed. Sig. Process. Control **21**, 157–168 (2015)
14. Leski, J.M.: Robust weighted averaging of biomedical signals. IEEE Trans. Biomed. Eng. **49**(8), 796–804 (2002)
15. Martens, S.M., Rabotti, C., Mischi, M., Sluijter, R.J.: A robust fetal ECG detection method for abdominal recordings. Physiol. Meas. **28**(4), 373 (2007)
16. Martinek, R., Kahankova, R., Nazeran, H., Konecny, J., Jezewski, J., Janku, P., Bilik, P., Zidek, J., Nedoma, J., Fajkus, M.: Non-invasive fetal monitoring: a maternal surface ECG electrode placement based novel approach for optimization of adaptive filter control parameters using the LMS and RLS algorithms. Sensors **17**(5), 1154 (2017)
17. Momot, A., Momot, M., Łęski, J.: Bayesian and empirical Bayesian approach to weighted averaging of ECG signal. Tech. Sci. **55**(4) (2007)
18. Silva, I., Behar, J., Sameni, R., Zhu, T., Oster, J., Clifford, G.D., Moody, G.B.: Noninvasive fetal ECG: the physionet/computing. In: Cardiology Challenge 2013, pp. 149–152 (2013)
19. Zarzoso, V., Nandi, A.K.: Noninvasive fetal electrocardiogram extraction: blind separation versus adaptive noise cancellation. IEEE Trans. Biomed. Eng. **48**(1), 12–18 (2001)

Computational Analysis of Induced Voltage on Implanted Cardiac Pacemaker's Lead by Mobile Phones

Maros Smondrk$^{(\boxtimes)}$, Mariana Benova, and Zuzana Psenakova

Department of Electromagnetic and Biomedical Engineering,
Faculty of Electrical Engineering, University of Zilina, Zilina, Slovakia
maros.smondrk@fel.uniza.sk

Abstract. The proposed paper deals with simulation and analysis of induced electric voltage in pacemaker lead model within the anatomical human body model due to the near-field exposure of dipole antennas covering carrier frequencies of both, GSM and UMTS mobile phone transmission technologies. The research was carried out using electromagnetic modelling based on the Finite Integration method and analysis was performed in terms of computing induced electric field distributions and induced electric voltage near to the pacemaker lead stimulation poles. The main objective was to compare levels of induced voltage on the pacemaker lead stimulation poles for both technologies, depending on the antenna distance from human torso model.

The numerical results have shown that closer proximity of antenna than the distance recommended by pacemaker manufacturers could not pose higher pacemaker interference risk. Additionally, the results of estimated induced voltage have revealed that the pacemaker interference risk of recent mobile phone transmission technology is lower compared to older ones.

Keywords: Pacemaker · Electromagnetic interference
Mobile phone · Numerical modelling · Induced voltage

1 Introduction

Many patients worldwide receive a pacemaker (PM) or implantable cardioverter defibrillator (ICD), implantable medical devices able to detect the heart's electrical activity and stimulate when this is insufficient. In general, pacemaker treats especially slow-rated arrhythmias and it is composed of a metallic case with electronic circuits and a battery inside while performing the electro-stimulation or detection in the heart via its leads. A technical services department of the leading PM manufacturer reports that they receive great number of calls per year from clinicians related to electromagnetic compatibility. Furthermore, 28% of all calls per month from patients are also related to electromagnetic compatibility issues [1,2]. According to a French survey conducted in 2014, 23% of 410

© Springer International Publishing AG, part of Springer Nature 2019
E. Pietka et al. (Eds.): ITIB 2018, AISC 762, pp. 325–336, 2019.
https://doi.org/10.1007/978-3-319-91211-0_29

questioned clinicians reported PM or ICD malfunction due to the electromagnetic interference (EMI) at least once a year [3]. These statistics briefly indicate increased concerns of patients and clinicians associated with PM electromagnetic interference as well as that the electromagnetic interference of PM are rare but represents serious issue. A one possible contribution to that could be increased use of wireless technologies to which PM patients are exposed over the last decade. These technologies as a source of high-frequency electromagnetic fields (EMFs) involve devices such as mobile phones, digital cordless phones, TERA transmitters, Bluetooth devices, Wi-Fi equipment, microwave ovens, electronic article surveillance devices, and so on. These devices, as the emitters of exogenous EMFs, could pose the risk of PM malfunction due to induced voltages in the human body and in the implanted leads, which may subsequently result in misinterpretation of recorded intracardiac electric potentials. Thus, leading to PM's oversensing with inhibition of pacing or inappropriate therapy [4,5].

Especially, increased concerns of PM patients and clinicians associated with EMI are related to mobile phones technology. Previous studies have shown EMI between mobile phones and implantable pacemakers [4–8]. Based on these studies and regulations of national authorities for testing PM's electromagnetic compatibility, all leading PM's manufactures recommend a safety distance of 15 cm between the implanted PM and mobile phone to prevent possible EMI [9,10]. However, technological advances of mobile phone technology have grown exponentially in the last decade and conducted studies primarily reflects EMI between PM and mobile phones using the GSM standard. The current mobile phones mostly use the UMTS standard. Moreover, a lot of metropolitan areas are covered by the newest LTE standard. These standards differ in signal properties such as the carrier frequency and the maximal permissible antenna power output. Furthermore, these studies mainly consider PM in a unipolar configuration which incidence is rare in current PM patients.

We therefore sought to evaluate the risk of EMI between PM and mobile phones. The aim of this study is to numerically calculate and analyse the electric field distribution within an anatomical human model including a PM model in bipolar configuration while exposed to near-field EMF radiation. The main objective is to compute and compare levels of induced voltages at the PM's lead tip for both, the GSM and UMTS communications bands. Furthermore, we evaluate levels of induced voltages with respect to the distance between the antenna and human body model. Both the electric field distributions and induced voltages are calculated by means of numerical electromagnetic simulations based on the Finite Integration Technique.

2   Materials and Methods

In this section we describe the methods employed for calculating and evaluating the induced voltage at the PM's lead tip within the numerical human body model. The characteristics of considered models is introduced as well.

2.1   Human Body and Pacemaker Model

As a numerical human body model, the AustinMan model was employed [11,12]. The AustinMan model, developed at The University of Texas, is a voxel-based model for electromagnetic simulations from the National Library of Medicine's Visible Human Project data set [13]. It is an anatomically realistic 3D model of a 38 years old adult male. Compared to the surface-based models, the voxel-based models are able to capture fine anatomical features and highly inhomogeneous tissues but suffer from staircased boundaries and higher computational costs. To reduce computational costs of numerical simulations while keep the sufficient spatial model resolution $(4 \times 4 \times 4\,\mathrm{mm}^3)$, we considered the upper body part cut through the transversal plane (at height of 1.27 m). The geometrical layout of a human body model with implanted PM model is depicted in Fig. 1. The AustinMan includes 80 anatomical features mapped by 47 different tissues. Their dielectric properties (i.e. relative permittivity and conductivity) were determined by the parametric model proposed by Gabriel et al. [14].

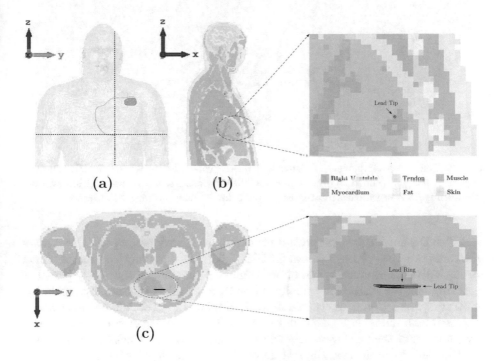

Fig. 1. (a) The geometrical layout of a used human body model with implanted PM model, in coronal plane. The dotted lines represent cutting planes in the transversal and sagittal planes used in the adjacent figures. (b), (c) The projections of numerical model in transversal and sagittal planes to emphasis the considered location of bipolar lead (lead ring is located in right ventricle and lead tip is located in myocardium)

The PM model represents a cylindrical structure whose shape and size were chosen to closely match real-life dimensions of most commonly implanted PMs, including a lead and connector part. Since the bipolar lead configuration is the most prevalent nowadays, the lead model was designed as a coaxial structure with inner and outer conductors separated by an inner insulation, and enclosed by an outer insulation. The PM's lead is terminated by the two stimulation/detection poles - ring and tip, separated by an insulation (Fig. 2). These poles are in a conductive contact with blood and myocardium in particular heart section (Fig. 1).

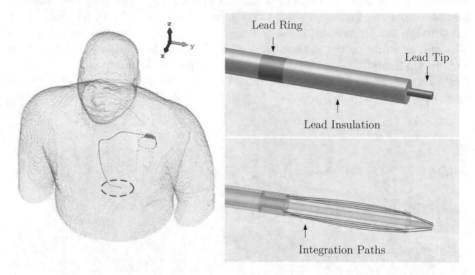

Fig. 2. The perspective view of numerical model with PM implanted in left pectoral region. Adjacent zoomed figures depict individual basics components of bipolar lead, where blue lines represent an integration path for induced voltage calculation

Since the geometrical properties of pacing leads vary among the PM's manufactures, we opted to use values 0.65, 1, 1.5, 2 mm for inner conductor, inner insulation, outer conductor, and outer insulation diameter, respectively [15]. The lead ring and tip length was equally set to 2 mm, while separated by insulation of 10 mm. The PM model was numerically implanted in the left pectoral region of AustinMan model in a particular manner, so that the lead is in contact with myocardium of the right ventricle and the lead trajectory tracks venous tree of AustinMan. We positioned the PM model in constant depth of 20 mm from air-tissue interface since the implant pocket location and implantation depth thereof are based upon physician preference and cannot be predicted. The dielectric and magnetic properties of the PM model are summarized in the Table 1. In addition, the simulation domain was extended to include the air domain in order to take into account the reflection that occurs at the air-skin boundary.

Table 1. The dielectric and magnetic properties of PM model, [15,16]

Part	Assigned Material	ε_r [-]	σ [S·m^{-1}]	μ_r [-]
PM case	Ti6Al4V	1	$0.562 \cdot 10^6$	1
PM cavity	Air	1	0	1
PM header	Polyurethane 80A	6	10^{-12}	1
Lead insulation	Polyurethane 80A	6	10^{-12}	1
Lead conductor	MP35N	1	$0.971 \cdot 10^6$	1

2.2 Source of Electromagnetic Exposure

A dipole antenna was considered as a sources of near-field RF exposure. A generalized tuned dipole antenna model was used since it is easy to model for specific resonant frequencies. Due to its form factor, its use in considered technologies is rare. Specifically, the planar inverted F-type antenna is most popular type of antenna suitable for hand-held devices. However, both of them have an omnidirectional radiation pattern [17–19]. Moreover, the dipole antennas are commonly used for testing PM's electromagnetic compatibility [20]. The dipole antenna was modelled as a long cylinder fed by a discrete port situated in the middle of longitudinal cylinder axis with a reference impedance of 50 Ω. Discrete port has been excited by an Gaussian shaped excitation signal with input powers of 1 and 0.25 W for 1800 (GSM) and 2100 MHz (UMTS) carrier frequency, respectively. The cylinder material was modelled as a perfect electric conductor. The geometrical parameters of tuned dipole antenna are summarized in the Table 2.

Table 2. Parameters of tuned dipole antennas

Parameter	Value	Unit
Carrier Frequency – f	1800 and 2100	MHz
Output Power	1 and 0.25	W
Speed of Light – c	299 792 458	m·s^{-1}
Wavelength – λ	$\frac{c}{f}$	m
Cylinder Length	$0.4325 \cdot \lambda$	m
Cylinder Radius	0.001	m

In all exposure scenarios, the antennas were placed directly over the PM model mimic the situation that patient wears the mobile phone in the pectoral pocket. The antennas were located in the air domain above the human body model and were rotated around frontal axis to be parallel to the body surface (Fig. 3). To analyse the effect of antenna distance from PM and human body model on the risk of EMI, the antenna distance from human body surface was varied from 0 mm to 450 mm. This provided a wide range of combinations that

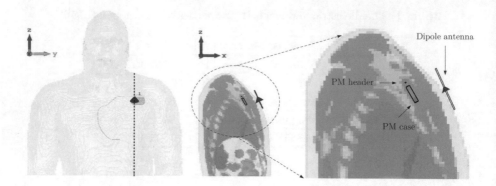

Fig. 3. The geometrical layout of a used human body model with implanted PM model, in coronal plane. The dotted line represents cutting line in the sagittal plane used in the adjacent figure. Red triangle depicts a discrete port of the dipole antenna

allowed us to analyse the electric field distribution inside human body model and calculate induced voltages in leads as a function of antenna distance.

2.3   Numerical Modelling

This study is based on electromagnetic modelling using the Finite Integration Technique implemented within a commercially available simulation software CST Microwave Studio. The time-domain solver based on the FIT was applied on the model which was discretized using a hexahedral mesh. In order to ensure accuracy of the obtained numerical results, the cell size inside the model space was set to fulfil the criterion requiring the maximum element size to be smaller than the recommended limit of 1/5 of the considered EMF wavelength. The problem addressed in this study was to calculate the electric field distribution $\boldsymbol{E}$ defined by the following equation

$$\nabla \times \mu_r^{-1}(\nabla \times \boldsymbol{E}) - k_0^2 \left(\varepsilon_r - \frac{j\sigma}{\omega \varepsilon_0} \right) \boldsymbol{E} = 0 \qquad (1)$$

where k_0 – is wave vector in free space [m^{-1}], ∇ – rotation vector operator, ε_r – relative permittivity, ε_0 – vacuum permittivity [F·m^{-1}], μ_r – relative permeability, σ – electrical conductivity [S·m^{-1}] and ω – angular wave frequency [rad·s^{-1}].

Knowing these EMF's quantities and parameters of exposed tissue, it is possible to calculate the spatial electric field distribution for every knot of the mesh. Subsequently, the electric potential difference between lead tip and lead ring within the human body model equals to total induced voltage (U_{ind}) due to the exogenous electric field emitted by the dipole antenna. This could be formulated as follows

$$U_{ind} = \varphi_{tip} - \varphi_{ring} = \int_{ring}^{tip} \boldsymbol{E} \, d\mathbf{s} \qquad (2)$$

where $\boldsymbol{E}$ is the electric field inside the human body model induced by the exogenous electric field emitted by the dipole antenna. Since the numerical domain has been discretized by hexahedral mesh, we implemented Eq. (2) in the following form

$$U_{ind} = \sum_{n=2}^{N} \frac{\boldsymbol{E}(n-1) + \boldsymbol{E}(n)}{2} ds \qquad (3)$$

where N is the number of points on the path form the lead ring to the tip and ds is the distance between two consecutive points on this path. In order to estimate induced voltage on the bipolar pacing lead we used the same methodology as the authors in [1,21]. However, we used a full-wave solver while their objective was to evaluate power-line frequency exposure utilizing electro-quasistatic assumptions. Furthermore, the integration paths between PM's ring and tip were not specified by these authors. We opted to use four lines and four spline paths in totally. Each integration path was oriented around coronal axis, connecting lateral edge of ring and lateral edge of tip (Fig. 2).

3   Computational Results and Discussion

To specify geometrical properties of the dipole antenna models, a plenty of parametric studies were firstly performed which allowed us thereafter to achieve optimal size while maintained good reflection coefficients in desired frequency bands. The frequency response of the simulated reflection coefficients are shown in Fig. 4, confirming that the designed antenna models are resonant at the desired frequencies.

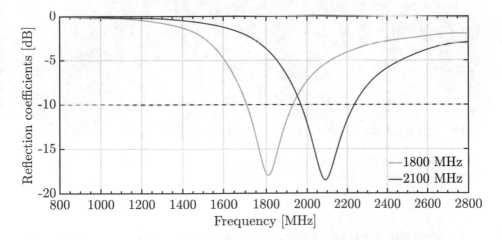

Fig. 4. Simulated reflection coefficients of designed dipole antennas. The reflection coefficients are plotted along the vertical axis with the blue and green curves representing the carrier frequency of 1800 MHz (GSM) and 2100 MHz (UMTS), respectively

The simulated reflection coefficients for desired frequencies were below the −10 dB, which is a voltage standing wave ratio of less than 2:1. This ratio describes how well the antenna input impedance is matched to the reference impedance.

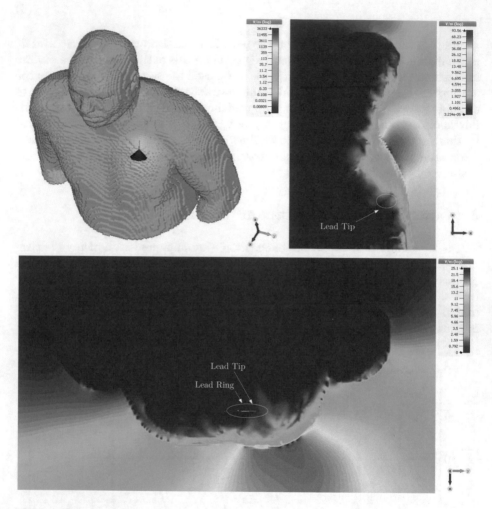

Fig. 5. The representative example of the spatial electric field distributions for one exposure configuration of numerical model. The surface distributions in the transversal and sagittal planes cross PM's lead tip

Subsequently, the spatial electric field distributions within the human body model including PM model in bipolar configuration were calculated considering both, GSM and UMTS mobile phone technology carrier frequency. The representative example of spatial electric field distributions for the UMTS carrier frequency exposure with antenna in the highest considered proximity from body surface is depicted in Fig. 5. Perspective view and surface distributions in transversal and sagittal planes revealed that the major part of electric field is located on the body surface around the antenna's discrete port. Due to the presence of air domain in front of the human body model, the majority of the electromagnetic energy is reflected back and only a minor part is transmitted towards the tissue. In general, the amount of incident EMFs that is reflected is proportional to dielectric and magnetic properties of the surrounding media at each boundary. While the EMF propagates trough the lossy tissue media, its energy or electric field amplitude gradually attenuates depending on the conductivity of each particular tissue layer. Considering anatomical structures (Fig. 1) related to the electric field distributions in the transversal and sagittal planes (Fig. 5), the EMF penetrates into heart region to some extent however the electric field amplitude progressively decrease.

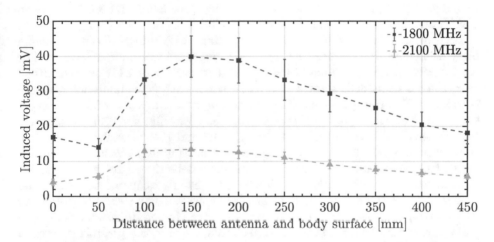

Fig. 6. Induced electric voltage between the lead ring and tip for the bipolar configuration of PM model implanted into human body model, due to the near-field exposure of dipole antennas (operating in the GSM and UMTS frequency bands) as a function of antenna distance from the body surface

The electric field distributions considering GSM and UMTS carrier frequencies were calculated as a function of antenna distance from the human body surface. The induced electric fields in the heart region were analysed by means of the numerical integration of the eight selected paths between lead ring and tip, thus estimating mean induced voltages on the PM lead. The results of mean induced voltages with reported standard deviation are depicted in Fig. 6. The calculated distributions of induced voltage revealed a high variability depending on the antenna distance. The maximal mean induced voltage achieved value of 39.9 mV (±5.9 mV) and 13.45 mV (±1.9 mV) for GSM and UMTS frequency bands, respectively. It represents a three-fold difference at antenna distance of 150 mm for both considered frequencies. The minimal mean induced voltage was 14 mV ($\pm$2.5 mV) and 4 mV ($\pm$0.9 mV) for GSM and UMTS frequency bands, respectively. The mean value of induced voltage revealed progressive increasing tendency while increasing antenna distance up to 150 mm. On contrary, the mean value of induced electric field has gradually shown declining tendency for antenna distance above this value. This is a result of near-field exposure where there are strong inductive and capacitive effects of antenna with surrounding tissue, thus modifying antenna performance. The boundary between near-field and far-field is proportional to the wavelength which is 166 mm and 143 mm for considered frequency of 1800 MHz and 2100 MHz, respectively. Comparing the results of mean induced voltage for both considered carrier frequencies regardless the antenna distance, the results revealed higher values of induced voltage for GSM compared to UMTS carrier frequency. The ratio of difference between them achieved value of 3.1 ($\pm$0.47). This tendency is caused by combination of two factors, a higher conductivity of human tissues for UMTS carrier frequency resulting in higher attenuation of incident EMF and 4 times smaller UMTS antenna power output compared to GSM.

In general, it is very difficult to measure internal EMF intensity in the human body using non-invasive methods or provide long-term recording of intra-cardiac electrogram utilizing implanted PM exposed to variety of EMF sources. However, the use of modelling tools such as an electromagnetic simulation software is well established way for quantitative and qualitative analysis of desired exposure scenarios. The current PMs encompass the input filters in order to suppress sensed signals different to intra-cardiac signals and their technical parameters such as the amplitude-frequency response are not publicly available. Similarly, the PM's manufactures have introduced the noise detection algorithms which differ from one to another PM model. However, the carrier frequencies of considered mobile phone standards are higher than frequency range of sensed biopotentials (0.1–300 Hz), but their modulation frequency is 8 Hz and 100 Hz for GSM and UMTS, respectively [15]. Thus, these technologies pose the possible sources of pacemakers EMI and could contribute to statistics reported in [2,3] to some extents. A set-up sensitivity of PM is another factor involved. It is a threshold value of sensed signal amplitude which is evaluated as the intra-cardiac signal. This value is set-up programmatically and vary within the range from 0.8 mV to 20 mV [22]. Thus, induced voltage in PM lead within this range could be possibly misinterpreted as a intrinsic cardiac activity. The proposed numerical model as well as the methodology to estimate induced voltage in PM lead provides quantitative estimate of EMI risk, due to the numerous factors involved. This limitation makes evident that more research has to be conducted by taking in to account mentioned parameters as well as verification of numerical outcomes with real-life measurements.

4   Conclusion

The proposed paper deals with simulation and analysis of induced electric voltage in pacemaker lead model within the anatomical high-resolution realistic human body model due to the near-field exposure of two dominant mobile phone transmission technologies. The computational results indicate that the risk of PM's EMI in bipolar configuration differs with respect to the mobile phone standard as well as to the antenna distance. Results from the near-field exposure have shown that the maximal values of mean induced voltage were estimated for antenna distance of 150 mm, concluding that higher antenna proximity to human body model could not cause higher induced electric field on the path between lead stimulating poles. Considering the recommended antenna distance of 150 mm as a worst-case scenario, the EMI risk decreases as the antenna proximity increases. Additionally, the results of estimated induced voltage have revealed that the PM interference risk of recent mobile phone transmission technology is lower compared to older ones. Two facts are involved, the higher attenuation of incident EMFs in the human body for the higher carrier frequency and the significantly lower power output of novel mobile phone transmission technologies.

Acknowledgement. This work has been supported by the Slovak Research and Development Agency (grant number APVV-16-0190). The authors acknowledge the Computational Electromagnetics Group at The University of Texas at Austin for developing and making the AustinMan Electromagnetic Voxels model available at http://bit.ly/AustinMan.

References

1. Gercek, C., Kourtiche, D., Nadi, M., Magne, I., Schmitt, P., Souques, M.: Bioengineering **4**(1), 19 (2017). https://doi.org/10.3390/bioengineering4010019
2. Medtronic. ResponseCare - Technical Services. http://www.responsecare.medtronic.com/technical-services/index.htm. Accessed 13 Sept 2017
3. Hours, M., Khati, I., Hamelin, J.: Pacing Clin. Electrophysiol. **37**(3), 290 (2014). https://doi.org/10.1111/pace.12269
4. Censi, F., Calcagnini, G., Triventi, M., Mattei, E., Bartolini, P.: Ann. Ist. Super. Sanita. **43**(3), 254 (2007)
5. Hekmat, K., Salemink, B., Lauterbach, G., Schwinger, R.H., Sudkamp, M., Weber, H.J., Mehlhorn, U.: Europace **6**(4), 363 (2004)
6. Hayes, D.L., Wang, P.J., Reynolds, D.W., Estes, N.M., Griffith, J.L., Steffens, R.A., Carlo, G.L., Findlay, G.K., Johnson, C.M.: N. Engl. J. Med. **336**(21), 1473 (1997). https://doi.org/10.1056/nejm199705223362101
7. Tandogan, I., Temizhan, A., Yetkin, E., Guray, Y., Ileri, M., Duru, E., Sasmaz, A.: Int. J. Cardiol. **103**(1), 51 (2005). https://doi.org/10.1016/j.ijcard.2004.08.031
8. Cecil, S., Neubauer, G., Rauscha, F., Stix, G., Müller, W., Breithuber, C., Glanzer, M.: Bioelectromagnetics **35**(3), 192 (2014). https://doi.org/10.1002/bem.21839
9. Calcagnini, G., Censi, F., Bartolini, P.: Ann. Ist. Super. Sanita. **43**(3), 268 (2007)
10. Medtronic. Patient Services Electromagnetic Compatibility Guide: For Implantation Cardiac Devices. http://www.medtronic.com/us-en/patients/electromagnetic-guide/communication-office.html. Accessed 11 Jan 2018

11. Massey, J.W., Yilmaz, A.E.: 2016 38th Annual International Conference of the IEEE Engineering in Medicine and Biology Society (EMBC). IEEE (2016). https://doi.org/10.1109/embc.2016.7591444
12. Massey, J.W., Prokop, A., Yilmaz, A.E.: 2017 39th Annual International Conference of the IEEE Engineering in Medicine and Biology Society (EMBC). IEEE (2017). https://doi.org/10.1109/embc.2017.8037283
13. Spitzer, V., Ackerman, M.J., Scherzinger, A.L., Whitlock, D.: J. Am. Med. Inform. Assoc. **3**(2), 118 (1996)
14. Gabriel, S., Lau, R.W., Gabriel, C.: Phys. Med. Biol. **41**(11), 2251 (1996)
15. David, P.A.F., Hayes, L., Asirvatham, S.J.: Cardiac Pacing, Defibrillation and Resynchronization: A Clinical Approach, 3rd edn. Wiley-Blackwell, Chichester (2013)
16. Cardarelli, F.: Materials Handbook. Springer, London (2008). https://doi.org/10.1007/978-1-84628-669-8
17. Psenakova, Z., Smondrk, M., Barabas, J., Sciuto, G.L., Benova, M.: 2016 ELEKTRO. IEEE (2016). https://doi.org/10.1109/elektro.2016.7512141
18. Psenakova, Z., Smondrk, M., Sciuto, G.L., Benova, M.: Advances in Intelligent Systems and Computing, pp. 245–254. Springer International Publishing, Cham (2016). https://doi.org/10.1007/978-3-319-39904-1
19. Islam, N.A., Arifin, F.: 2016 3rd International Conference on Electrical Engineering and Information Communication Technology (ICEEICT). IEEE (2016). https://doi.org/10.1109/ceeict.2016.7873145
20. International Organization for Standardization, Active implantable medical devices - electromagnetic compatibility - EMC test protocols for implantable cardiac pacemakers, implantable cardioverter defibrillators and cardiac resynchronization devices. Standard 14117:2012, ISO, Geneva, Switzerland (2012)
21. Seckler, T., Stunder, D., Schikowsky, C., Joosten, S., Zink, M.D., Kraus, T., Marx, N., Napp, A.: Europace, p. euv458 (2016). https://doi.org/10.1093/europace/euv458
22. Medtronic. Dual Chamber Temporary Pacemaker Model 5388 - Technical Manual. https://goo.gl/tb72na. Accessed 18 Jan 2018

Influence of Gravitational Offset Removal on Heart Beat Detection Performance from Android Smartphone Seismocardiograms

Szymon Sieciński[✉] and Paweł Kostka

Faculty of Biomedical Engineering, Department of Biosensors
and Biomedical Signals Processing, Silesian University of Technology, Zabrze, Poland
szymon.siecinski@polsl.pl

Abstract. Seismocardiography (SCG) is a non-invasive method of analyzing and recording cardiovascular vibrations on the chest wall. Mobile devices offer the possibility to monitor cardiac activity. Accelerometers used in such analysis register gravitational offset because the effects of gravity on an object are indistinguishable from acceleration. Our aim is to investigate the influence of gravitational offset removal on heart beat detection from smartphone seismocardiograms.

We registered SCG signals from two subjects (male and female) in supine position before and after enabling gravitational offset removal to analyze its influence on beat detection algorithm performance. Our algorithm consists of signal preprocessing, calculating analytical envelope and RMS envelope and peak finding.

The influence of gravitational offset on heart beat detection is insignificant due to band-pass filtration. Offset removal slightly increased PPV for male subject and sensitivity for female subject. We observed beat detection quality improvement when using RMS envelope. The best performance was achieved using RMS envelope on signal from male subject.

This study proves insignificant influence of gravitational offset on our heart beat detection algorithm. Very high performance on analyzed signals ($Se = 0.990$, $PPV = 0.948$ for all beats, $Se = 1.000$, $PPV = 0.962$ for the best case) encourages studies on another SCG data sets or experiment set-ups.

Keywords: Seismocardiography · Heart beat detection
Gravitational offset · Smartphone

1 Introduction

Development of high quality, sensitive and inexpensive MEMS accelerometers in the last decade in combination with low cost computational power provided the reasons for reconsidering analysis of cardiovascular vibrations in clinical practice [4,21]. Accelerometers used in such analysis register gravitational offset because

© Springer International Publishing AG, part of Springer Nature 2019
E. Pietka et al. (Eds.): ITIB 2018, AISC 762, pp. 337–344, 2019.
https://doi.org/10.1007/978-3-319-91211-0_30

of Einstein's equivalence principle [12], which states the effects of gravity on an object are indistinguishable from acceleration.

Seismocardiography (SCG) is a non-invasive method of recording and analyzing vibrations generated by the cardiovascular system to the chest wall [7]. Recordings are performed on subjects in supine position with the accelerometer placed on the sternum, using the ultra-low frequency acceleration transducer with linear response from 0.1 to 800 Hz and a sensitivity of 1.0 V/g [19,20]. Availability of low cost MEMS accelerometers and portable devices including smartphones makes seismocardiography cost-effective and powerful tool for examining cardiac activity [13,14,17]. SCG found its use in heart rate variability analysis, detecting heart arrhythmias, myocardial ischemia [5,6,21].

SCG signal consists of the following fiducial points: mitral valve closure (MC), aortic valve opening (AO), onset of rapid enjection (RE), aortic valve closure (AC), mitral valve opening (MO), the peak of rapid filling (RF) and atrial systole (AS) [20]. Because aortal valve opening (AO) has the highest amplitude [16], we considered the time of its ocurrence as the occurence of heart beat. Figure 1 presents a SCG cycle with annotated fiducial points.

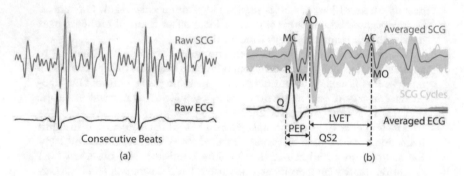

(a)   (b)

Fig. 1. SCG vs. ECG by Ghufran Shafiq et al. Image retrieved from [16]. License: CC-BY 4.0. Part (a) shows raw SCG signal (above) and ECG signal (below). Part (b) presents annotated SCG and ECG ensemble averages (dark lines) and superimposed SCG and ECG beats (light shades)

Our aim is to investigate the influence of gravitational offset removal on heart beat detection from 3-axis Android smartphone seismocardiograms without concurrent ECG registration.

2 Methods

2.1 Experiment Protocol

The experiment was conducted on 2 subjects: 25 year old male subject with no diagnosed cardiovascular disease and a 63 year old female subject with hypertension. Each subject was lying down in supine position at rest. We used LG

H340n smartphone furnished with Bosch Sensortec BMA255 accelerometer and Accelerometer Analysis mobile application available on Google Play to register SCG. This application can record acceleration without gravitational offset using online high-pass filter implementation shown in Android API Guide [1] as described further.

High-pass filter was implemented as subtraction of low-pass filter output from current acceleration value. Difference equation describing low-pass filter is shown in the Eq. (1).

$$y[n-1] = \alpha y[n-1] + (1-\alpha)y[n] \tag{1}$$

where $y[n]$ is the current signal value, $y[n-1]$ is the previous signal value and α is calculated as in the Eq. (2):

$$\alpha = \frac{t}{t + dT} \tag{2}$$

where t is time constant and dT acceleration value fetching rate. We assume $\alpha = 0.1$.

During the experiment the smartphone was placed loosely on sternum according to Fig. 2. Subjects were asked to stay still during the signal recording to minimize motion artifacts and to secure the position of smartphone.

We performed two recordings on each subject without concurrent ECG acquisition. During the first recording we enabled gravitational offset removal in the mobile application. The second recording was performed with that option disabled. Each recording lasted about 3–4 min.

The authors acquired SCG recording with sampling frequency $f_s = 100$ Hz. Technical specifications of accelerometer embedded in mobile device used for signal acquisition are shown in Table 1.

Table 1. Accelerometer technical specifications acquired by Sensor Multitool mobile application [15] (above) and selected parameters listed in BMA255 Datasheet [2] (below)

Sensor name	LGE accelerometer sensor
Vendor	BOSCH
Current consumption	0.13 mA
Resolution	0.00958 m/s^2
Maximum range	156.88 m/s^2
Total supply current in normal mode	130 µA = 0.13 mA
Resolution	0.98 mg $\approx$ 0.0096138 m/s^2 [3]
Sensitivity (g$_{FS16g}$, $T_A = 25°C$)	128 LSB/g
Zero-g offset	±60 mg
Maximum bandwidth	1000 Hz
Maximum range	16 g $\approx$ 156.96 m/s^2

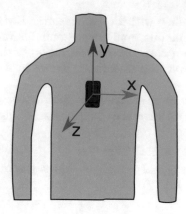

Fig. 2. Smartphone placement and coordinate system

2.2 Signal Processing

The SCG signal registered by a smartphone consists of three orthogonal components X, Y, Z. Recordings were exported to text files and analyzed off-line using MATLAB software (The Mathworks, Inc., Natick, MA, USA).

First, each registered acceleration component of the signal is band-pass filtered using FFT filtering. We used frequency bands described in the Table 2. The authors chose cut-off frequencies for X and Z axis proposed by Landreani et al. [8,9] to filter out out-of-band noise and artifacts due to respiratory movements.

Then, we computed upper RMS envelope with 50 samples window of each component. Segments with values over the standard deviation of upper RMS envelope or the mean RMS envelope times two were zeroed out.

We analyze two methods of extracting heart beats intervals (AO points) on three components X, Y and Z: upper signal envelope (as the magnitude of analytic signal of Hilbert transform [10]) and upper RMS envelope with 10-sample window. Then, we find peaks separated by at least 50 samples and with an amplitude of at least the mean of the envelope.

Table 2. Frequency bands chosen for band-pass filter

Component	Frequency band
X	1–25 Hz
Y	3–25 Hz
Z	5–25 Hz

3   Results

To assess the performance of heart beat detection algorithm, we annotated manually the heart beats based on SCG curve annotation presented in [20] and calculated the true positives (TP), false positives (FP), false negatives (FN). True positive is defined as the AO point detected correctly. False negative is considered if proposed algorithm omits the AO point and false positive is determined for misclassified AO points. Sensitivity (Se) is defined as $Se = \frac{TP}{TP+FN}$ and positive predictive value (PPV) is defined as $PPV = \frac{TP}{TP+FP}$. The number of beats is the sum of TP and FN. Tables 3 and 4 show number of TPs, FPs, FNs, beats and calculated values of Se and PPV for two variants of heart beat detection algorithm: variant 1 (analytical envelope) and variant 2 (RMS envelope). Table 5 shows aggregated results as the sum of TPs, FPs, FNs and calculated Se and PPV. Enabling gravitational offset removal slightly improves beat detection performance for signals acquired from subject 1 for two tested envelope types. For signals acquired from subject 2, removing gravitational offset slightly improves PPV and worsens Se.

For signal acquired with gravitational offset removal from subject 1, the best performance was achieved on Y axis for both variants, however, the differences between the performance on different axes are small. For signal acquired without gravitational offset removal for the same subject the best performance was achieved for X axis for both analyzed variants. The best performance of variant 1 heart beat detection algorithm of signal from subject 2 registered without gravitational offset removal was achieved for Z axis. For variant 2 the best performance was achieved for X axis of signal registered with gravitational offset removal.

Table 3. Heart beat detector performance for variant 1 (signal upper envelope)

Subject	Gravitational offset removal	Signal length [s]	Axis	TP	FP	FN	Beats	Se	PPV
1	Yes	236.123	X	252	15	0	252	1.000	0.944
			Y	252	11	0	252	1.000	0.958
			Z	252	14	0	252	1.000	0.947
	No	191.39	X	193	12	0	193	1.000	0.944
			Y	192	17	1	193	0.995	0.919
			Z	193	15	0	193	1.000	0.928
2	Yes	133.64	X	158	17	2	160	0.988	0.903
			Y	158	9	2	160	0.988	0.946
			Z	158	13	2	160	0.988	0.924
	No	194.315	X	223	9	3	226	0.987	0.961
			Y	223	8	3	226	0.987	0.965
			Z	223	0	3	226	0.987	1.000

Table 4. Heart beat detector performance for variant 2 (signal upper RMS envelope)

Subject	Gravitational offset removal	Signal length [s]	Axis	TP	FP	FN	Beats	Se	PPV
1	Yes	236.123	X	252	13	0	252	1.000	0.951
			Y	252	10	0	252	1.000	0.962
			Z	252	11	0	252	1.000	0.958
	No	191.39	X	184	11	0	184	1.000	0.944
			Y	184	15	0	184	1.000	0.925
			Z	184	23	0	184	1.000	0.889
2	Yes	133.64	X	159	13	1	160	0.994	0.952
			Y	158	10	2	160	0.988	0.969
			Z	153	0	7	160	0.956	1.000
	No	194.315	X	220	25	6	226	0.973	0.898
			Y	217	5	9	226	0.960	0.977
			Z	223	3	3	226	0.987	0.987

Table 5. Aggregated heart beat detector performance

Subject	Envelope type	Gravitational offset removal	TP	FP	FN	Beats	Se	PPV
1	Analytical	Yes	756	40	0	756	1.000	0.950
		No	579	44	1	252	0.998	0.929
	RMS	Yes	756	34	0	756	1.000	0.957
		No	552	49	0	552	1.000	0.918
2	Analytical	Yes	474	39	6	252	0.988	0.924
		No	669	17	9	678	0.987	0.975
	RMS	Yes	470	13	10	480	0.979	0.973
		No	660	33	18	678	0.973	0.952
Total			4160	229	44	4204	0.990	0.948

For variant 2 we achieved slightly better performance of heart beat detection algorithm than for variant 1 (for both subjects) because of smaller number of false positives and small negatives. Due to lower FN number the sensitivity of proposed algorithm is higher for subject 1 (male) than female (subject 2).

4   Conclusion and Discussion

There are no significant differences between beat detection algorithm performance between three analyzed axes X, Y and Z for all signals. We observed insignificant influence of gravitational offset removal on proposed beat detection algorithm due to the use of band-pass filtering before further analysis.

This indicates that proposed beat detection algorithm may be used on any available axis and is insensitive to gravitational offset. Using variant 2 (RMS envelope) improves the performance of proposed algorithm, which makes RMS envelope viable option for next studies.

Heart beat detection quality is very high on analyzed signals ($Se = 0.990$, $PPV = 0.948$ for all beats, $Se = 1.000$, $PPV = 0.962$ for the best case), which encourages studies of performance on another SCG data sets. The result is similar to that reported by Jafari Tadi et al. [6], Li et al. [11] and Xu et al. [18] for supine position. Achieved performance encourages to repeat the study of beat detection algorithm for another SCG data set.

The main limitations were very limited number of patients and examining only one case: patient lying still on supine position at rest. Different patient positions and activities should be examined in future. Next studies should include comparison of heart beat detection performance on SCG signals registered by smartphone and high precision accelerometer, tests on other mobile devices and processing time measurements.

References

1. Google and Open Handset Alliance (n.d). Sensors Overview. Android API Guide. https://developer.android.com/guide/topics/sensors/sensors_motion.html#sensors-motion-accel. Accessed 21 Jan 2018
2. Sensortec, B.: BMA255, Digital, Triaxial Accelerometer. BMA255 Datasheet, 1 August (2014)
3. Sensortec, B.: BMA255 (n.d.). https://www.bosch-sensortec.com/bst/products/all_products/bma255. Accessed 24 Jan 2018
4. Castiglioni, P., Meriggi, P., Rizzo, F., Vaini, E., Faini, A., Parati, C., Merati, G., Di Rienzo, M.: Cardiac sounds from a wearable device for sternal seismocardiography. In: Annual International Conference of the IEEE Engineering in Medicine and Biology Society, pp. 4283–4286 (2011)
5. Inan, O.T., Migeotte, P.F., Park, K.S., Etemadi, M., Tavakolian, K., Casanella, R., Zanetti, J., Tank, J., Funtova, I., Prisk, G.K., Di Rienzo, M.: Ballistocardiography and seismocardiography: a review of recent advances. IEEE J. Biomed. Health Inform. **19**(4), 1414–27 (2015)
6. Tadi, M.J., et al.: A real-time approach for heart rate monitoring using a Hilbert transform in seismocardiograms. Physiol. Meas. **37**, 1885 (2016)
7. Korzeniowska-Kubacka, I.: Sejsmokardiografia - nowa nieinwazyjna metoda oceny czynności lewej komory w chorobie niedokrwiennej serca. Folia Cardiol. **10**(3), 265–268 (2003). (in Polish)
8. Landreani, F., et al.: Beat-to-beat heart rate detection by smartphone's accelerometers: validation with ECG. In: 38th Annual International Conference of the IEEE Engineering in Medicine and Biology Society (EMBC), pp. 525–528, Orlando, FL (2016)
9. Landreani, F., et al.: Ultra-short-term heart rate variability analysis on accelerometric signals from mobile phone. In: 2017 E-Health and Bioengineering Conference (EHB), Sinaia, pp. 241–244 (2017). https://doi.org/10.1109/EHB.2017.7995406

344   S. Sieciński and P. Kostka

10. MathWorks, Natick, MA, USA. Envelope in: MATLAB R2017b Documentation. https://www.mathworks.com/help/signal/ref/envelope.html?s_tid=doc_ta#buv7i14-1. Accessed 13 Oct 2017
11. Li, Y., Tang, X., Xu, Z.: An approach of heartbeat segmentation in seismocardiogram by matched-filtering. In: 2015 7th International Conference on Intelligent Human-Machine Systems and Cybernetics, Hangzhou, pp. 47–51 (2015)
12. Penrose, R.: 17.4 the principle of equivalence. In: The Road to Reality, pp. 393–394. Knopf, New York (2005). ISBN 0-470-08578-9
13. Ramos-Castro, J., Moreno, J., Miranda-Vidal, H., Garcia-Gonzalez, M., Fernandez-Chimeno, M., Rodas, G., Capdevila, L.: Heart rate variability analysis using a seismocardiogram signal. In: 2012 Annual International Conference of the IEEE on Engineering in Medicine and Biology Society (EMBC), pp. 5642–5645 (2012)
14. Rienzo, M.D., Vaini, E., Castiglioni, P., Merati, G., Meriggi, P., Parati, G., Faini, A., Rizzo, F.: Wearable seismocardiography: towards a beat-by-beat assessment of cardiac mechanics in ambulant subjects. Auton. Neurosci. **178**, 50–59 (2013)
15. Wered Software: Sensor Multitool (Version 1.3.0) (2017). https://play.google.com/store/apps/details?id=com.wered.sensorsmultitool&hl=pl. Accessed 23 Jan 2018
16. Shafiq, G., et al.: Automatic identification of systolic time intervals in seismocardiogram. Sci. Rep. **6**, 37524 (2016). https://doi.org/10.1038/srep37524
17. Tavakolian, K., Khosrow-khavar, F., Kajbafzadeh, B., Marzencki, M., Rohani, S., Kaminska, B., Menon, C.: Seismocardiographic adjustment of diastolic timed vibrations. In: 2012 Annual International Conference of the IEEE Engineering in Medicine and Biology Society (EMBC), pp. 3797–3800 (2012)
18. Xu, W., Sandham, W.A., Fisher, A.C., Conway, M.: 18th Annual International Conference of the IEEE Engineering in Medicine and Biology Society, Amsterdam (1996)
19. Zanetti, J.M., Salerno, D.M.: Seismocardiography: a technique for recording precordial acceleration. In: Proceedings of Fourth Annual IEEE Symposium of Computer-Based Medical Systems, Baltimore, MD, USA, pp. 4–9 (1991)
20. Zanetti, J.M., Poliac, M.O., Crow, R.S.: Seismocardiography: waveform identification and noise analysis. In: Computers in Cardiology, Venice, Italy, pp. 49–52 (1991)
21. Zanetti, J.M., Tavakolian, K.: Seismocardiography: past, present and future. In: Proceedings of 35th Annual International Conference of the IEEE EMBS, Osaka, Japan, 3–7 July (2013)

Transfer Entropy in Quantifying the Interactions in Preterm Labor

Marta Borowska[1]([✉]) and Paweł Kuć[2]

[1] Faculty of Mechanical Engineering, Bialystok University of Technology,
Wiejska 45C, 15-351 Białystok, Poland
m.borowska@pb.edu.pl
[2] Faculty of Medicine, Department of Perinatology, Medical University of Bialystok,
M. Curie-Skłodowskiej 24A, 15-276 Białystok, Poland

Abstract. Evidence of the relationships between physiological data has
been found in previous studies. However there is still limited knowledge about underlying mechanisms and patterns of the preterm birth
and direction of propagating uterine contraction. In this paper we
study transfer entropy (TE) that is widely used to quantify interactions
between biomedical time series. We are searching for indices that could
detect preterm labor using 112 contractions extracted from differentiated
electrohysterographical (EHG) signals. Transfer entropy was considered
as a bivariate approach to quantify the bidirectional information flow
from channel 1 to channel 4. TE values for women delivering after 7
days from presenting of threatened preterm labor symptoms were significantly higher than those delivering within 7 days ($p < 0.01$). The parameters used in this study help to estimate the potential of premature labor
as it progresses. Therefore, they may be useful as early risk markers of
preterm birth.

Keywords: Transfer entropy · Preterm birth · Electrohysterography

1 Introduction

In multivariate time series analysis, it is often a challenge to present information
exchange between signals at different time scales in order to extract important knowledge about the structure and functions of the analyzed dynamics.
The components of the analyzed data often interact in a nonlinear manner and
the mechanisms that cause them are not fully known. Therefore, best when
the method of analyzing interactions between components is not based on any
model or assumption about the nature of the data and their interactions. One
of the promising asymmetric measures to quantify the orientation of dynamic
association is the transfer entropy. This method can be useful in the analysis of
complex nonlinear systems whose knowledge is incomplete. Transfer of entropy
was introduced by Schreiber [17]. However, the popularity of this measure has
increased after explaining its relationship to Granger's concept of causality [2].

© Springer International Publishing AG, part of Springer Nature 2019
E. Pietka et al. (Eds.): ITIB 2018, AISC 762, pp. 345–352, 2019.
https://doi.org/10.1007/978-3-319-91211-0_31

TE is increasingly being used to assess the transfer of information in physiological systems. In neurophysiology it has been used for electroencephalograms and magnetoencephalograms to elucidate complex neuronal conditions during anesthesia [1], in a simple motor task [18], in short-term memory experiment [19], in comparison of connectivity for resting state in eyes open and eyes closed [15]. In cardiovascular physiology, causal relationships in cerebral hemodynamics are explained [6]. In cardiology to analyze heart rate (HR), respiratory variability and their interrelationship in different sleep states (active vs. quiet) [10], to assess the aging-related changes in contribution of respiration and blood pressure [14]. TE was used also to quantifying the interactions between maternal and fetal heart rates [11].

Understanding the mechanism of physiological processes during the exchange of information between time series representing the contraction of the uterus in preterm labor is important for the development of methods for controlling uterine function. Current methods of assessing uterine function in preterm labor are insufficient. In recent years, several non-invasive methods have been developed to evaluate uterine function based on the registration of electrical signals from the abdominal surface of a pregnant woman - electromyography (EMG). Studies show that the EMG of the uterus, also called electrohysterography (EHG), can be used to monitor condition during both gestation and labor. Important advantages of the proposed method include: reducing the risk of preterm labor, improving perinatal care, monitoring the treatment process, and the possibility of carrying out tests to understand the function of the uterus. EMG can supplement or replace commonly used methods of evaluation uterine function such as cardiotocography, ultrasound cervical length measurement [5, 16], selected biochemical and molecular markers detected in serum or urine of pregnant patients [7,8]. Until now, methods of monitoring births are only subjective and do not provide a clear distinction between true and false birth or knowledge about when the birth will occur.

Labor is a physiological process in which regular contractions accompanying cervical dilatation occur. At the time of delivery, biochemical changes in the cervical total tissue cause contraction and cervical dilatation. The sequence of contractility and relaxation of uterine muscle is due to the depolarization and repolarization of the muscle cell membrane. Spontaneous electrical discharge from uterine myocardium consists of intermittent series of action potentials initiating contraction. Timely correlation between electrical events and contractions has been demonstrated. Preterm labor defined as delivery between 27th and 37th weeks of gestation occurs in approximately 20% of pregnant women. There are many complications associated with it, namely the high mortality rate of newborns, the high number of neurological diseases in patients who have survived. Therefore, the detection and prediction could be the key to treating premature labor.

The aims of this study were: (1) evaluating the performance of transfer entropy to predict the risk of threatening preterm birth; (2) to assess the usefulness of EHG in the quantifying preterm delivery. The hypothesis of our research is that preterm labor is associated with a sequential activation of different muscle components that generate efficient contractions in order to push the baby out. Our approach allows to characterize EHG signals in the preterm delivery. It consists of the following steps, which represented in block diagram on Fig. 1.

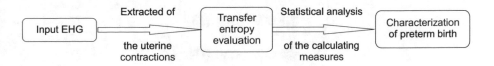

Fig. 1. The scheme of the calculation process

2   Materials and Methods

2.1   Data Collection

The recording of EHG signals was performed at Department of Perinatology Medical University of Bialystok [9]. Material of the study was obtained from 100 patients with threatened preterm labor between the 24th and the 36th week of pregnancy. Patients included to the study had a shortened cervix (<25 mm) without regular uterine contractions on cardiotocography (CTG). Material of the study consists of 112 uterine contractions extracted from EHG signals received from patients with threatened preterm labor between the 24th and the 36th week of pregnancy. The women were divided into two groups: those delivering within 7 days from presenting of threatened preterm labor symptoms — Group A and women delivering after 7 days — Group B. In the research, for recording of uterine activity a custom created system was used (Neuron-Spectrum 5, Neurosoft Ltd, Russia). The system allowed 8-channel signal registration in 8 different points of abdominal wall over the pregnant uterus (Fig. 2). The sampling frequency was 500 Hz. The analysis concerned the differentiated signals from the electrode 1 and electrode 4 (Fig. 3).

2.2   Transfer Entropy Measure

Transfer entropy is a measure of effective connectivity based on information theory. Transfer entropy is a model-free measure which is designed as the Kullback-Leibler divergence of transition probabilities. With very little assumptions this approach allows to quantify information transfer without being restricted to linear dynamics.

These promising methods of the coupling strength between two time series $X = x_1, x_2, ..., x_n$ and $Y = y_1, y_2, ..., y_n$ on Y to X direction is transfer entropy [1] defined by:

$$T_{Y \to X} = \sum p(x_{n+1}, x_n^{(k)}) \log \frac{p(x_{n+1}|x_n^{(k)}, y_n^{(l)})}{p(x_{n+1}|x_n^{(k)})} \qquad (1)$$

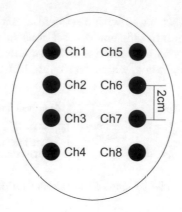

Fig. 2. Localization of the 8 different points of abdominal wall over the pregnant uterus; the distance between the electrodes is $2\,\mathrm{cm} \pm 0.5\,\mathrm{cm}$

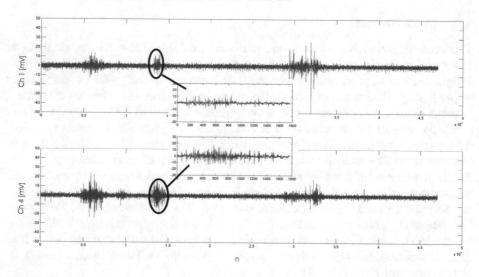

Fig. 3. Electrohysterogram patient of channels 1 and 4 at risk of preterm birth (labor within 7 days of admission to the hospital)

where k and l are the lengths of the blocks containing the past values of receiving system X and the driver/sender system Y, respectively. The conditional probabilities in Eq. 1 are conditioned on $x_n^{(k)} = (x_n, x_{n+1}, ..., x_{n+k+1})$ and $y_n^{(l)} = (y_n, y_{n+1}, ..., y_{n+l+1})$. The transfer entropy is a non-negative measure of the reduction in uncertainty of x_i given $x_n^{(k)}$ and $y_n^{(l)}$, compared to given only $x_n^{(k)}$. TE measures the amount of directed information flow from Y to X.

The TE measure is a useful tool for detecting non-linear interactions and deals with various interactions delays. It also does not require a specific assumption of a model describing the dynamics of the system and the interactions occurring in it. Despite these advantages it requires the approximation of infinite-dimension variables representing a history of processes, that is, the past dynamics of the system is represented by the processes of Y and X in relation to the Y process. The resulting vector consists of significant variables affecting the current state of the system. Two embedding schemes uniform and non-uniform of reconstruction the past of system dynamics are applied [13]. In uniform embedding scheme, components of embedding vectors are selected a priori and separately for each time series. In non-uniform embedding scheme is applied a progressive selection technique to identify the most significant variable affecting the current state of the system using all ranges to the maximum lag. Choice of appropriate embedding procedure is associated with the issue of dimensionality [10]. In order to calculate transfer entropy, three different methods of estimation the joint probability distribution to estimate conditional entropies: linear estimator (LIN), a fixed state space partitioning estimator (BIN) and the K-Nearest Neighbor technique estimator (NN) can be applied [13]. The main steps for TE estimation procedure are presented in Fig. 4.

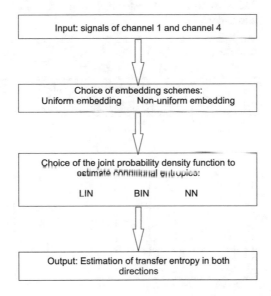

Fig. 4. Scheme of the main steps of calculation TE: (1) Selection of the two signals used to calculation of TE in the direction of channel 1 → channel 4 and vice versa, (2) Choice of the method to approximate the infinite-dimension past states of the systems, (3) Choice of Conditional Entropy estimator (LIN vs. BIN vs. NN) and TE estimation

3   Results

Selection of the appropriate parameters such as the embedding dimension, time delay and the estimator of the probability density function is required to calculate TE. In the literature, several methods of selection embedding dimension and selection time delay were studied. The time delay and embedding dimension were obtained from the first zero of the autocorrelation function [3] and the Cao criterion [4], which is based on the search for false neighbors. For this purpose, the OpenTSTOOL toolbox [12] was used. The non-uniform embedding was chosen since this order was suggested to have high sensitivity and specificity both for linear and non-linear systems - in the sense of predictive information. The probability distribution was estimated using binning estimator based on performing uniform quantization of the time series and estimation of the conditional entropy with the frequency of visitation of the quantized states (in our case six levels). TE were calculated using the MuTE Toolbox (http://mutetoolbox.guru/) [13]. Transfer entropy for Group B was significantly higher than for Group A, both with respect to direction Ch1 – Ch4 and Ch4 – Ch1, as shown in Fig. 5. Comparing the two directionalities, there was no clear difference both in Group A and in Group B (Table 1).

Table 1. Transfer entropy values (mean±SD) for 112-contraction segments, for Group A and Group B. Statistical analysis was performed by means of nonparametric Mann-Whitney test for unpaired data ($p < 0.05$)

Transfer entropy	Group A	Group B	p-values
	N = 36	N = 76	
Ch1–Ch4	0.068 ± 0.060	0.121 ± 0.095	<0.01
Ch4–Ch1	0.061 ± 0.056	0.107 ± 0.080	<0.001

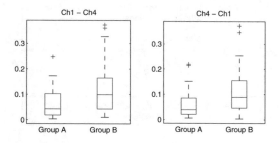

Fig. 5. Boxplot of TE values in Group A and Group B in the direction of channel 1 ⟶ channel 4 and vice versa

4   Conclusion

This paper shows a novel technique to characterize uterine behavior during preterm birth. The main aim is to use a parameter named transfer entropy in quantifying the flow of information between different points of abdominal wall over the pregnant uterus. Only two signals were used to detect differences in the transmission of information during preterm birth using binning estimator with the non-uniform embedding. The chosen approach has the ability to detect both linear and non-linear interactions, whereby detection of effective connectivity was possible without specifying an a priori model. The analysis of electrophysiological data of the uterus revealed differences in the interactions of signals in Group A compared to patients in Group B. More information is transferred between the EHG signals in patients delivering after 7 days from presenting of threatened preterm labor symptoms. Comparing the two directionalities, there was no clear difference both for Group A and Group B between Ch1→Ch4 and Ch4→Ch1. The next step of our research is to extend the analysis of multidimensional data. TE is a useful tool for quantifying information transmitted between variables represented by time series.

Compliance with Ethical Standards. The study protocol was approved by the Local Ethical Committee of Medical University of Bialystok, Poland, and an informed consent was obtained from each patient.

Conflicts of Interest. The authors declare that there are no financial or personal relationships with other people or organizations that could inappropriately influence this study.

Acknowledgement. Research for female patients was supported by Grant no. N N407 598338 from the National Science Center. The research was performed as a part of the projects S/WM/1/2017 and was financed with the founds for science from the Polish Ministry of Science and Higher Education.

References

1. Alkire, M.T., Hudetz, A.G., Tononi, G.: Consciousness and anesthesia. Science **322**(5903), 876–880 (2008)
2. Barnett, L., Barrett, A.B., Seth, A.K.: Granger causality and transfer entropy are equivalent for gaussian variables. Phys. Rev. Lett. **103**(23), 238701 (2009)
3. Bassingthwaighte, J.B., Liebovitch, L.S., West, B.J.: Fractal Physiology. Springer (2013)
4. Cao, L.: Practical method for determining the minimum embedding dimension of a scalar time series. Physica D: Nonlinear Phenomena **110**(1–2), 43–50 (1997)
5. Gomez, R., Romero, R., Nien, J.K., Chaiworapongsa, T., Medina, L., Kim, Y.M., Yoon, B.H., Carstens, M., Espinoza, J., Iams, J.D., et al.: A short cervix in women with preterm labor and intact membranes: a risk factor for microbial invasion of the amniotic cavity. Am. J. Obstet. Gynecol. **192**(3), 678–689 (2005)
6. Katura, T., Tanaka, N., Obata, A., Sato, H., Maki, A.: Quantitative evaluation of interrelations between spontaneous low-frequency oscillations in cerebral hemodynamics and systemic cardiovascular dynamics. Neuroimage **31**(4), 1592–1600 (2006)
7. Kuć, P., Laudański, P., Kowalczuk, O., Chyczewski, L., Laudański, T.: Expression of selected genes in preterm premature rupture of fetal membranes. Acta obstetricia et gynecologica Scandinavica **91**(8), 936–943 (2012)

8. Laudanski, P., Raba, G., Kuc, P., Lemancewicz, A., Kisielewski, R., Laudanski, T.: Assessment of the selected biochemical markers in predicting preterm labour. J. Matern. Fetal Neonatal Med. **25**(12), 2696–2699 (2012)

9. Lemancewicz, A., Borowska, M., Kuć, P., Jasińska, E., Laudański, P., Laudański, T., Oczeretko, E.: Early diagnosis of threatened premature labor by electrohystero-graphic recordings-the use of digital signal processing. Biocybern. Biomed. Eng. **36**(1), 302–307 (2016)

10. Lucchini, M., Pini, N., Fifer, W.P., Burtchen, N., Signorini, M.G.: Entropy information of cardiorespiratory dynamics in neonates during sleep. Entropy **19**(5), 225 (2017)

11. Marzbanrad, F., Kimura, Y., Palaniswami, M., Khandoker, A.H.: Quantifying the interactions between maternal and fetal heart rates by transfer entropy. PloS one **10**(12), e0145672 (2015)

12. Merkwirth, C., Parlitz, U., Wedekind, I., Engster, D., Lauterborn, W.: Opentstool user manual. Drittes Physikalisches Institut, Universität Göttingen, Göttingen (2009)

13. Montalto, A., Faes, L., Marinazzo, D.: Mute: a Matlab toolbox to compare established and novel estimators of the multivariate transfer entropy. PloS one **9**(10), e109462 (2014)

14. Nemati, S., Edwards, B.A., Lee, J., Pittman-Polletta, B., Butler, J.P., Malhotra, A.: Respiration and heart rate complexity: effects of age and gender assessed by band-limited transfer entropy. Respir. Physiol. Neurobiol. **189**(1), 27–33 (2013)

15. Olejarczyk, E., Marzetti, L., Pizzella, V., Zappasodi, F.: Comparison of connectivity analyses for resting state EEG data. J. Neural Eng. **14**(3), 036017 (2017)

16. Romero, R., Kalache, K., Kadar, N.: Timing the delivery of the preterm severely growth-restricted fetus: venous doppler, cardiotocography or the biophysical profile? Ultrasound Obstet. Gynecol. **19**(2), 118–121 (2002)

17. Schreiber, T.: Measuring information transfer. Phys. Rev. Lett. **85**(2), 461 (2000)

18. Vicente, R., Wibral, M., Lindner, M., Pipa, G.: Transfer entropy - a model-free measure of effective connectivity for the neurosciences. J. Comput. Neurosci. **30**(1), 45–67 (2011)

19. Wibral, M., Rahm, B., Rieder, M., Lindner, M., Vicente, R., Kaiser, J.: Transfer entropy in magnetoencephalographic data: quantifying information flow in cortical and cerebellar networks. Prog. Biophys. Mol. Biol. **105**(1), 80–97 (2011)

Dynamic Resource Allocation of Switched Ethernet Networks in Embedded Real-Time Systems

Michael Schmidt[✉], Roman Obermaisser, and Christian Wurmbach

Chair for Embedded Systems, University of Siegen,
Hölderlinstr. 3, 57068 Siegen, Germany
michael.schmidt@eti.uni-siegen.de
http://www.uni-siegen.de

Abstract. Manual reconfiguration of a distributed real-time communication system by humans is error-prone and time consuming. To avoid
errors, which may result in latter failures of the system, the reconfiguration of the communication resources should be carried out automatically
by the system itself. This paper introduces a new broker model which
enables the system to respond dynamically to changes in the system composition, like newly added network nodes or services. Further, we introduce a new client model that implements protocols for the agreement and
coordination of the reconfiguration phases of the network nodes. Besides
the support for ARINC 615A-3 (ARINC615A), the client model also
provides a new way for data loading for devices that are not compatible
with this standard. Our introduced models are finally implemented and
evaluated within an experimental setup for TTEthernet. The main contribution of our approach is to adapt to both changes within the system's
service compositions (e.g., now services, changed timing requirements)
and changes within the network composition (e.g., newly added switches
or nodes).

Keywords: Ambient-Assisted Living (AAL)
Dynamic resource allocation · TTEthernet
Time Sensitive Networking (TSN) · Real-time communication

1 Introduction

Typically, systems with hard real-time requirements have a fixed network topology and are scheduled in advance. Predefined schedules provide determinism
and good analysis facilities. Though, there is no possibility to integrate new
components and to reconfigure the schedule at run-time. However, systems with
predefined schedules do not cope with the requirements for a dynamic change of
the system composition. For example, medical AAL applications may require a
dynamic integration of new devices at run-time. This openness of the AAL system, where devices and applications have to be dynamically integrated, implies

© Springer International Publishing AG, part of Springer Nature 2019
E. Pietka et al. (Eds.): ITIB 2018, AISC 762, pp. 353–364, 2019.
https://doi.org/10.1007/978-3-319-91211-0_32

a dynamic scheduling of network traffic where it is not feasible to prepare communication schedules beforehand. Another application area is for example biomedicine, where medical control loops enforce hard real time requirements both for end-systems and communication networks in order to be reliable and stable. This implies bounded message-transport latency and jitter at the communication networks. Time-triggered networks such as TTEthernet [1] or the evolving Time Sensitive Networking (TSN) [2] standard are well suited to satisfy these timing requirements and provide temporal partitioning. When time-triggered protocols like TTEthernet are employed, a global time base [3] must be available for every part of the communication network to ensure a common view of time among all communication participants.

Manual reconfiguration of the system by humans is error-prone and time consuming. To avoid errors, which may result in later failures of the system, the reconfiguration should be done automatically by the system itself. Self-adaptation of real-time systems has already been addressed in prior work [4–7]. Though, the self-adaptation focuses today on the reconfiguration of resources within a fixed network topology. To our knowledge, there is no solution in the state-of-the art for a self-adaptable real-time system, that considers changes within the network composition. Zowda et al. [8] introduced the concept of a dynamic time-triggered platform based on TTEthernet where the bandwidth of pre-defined Virtual Links (VL) is allocated dynamically. However this concept does not support the introduction of new devices in the network. Thus, the system is restricted to the dynamic integration of new software components. Our approach will extend the state-of-the-art by introducing a central authority for real-time communication resources that allows the dynamic integration of new software components and network nodes at run-time of the system.

At present, real-time communication systems become increasingly important for the field of biomedicine. For example, consider the future where robotic systems for surgery will grow in importance. According to [9], it will be possible to perform surgical procedures that are limited only by available communication technologies even at extreme distances between the surgeon and the patient by computerized mediation of the surgeon's actual hand motions to the surgical instruments affecting the patient's tissue. Referring to this, the underlying communication technologies must fulfill several prerequisites:

Real-time: Real-Time communication is of utmost importance in the operation room of the future. Time-triggered communication networks provide bounded latencies which will ensure stable control loops between the operating controls and the surgical instruments.

Fault-Tolerance: Without fault-tolerance, the failure of a single component can lead to a catastrophic system failure which can even lead to dangerous situations for the patients. Further, fault-tolerance is for example required to prevent malicious devices to jeopardize the network and thus lead to unstable control loops.

Openness: The operation room of the future must adapt to the needs of the patients and their different diseases. Precisely, sensors, actuators or monitoring devices will change with every patient. This requires the underlying communication network to be also highly adaptable, which must allow the dynamic integration of new devices even at run-time.

2 Background

2.1 Traffic Classes

Many systems with hard-real time requirements are based on time-triggered communication protocols where messages are sent at predefined instants of time. In order to prevent collisions, the local clocks of all network nodes have to be synchronized with a global time base. Many real-time communication protocols support further traffic classes. For example, TTEthernet classifies the network traffic into three different classes: Time-Triggered (TT), Rate-Constrained (RC) and Best-Effort (BE) [10]. TT messages are sent at predefined instant of times and can be used when tight latencies with minimal and bounded jitter are required. Unlike TT messages, RC messages are not sent by a predefined schedule. Instead, sufficient bandwidth is allocated in order to provide upper bounds for latency and jitter [10]. However, these bounds are larger than those which are provided by the TT message class. Finally, BE messages use the remaining bandwidth and do not provide guarantees for delivery or timeliness.

2.2 Network Description

The scheduling of time-triggered networks requires knowledge about the network structure and communication requirements of the services running on the end systems. This knowledge is typically represented in a network description document. Ideally, the network description is available in a machine-readable markup language like XML which can be automatically checked for syntactical (document is well-formed) and semantical (document is valid) correctness. The network description should abstract from the specific hardware and must define global properties like the topology of the network which includes all network nodes (switches and end systems), the cabling and the properties of the communication links. Further, the network description may contain information about redundancy and fault-tolerance requirements of the network nodes.

3 Challenges

In this section we introduce two scenarios in order to show the challenges that derive from dynamic resource allocation in self-adaptable switched real-time Ethernet networks. The first scenario covers a fixed network topology as typically found in airplanes or cars. In a fixed topology, all network nodes (switches and end systems) are known a-priori and do not change at runtime. The second scenario follows an open-world assumption where network nodes can enter and leave at runtime. In both scenarios, the location and composition of services is not fixed and can change at runtime. Additionally we assume, that the mentioned services are real-time services.

3.1   Fixed Network Topology

For the first scenario we assume a fixed network topology where all end systems, switches and interconnections are known a-priori. Within this topology, services are distributed among the end systems. A service is registered at a global service management where it can be discovered by other services. This enables dynamic service compositions where services can use other services in order to fulfill their own task. Further, the global service management must have a global view on the communication resources of the network and their usage by services. To establish and maintain this global view, services have to send a request to the global service management in order to bind and use other services. This provides the global service management with the capability to decide whether sufficient communication resources are available to fulfill the pending service usage request. If sufficient resources are available, the global service management can calculate a new communication schedule that has to be distributed to all network nodes.

3.2   Dynamic Network Topology

In the second scenario we assume a dynamic network topology where network nodes can enter and leave dynamically during the run-time of the system. This may require new schedules for the communication resources and can affect already composed services, e.g. when a node is removed that runs a service which is required by another service. In this case, the composed service has to find an alternative for the missing service and, if available, will send a request to the global service management in order to bind and use the alternative service.

The integration of a network node can either be introduced manually or be automatically detected by a management component. Ideally, this should happen automatically to avoid faults due to human failures. Though, this requires topology discovery mechanisms in order to update automatically the global view of all available communication resources and services.

3.3   Reconfiguration of Network Nodes

In order to integrate new nodes into the network, a new communication schedule has to be calculated and distributed to all network nodes. Distributing the schedules among the nodes manually is error-prone, time consuming and does not allow the system to automatically adopt to new services and nodes. Ideally, this task should to be automatized. After the new schedule is distributed to all nodes, it has to be activated at the same instant of time.

4   System Model

As introduced in Sect. 3, several challenges have to tackled in order to establish a system that is capable of conducting an automatic reconfiguration of its real-time communication resources (e.g. in case of changes within the network infrastructure). First, it has to maintain detailed information about the network topology and has to keep this view always up-to-date. Second, it must adopt to changes within the communication network and the composition of services. Third, it must be capable of carrying out a re-scheduling of all communication resources and further being able to distribute the new schedules among all nodes.

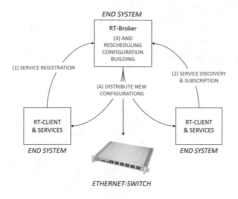

Fig. 1. System model

As illustrated in Fig. 1, our system model distinguishes between two types of software components in a distributed real-time system: the Real-Time Broker (RT-Broker) and the Real-Time Client (RT-Client). Both components are introduced in detail in Sects. 4.1 and 4.2. Generally, the RT-Broker is responsible for topology and service management, scheduling, configuration building and distribution. The RT-Broker is designed as a central instance and therefore exists only once in the network. The counterpart of the RT-Broker is the RT-Client, which is installed on every end system in the real-time network. The RT-Client is responsible for the management of the services running on the corresponding node. It manages all services that are offered by the end-system and it announces to the RT-Broker, which services want to use the real-time communication services of the network. The RT-Client also provides a data loading interface for the RT-Broker in order to push new network configurations to the end system.

Figure 1 shows a high level overview of the intended behavior and responsibilities of the RT-Broker and RT-Client. As depicted, the RT-Broker waits for service offer and service usage requests of the Real-Time Clients (RT-Clients). Service offer requests are sent by the RT-Client of the nodes that offer real-time services. Service offer requests also contain information about the communication requirements of the offered real-time service. In contrast, service usage request are sent by the nodes that wants to use a real-time service. Whenever a service usage request arrives at the RT-Broker and real-time communication resources are available, a new communication schedule is calculated that includes the new service usage. After distributing the new schedules to the switches and the end systems, the RT-Broker and the RT-Clients run an agreement protocol to negotiate about the restarting phase of the network. An detailed view on the internal structure and tasks of the RT-Broker and RT-Client is given in Fig. 2.

4.1   Real-Time Broker

The RT-Broker fulfills various tasks in order to establish an automatic and self-reconfigurable real-time network. The RT-Broker is designed as a server component and therefore exists only once in the network. The RT-Broker can be realized as a dedicated management server or in any end-system of the network. The following sections explain in detail the different modules and the underlying concepts.

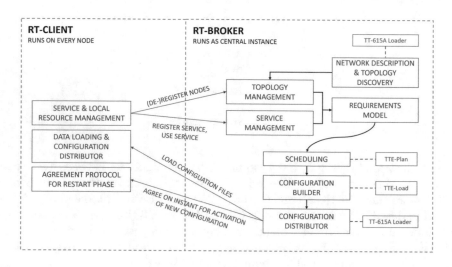

Fig. 2. RT-Broker and RT-Client

Topology Management. Information about the network topology and details about the network nodes is maintained by the topology management component. In order to keep this view up-to-date, it has several functions that are as follows.

The RT-Broker can automatically detect network devices that support the ARINC 615A-3 standard, like the TTEthernet switch (TTE Switch A664 Lab [11]) used in our experimental setup (cf. Sect. 5). ARINC 615A is an avionics standard that defines a Data Loading Protocol (DLP) which can be used to load software into network switches or end-system. If a node has to be integrated into the network, that does not support the ARINC 615A-3 standard, the RT-Broker and the RT-Client implement a DLP. The integration process is initiated by the RT-Client and must contain the relevant informations about the device and has to be configured beforehand in the RT-Client. In case of TTEthernet as the underlying communication protocol, the following parameters are mandatory:

- *name*: name of the device (unique, used for identification)
- *type*: device type (e.g. end-system or switch)
- *sync-role*: define the role of the device regarding clock synchronization (e.g. synchronization or compression master)
- *ports*: a list of the physical ports of the device (including informations like type or MAC-address)
- *links*: a list of all physical links (including informations like media type or cable length)

In the following, the RT-Broker decides depending on the device type which action has to be performed. In case of a switch, a new schedule will be calculated and distributed to all switches and end systems. This reconfiguration is required because new redundancy levels might be available in the system that are required by services. In case of an end system, an immediate reconfiguration is not required because no services of the newly integrated node are yet registered or used.

Service Management. The RT-Broker maintains informations about all real-time services in the network. This is required to establish knowledge the communication requirements and location of the services in the network. Services can either be (de-)registered or requested by the RT-Clients by sending service offer or service usage requests to the RT-Broker.

Service Registration: Services have to be registered at the RT-Broker by providing the following information:

- *name*: Name of service (unique, used for identification)
- *device*: Device name (unique name of corresponding end-system)
- *messages*: Messages sent by the service
  - *name*: Name of the message
  - *type*: Message type (Time-Triggered or Rate-Constrained)
  - *frame-size*: Maximum frame size
  - *redundancy-level*: Desired redundancy level
  - *payload-size*: Maximum payload size

Additionally, for time-triggered messages, the *period* has to be provided, in which the time-triggered message are sent. For rate-constrained messages, the following additional informations have to be provided: the *maximum allowed jitter* and the *bandwidth allocation gap* which defines the Minimum Inter-Arrival Time between two subsequent rate-constrained messages.

Requesting for Services: Services can request other services by using the RT-Client, which will in turn send a service usage request to the RT-Broker. The RT-Broker first checks if a service is registered with the desired properties. If a corresponding service is found, the RT-Broker registers the service usage and carries out the rescheduling and reconfiguration of the network nodes. If no corresponding service is found, the RT-Client is asked by the RT-Broker if the service wants to wait for a registration of the desired service in future. If this is the case, the RT-Broker will store the service usage request. Whenever the requested service is registered in the future, the RT-Broker will conduct the rescheduling and reconfiguration of the network nodes. Of course, the RT-Client can revoke the pending service usage request at any time.

De-registration of Services: If a service can no longer be provided, services can be de-registered at the RT-Broker by using the RT-Client. The RT-Broker will inform all services about this event so that they can react to the withdrawn service. In this case, the RT-Broker will not start a rescheduling and reconfiguration process in order to avoid downtime of the communication infrastructure due to the restart phase after activating a new schedule in the network nodes. Of course, the freed resources are made available for future scheduling processes. Although no rescheduling is triggered by the RT-Broker at this moment, the rescheduling is most likely to take place because of changing service usages due to the withdrawn service.

Revoking of Service Usages: A service usage can be revoked at any time using the RT-Client. The RT-Broker will not conduct a scheduling and reconfiguration due to the same reasons as during the de-registration of services.

Scheduler. The scheduling is performed on the basis of the requirements model, that is established with the information of the topology and service management. In most cases, the integration of a scheduler that is specific for the underlying communication protocol is the reasonable choice. For example, in case of our experimental setup we used the scheduler for TTEthernet that was provided by the manufacturer TTTech.

Configuration Builder and Distributor. After the new communication schedule is calculated, the configuration of the network devices is generated, based on the individual device information in the RT-Broker. This is done by the configuration builder component of the RT-Broker. After the generation, the configuration is distributed to the network nodes by the configuration distributor component. Similar to the topology management in Sect. 4.1, the configuration distributor can load the configuration in two ways: the RT-Client and ARINC 615A. If the node does not support the ARINC 615A standard for loading new configurations, the node can use the RT-Client as data loading provider. For this purpose, the RT-Client implements a data loading service. In the experimental setup, the data loading service uses Secure Copy (SCP) as the underlying technology. However, any other data transfer protocol like Trivial File Transfer Protocol (TFTP) can be used.

4.2   Real-Time Client

The counterpart of the RT-Broker is the RT-Client, which is running on every node in the network that wants to run services that require real-time communication resources. Most features have already been introduced in the context of the RT-Broker. Besides this functionality, the RT-Client is mainly responsible for the management of the local services. In this context, the RT-Client for example registers and starts all services, which are offered by the end system.

5   Implementation and Evaluation

For the implementation and evaluation, we used TTEthernet as underlying real-time communication protocol. However, the concepts and the models introduced within this paper can be adopted to other technologies, like for example the upcoming IEEE 802.1 standard Time Sensitive Networking (TSN) [2].

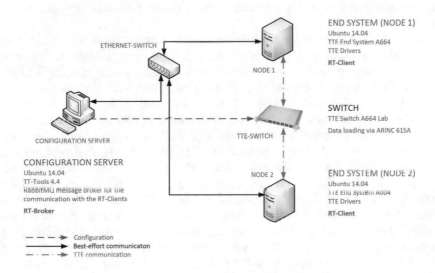

Fig. 3. Experimental setup for the implementation

Figure 3 shows the experimental setup used for the implementation of our model. As depicted, the real-time communication network consists of two end systems equipped with TTEthernet network cards (TTE End System A664 [12]) and one TTEthernet switch (TTE Switch A664 Lab [11]). These end systems are running each a RT-Client and are supposed to offer services or to use services. Additionally, our setup comprises a management network based on Ethernet, that is used for the communication between the RT-Broker and the RT-Clients and for the monitoring of the end systems during the reconfiguration phases of the real time network. Though, the communication between the RT-Broker and the RT-Clients could also be implemented by exploiting the BE message class of

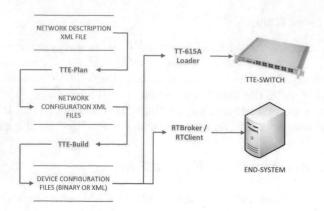

Fig. 4. TTEthernet-Toolchain

TTEthernet. The RT-Broker is running on a third end system, the configuration
server.

Due to TTEthernet as the underlying communication protocol, we integrated
the TTEthernet-Toolchain [13] shown in Fig. 4 into the RT-Broker implementation. The assignment of the RT-Broker components to the specific TTEthernet tools is depicted in Fig. 2. The TTEthernet-Toolchain also uses a network
description (see also Sect. 2.2) to define the topology of the network. Further,
the TTEthernet network description contains information about the logical connections, which are called Virtual Links (VLs). According to the traffic classes
introduced in Sect. 2.1, there are VLs for TT, RC and BE messages available.
The endpoints of the VLs are called Data Ports. As VLs are unidirectional, a
Virtual Link (VL) always has one sending Data Port and has one or multiple
receiving Data Ports. The definition of a VL in the network description also
includes the properties of the messages, like maximum message size and period
in which the data frames are transmitted. Further, the network definition defines
the network periods, that are required for the establishment of the cluster cycles
and the VLs. For TT messages, the TTEthernet network description additionally
defines a synchronization domain that further specifies the behavior of the clock
synchronization within the network. By implementing a parser for the TTEthernet network description, the RT-Broker can use an existing network description
from the TTEthernet-Toolchain as a starting point for the network topology
management. If a new communication schedule has to be calculated (e.g. due
to new network nodes or service usages), the broker uses the scheduler of the
TTEthernet-Toolchain, which is included in the tool TTE-Plan. The outputs
of this tool are configuration files for each TTEthernet device in the network.
Since our experimental setup is based on TTEthernet, a further step is necessary
in order to load the configurations on the devices. The configuration files have
to be transformed with the tool TTE-Build into binaries that can be uploaded
to the devices. The TTEthernet switches (TTE Switch A664 Lab) used for the
experimental setup support the ARINC615A standard. Therefore the RT-Broker

uses the TT-615A-Loader of the TTEthernet-Toolchain in order to load the configuration on the switch. The situation for the end systems (TTE End System A664) is different, because these devices do not the support ARINC615A for data loading. As introduced in the model, the RT-Broker uses in this case the data loading feature of the RT-Client. During the execution of the data loading protocol, the RT-Broker transfers the device configuration files using SCP. Second, the RT-Client distributes the configuration files to the corresponding services. Since the IDs of the VLs are assigned dynamically during the scheduling with the tool TTE-Plan, the services cannot use directly the IDs of the VLs as virtual communication links. For this purpose, the RT-Client implements a link manager that must be used by the services in order to find their corresponding VL. The required informations in the link manager is also updated by the RT-Broker during the execution of the data loading protocol. Finally, after the configuration files are distributed, the RT-Broker and the RT-Client run an agreement protocol to negotiate about the restarting phase of the network.

Table 1. Reconfiguration times

Action	Minimum	Maximum	Average
(1) Arinc 615A discovery	2.811	4.598	4.252
(2) Generation of network definitions	0.007	0.482	0.060
(3) TTE-Plan	3.944	14.598	5.906
(4) TTE-Build	10.959	34.464	14.949
(5a) Preparation of configuration files	0.644	2.296	1.109
(5b) Generation of loading files	0.001	0.022	0.002
(6) Arinc 615A loading	50.842	65.391	53.622
(7) Loading of end systems	0.997	46.767	15.218
Total time	74.903	122.845	95.178

In our experimental setup, the rescheduling and the distribution of the device configuration files takes in average about 90 s in total (end system with Intel Core i5-5200U and 4GB memory). During this time, the real time network is still fully operational. A downtime will first occur when the end systems and the switches adopt the new configurations. Table 1 show the measured times during the reconfiguration phase. The measured minimum, maximum and average times are based on 100 reconfiguration cycles.

6   Conclusion and Future Work

Within this paper we introduced a broker model for the automatic reconfiguration of real-time communication resources in a distributed real-time network. The implementation of the RT-Broker and RT-Client was done experimentally for TTEthernet. Though, the introduced concepts can be adopted to other technologies, like for example the upcoming IEEE 802.1 standard TSN. We are currently extending our approach in order to include the results of Owda et al. [8] into our model in order to provide dynamic communication resource allocation based on VLs. This would decrease the total amount of reconfiguration phases in case of new service offers and requests resulting in reduced downtime of the communication network.

References

1. Kopetz, H., Ademaj, A., Grillinger, P., Steinhammer, K.: Eighth IEEE International Symposium on Object-Oriented Real-Time Distributed Computing, ISORC 2005, pp. 22–33 (2005). https://doi.org/10.1109/ISORC.2005.56
2. IEEE Time-Sensitive Networking Task Group: Time Sensitive Networking (TSN) (2016). http://www.ieee802.org/1/pages/tsn.html. Accessed 14 Jan 2016
3. Kopetz, H.: Proceedings of the 12th International Conference on Distributed Computing Systems, pp. 460–467. IEEE (1992)
4. Höftberger, O., Obermaisser, R.: 16th IEEE International Symposium on Object/Component/Service-Oriented Real-time Distributed Computing (ISORC 2013), pp. 1–9 (2013). https://doi.org/10.1109/ISORC.2013.6913205
5. Brinkschulte, U., Schneider, E., Picioroaga, F.: Eighth IEEE International Symposium on Object-Oriented Real-Time Distributed Computing (ISORC 2005), pp. 174–181 (2005). https://doi.org/10.1109/ISORC.2005.25
6. Prehofer, C., Zeller, M.: Proceedings of 2012 IEEE 17th International Conference on Emerging Technologies Factory Automation (ETFA 2012), pp. 1–8 (2012). https://doi.org/10.1109/ETFA.2012.6489585
7. Rasche, A., Poize, A.: 10th IEEE International Workshop on Object-Oriented Real-Time Dependable Systems, pp. 347–354 (2005). https://doi.org/10.1109/WORDS.2005.31
8. Owda, Z., Abuteir, M., Obermaisser, R., Dakheel, H.: 2014 8th International Symposium on Medical Information and Communication Technology (ISMICT), pp. 1–5. IEEE (2014)
9. Kopelman, Y., Lanzafame, R.J., Kopelman, D.: Trends in evolving technologies in the operating room of the future. JSLS J. Soc. Laparoendosc. Surg. **17**, 171 (2013)
10. Obermaisser, R.: Time-Triggered Communication. CRC Press, Boca Raton (2011)
11. TTTech: TTE Switch A664 Lab (2017). https://www.tttech.com/products/aerospace/development-test-vv/development-switches/tte-switch-a664-lab/. Accessed 11 Dec 2017
12. TTTech: TTE End System A664 Lab (2017). https://www.tttech.com/products/aerospace/development-test-vv/development-end-systems/tte-end-system-a664-lab/. Accessed 11 Dec 2017
13. TTTech: TTE Development Tools (2017). https://www.tttech.com/products/aerospace/development-test-vv/development-tools/. Accessed 11 Dec 2017

Brute Force ECG Feature Extraction Applied on Discomfort Detection

Guillermo Hidalgo Gadea[1,2(✉)], Annika Kreuder[1], Carsten Stahlschmidt[1], Sebastian Schnieder[1,2,3], and Jarek Krajewski[1,2,4]

[1] Institute of Experimental Psychophysiology, Duesseldorf, Germany
g.hidalgo@ixp-duesseldorf.de
[2] Institute of Safety Technology, University of Wuppertal, Wuppertal, Germany
[3] Engineering Psychology, HMKW Berlin, Berlin, Germany
[4] Human-Technology-Interaction, Rhenish University of Applied Science Cologne, Cologne, Germany

Abstract. This paper presents the idea of brute force feature extraction for Electrocardiography (ECG) signals applied to discomfort detection. To build an ECG Discomfort Corpus an experimental discomfort induction was conducted. 50 subjects underwent a 2 h (dis-)comfort condition in separate sessions in randomized order. ECG and subjective discomfort was recorded. 5 min ECG segments were labeled with corresponding subjective discomfort ratings, and 6365 brute force features (65 low-level descriptors, first and second order derivatives, and 47 functionals) and 11 traditional heart rate variability (HRV) parameters were extracted. Random Forest machine learning algorithm outperformed SVM and kNN approaches and achieved the best subject-dependent, 10-fold cross-validation results ($r = .51$). With this experiment, we are able to show that (a) brute force ECG feature sets achieved better discomfort detection than traditional HRV based ECG feature set; (b) cepstral and spectral flux based features appear to be the most promising to capture HRV phenomena.

Keywords: Affective computing · ECG · HRV
Brute force feature extraction · Machine learning
Low-level descriptors · Functionals

1 Introduction

Affective and behavioral computing is an emerging field of research that enables algorithms to detect and predict human emotions and actions. With this aim, an interdisciplinary research field spanning computer science and psychology is consolidating to foster multimodal signal analysis [21]. An increasing number of research groups is making use of biosignals - besides video imaging and individual speech patterns - to enhance performance and accuracy in emotion recognition.

© Springer International Publishing AG, part of Springer Nature 2019
E. Pietka et al. (Eds.): ITIB 2018, AISC 762, pp. 365–376, 2019.
https://doi.org/10.1007/978-3-319-91211-0_33

While strong sentiments and emotions like joy and fear, sadness and disgust [10], fatigue [9] and depression [26] usually take center stage in affective computing research, others like discomfort have been mostly neglected. However, comfort is a very important component of daily life quality, and many interventions by health professionals are focused on avoiding and mitigating discomfort [19]. Discomfort is therefore an important aspect of patient care oriented affective computing for assisted living and computer assisted diagnosis.

Few reliable approaches to measure objective (dis-)comfort using Electromyography (EMG) and video- or pressure-sensor based body movement [18] fail to operationalize comfort by taking the impact of physical, emotional and environmental factors into account [19]. Electrocardiography (ECG) can describe autonomic nervous system (ANS) activity in ambulatory assessment and is not tied to postural expression of discomfort, as measured by body movement and posture changes with video data, EMG or pressure sensors. We hypothesize that the association between ECG and negative emotions [11] should be useful to capture discomfort from a psychophysiological perspective.

This paper aims to examine the feasibility of a multipurpose biosignal processing approach on an ECG data corpus to detect discomfort. In the following pages we propose a brute force feature extraction method to train machine learning classifiers on a discomfort target. Benefits of the proposed method over standard heart rate variability (HRV) based ECG analysis will be shown and brute force feature extraction techniques will be addressed. Section 2 will summarize discomfort induction, data collection, data processing and model training. Finally, performance results of both approaches will be compared in Sect. 3. Section 4 of this paper will show the main added value of the proposed approach through: (1) the introduction of brute force feature extraction schema using low-level descriptors (LLD), derivatives and functionals, (2) the analysis of several new or rarely used spectral and cepstral coefficients.

1.1   Standard Heart Rate Variability Based ECG Analysis

ECG signals represent electric potential alterations on the skin caused by the depolarizing and re-polarizing pattern of the heartbeat. This data can be used to identify cardiac arrhythmia and atrial fibrillations in patients prior to onset of acute heart diseases [27], but can also be used to objectively measure pain [12], cognitive performance [22], and to analyze psychological states as fatigue [9] and thermal comfort [17].

Typical ECG analysis approaches use (1) morphological ECG features (characteristic voltage peaks and lows in the ECG waveform as displayed in Fig. 2), (2) HRV features (time variations between heartbeats e.g. HR, pNN50%, RMSSD, Sd1, Sd2, SDNN), (3) frequency features (specific bands from the power density spectrum e.g. Hf, Lf) and (4) statistical features (e.g. linear predictive coefficients). Nevertheless only time and frequency domain HRV features are most widely applied [14].

Heart rate variability reflects the balance between sympathetic and parasympathetic activity in the autonomic nervous system. High energies in low frequency bands of the power spectral density (Lf) indicate increased sympathetic activity, an indicator of wakefulness, while high spectral energy in high frequency bands (Hf) indicate lower sympathetic and increased parasympathetic activity, an indicator of sleepiness [15].

Several scientific challenges like PhysioNet and Computing in Cardiology [16] have provided different approaches to overcome the ECG feature shortage with various analysis attempts. These ECG feature extraction approaches extending the traditional HRV measures have used cepstral and spectral features [2,4], or dual tree complex wavelet transformation [25], to name a few. However, most do not aim to provide an extensive brute force solution. We present a brute force feature extraction approach including LLDs, ΔLLDs, $\Delta\Delta$LLDs and functionals applied on ECG data. Due to its high degree of abstraction, this approach can also be used to capture the concept of heart rate variability to a much finer-grained extend than traditional feature extraction methods.

1.2   Brute Force Feature Extraction

A promising approach used in e.g. computational paralinguistics is to outperform theoretically driven parameters with brute force feature extraction for machine learning applications [24]. Brute force feature extraction exploits the feature space by decomposing the raw signal in many descriptive coefficients with a high degree of abstraction [6]. This (over)generates a large, highly diversified feature set combining frame wise low-level descriptors (LLD) with temporal contour describing functionals to achieve an exhaustive description of the raw data.

The general procedure of brute force feature extraction runs as follows: Signals are framed to a usually sort frame length of about 500 ms with overlapping windows (i.e. Hamming) to calculate about 10 to 60 low-level descriptors (e.g. spectral flux, spectral entropy, cepstral coefficients, zero crossing rates) per segment. LLDs are smoothed by simple moving average (sma) low-pass filtering with a window length of three frames. Next, their first and second order delta coefficients are computed for each LLD time series. Then, the time course describing 20–80 functionals (e.g. percentiles, inter quartile rates, bandwidth of peaks distance) are applied to all LLDs, ΔLLDs and the $\Delta\Delta$LLDs - resulting in typically several thousand features ([LLDs + ΔLLDs + $\Delta\Delta$LLDs] · number of functionals). The simplified workflow of brute force feature extraction is represented in Fig. 1. Further feature description is provided in Sect. 2.4, and an overview on LLDs and functionals is provided in Table 2.

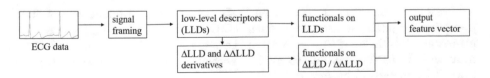

Fig. 1. Simplified brute force feature extraction in ECG signal processing

2   Methods

2.1   Experimental Discomfort Corpus Engineering

To test the proposed approach on ECG data analysis for discomfort classification, a study was conducted to monitor ECG signals while inducing discomfort. A total of 50 subjects were tested in a within-subject design undergoing both experimental conditions (comfort and discomfort induction) in randomized order. (Dis-)comfort was induced, manipulating key seat qualities compared to the baseline seat. Living space, material and hardness was manipulated to up- or downgrade seat quality in respecting conditions.

Subjective discomfort was assessed during baseline, after 40 min, 80 min and 120 min of experimentally manipulated sitting. Different ergonomic seat quality factors were considered to generate an overall discomfort score ranging from 1 = very comfortable to 8 = very discomfortable. A mean difference of 15% in subjectively rated discomfort induction was reached between conditions through experimental manipulation ($p < .001$).

The resulting experimental discomfort corpus combines a total of 6376 features for 92 ECG intervals of 300 s length from 30 different subjects. All instances contain standard heart rate variability and brute force extracted features, labeled for subjectively rated discomfort on a 8-point Likert scale (ranging from 1 = lowest discomfort to 7 = highest discomfort). Corpus descriptives are summarized in Table 1.

Table 1. Descriptives of experimental discomfort corpus

	Age	Height	Weight	BMI	Discomfort
M	25.90	170.62	66.21	22.66	2.92
SD	7.35	7.33	12.26	3.05	1.13
min	18	156	48	18	1.25
max	45	188	95	29	5.57

Note: Mean, standard deviation, minimum and maximum of age, height, weight, body mass index and discomfort.

2.2   Data Pre-processing

Analysis intervals were extracted from ECG signal with a frame length of 300 s preceding subjective discomfort ratings. ECG recordings were digitally upsampled from 1024 Hz to 16 kHz as .wav file to meet processing criteria needed for brute force feature extraction. Exemplary sections of analysis intervals extracted from ECG signal can be seen in Fig. 2.

ECG intervals were manually inspected and excluded if data quality criteria were not fulfilled. Corrupted signals showing no periodic QRS-complex pattern, see Fig. 2(e) and (f), were excluded from further analysis. Analysis intervals with less than 20% corrupted QRS-complexes, see Fig. 2(a)–(d), fell under a tolerable artifact range and were still considered for analysis.

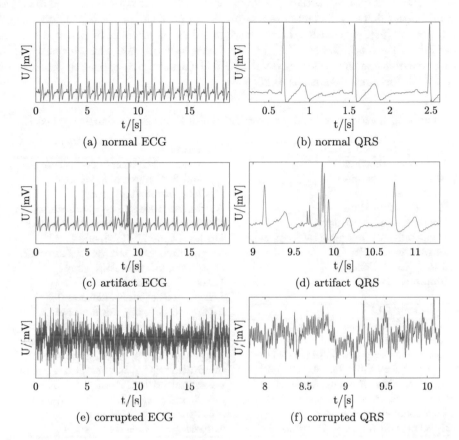

Fig. 2. Exemplary analysis intervals extracted from ECG signal for manual data quality inspection during pre-processing

2.3   Standard ECG Feature Extraction

Raw ECG signals were firstly analyzed with DataAnalyzer (movisens GmbH). Heart rate variability parameters in time and frequency domain (i.e. RMSSD, pNN50%, SDNN, Sd1, Sd2, Sdsd, Sd2Sd1, Hf, Lf, LfHf and HR) were calculated for 10 s analysis windows and averaged for the entire analysis interval [7]. The resulting output feature vectors were aggregated to a HRV_ECG feature set of 11 standard HRV parameter.

2.4   Brute Force ECG Feature Extraction

Raw ECG Signals are windowed at a 390 ms frame length with 40% overlapping windows (i.e. Hamming) to calculate 65 low-level descriptors (e.g. spectral flux, spectral entropy, cepstral coefficients, zero crossing rates; see Table 2) per frame. The frame-wise computed series of LLDs is smoothed by simple moving average (sma) low-pass filtering with a window length of three frames. Next, the first and second order delta coefficients are computed for each series of LLD. Then, the 47 functionals (e.g. percentiles, inter quartile rates, bandwidth of peaks distance; see Table 2) are applied to all LLDs, Δ LLDs and the $\Delta\Delta$ LLDs - resulting in 6365 features for each 300 s interval of ECG (brute force extracted feature set BF_ECG; for more details see [6,23]).

Table 2. Overview of low-level descriptors (LLDs) and functionals applied [5]

Energy related LLD	Fuctionals
Loudness spectrum	Quartiles 1-3, 3 inter-quartile ranges
Modulation loudness	1% and 99% percentile, range
RMS Energy	Position of min/max, range
Zero-Crossing Rate	Arithmetic mean, root quadratic mean
Fundamental frequency	Flatness, std.dev., skewness, kurtosis
Probability of fundamental frequency	Up-level time 25,50,75,90%
Logarithmic HNR	Mean, max, min, std. dev. of segment
Jitter (local, delta)	Rise time, left curvature time
Shimmer (local)	Linear Prediction gain
	Linear Prediction coefficients 0-4
Spectral LLD	Mean/std.dev. of peak distances
RASTA bands 0-25 (0-8kHz)	Mean/std.dev. of rising/falling slopes
MFCC 1-14	mean/std.dev. of inter max. distances
Spectral energy 250-650Hz, 1-4kHz	linear reg.: slope, offset, quad. error
Spectral Roll Off (.25, .50, .75, .90)	quadratic reg.: a, b, offset, quad. error
Spectral Flux, Entropy, Variance	mean and arithm. mean value of peaks
Spectral Skewness, Kurtosis, Slope	amplitude mean of maxima/minima
Psychoacoustic Sharpness	amplitude range of maxima
Spectral Harmonicity, Centroid	percentage of non-zero frames

Some of the most promising LLDs used were mel frequency cepstrum coefficient (mfcc), the root-mean-square of signal frame energy (RMSenergy), spectral flux, spectral entropy and spectral slope, the frequency bands reduction from the power spectrum to auditory frequency scale (audSpec) and the RASTA-style filtered spectrum (Rfilt) [6]. The central LLDs group of the proposed ECG brute force feature extraction are based on cepstral analysis.

The ECG signal has quasi-periodic characteristics as a result of the convolution between the excitation (heart beat rate) and the system response (ECG waveform shapes). Thus, in this work, we use cepstral features, that allow to separate such convolutive effects by simple linear filtering to model the frequency information of the native ECG. Standard formulas used to calculate several features are listed below:

The mfcc used, $C^{(mel)'}(k)$, is computed from a linear scale magnitude or power spectrum using triangular filters and 50% overlap. After logarithm is applied and a discrete cosine transformation type-II is performed, filtered coefficient is expressed as follows:

$$C^{(mel)'}(k) = C^{(mel)}(k)\left(1 + \frac{L}{2}\sin\frac{\pi k}{L}\right).$$ (1)

The Root Mean Square (RMS) energy for a normalized signal $x(n)$ is defined as:

$$E_{rms} = \sqrt{\frac{1}{N}\sum_{n=0}^{N-1} x^2(n)}.$$ (2)

The spectral flux S_{flux} represents a quadratic, normalized version of the simple spectral difference. With general normalization coefficient μ_k the definition of spectral flux is:

$$S_{flux}^{(k)} = \sum_{m=m_l}^{m_u}\left(\frac{X^{(k)}(m)}{\mu_k} - \frac{X^{(k-1)}(m)}{\mu_{k-1}}\right)^2.$$ (3)

The spectral entropy relates to the peakedness of the spectrum. $S_{entropy}$ is defined as:

$$S_{entropy} = -\sum_{m=m_l}^{m_u} px(m) \cdot \log_2 px(m).$$ (4)

The overall shape of a spectrum $X(m)$ expressed by its linear slope $\hat{y} = ax + b$ with $y = X$ and $x = m$ leads to:

$$a = \frac{N\sum_{i=0}^{N-1} x_i y_i - \sum_{i=0}^{N-1} x_i \sum_{i=0}^{N-1} y_i}{N\sum_{i=0}^{N} x_i^2 - \left(\sum_{i=0}^{N-1} x_i\right)^2}.$$ (5)

The predicted value in linear predictive coding can be calculated from:

$$\hat{x}(n) = -\sum_{i=1}^{p} a_i x(n-i).$$ (6)

Linear predictive coding has been used extensively in speech recognition because of its ability to detect poles. Even though the ECG signal is not speech, it shows similar quasi-periodic properties to a phonetic segment of speech. LPC is a technique of time series analysis used to predict future values of a signal as a linear function of previous samples.

2.5 Classifiers

For the sake of transparency and reproducibility, standard algorithms implemented in an open source data mining tool (WEKA 3; [8]) were used. Support Vector Machines (SVM), Random Forests and k-Nearest Neighbors (kNN) were used as machine learning paradigms to explore different classification performances. WEKA's SVM implementation with linear kernels was used with the sequential minimal optimization algorithm (SMO) for training [20], together with Random Forest [3] and kNN [1]. Predictive performance was assessed using a 10-fold stratified cross-validation procedure.

3   Results

3.1   Standard Heart Rate Variability Based ECG Analysis

Spearman rank correlations show high intercorrelations between all heart rate variability parameters ($|r| = .40 - .99$) at a $p < .001$ significance level, but no significant correlation between discomfort, thus any HRV parameter was able to identify affective conditions. Frequency domain parameters Lf and Hf correlated with $r = .04$ and $r = .06$ with discomfort, while SDNN, RMSSD and Sd2Sd1 correlated with $r = .10$, $r = .11$ and $r = -.12$, respectively. Neither nonparametric Mann-Whitney U test accomplishes to differentiate discomfort states out of any standard HRV parameter.

3.2   Brute Force ECG Feature Performance

Over 100 different features of the highly diversified BF_ECG feature subset are correlated with discomfort $|r| = .29 - .45$, outperforming standard heart rate variability analysis (see Table 3).

Table 3. Best Brute Force extracted Features correlated to discomfort

Brute force features	r
mfcc_sma[9]_iqr2-3	.43
mfcc_sma[7]_lpc4	−.39
RMSenergy_sma_de_leftctime	.41
RMSenergy_sma_de_risetime	−.31
fftMag_spectralFlux_sma_risetime	.29
fftMag_spectralFlux_sma_leftctime	−.40
fftMag_spectralEntropy	.30
fftMag_spectralEntropy_sma_risetime	−.31
fftMag_spectralSlope_sma_de_leftctime	−.31
audSpec_Rfilt_sma_de[0]_lpc0	.30
audSpec_Rfilt_sma_de[3]_risetime	−.45

Note: The naming of all features is documented in [6].

The inter-quartile range of the smoothed time series of mfcc 9 correlates with $r = .43$ (mfcc_sma[9]_iqr2-3), and the linear predictive coding coefficient 4 of the

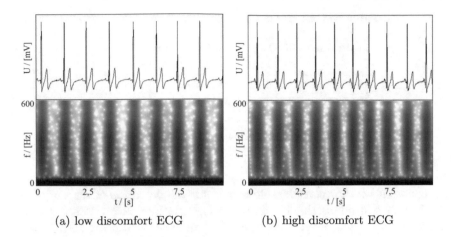

(a) low discomfort ECG   (b) high discomfort ECG

Fig. 3. Exemplary spectral analysis on ECG intervals with low ($<$ 2) and high ($>$ 5) subjective discomfort

smoothed time series of mfcc 7 correlates with $r = -.39$ (mfcc_sma[7]_lpc4) to discomfort. The time during which the first derivative of the smoothed root mean square energy has a left curvature (RMSenergy_sma_de_leftctime) is correlated to discomfort with $r = .41$, while the time during which the first derivative of the smoothed signal energy is rising (RMSenergy_sma_de_risetime) shows a correlation coefficient of $r = -.31$, to name a few.

Further frequency parameters describing spectral flux, entropy and slope reach a medium size correlation, higher than twice the correlation reached with the best performing standard HRV parameter. An exemplary spectral energy profile of two distinct analysis intervals is shown in Fig. 3.

3.3   Machine Learning Performance

Classification performance of all trained models is summarized in Table 4. Combination of different feature subsets trained with different classifiers resulted in nine different models tested in 10-fold cross validation. Random forest classification reached highest correlations and least mean absolute errors over all feature subsets, compared to k-nearest neighbors (kNN) and sequential minimal optimization (SMO).

Best discomfort prediction model based on standard HRV parameters outperformed simple statistical analysis, see Table 4, with a $r = .25$ correlation between prediction and target, and a mean absolute error of 0.89 (in a 8-point Likert scale). The brute force extracted feature subset reached the highest correlation ($r = .57$, MAE $= 0.80$), while predictions of the combined feature set of standard and brute force extracted features were correlated to discomfort targets with $r = .50$ and a mean absolute error of 0.81.

Table 4. Classifier performance in different feature sets

Feature sets	SMOreg		Random forest		kNN	
	r	MAE	r	MAE	r	MAE
HRV_ECG	.18	0.91	.25	0.89	.20	1.11
BF_ECG	.50	0.80	.57	0.80	.47	0.91
Total_ECG	.30	0.91	.51	0.81	.43	0.89

Note: Predictive performance by correlation and mean absolute error.

4   Discussion

This paper shows that considerable results for the detection of discomfort from ECG Signals can be obtained with brute force feature extraction and machine learning classification, even when statistical analysis with heart rate variability data fails to show any notable effects. As seen in Sect. 3.1, heart rate variability based ECG features fail to detect discomfort differences from the ECG signal. While best HRV based ECG features reached correlations of $r = |.12|$ with discomfort, over 100 brute force extracted features outperformed $r = |.29| - |.45|$ correlations, showing the added value of the proposed approach. Some of the most effective features for discomfort detection using ECG signal processing were based especially on cepstral coefficients, spectral entropy and spectral flux measures (see Table 3). Obviously, these LLDs capture the physiological concept of heart rate variability (HRV) to a more specified extend than the traditional HRV feature approaches.

After applying the extended concept of brute force feature extraction standard machine learning approached are trained. Random Forest outperformed SMO and kNN classifying discomfort in all feature subsets. A prediction performance of $r = .57$ was achieved with the brute force feature subset, slightly better than the combined feature set performance of $r = .51$. Model performance could be enhanced in future research by using more meticulous data pre-processing (e.g. blind source separation applying non-negative matrix factorization and independent component analysis) and identifying optimal frame length for the extraction of specific LLDs. Moreover non-linear dynamics feature extraction methods could be used, as reconstructed phase space features, fractal features (e.g. largest Lyapunov exponent, fractal dimension spectrum, minimum embedding dimension), and entropy features assessing regularity or randomness of ECG signal fluctuations [13]. Moreover, subsequent feature selection methods (e.g. sequential forward floating search) and ensemble meta classification methods (e.g. bagging, boosting) should be tested.

To overcome limitations in internal and external validity expanding the robustness of used data, a larger highly diversified discomfort corpus is needed: a higher number of instances and participants with a balanced variability in gender, age, and physical condition. Limitations of the collected corpus are restrictions in age (missing elderly subjects), health state (no subjects in need of care), discomfort range (no extreme (dis-)comfort values), and a disbalanced gender distribution (83% female).

References

1. Aha, D.W., Kibler, D., Albert, M.K.: Instance-based learning algorithms. Mach. Learn. **6**(1), 37–66 (1991). https://doi.org/10.1023/A:1022689900470
2. Boussaa, M., Atouf, I., Atibi, M., Bennis, A.: ECG signals classification using MFCC coefficients and ANN classifier. In: Proceedings of 2016 International Conference on Electrical and Information Technologies, ICEIT 2016, pp. 480–484, May 2016. https://doi.org/10.1109/EITech.2016.7519646
3. Breiman, L.: Random forests. Mach. Learn. **45**(1), 5–32 (2001). https://doi.org/10.1023/A:1010933404324
4. Datta, S., Puri, C., Mukherjee, A., Banerjee, R., Choudhury, A.D., Singh, R., Ukil, A., et al.: Identifying Normal, AF and other Abnormal ECG Rhythms using a cascaded binary classifier. Comput. Cardiol. **44**, 2–5 (2017). https://doi.org/10.22489/CinC.2017.173-154
5. Eyben, F.: Real-time Speech and Music Classification by Large Audio Feature Space Extraction (2016). https://doi.org/10.1007/978-3-319-27299-3
6. Eyben, F., Wöllmer, M., and Schuller, B.: Opensmile: the munich versatile and fast open-source audio feature extractor. In: Proceedings of ACM Multimedia, pp. 1459–1462 (2010). https://doi.org/10.1145/1873951.1874246
7. movisens GmbH: Data analyzer sensor data analysis. Technical report (2018)
8. Hall, M., National, H., Frank, E., Holmes, G., Pfahringer, B., Reutemann, P., Witten, I.H.: The WEKA data mining software: an update. ACM SIGKDD Explor. Newslett. **11**(1), 10–18 (2009). https://doi.org/10.1145/1656274.1656278
9. Hidalgo Gadea, G.: Fatigue detection based on multimodal biosignal processing. Thesis. Bergische Universität Wuppertal (2017). https://doi.org/10.13140/RG.2.2.29666.63684
10. Jang, E.H., Cho, H.Y., Kim, S.H., Eum, Y., Sohn, J.H.: Reliability of physiological signals induced by sadness and disgust. In: HUSO 2015: The First International Conference on Human and Social Analytics, pp. 35–36. IARIA (2015)
11. Koelstra, S., Muhl, C., Soleymani, M., Lee, J.-S., Yazdani, A., Ebrahimi, T., Pun, T., et al.: DEAP: a database for emotion analysis; using physiological signals. IEEE Trans. Affect. Comput. **3**(1), 18–31 (2012). https://doi.org/10.1109/T-AFFC.2011.15
12. Koenig, J., Jarczok, M., Ellis, R., Hillecke, T., Thayer, J.: Heart rate variability and experimentally induced pain in healthy adults: a systematic review. Eur. J. Pain **18**(3), 301–314 (2014). https://doi.org/10.1002/j.1532-2149.2013.00379.x
13. Krajewski, J., Schnieder, S., Sommer, D., Batliner, A., Schuller, B.: Applying multiple classifiers and non-linear dynamics features for detection sleepiness from speech. Neurocomputing 84, 65–75 (2012). https://doi.org/10.1016/j.neucom.2011.12.021
14. Laborde, S., Mosley, E., Thayer, J.F.: Heart rate variability and cardiac vagal tone in psychophysiological research - recommendations for experiment planning, data analysis, and data reporting. Front. Psychol. **8**, 1–18 (2017). https://doi.org/10.3389/fpsyg.2017.00213
15. Michail, E., Kokonozi, A., Chouvarda, I., Maglaveras, N.: EEG and HRV markers of sleepiness and loss of control during car driving. In: 30th Annual International Conference of the IEEE Engineering in Medicine and Biology Society, pp. 2566–2569 (2008). https://doi.org/10.1109/IEMBS.2008.4649724
16. Moody, G.B., Mark, R.G., Goldberger, A.L.: PhysioNet: a web-based resource for the study of physiologic signals. IEEE Eng. Med. Biol. Mag. **20**(3), 70–75 (2001). https://doi.org/10.1109/51.932728

17. Nkurikiyeyezu, K.N., Suzuki, Y., Lopez, G.F.: Heart rate variability as a predictive biomarker of thermal comfort. J. Ambient Intell. Humaniz. Comput. (2017). https://doi.org/10.1007/s12652-017-0567-4

18. Parent, F., Dansereau, J., Lacoste, M., Aissaoui, R.: Evaluation of the new flexible contour backrest for wheelchairs. J. Rehabil. Res. Dev. **37**(3), 325–333 (2000)

19. Pearson, E.J.M.: Comfort and its measurement - a literature review. Disabil. Rehabil. Assistive Technol. **4**(5), 301–310 (2009). https://doi.org/10.1080/17483100902980950

20. Platt, J.: Probabilistic outputs for support vector machines and comparisons to regularized likelihood methods. Adv. Large Margin Classifiers **10**(3), 61–74 (1999). http://citeseerx.ist.psu.edu/viewdoc/summary?doi=10.1.1.41.1639

21. Poria, S., Cambria, E., Bajpai, R., Hussain, A.: A review of affective computing: From unimodal analysis to multimodal fusion. Inf. Fusion **37**, 98–125 (2017). https://doi.org/10.1016/j.inffus.2017.02.003

22. Prinsloo, G.E., Rauch, H.G.L., Lambert, M.I., Muench, F., Noakes, T.D., Derman, W.E.: The effect of short duration heart rate variability (HRV) biofeedback on cognitive performance during laboratory induced cognitive stress. Appl. Cogn. Psychol. **25**(5), 792–801 (2011). https://doi.org/10.1002/acp.1750

23. Schuller, B., Steidl, S., Batliner, A., Vinciarelli, A., Scherer, K., Ringeval, F., Chetouani, M., et al.: The INTERSPEECH 2013 computational paralinguistics challenge: Social signals, conflict, emotion, autism. In: Proceedings of the Annual Conference of the International Speech Communication Association, pp. 148–152 (2013)

24. Steidl, S., Batliner, A., Bergelson, E., Krajewski, J., Janott, C., Amatuni, A., Casillas, M., et al.: The computational paralinguistics challenge. In: Interspeech 2017, pp. 1–5 (2017). https://doi.org/10.21437/Interspeech.2017-43

25. Sudarshan, V.K., Acharya, U., Oh, S.L., Adam, M., Tan, J.H., Chua, C.K., Chua, K.P., et al.: Automated diagnosis of congestive heart failure using dual tree complex wavelet transform and statistical features extracted from 2 s of ECG signals. Comput. Biol. Med. **83**, 48–58 (2017). https://doi.org/10.1016/j.compbiomed.2017.01.019

26. Valstar, M., Gratch, J., Schuller, B., Ringeval, F., Lalanne, D., Torres, M.T., Scherer, S., et al.: AVEC 2016 - Depression, Mood, and Emotion Recognition Workshop and Challenge (2016). https://doi.org/10.1145/2988257.2988258

27. Wachter, R., Gröschel, K., Gelbrich, G., Hamann, G.F., Kermer, P., Liman, J., Seegers, J., et al.: Holter-electrocardiogram-monitoring in patients with acute ischaemic stroke: an open-label randomised controlled trial. Lancet Neurol. **16**(4), 282–290 (2017). https://doi.org/10.1016/S1474-4422(17)30002-9

Bioinformatics

Semantic Segmentation of Colon Glands in Inflammatory Bowel Disease Biopsies

Zhaoxuan Ma[1,2], Zaneta Swiderska-Chadaj[5], Nathan Ing[1,3], Hootan Salemi[3], Dermot McGovern[1,4], Beatrice Knudsen[1,3], and Arkadiusz Gertych[2,3(✉)]

[1] Department of Biomedical Sciences, Cedars-Sinai Medical Center,
Los Angeles, CA 90048, USA
[2] Department of Pathology and Laboratory Medicine,
Cedars-Sinai Medical Center, Los Angeles, CA 90048, USA
arkadiusz.gertych@cshs.org
[3] Department of Surgery, Cedars-Sinai Medical Center,
Los Angeles, CA 90048, USA
[4] Department of Medicine, Cedars-Sinai Medical Center,
Los Angeles, CA 90048, USA
[5] Faculty of Electrical Engineering, Warsaw Technical University, Warsaw, Poland

Abstract. Robust delineation of tissue components in hematoxylin and eosin (H&E) stained slides is a critical step in quantifying tissue morphology. Fully convolutional neural networks (FCN) are ideally suited for automatic and efficient segmentation of tissue components in H&E slides. However, their performance relies on the network architecture, quality and depth of training. Here we introduce a set of 802 image tiles of colon biopsies from 2 subjects with inflammatory bowel disease (IBD) annotated for glandular epithelium (EP), gland lumen together with goblet cells (LG), and stroma (ST). We either trained the FCN-8s de-novo on our images (DN-FCN 8s) or pre-trained on the ImageNet dataset and fine-tuned on our images (FT-FCN-8s). For comparison, we used the U-Net trained de-novo. The training involved 700/802 images, leaving 102 images as a testing set. Ultimately, each model was validated in an independent digital biopsy slide. We also determined how the number of images used for training affects the performance of the model and observed a plateau in trainability at 700 images. In the testing set, U-Net and FT-FCN-8s achieved accuracies of 92.30% and 92.26% respectively. In the independent biopsy slide, U-Net demonstrated a segmentation accuracy of 88.64%, with F1-scores of 0.74 (EP), 0.92 (LG), and 0.93 (ST). The performance of the FT-FCN-8s was slightly worse, but the model required fewer images to reach a high classification performance. Our data demonstrate that all 3 FCNs are appropriate for segmentation of glands in biopsies from patients with IBD and open the door for quantification of IBD associated pathologies.

Keywords: Semantic tissue segmentation · Deep learning
Convolutional neural networks · Colon biopsy
Inflammatory bowel disease

© Springer International Publishing AG, part of Springer Nature 2019
E. Pietka et al. (Eds.): ITIB 2018, AISC 762, pp. 379–392, 2019.
https://doi.org/10.1007/978-3-319-91211-0_34

1   Introduction

Deep learning (DL) tools have recently become in high demand for development of complex computer vision applications in medicine. Digital pathology is one of the areas that has been impacted the most [3,14,15]. To date, DL-based solutions have been shown to reduce intra- and inter-observer biases and to improve the accuracy and speed of quantitative measurements. However, despite these advances in digital image analysis, the vast majority of slides are still evaluated manually using the light microscope.

Microscopic evaluation of colon biopsies stained with hematoxylin and eosin (H&E) is the standard of care and a routine workup for patients with a wide spectrum of colon diseases [6,20]. The procedure includes visual assessment of glandular architecture, as well as of the immune infiltrate in the stroma. At present, this assessment is performed by the pathologist through the microscope. However, DL tools have the potential to dramatically change the workflow. The utility of DL tools, including convolutional neural networks (CNN) that are trained to generate a binary map separating tissues into glandular versus non-glandular components has been shown in [2,11,13]. In these applications, the first tissue category consists of glandular epithelium and gland lumen. The epithelial lining of the glands consists in part of goblet cells with large, cytoplasmic, mucin filled vacuoles. Glands in the foreground can be readily distinguished from stroma and artifacts in the background. The CNNs were trained based on the Warwick-QU dataset [19] that contains 165 images of normal/benign (n = 74) and cancer colon glands (n = 91) from colorectal cancer patients. Images in this set were hand-annotated by a pathologist who distinguished foreground from background components. The Warwick-QU set is sufficient to train models to first delineate glands [2,13] and then subsequently separate them into benign or malignant categories [11].

The CNNs in [2,13] harnessed a sliding window approach to classify image patches. In the sliding window technique, tissue in the window is classified into one of the labeled categories and the result is assigned to the central pixel in the window. This approach is slow, but can be performed faster using fully convolutional neural networks (FCN) that directly classify all pixels in the window [8], without sliding.

In this work we highlight the need for computer-based analysis of colon specimens in gastrointestinal pathology. The information that is extracted from colon biopsies goes beyond the delineation and classification of glands and is critical for the acute and chronic treatment and management of patients. To address this need we postulate that the DL model should be able to distinguish several tissue categories, and suggest that epithelial lining, cytoplasm and goblets, and stroma are included as separate tissue categories for segmentation. Our work has two aims. First, we propose to augment the Warwick-QU dataset by introducing a new pathologist-annotated set of colon biopsy images from inflammatory bowel disease (IBD) patients. We will use this new set to train and assess the performance of several state-of-the-art FCNs for semantic segmentation. Second, we want to investigate the influence of the training set size on the performance of

FCNs. Our overarching goal is to determine whether the collected set of images and the models can aid in the evaluation of histologic features in colonic mucosa from individuals afflicted by IBD.

2 Materials and Methods

2.1 Image Data

Four hematoxylin and eosin (H&E) stained slides of colon biopsy from two patients with confirmed IBD were obtained from the Inflammatory Bowel Disease Consortium (Cedars-Sinai repository). One slide originated from ascending colon, one from descending colon (Patient 1), and two from rectum (Patient 1 and 2 respectively). The slides were digitized at 40× magnification using an Aperio Turbo AT (Leica Biosystems, Vista CA) whole slide scanner. Virtual slides outputted from the scanner were encoded as high-resolution RGBA matrices with pixel size of $0.244\,\mu m \times 0.244\,\mu m$.

To train and test our FCN models, a set of 802 non-overlapping image tiles, each 600×600 pixels large, were extracted from randomly picked areas in virtual slides (Table 1). Using a lab-developed graphical user interface [7], glandular epithelium (EP), glandular lumens plus mucin-filled intraepithelial goblets (LG), and stroma (ST) were manually delineated by a pathologist (Fig. 1). This set of images was shuffled and then randomly divided into training ($n = 700$) and test ($n = 102$) sets. The training set was further split into sub-sets containing respectively 700, 600, 500, 400, 300, 200, 100, 75, 50, 20, and 10 images. After down-sizing to 256×256 pixels, the number of images in each sub-set was augmented through a product of image rotation ($0, 90, 180$ and $270°$) and diagonal flipping (original + flipped), and thus yielding in total 8× more images in each sub-set.

To validate the performance of FCNs, one virtual (H&E) slide with rectal biopsy (Fig. 1(a)) (IBD Consortium, Johns Hopkins Hospital repository) was annotated by the pathologist who, by means of Aperio slide viewer, manually traced lines around EP, LG, and ST components directly on the virtual slide (Fig. 1(b)).

Table 1. Quantities of H&E colon biopsy images for FCN models testing and training

Image set	Patient 1			Patient 2	Total
	Ascending colon	Descending colon	Rectum	Rectum	
Training	200	244	66	190	700
Test	37	33	7	25	102

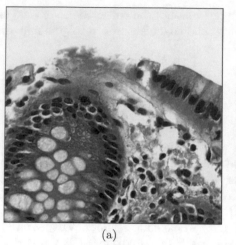 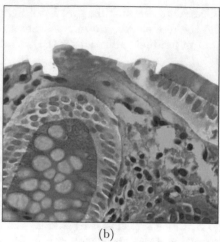

(a)   (b)

Fig. 1. Example manual ground truth annotations of colon biopsy images: (a) original H&E image, (b) manual ground truth overlaid on the H&E image (red – glandular lumens plus mucin-filled intraepithelial goblets (LG), green – glandular epithelium (EP), blue – stroma (ST), white – background pixels)

2.2 FCN Training

For our project, we chose a fully convolutional network with 8× upsampled prediction (FCN-8s) [16,18], and U-Net – a network with three up- and down-sampling layers for fast segmentation [17]. Both are state-of-the-art models for semantic segmentation and have achieved very good performance in the analysis of medical images [17,23].

The networks were trained as follows: we fine-tuned an existing pre-trained FCN-8s (FT-FCN-8s) and trained one de-novo (DN-FCN-8s). The fine tuning was done on the FCN-8s pretrained on the Pascal-VOC 2011 dataset [5]. To work with our data set of labeled images, one additional convolutional layer was appended to both FT-FCN-8s and DN-FCN-8s to reduce the output to the 4 desirable categories: LG, EP, ST and background. FT-FCN-8s was trained in Caffe environment [10] and the DN-FCN-8s using Keras [4] with a TensorFlow backend [1], both with a stochastic gradient descent (SGD) optimizer. The learning rate (lr) hyperparameter was originally set to 0.0001 and then decreased for every epoch with the exponential decay γ set to 0.95. The batch size was 1 per iteration.

The original U-Net network [17] has been extended by adding dropout layers between the convolutional layers. This modification reduces the chance of over-fitting in a case of limited number of training image data. Based on the existing literature and our own experience the dropout factor has been experimentally set to 0.5, and the SGD optimizer applied to adjust the parameters of the network. The lr was changed using a scheduler; the initial value of lr was 0.05 and after every 10 iterations the lr was gradually reduced 2×. The batch size was

= 2. Such approach usually leads to a fast and precise training of this model. U-Net was trained from randomly initialized weights using Keras [4] with a TensorFlow backend [1]. The training stopped when the accuracy in the validation set plateaued or if the number of epochs reached 35. Training of DN-FCN-8s and U-Net began after random initialization of network's weights. The accuracy of validation dataset was automatically calculated, recorded and outputted after every training epoch until the end-of-training criterion was met. The training was carried out on workstations with NVIDIA GPU support.

2.3   Evaluation

To investigate whether a random initialization of weights in a model has any effect the network's performance, the DN-FCN-8s and U-Net were trained from scratch 5× for each training set size. After training, the average accuracy and standard deviations were plotted for comparison. This experiment was not performed for FT-FCN-8s because it has-been previously pre-trained.

In the next step, we assessed the performance of FCNs by recording trends of classification accuracy using a model that yielded best accuracy, one accuracy trend line for each of the training sets was created. In each case the accuracy was determined in the test set of 102 images. To calculate the accuracy, pixel-level predictions were juxtaposed with ground truth labels in the 4×4 confusion matrix (refer to 4 annotated categories in Fig. 1).

Subsequently, after discarding background category we used 3×3 confusion matrices (3-class classification scheme) to calculate overall classification accuracy and F1-scores for the EP, LG, and ST. The goal was to determine if there is a difference in classification performance of individual tissues for different training data sets. Next, a 2-class classification (2×2 confusion matrix) scheme was introduced. In this scheme, the LG and EP categories were merged under one category (glands) whereas ST was the second category. The purpose of this experiment was to compare the performance of gland segmentation performed by our FCNs to the performance of gland segmentation methods described in [11,13].

For the three- and two-class classifications, we took into consideration the best U-Net, DN-FCN-8s and FT-FCN-8s that were trained with augmented subset of 700 training images. Results of this evaluation were collected in tables that show values of accuracy and F1-scores. The accuracy was calculated as: $\mathrm{ACC} = (\sum(tp) + \sum(tn))/(\sum(tp) + \sum(tn) + \sum(fp) + \sum(fn))$, with: tp, tn, fp, and fn representing respectively true positive, true negative, false positive and false negative pixel classifications, and with the $\sum$ symbol indicating the summation of pixels in a labeled category over all images in the test set. The F1-score was calculated as follows: $\text{F1-score} = 2 \cdot (pr \cdot re)/(pr + re)$. Where the precision ($pr$) is defined as: $pr = tp/(tp + fp)$ and the recall (re) as: $re = tp/(tp + fn)$.

Finally, to evaluate the performance of FCNs in the virtual slide, we plugged them into our existing whole slide processing pipelines [8,21]. They automate the segmentation of a gigapixel image pyramids by retrieving, color-normalizing, down-sizing and classifying consecutive image tiles, and then stitching the classified tiles together for a final tissue map and visualization.

3   Results

3.1   Effect of Training Set Size on FCNs Performance

Figure 2 shows how the segmentation accuracy of U-Neat and DN-FCN-8s changes when the model is trained de-novo each time beginning with a random initialization of network's weights. Note, that FT-FCN-8s reaches the same accuracy level for each initialization. One box plot represents the mean and standard deviation of accuracy in recognizing 4 image categories by five models each trained with a training set of a predefined size. Table 2 shows the segmentation accuracy as a function of the training set size. Results included in this table originate from models that scored highest accuracy when trained with a fixed number of training images.

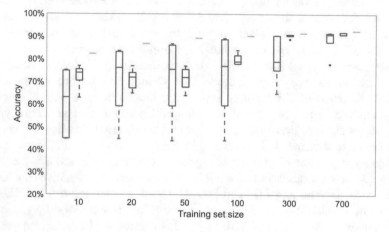

Fig. 2. Box plots of FCNs' segmentation accuracy. Each model was trained 5 times using a training set of a fixed size, and then tested on 102 images. The tops and bottoms of each box are respectively the 25th and 75th percentiles of the sample. The line in the middle of each box is the median, and the whiskers are the max and min of the sample. FT-FCN-8s (yellow), DN-FCN-8s (blue), and U-Net (orange) red dots – outliers

Table 2. Segmentation accuracy in the test (n = 102) as a function of the training set size

Model	Training set size				
	10	20	50	75	100
FT-FCN-8s	**82.39**	**86.88**	**89.32**	**89.93**	**90.30**
DN-FCN-8s	76.09	84.06	87.11	88.72	89.24
U-Net	80.15	83.50	88.83	85.68	88.47

Model	Training set size				
	200	300	400	500	600	700
FT-FCN-8s	90.92	91.64	91.94	92.04	92.54	**92.59**
DN-FCN-8s	90.25	90.58	90.91	91.18	91.52	91.74
U-Net	**91.72**	**92.00**	**92.78**	**92.80**	**92.66**	92.26

Figures 3(a), (c) and (e) illustrate the fluctuation and trend of classification accuracy across training epochs. Note, that for the FT-FCN-8s model trained with 100 images or more, the accuracy reaches a plateau after just 10 epochs.

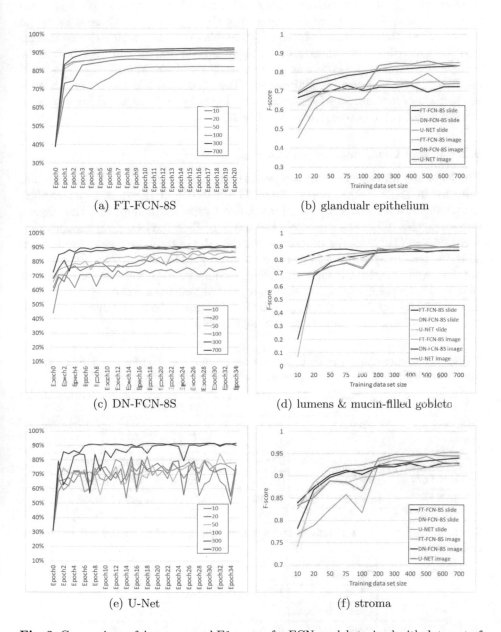

(a) FT-FCN-8S

(b) glandualr epithelium

(c) DN-FCN-8S

(d) lumens & mucin-filled goblets

(e) U-Net

(f) stroma

Fig. 3. Comparison of Accuracy and F1-scores for FCN models trained with datasest of different size. The classification performance is evaluated for three tissue components. Left column: Accuracy in the test set. Right column: F1-scores for different tissue categories

The DN-FCN-8s and U-Net models required 3 times as many epochs to train. Also, these two models needed at least 300 images to train to reach their top training accuracy. Accuracy flucuations observed in models trained with small dataset size may be indicative of insufficient model training and poor generalization. Figures 3(b), (d) and (f) report the F1-scores for the three-class tissue classification. Results were obtained for models evaluated with the test images and the validation slide. Interestingly, there is a discrepancy in performance in recognizing luminal and goblet areas between FT-FCN-8s and DN-FCN-8s models trained with a dataset ≤ 100 images. The difference is associated with poor recognition of stroma, implying that larger training set is required for a reliable distinction of these two region types (Fig. 3(f)).

3.2   Tissue Classification Performance

The F1-scores and accuracy for top performing models trained on 700 images are collected in Table 3. On average, the ACC was 4.51% higher in test images than in the validation slide, and the ability to recognize epithelium had the biggest impact on this difference regardless the model. When the two-class classification is considered (Table 4), the difference between the performance in the validation slide and test images diminishes to approximately 3.11%. Note, that whole glands are very well separated from surrounding stroma (Fig. 4) and one from another (Fig. 5). Our pipelines for whole slide analysis can process a gigapixel virtual slide in about 30 min and output a map with EP, LG and ST components highlighted for visualization and performance evaluation (Fig. 6).

Table 3. F1-score and accuracy in test set and validation slide for the 3-class classification: epithelium (EP), gland lumen with goblets (LG), and stroma (ST)

Model	Test set				Virtual slide			
	F1-score			Accuracy %	F1-score			Accuracy %
	EP	LG	ST		EP	LG	ST	
FT-FCN-8S	**0.86**	0.89	**0.97**	92.26	0.72	0.87	**0.93**	86.67
DN-FCN-8S	0.84	0.90	0.95	91.36	**0.75**	0.89	0.92	87.53
U-NET	0.84	**0.92**	0.96	**92.30**	0.74	**0.92**	**0.93**	**88.64**

Table 4. F1-score and accuracy in test set and validation slide for the 2-class classification scheme

Model	Test set		Virtual slide		
	F1-score		Accuracy %	F1-score		Accuracy %
	Gland	Stroma		Gland	Stroma	
FT-FCN-8S	**0.96**	**0.97**	**96.22**	**0.92**	**0.93**	**92.54**
DN-FCN-8S	0.94	0.95	94.74	0.92	0.92	92.09
U-NET	0.95	0.96	95.29	0.92	0.93	92.31

| U-Net | DN-FCN-8s | FT-FCN-8s | GT | H&E |

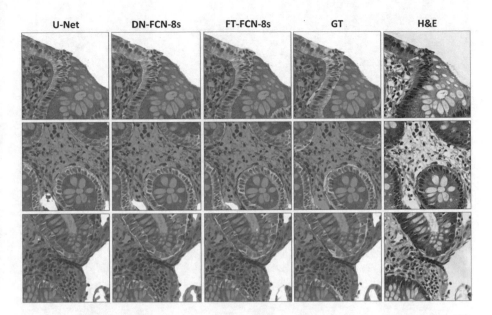

Fig. 4. Example semantic segmentation results by three FCNs for three different regions. GT – ground truth pathologist annotations

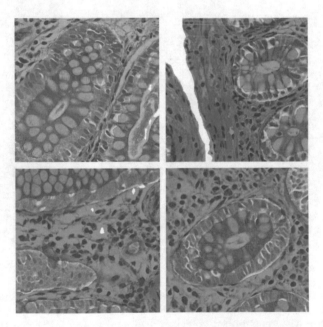

Fig. 5. Segmentation of closely adjacent glands in tiles from the test set. Results are obtained from FT-FCN-8s

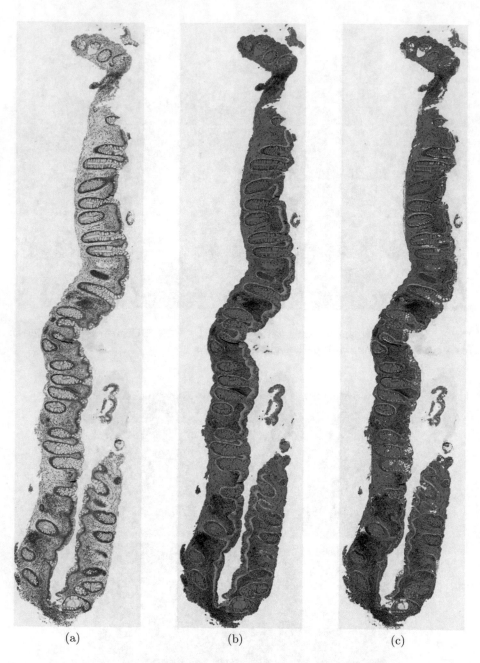

(a)   (b)   (c)

Fig. 6. Semantic segmentation of rectal biopsy: (a) original H&E image, (b) ground truth delineations, (c) result outputted by the FT-FCN-8s model: blue – stroma, red – lumens together with mucin-filled goblets, green – epithelium. For clarity, the area in the figure (5000 × 22300 pixels) shows one tissue fragment. The virtual slide contains 5 more similarly looking tissue pieces from biopsy

4   Discussion

Promising advancements have been made in digital pathology to automatically detect and delineate objects of interest (tumor areas, glands, glomeruli, blood vessels, nuclei etc.) in images of H&E stained tissues. To segment glands in biopsies obtained from the colon, a commonly used approach is a CNN-based tool that exports a window-wise likelihood map for the presence or absence of the objects of interest. As described in [11,13,19], to perform a semantic segmentation of colon tissues by a CNN, a scanning window is centered at each pixel and the likelihood of the pixel belonging to one of the objects of interest is recorded. This approach suffers a computational penalty since an FCN of similar complexity may process up to window size^2 times more area per iteration, a factor that is of utmost importance in whole slide processing.

Obtaining the pixel-level ground-truth annotations in multiple images is costly and time consuming [7,9]. For this reason, it is worth investigating how much image data is needed to train a model that performs an accurate semantic segmentation. Towards this goal we trained three semantic FCNs, compared their performances and confirmed them in an independent validation slide. As expected, the average performance as determined by accuracy and F1-score, gradually increased with the number of images in the training set. For the largest training set, U-Net (ACC = 88.64%) and DN-FCN-8s (ACC = 87.53%) were best in classifying 3 tissue categories in the validation slide, but FT-FCN-8s achieved only a marginally lower accuracy (ACC = 86.67%). However, interestingly, FT-FCN-8S when trained using only 100 images reached an ACC of 90% in the test set, suggesting that a training set of this size may be enough to obtain a baseline FCN model for colon tissue segmentation. We expect the necessary size of training data is proportional to the complexity of tasks, network perplexity, and the optimization procedure. Since the FT-FCN-8s was pre-trained and since we expected similarities between features in natural and histology image, as little as 10 training epochs were sufficient to fine tune the weights and obtain stable performance. The other two models required at least 30 epochs to arrive at the same performance level.

Through our experiments in (Fig. 2) we learned that training a FCN model de-novo several times with a fixed set of training images gives a good estimation of the model's average performance, allows selecting the best performing model, and helps assess the number of images that are needed to fully train the model.

For the FT-FCN-8s and DN-FCN-8s models trained on 700 and tested on 102 images, F1-scores obtained for the lumen or stroma were higher than for the epithelium (Fig. 3), suggesting that the epithelial layer is the hardest to be segmented properly. The effect of misclassifying the epithelial layer as a lumen or goblet cell is seen in Fig. 4. This error appears related to spatial saliency in semantic segmentation, a known source of error in multiple approaches including conditional random fields [22], and approximate Bayesian inference [12]. Despite this error, F1-score values remained high for epithelium: 0.72–0.75, lumen+ goblets: 0.87–0.89 and stroma: 0.92–0.93 in the validation digital slide (Fig. 6(c), Table 3), collectively indicating excellent tissue recognition performance.

When two of the models were evaluated in a binary tissue classification (glands versus stroma), the F1-scores of the FT-FCN-8s and DN-FCN-8s models (Table 4) surpassed the scanning window CNN models by at least 0.15 [11, 13]. The ability to segment glands separated by a single layer of fibroblasts is illustrated in Fig. 5. Hence, we postulate that the FCNs are better tools for colon gland segmentation.

In contrast to CNN models reported in [11, 13] trained on the Warwick-QU datasest [19], our experiments involved semantic segmentation models trained on data solely from IBD specimens. After an initial validation our models can readily provide excellent predictions for three tissue categories. This opens up the possibility for an in depth-quantification of the tissue architecture in heavily inflamed colon biopsies from individuals with IBD. The segmented images can be used for measurements of gland size, diameter, architectural distortion and bifurcation, area and distances between glands, as well as thicknesses of the glandular epithelium. These measurements can eventually lead to an automated and reproducible assessment of the severity of the disease and the risk of relapse and can be tested in the future for improving the management of individuals with IBD.

5 Conclusions

Towards the primary goal, our team collected and finely annotated a new set of colon images. In contrast to the set described in [19], delineations of additional components are provided through our data set. Essentially, our set complements the set from [19] and allows training models for tasks that go beyond gland segmentation. The set of collected images appears to be sufficiently large to reliably train FCN models for semantic segmentation of colon tissue from IBD specimens. Our experiments suggest that with this newly collected set of images, three tissue classes: namely glandular epithelium, glandular lumens and mucin-filled intraepithelial goblets, and stroma can be successfully distinguished by two state-of-the-art semantic FCN models. FCN-8s trained from scratch required all available images to train, whereas fine-tuning of the pre-trained FCN-8s required only 100 images to train to achieve similar performance. Essentially, the performance of all three models is comparable.

Acknowledgement. This work was in part funded by seed grants from the Department of Surgery, The Biobank & Translation Research Core at Cedars-Sinai Medical Center, in part by Cedars-Sinai in support of CTSI grant UL1TR001881-01, and in part by the National Science Center (Poland) by the grant UMO-2016/23/N/ST6/02076. The authors would also like to thank The Inflammatory Bowel Disease Consortium for digital slides of colon specimens.

References

1. Abadi, M., Agarwal, A., Barham, P., Brevdo, E., Chen, Z., Citro, C., Corrado, G.S., Davis, A., Dean, J., Devin, M., Ghemawat, S., Goodfellow, I., Harp, A., Irving, G., Isard, M., Jia, Y., Jozefowicz, R., Kaiser, L., Kudlur, M., Levenberg, J., Mané, D., Monga, R., Moore, S., Murray, D., Olah, C., Schuster, M., Shlens, J., Steiner, B., Sutskever, I., Talwar, K., Tucker, P., Vanhoucke, V., Vasudevan, V., Viégas, F., Vinyals, O., Warden, P., Wattenberg, M., Wicke, M., Yu, Y., Zheng, X.: TensorFlow: large-scale machine learning on heterogeneous systems (2015)
2. BenTaieb, A., Hamarneh, G.: Topology aware fully convolutional networks for histology gland segmentation, pp. 460–468. Springer International Publishing, Cham (2016)
3. Bueno, G., Fernández-Carrobles, M.M., Deniz, O., García-Rojo, M.: New trends of emerging technologies in digital pathology. Pathobiology **83**(2–3), 61–69 (2016)
4. Chollet, F., et al.: Keras (2015)
5. Everingham, M., Van Gool, L., Williams, C.K.I., Winn, J., Zisserman, A.: The PASCAL visual object classes challenge 2011 (VOC2011) results. http://www.pascal-network.org/challenges/VOC/voc2011/workshop/index.html
6. Feakins, R.M.: Inflammatory bowel disease biopsies: updated british society of gastroenterology reporting guidelines. J. Clin. Pathol. **66**(12), 1005–1026 (2013)
7. Gertych, A., Ing, N., Ma, Z., Fuchs, T.J., Salman, S., Mohanty, S., Bhele, S., Velásquez-Vacca, A., Amin, M.B., Knudsen, B.S.: Machine learning approaches to analyze histological images of tissues from radical prostatectomies. Comput. Med. Imaging Graph. **46**(Part 2), 197–208 (2015)
8. Ing, N., Ma, Z., Li, J., Salemi, H., Arnold, C., Knudsen, B., Gertych, A.: Semantic segmentation for prostate cancer grading by convolutional neural networks. In: Proceedings of the SPIE Medical Imaging, vol. 10581, pp. 10581-1–10581-13 (2018). https://doi.org/10.1117/12.2293000
9. Ing, N., Salman, S., Ma, Z., Walts, A., Knudsen, B., Gertych, A.: Machine learning can reliably distinguish histological patterns of micropapillary and solid lung adenocarcinomas. In: Piętka, E., Badura, P., Kawa, J., Wieclawek, W. (eds.) Proceedings of the Information Technologies in Medicine: 5th International Conference, ITIB 2016, Kamień Śląski, Poland, 20–22 June 2016, vol. 2, pp. 193–206. Springer International Publishing, Cham (2016)
10. Jia, Y., Shelhamer, E., Donahue, J., Karayev, S., Long, J., Girshick, R., Guadarrama, S., Darrell, T.: Caffe: convolutional architecture for fast feature embedding. arXiv preprint arXiv:1408.5093 (2014)
11. Kainz, P., Pfeiffer, M., Urschler, M.: Segmentation and classification of colon glands with deep convolutional neural networks and total variation regularization. PeerJ **5**, e3874 (2017)
12. Kendall, A., Gal, Y.: What uncertainties do we need in Bayesian deep learning for computer vision? arXiv preprint arXiv:1703.04977 (2017)
13. Li, W., Manivannan, S., Akbar, S., Zhang, J., Trucco, E., McKenna, S.: Gland segmentation in colon histology images using hand-crafted features and convolutional neural networks, June 2016, pp. 1405–1408. IEEE (2016)
14. Litjens, G., Sánchez, C.I., Timofeeva, N., Hermsen, M., Nagtegaal, I., Kovacs, I., van de Kaa, C.H., Bult, P., van Ginneken, B., van der Laak, J.: Deep learning as a tool for increased accuracy and efficiency of histopathological diagnosis. Sci. Rep. **6**, 26286 (2016)

15. Litjens, G.J.S., Kooi, T., Bejnordi, B.E., Setio, A.A.A., Ciompi, F., Ghafoorian, M., van der Laak, J.A.W.M., van Ginneken, B., Sánchez, C.I.: A survey on deep learning in medical image analysis. CoRR abs/1702.05747 (2017)
16. Long, J., Shelhamer, E., Darrell, T.: Fully convolutional networks for semantic segmentation. In: The IEEE Conference on Computer Vision and Pattern Recognition (CVPR) (2015)
17. Ronneberger, O., Fischer, P., Brox, T.: U-net: convolutional networks for biomedical image segmentation. CoRR abs/1505.04597 (2015). http://arxiv.org/abs/1505.04597
18. Shelhamer, E., Long, J., Darrell, T.: Fully convolutional networks for semantic segmentation. CoRR abs/1605.06211 (2016). http://arxiv.org/abs/1605.06211
19. Sirimukunwattana, K., Pluim, J.P.W., Chen, H., Qi, X., Heng, P.A., Guo, Y.B., Wang, L.Y., Matuszewski, B.J., Bruni, E., Sanchez, U., Böhm, A., Ronneberger, O., Cheikh, B.B., Racoceanu, D., Kainz, P., Pfeiffer, M., Urschler, M., Snead, D.R.J., Rajpoot, N.M.: Gland segmentation in colon histology images: the glas challenge contest. Med. Image Anal. **35**, 489–502 (2017)
20. Stewart, S.L., Wike, J.M., Kato, I., Lewis, D.R., Michaud, F.: A population-based study of colorectal cancer histology in the united states, 1998–2001. Cancer **107**(S5), 1128–1141 (2006)
21. Swiderska-Chadaj, Z., Markiewicz, T., Grala, B., Lorent, M., Gertych, A.: A deep learning pipeline to delineate proliferative areas of intracranial tumors in digital slides, pp. 448–458. Springer International Publishing, Cham (2017)
22. Zheng, S., Jayasumana, S., Romera-Paredes, B., Vineet, V., Su, Z., Du, D., Huang, C., Torr, P.H.: Conditional random fields as recurrent neural networks. In: Proceedings of the IEEE International Conference on Computer Vision, pp. 1529–1537 (2015)
23. Zhou, Y., Xie, L., Fishman, E.K., Yuille, A.L.: Deep supervision for pancreatic cyst segmentation in abdominal CT scans, pp. 222–230. Springer International Publishing, Cham (2017)

Color Normalization Approach to Adjust Nuclei Segmentation in Images of Hematoxylin and Eosin Stained Tissue

Adam Piórkowski[1(✉)] and Arkadiusz Gertych[2]

[1] Department of Geoinformatics and Applied Computer Science,
AGH University of Science and Technology, A. Mickiewicza 30 Av.,
30–059 Cracow, Poland
pioro@agh.edu.pl

[2] Department of Surgery, Department of Pathology and Laboratory Medicine,
Cedars-Sinai Medical Center, Los Angeles, CA 90048, USA

Abstract. Lack of standards in hematoxylin and eosin (H&E) tissue staining across laboratories is one of the reasons for differences in appearance of specimens under the microscope. It also negatively impacts the performance of digital image analysis algorithms, including nuclei segmentation that is deemed to be affected the most. To alleviate this problem, we searched through the color space to find color targets to which coloration of the original H&E image can be transferred with the goal to improve performance of a baseline nuclear segmentation method. Color targets that we found were plugged into the Reinhard's color normalization algorithm to transfer the original H&E image to a new color space. The color-transferred images were then processed by two proposed approaches that subtract and subsequently threshold red and blue color channels. Implementation of these steps improved the amount of false positive pixels and splitting of clustered nuclei in the nuclear mask generated by the baseline method. The pixel-based segmentation accuracy was 94% in selected images. The performance was assessed in heterogeneous images of colon with manually delineated nuclei.

Keywords: Edge detection · Nuclei segmentation · Cell counting
Image processing · Color transfer · Microscopy images

1 Introduction

Hematoxylin and eosin (H&E) are dyes that are commonly used in tissue staining for histological evaluation. H&E staining cocktail is largely not standardized and often inconsistent across laboratories. The inconsistency that is caused by different quality and freshness of the staining reagents can create variability in contrast and coloration that is an impediment to quantitative digital imaging.

The lack of standardized protocols for H&E staining results in profound differences in coloration of specimens. Depending on reagents' concentration, the

© Springer International Publishing AG, part of Springer Nature 2019
E. Pietka et al. (Eds.): ITIB 2018, AISC 762, pp. 393–406, 2019.
https://doi.org/10.1007/978-3-319-91211-0_35

appearance of cell nuclei can range from pale to dark blue. Likewise, discrepancies in concentration of eosin will result in cytoplasm staining with a wide range of pink, red, violet or orange. The issue of differences in tissue coloration negatively affects performance of nuclei segmentation algorithms [22].

Despite this disadvantage, the majority of approaches targeting the segmentation of nuclei in images of H&E stained tissues is based on the analysis of blue image channel because blue color approximates the location of hematoxylin and it is easy to work with. More sophisticated approaches utilize red and blue color ratio [1], a gray-level image representation [9,12], or ad-hoc color standardization [7]. In [23] the authors concluded that a substantial overlap exists in the color un-normalized images, but the normalization helps to discern images components such as nuclei, cytoplasm and background. However, no quantitative data was shown that color normalization improves analytically routines such as for example segmentation of nuclei.

Other methods put more emphasis on color normalization in the image followed by the deconvolution of hematoxylin, eosin or other stains, and then use the hematoxylin image as a starting point for nuclear segmentation [3,8,18]. Color normalization methods have been developed to alleviate the problem of inconsistencies in the preparation of histology slides. The goal is to bring images of slides that were processed under different conditions into unified space to enable robust quantitative tissue analysis. Reinhard's [19], Macenko's [11], and Li's [10] color normalization methods that were compared in [8] seem to be most commonly used. A review of these and other state-of-the-art color normalization methods can be found in [16].

With regards to nuclei segmentation methods that utilize blue, red, or both channels for input, as well as color-normalization in the image processing pipeline, there seems to be an unexplored opportunity in manipulating basic color channels that could lead to a more optimal separation of dyes in the image. In this work, we propose three computationally inexpensive approaches for finding optimal vectors of Lab color space to which original image colors can be transferred by means of the Reinhard's algorithm [19]. We check whether the analytically determined vectors have the potential to separate tightly packed nuclei which a baseline segmentation has difficulties to deal with.

Segmentation of cell nuclei in tissues with clusters of heterogeneous cells is a long-standing problem in quantitative image analysis [14]. For our research, we chose colon tissue because epithelial cells in colon crypts are tightly packed and have elliptical or cone shapes. In addition, stroma that surrounds the crypts, consists of fibroblasts, nerve and blood vessel cells, and cells of immune system that all have different size and morphology.

2   Materials

One glass slide with normal colon specimen was retrieved from the Biobank at Cedars-Sinai Medical Center, then stained with hematoxylin and eosin (H&E) and subsequently digitized with Aperio AT Turbo (Leica Biosystems, Vista CA) whole slide scanner. The scanning magnification was set to 40x and the pixel size was $0.244\,\mu m \times 0.244\,\mu m$. Next, the digital slide outputted by the scanner was reviewed by a pathologist who identified heterogenous tissue areas containing epithelium with adjacent stroma and immune cells. Then, square tiles (n = 80) with the tile length of 1000 pixels were manually selected and extracted from the digital slide, and saved as 8-bit encoded RGB matrices for further analysis.

3 Methods

3.1 Baseline Segmentation of Nuclei

H&E images (Fig. 1(a)) were subjected to Reinhard's color normalization [19], and then color-deconvoluted to obtain a gray scale image of the hematoxylin staining (Fig. 1(b)). We chose the Reinhard's method over other methods available from the literature due to its low computational complexity. The hematoxylin image was subsequently filtered with a circular averaging filter (pillbox) with an experimentally adjusted radius = 5 to attenuate noise and remove small non-nuclear objects. The image was automatically binarized using the statistical dominance algorithm (SDA) [15,17]. In this method, the intensity threshold and the radius parameters were respectively set to 90 and 50. Separately, the filtered hematoxylin image was processed by the fast radial symmetry transform (FRST) to yield an intensity image in which nuclear centers are marked by high-intensity peaks. Next, the FRST image was thresholded to obtain a binary mask of nuclear markers, and a marker-controlled watershed transform was applied to separate clustered and closely positioned nuclei (Fig. 1(c)). The watershed lines were traced within the mask of nuclei using the hematoxylin image that served as an intensity landscape to find ridge lines between marked nuclei similarly to the procedure described in [6]. Parameters for the FRST were set as described in [5]. All other parameters were determined experimentally to render best nuclear delineation performance. In the next step, original images with superimposed segmentation results (Fig. 2(a)) were shown to a pathologist who reviewed and then manually corrected the contours of segmented nuclei. This activity was limited only to correcting over- and under-segmentations (Fig. 2(b)). This manually corrected mask served as a ground truth for evaluation of methods discussed in the subsequent sections.

3.2 Analysis of Dependencies Between Colors in H&E Stained Images

To highlight the possibilities of improving segmentation performance through the analysis of color channels, one can consider an example in Fig. 3 that shows the color intensity along profiles in the original image (Fig. 3(a)) and the same image normalized using Reinhard's method [19] (Fig. 3(b)). In this example, the set of normalization parameters in the Lab space, calculated from the RGB space is as follows (mean,std): (L = (198,78), a = (120,9), b = (185,3)). The profiles show

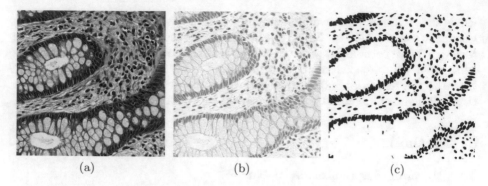

Fig. 1. Processing steps of baseline segmentation of nuclei: (a) original H&E image, (b) color-deconvoluted hematoxylin channel, and (c) baseline mask of nuclei

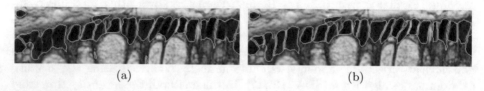

Fig. 2. A closeup view of nuclear segmentation results: (a) baseline method, (b) manual refinement of the baseline segmentation

color brightness values in each color channel. One can note that in the original image blue is the most intense color in cell nuclei, but this is not the case for the color-normalized image in which blue color in nuclei has reduced intensity.

However, one can notice that the difference in pixel intensities between red and blue channels is the most prominent at the edge between the nucleus and surrounding cytoplasm. More specifically, examining the relationships between intensities in the red (R) and blue (B) channels opens up the possibility of detecting nuclear boundaries, for instance by applying the following formula:

$$V_1(x, y) = |R(x, y) - B(x, y)| \tag{1}$$

This concept is visualized in Fig. 4(b). Following this idea, pixels that are located at nuclear edges visualized through Eq. (1) can be considered as local image minima.

Unfortunately, the obtained result in Fig. 4(b) may be difficult to use for extracting nuclear borders due to poor foreground to background ratio. Instead, full nuclei can be marked, taking into account only those areas in which the intensity of the red color dominates over the blue color. This leads to an extended version of formula Eq. (1) defined as follows:

$$V_2(x, y) = \max\left(0, R(x, y) - B(x, y)\right) \tag{2}$$

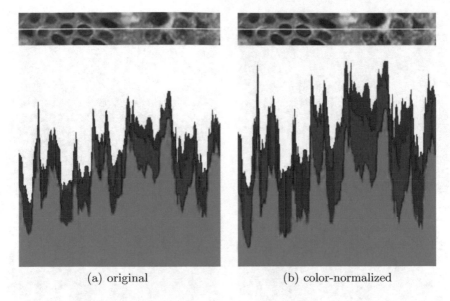

(a) original   (b) color-normalized

Fig. 3. Image profiles across the original and color normalized H&E images. The normalization enhances blue and red colors and attenuates the green color. Note that red and blue colors are much more intense than the green color. Interestingly, the color normalization reduced the intensity of blue color which in some areas is less intense than red color. Intensity value is reflected vertically

3.3   Seeking Optimal Color-Normalization Parameters Through a Random Guess

A test was carried out to evaluate approach described by Eq. (?). Three randomly selected original H&E images of colon tissue (see Sect. 2), marked here as P1, P2 and P3, were color-normalized each using 100,000 randomly generated vectors with mean and stds of Lab color space components, and colors in the original image were transferred accordingly. The ranges of color means ranged from 0 to 255, and the std deviation from 0 to 500. Following this step, a nuclear mask was obtained by thresholding of the image $V_2(x,y)$ (Fig. 4(c)) with a threshold of $t = 1$ separating nuclei (values under the threshold) from other components. Example result is show in Fig. 5(b). Then, the nuclear mask was overlaid onto the corresponding ground-truth image to assess the segmentation accuracy.

The segmentation performance of this approach was examined using the following measures: Dice coefficient (known also as F1 score), accuracy (ACC), and accuracy with 5× penalty rate for FP detections (FPEN5) see Table 1. The FPEN5 is a modification of the original ACC measure, and is defined solely for the purpose of this project. It penalizes stronger the presence of FP pixels in the output mask. Thus, FPEN5 is helpful in finding Lab parameters that lead to a reduces number of FP instances. The measures were calculated using the ground truth and the output mask based on a 2×2 confusion matrix.

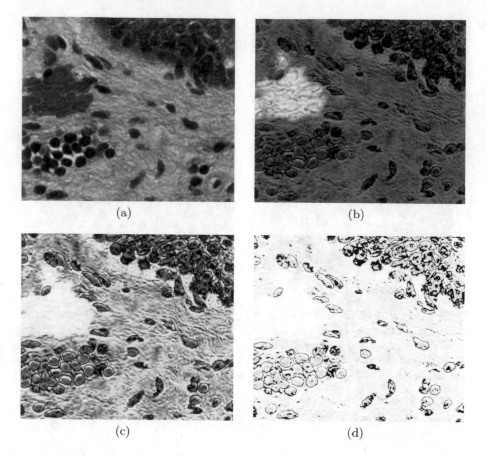

Fig. 4. Example output from the method described by Eq. (1). After processing the original H&E image from (a), the output in (b) is histogram stretched (c), and additionally gamma-corrected ($\gamma = 4.5$) (d) to visualize edges between nuclei and cytoplasm (black lines) that the Eq. (1) enhances

This method selects Lab vectors that maximize the measures of accuracy. However, its main disadvantage is the high computational cost. This cost is predominantly associated with transferring colors in the original image to the new space (100,000 iterations), and then generating the nuclear mask. This process took 8 h for a code written in Matlab R2017a (Matlab, Natick MA). Nevertheless, the search through a random guess provides some hints that Lab parameters leading to a high segmentation accuracy can be found experimentally. In the future studies we will implement an approach that determines optimal Lab parameters analytically. Preliminary results included in Table 2 are quite diverse, and suggest that the range of vector components is rather wide - spreading nearly through the entire range of possible values of the mean in each channel (0–255).

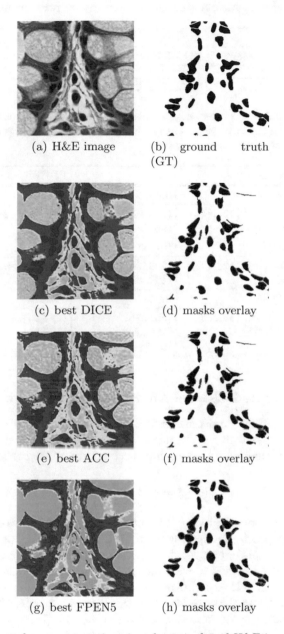

(a) H&E image

(b) ground truth (GT)

(c) best DICE

(d) masks overlay

(e) best ACC

(f) masks overlay

(g) best FPEN5

(h) masks overlay

Fig. 5. Example nuclear segmentations in color transferred H&E images. The original image from (a) was color-transferred using three different Lab vectors and subsequently segmented using Eq. (2). Each of the Lab vectors maximizes respectively the DICE (b), ACC (c) and FPEN5 (d) performance segmentation measures. The difference between ground truth (GT) nuclear mask in (e) and the segmentation results for each measure is respectively shown in (f), (g), and (h). TP pixels are black, FP red, and FN blue

Table 1. Measures of nuclei segmentation performance

Abbr.	DICE	ACC	FPEN5
Name	DICE Coefficient	ACCURACY	FP PENALTY 5
Formula	$\dfrac{2 \cdot TP}{2 \cdot TP + FP + FN}$	$\dfrac{TP + TN}{TP + TN + FP + FN}$	$\dfrac{TP + TN}{TP + TN + 5 \cdot FP + FN}$

Table 2. Performance of nuclear segmentation by method Eq. (2) with color transfer parameters (ctv) in the Lab space determined by a random guess. Best parameters are presented along the performance measures

Image	DICE	ACC	FPEN5
P1	0.8734	0.9615	0.9385
@ctv	(31,488), (15,281), (135,341)	(249,120), (99,474), (242,44)	(244,30), (245,142), (215,122)
P2	0.8676	0.9453	0.9134
@ctv	(220,29), (123,490), (46,79)	(220,29), (123,490), (46,79)	(234,6), (90,23), (123,56)
P3	0.8995	0.9537	0.9119
@ctv	(255,20), (48,275), (227,228)	(251,10), (196,117), (97,261)	(252,54), (235,40), (100,51)

3.4 Analysis of Red Channel After Custom Color Transformations

In the previous section we demonstrated the feasibility of the experiments and provide a proof of concept for the method. In this section we narrow down our analysis to the R channel by taking into account the following function:

$$V_3(x,y) = \begin{cases} 0, & R(x,y) > 0 \\ 1, & R(x,y) = 0 \end{cases} \tag{3}$$

To assess the applicability of this method, we used the color-transformed images from the previews experiment and then applied Eq. (3) to obtain the nuclear mask. Example images for the highest measures of accuracy are presented in Fig. 6. The highest measures with the corresponding Lab vectors are included in Table 3. Based on this experiment, we conclude that this method yields very similar results to those that are based on the $V_2(x,y)$ output. However, we find that segmentation results from the method based on $V_3(x,y)$ not only rank among the best, but they also lead to a single and generally applicable Lab vector = ((255, 400) (0, 0) (0, 20)) found for the P3 image (Tables 4 and 5).

Figure 7 shows example results of nuclear mask outputted by $V_3(x,y)$ for the images color-normalized with these Lab parameters to arrive at highest FPEN5, ACC, and Dice measures. Figure 7(d) shows that objects in the outputted mask and ground-truth mask overlap (black color). Discordant pixels are marked with blue (FN) or red colors (FP) respectively. Interestingly, when we take a closer

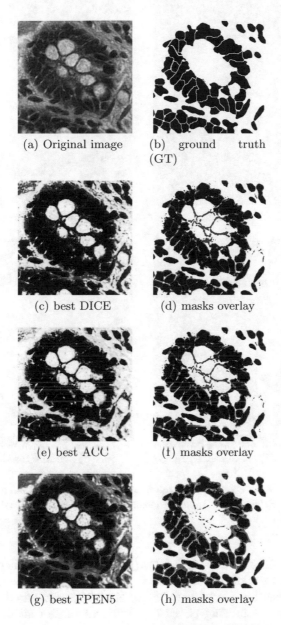

(a) Original image

(b) ground truth (GT)

(c) best DICE

(d) masks overlay

(e) best ACC

(f) masks overlay

(g) best FPEN5

(h) masks overlay

Fig. 6. Example nuclear segmentations in color transferred H&E images. The original image from (a) was color-transferred using three different Lab vectors and subsequently segmented using Eq. (3). Each of the Lab vectors maximizes respectively the DICE (b), ACC (c) and FPEN5 (d) performance segmentation measures. The difference between ground truth (GT) nuclear mask in (e) and the segmentation results for each measure is respectively shown in (f), (g), and (h). TP pixels are black, FP red, and FN blue

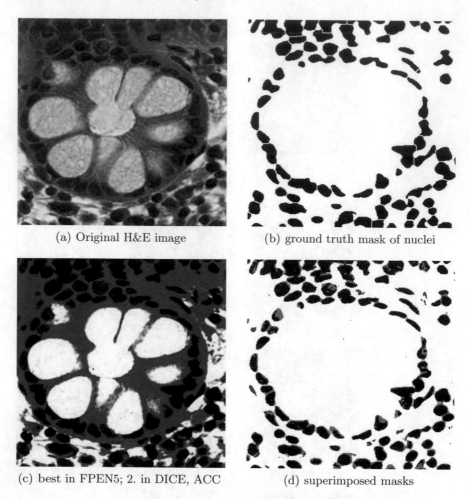

(a) Original H&E image   (b) ground truth mask of nuclei

(c) best in FPEN5; 2. in DICE, ACC   (d) superimposed masks

Fig. 7. An example of manual adjustment of color-transfer parameters to maximize DICE, ACC and FPEN performance measures. The meaning of colors in (a) is the same as in Figs. 5 and 6

look at the red lines in Figs. 6(d), (f), (g) we notice that they divide closely adjacent nuclei. In addition, blue areas - nuclei or their fragments that were removed by the baseline method are highlighted. This suggests that the proposed method incorporates missing pixels and removes those that do not belong to nuclei.

From results in Tables 4 and 5, we glean that both manual and automated methods overlap in a narrow range color transfer vectors. Interestingly, the mean and std values for the component a of the Lab color space, as well as the mean for the component b can be set to 0. This observation can be helpful in implementation of less complex algorithms that seek optimal color transfer vectors.

Table 3. Performance of nuclear segmentation by method Eq. (3) with color transfer parameters (ctv) in the Lab space determined by a random guess. Best parameters are presented together with corresponding the measures

Image	DICE	ACC	FPEN5
P1	0.8657	0.9579	0.9298
@ctv	(213,460), (223,80), (68,21)	(248,485), (63,80), (14,22)	(94,131), (2,6), (132,5)
P2	0.8723	0.9448	0.9036
@ctv	(213,452), (120,145), (78,31)	(125,238), (87,48), (157,16)	(208,237), (54,3), (207,19)
P3	0.8981	0.9528	0.9117
@ctv	(231,432), (194,137), (26,30)	(222,385), (188,154) (182,27)	(251,336), (31,107), (130,14)

Table 4. Performance of the baseline nuclear segmentation method preceded by the manual adjustment of color transfer vectors. Note, that it is possible to find more than one vector that leads to high values of DICE, ACC, and FPEN5. These vectors rank in the top 30 vectors out of 100,000 that were found by a random guess

Image	Color transfer vector	Dice	ACC	FPEN5
P1	(255,400), (0,0), (0,20)	0.8284	0.9513	0.9272 (22 of 100 000)
P1	(255,320), (0,0), (0,20)	0.7609	0.9371	0.9260 (38 of 100 000)
P2	(255,300), (0,0), (0,20)	0.7885	0.9226	0.9031 (3 of 100 000)
P2	(255,300), (0,0), (0,30)	0.8161	0.9304	0.9028 (8 of 100 000)
P3	(255,360), (0,0), (0,25)	0.8579	0.9403	0.9104 (28 of 100 000)
P3	(255,360), (0,0), (0,20)	0.8428	0.9352	0.9103 (30 of 100 000)

4   Summary

Challenges of nuclei segmentation in colon tissue have previously been recognized in [2,4,13,18,20–22]. For our research, we chose colon tissue because epithelial cells in colon crypts are tightly packed and have elliptical or cone shapes. In addition, stroma that surrounds the crypts, consists of fibroblasts, nerve and blood vessel cells, and cells of the immune system that have different size and morphology.

Our experiments were conducted using a lab-grown nuclei segmentation algorithm applied to high-resolution images of colon crypts that were supplemented with pathologist ground truth annotations. For three images that we randomly selected from our data set, our experimental approaches yielded target Lab color space vectors to which the images were normalized with and lead to a more accurate nuclei segmentation as compared to a method (see Materials) that has implemented an ad hoc color normalization vector. Our color normalization

Table 5. Performance of the baseline nuclear segmentation method preceded by the manual adjustment of color transfer vectors for a single image in a selected range of values. Results from row 10 are visualized in Fig. 7

Image	Color transfer vector	Dice	ACC	FPEN5
P3	(255,300), (0,0), (0,10)	0.6586	0.8814	0.8770
P3	(255,300), (0,0), (0,15)	0.7336	0.9015	0.8934
P3	(255,300), (0,0), (0,20)	0.7809	0.9155	0.9035
P3	(255,300), (0,0), (0,25)	0.8133	0.9256	0.9087
P3	(255,300), (0,0), (0,30)	0.8350	0.9326	0.9095
P3	(255,360), (0,0), (0,5)	0.7440	0.9043	0.8931
P3	(255,360), (0,0), (0,10)	0.7915	0.9185	0.9027
P3	(255,360), (0,0), (0,15)	0.8226	0.9285	0.9086
P3	(255,360), (0,0), (0,20)	0.8428	0.9352	<u>0.9103</u>
P3	(255,360), (0,0), (0,25)	<u>0.8579</u>	<u>0.9403</u>	**0.9104**
P3	(255,400), (0,0), (0,20)	**0.8650**	**0.9425**	0.9064
P3	(255,400), (0,0), (0,100)	0.7317	0.8471	0.5577
P3	(255,520), (0,0), (0,100)	0.8470	0.9230	0.7478
P3	(255,520), (0,0), (0,120)	0.7228	0.8362	0.5282
P3	(255,520), (0,0), (0,140)	0.6545	0.7742	0.4227

approaches relied on the Reinhard's method which has low computational complexity and allows manipulating components of the Lab color spaces. The ability to directly manipulate Lab parameters is the main advantage of the proposed methods over many others published to date.

Following the normalization, the images were processed by the proposed approaches that in principle subtract one color channel from another or threshold the red channel in post-normalized images. These experiments led to a segmentation accuracy of 94% or better depending on the method.

5 Further Work

Our results indicate that by manipulating color spaces in the image is advantageous for the nuclei segmentation procedure. We found numerous vectors that led to highly accurate segmentation. However, finding one common Lab vector or a small set of vectors for all images would be the ultimate goal. Further work should consider a more thorough search of Lab vectors, particularly for the methods described with Eqs. (2) and (3) because they have the highest potential of separating clustered cells.

Acknowledgement. This work was financed by the AGH – University of Science and Technology, Faculty of Geology, Geophysics and Environmental Protection as a part of a statutory project. The authors would like to thank Dr. Karolina Nurzynska for using her software to generate data for this research.

References

1. Chang, H., Han, J., Borowsky, A., Loss, L., Gray, J.W., Spellman, P.T., Parvin, B.: Invariant delineation of nuclear architecture in glioblastoma multiforme for clinical and molecular association. IEEE Trans. Med. Imaging **32**(4), 670–682 (2013)
2. Chen, J.M., Li, Y., Xu, J., Gong, L., Wang, L.W., Liu, W.L., Liu, J.: Computer-aided prognosis on breast cancer with hematoxylin and eosin histopathology images: a review. Tumor Biol. **39**(3), 1010428317694550 (2017)
3. Cui, Y., Hu, J.: Self-adjusting nuclei segmentation (SANS) of hematoxylin-eosin stained histopathological breast cancer images. In: IEEE International Conference on Bioinformatics and Biomedicine (BIBM 2016), pp. 956–963. IEEE (2016)
4. Eramian, M., Daley, M., Neilson, D., Daley, T.: Segmentation of epithelium in H&E stained odontogenic cysts. J. Microsc. **244**(3), 273–292 (2011)
5. Gertych, A., Joseph, A.O., Walts, A.E., Bose, S.: Automated detection of dual p16/ki67 nuclear immunoreactivity in liquid-based Pap tests for improved cervical cancer risk stratification. Ann. Biomed. Eng. **40**(5), 1192–1204 (2012)
6. Gertych, A., Ma, Z., Tajbakhsh, J., Velásquez-Vacca, A., Knudsen, B.S.: Rapid 3-d delineation of cell nuclei for high-content screening platforms. Comput. Biol. Med. **69**(Suppl. C), 328–338 (2016)
7. Kłeczek, P., Dyduch, G., Jaworek-Korjakowska, J., Tadeusiewicz, R.: Automated epidermis segmentation in histopathological images of human skin stained with hematoxylin and eosin. In: Medical Imaging 2017: Digital Pathology, vol. 10140, p. 101400M. International Society for Optics and Photonics (2017)
8. Kłeczek, P., Mól, S., Jaworek-Korjakowska, J.: The accuracy of H&E stain unmixing techniques when estimating relative stain concentrations. In: Polish Conference on Biocybernetics and Biomedical Engineering, pp. 87–97. Springer (2017)
9. Kowal, M., Filipczuk, P., Obuchowicz, A., Korbicz, J., Monczak, R.: Computer-aided diagnosis of breast cancer based on fine needle biopsy microscopic images. Comput. Biol. Med. **43**(10), 1563–1572 (2013)
10. Li, X., Plataniotis, K.N.: A complete color normalization approach to histopathology images using color cues computed from saturation-weighted statistics. IEEE Trans. Biomed. Eng. **62**(7), 1862–1873 (2015)
11. Macenko, M., Niethammer, M., Marron, J., Borland, D., Woosley, J.T., Guan, X., Schmitt, C., Thomas, N.E.: A method for normalizing histology slides for quantitative analysis. In: IEEE International Symposium on Biomedical Imaging, ISBI 2009, pp. 1107–1110. IEEE (2009)
12. Mazurek, P., Oszutowska-Mazurek, D.: From the slit-island method to the ising model: analysis of irregular grayscale objects. Int. J. Appl. Math. Comput. Sci. **24**(1), 49–63 (2014)
13. Nawandhar, A.A., Yamujala, L., Kumar, N.: Image segmentation using thresholding for cell nuclei detection of colon tissue. In: International Conference on Advances in Computing, Communications and Informatics (ICACCI 2015), pp. 1199–1203. IEEE (2015)
14. Nurzynska, K.: Deep learning as a tool for automatic segmentation of corneal endothelium images. Symmetry **10**(3), 60 (2018)

15. Nurzynska, K., Mikhalkin, A., Piorkowski, A.: CAS: cell annotation software - research on neuronal tissue has never been so transparent. Neuroinformatics **15**, 365–382 (2017)

16. Onder, D., Zengin, S., Sarioglu, S.: A review on color normalization and color deconvolution methods in histopathology. Appl. Immunohistochem. Mol. Morphol. **22**(10), 713–719 (2014)

17. Piorkowski, A.: A statistical dominance algorithm for edge detection and segmentation of medical images. In: Information Technologies in Medicine. Advances in Intelligent Systems and Computing, vol. 471, pp. 3–14. Springer (2016)

18. Qin, Y., Walts, A.E., Knudsen, B.S., Gertych, A.: Computerized delineation of nuclei in liquid-based pap smears stained with immunohistochemical biomarkers. Cytometry Part B Clin. Cytometry **88**(2), 110–119 (2015)

19. Reinhard, E., Adhikhmin, M., Gooch, B., Shirley, P.: Color transfer between images. IEEE Comput. Graph. Appl. **21**(5), 34–41 (2001)

20. Rogojanu, R., Bises, G., Smochina, C., Manta, V.: Segmentation of cell nuclei within complex configurations in images with colon sections. In: IEEE International Conference on Intelligent Computer Communication and Processing (ICCP 2010), pp. 243–246. IEEE (2010)

21. Tosta, T.A.A., Neves, L.A., do Nascimento, M.Z.: Segmentation methods of H&E-stained histological images of lymphoma: a review. Inform. Med. Unlocked **9**, 35–43 (2017)

22. Veta, M., van Diest, P.J., Kornegoor, R., Huisman, A., Viergever, M.A., Pluim, J.P.: Automatic nuclei segmentation in H&E stained breast cancer histopathology images. PLOS ONE **8**(7), e70221 (2013)

23. Zarella, M.D., Yeoh, C., Breen, D.E., Garcia, F.U.: An alternative reference space for H&E color normalization. PLOS ONE **12**(3), 1–14 (2017)

Cell Nuclei Segmentation Using Marker-Controlled Watershed and Bayesian Object Recognition

Marcin Skobel[✉], Marek Kowal, Józef Korbicz, and Andrzej Obuchowicz

Institute of Control and Computation Engineering, Faculty of Computer,
Electrical and Control Engineering, University of Zielona Góra,
ul. Licealna 9, 65-417 Zielona Góra, Poland
M.Skobel@issi.uz.zgora.pl

Abstract. Computer-assisted image analysis cytology play an important function in modern cancer diagnostics. A crucial task of such systems is segmentation of cell nuclei. Automatic procedure have to locate their exact position in cytological preparation and determine precise edges in order to extract morphometric features. Unfortunately, segmentation of individual nuclei is a huge challenge because they often creates complex clusters without clear edges. To deal with this problem we are proposing to combine Bayesian object recognition approach to approximate nuclei by circles with marker-controlled watershed employed to determine their exact shape. Watershed segmentation can reconstruct a precise shape of nuclei but only if their approximate location is known. On the other hand, Bayesian object recognition approach allows to isolate single nuclei even in complex nuclei structures but without determining their exact shape. Thus, we used Bayesian object recognition to generate markers required to form a topographic map for a watershed method. The effectiveness of the proposed approach was examined using artificially generated images and real cytological images of breast cancer. Tests carried out have shown that the proposed version of the marked-controlled watershed can be used with success to segment elliptic-shaped objects.

Keywords: Stochastic geometry · Watershed segmentation
Nuclei segmentation · Breast cancer

1 Introduction

Cancer diagnosis very often requires direct intervention in diseased tissue in order to collect diagnostic material. Next, pathomorphologists analyze visually collected material under a microscope, Unfortunately, interventions in tissue always carry a certain risk to a patient, which grows if the intervention is larger. Therefore, reducing the size of medical interventions reduces the risk of post-surgery complications. Fine-needle biopsy method is one of the best regarding

© Springer International Publishing AG, part of Springer Nature 2019
E. Pietka et al. (Eds.): ITIB 2018, AISC 762, pp. 407–418, 2019.
https://doi.org/10.1007/978-3-319-91211-0_36

low invasiveness. Due to the lack of the possibility of direct visual control over the course of the biological material extraction process, a imaging method (e.g. ultrasonography, radiography) is used during a fine needle biopsy. Another essential stage of sample preparation is fixing and staining of biological material. The resulting glass slide is then scanned and stored as a digital image.

Breast cancer diagnosis is mainly based on analysis of cell nuclei morphometric and topological features. Thus, automatic detection and segmentation of nuclei is a crucial issue in computer-assisted image analysis cytology [5]. A number of scientific centers conduct an intensive research to develop accurate algorithms to object segmentation [2–4,12,18]. The most common approaches are primarily based on intensity thresholding, deep learning, watershed transform, region growing, deformable models and morphological mathematics.

For cytological images, we first subject them to deconvolution to determine for each pixel the amount of deposited hematoxylin (this dye is deposited mainly in the cell nuclei). Next, hematoxylin intensity image is binarized using thresholding method. The segmentation of the image into two regions makes it possible to distinguish cell nuclei from a background, cytoplasm and red blood cells.

Nuclei have tendency to clump and overlap each other. However, to determine their morphometric features, they must be separated. Intensity thresholding is usually ineffective if nuclei create clusters. To deal with this problem, we can use the watershed method to separate overlapping or touching nuclei [10,16,19]. Unfortunately, the method suffers from the problem of over-segmentation. It usually generates an excess number of objects [19]. To overcome this problem the marker-controlled watershed was proposed [16,19]. The method to work requires the approximate centers of prospective objects. They are used to modify the topographic surface of watershed to prevent over-segmentations. The effectiveness of this approach is strongly dependent on the accuracy of markers. Unfortunately, finding the markers of nuclei is not much simpler than the segmentation of the nuclei itself. To deal with this problem, we are proposing Bayesian object recognition approach to estimate the actual underlying object configuration by the configuration of prototype objects [6]. To simplify the problem, we are assuming that nuclei can be approximated precisely enough by circles of various sizes. Then we are searching for the configuration of circles that describes the best the silhouette of nuclei region. For this purpose, we use the Iterated Conditional Modes algorithm for a marked point process. The marked point process is constructed in such a way that it prefers to generate a configuration of circles consistent with the analyzed image. Resulting circle configuration is then combined with the original topographic map to improve the segmentation results of watershed.

To verify the effectiveness of the proposed segmentation method, it was applied to segment artificially generated overlapping disks and then to segment nuclei in cytological images of breast cancer. We compared our approach with the manual segmentation and with classical watershed transform. The obtained results indicate that proposed approach outperforms classical watershed in nuclei segmentation.

The rest of this paper is organized as follows. Section 2 presents materials used for the experiment. Section 3 describes the approaches used in experiment. Section 3 have the three sub-sections describing image preprocessing, Bayesian object recognition and watershed segmentation. Then there is a Sect. 4 with results and finally conclusions in Sect. 5.

2   Materials

We have prepared two types of test images to verify the accuracy of proposed nuclei segmentation algorithm. One set contains artificially generated images of disks and the other a real images of cell nuclei.

In the preliminary studies, we used artificially generated images of touching or overlapping disks. Nine different disk configurations composed of 2, 3 and 4 disks with various overlapping ratios were generated (see Fig. 3). Values of pixel intensities are generated randomly with normal distributions. Foreground pixels (disks) have lower mean value than background pixels, thus disks are darker than background.

The second test set consist of 10 cytological images of breast cancer. Cellular material for these images was collected at the University Hospital in Zielona Góra, Poland from patients with benign and malignant lesions. It was acquired from affected breast tissue using 0.5-mm- diameter needle under the control of an ultrasonograph. Next, the material was fixed with Cellfix (Shadon) fixative spray and dyed with hematoxylin and eosin. Cytological preparations were digitized into virtual slides using the Olympus VS120 Virtual Microscopy System. Ten fragments of these slides (size 500×500 pixels) selected by pathologists were used to carry out segmentation experiments (see Fig. 4).

3   Method

3.1   Image Preprocessing

Cell nuclei are crucial diagnostic objects in cytology. Therefore, it seems to desirable to preprocess the image to filter out cytoplasm and red blood cells and leave nuclei. The cellular material is dyed with hematoxylin and eosin. Hematoxylin is mainly absorbed by nuclei and eosin by cytoplasm. As the result, nuclei have blue color and cytoplasm is red. However nuclei structures also deposite eosin to some extent. Absorption spectra of hematoxylin and eosin overlap in RGB space, but color deconvolution allows us to some extent evaluate the contribution of hematoxylin and eosin at each pixel [14]. Three separate intensity images are created as a result of deconvolution, the first represents the hematoxylin density, second eosin density, and third residuals. For further processing, we are using images of hematoxylin density. They emphasize nuclei and suppress cytoplasm and red blood cells which absorbs mainly eosin (see Fig. 1).

Next step is carried out to determine binary mask of hematoxylin area. Hematoxylin density image is subjected to intensity thresholding using Otsu

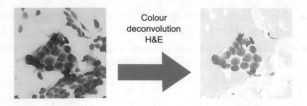

Fig. 1. Example of colour deconvolution

method [9]. As a result, we obtain binary mask which indicates where nuclei are located. Unfortunately, such binarization often leads to the creation of artifacts. These artifacts take the form of tiny objects that are not nuclei, huge objects that often represents nuclei clusters and holes in objects.

To deal with these problems we annotated manually 4500 nuclei to determine their area distribution. Based on this knowledge, we can conclude that typical nuclei have area in the range from 500 to 4000 pixels. Thus, we decided to eliminate from further processing small objects with the area lower than 300 pixels. Moreover, we filled all holes of the size lower than 50 pixels. Such modified nuclei mask was subjected to euclidean distance transform to determine topographic map for watershed algorithm. Next, classical watershed was applied to pre-segment image (see Sect. 3.3).

3.2 Bayesian Circle Recognition

Bayesian object recognition approach is applied to extract markers for watershed. The task boils down to find the configuration of circles $\mathbf{x} = \{x_1, \ldots, x_n\}$ varying in size, location, and orientation which approximates real nuclei. Silhouettes of circles must cover appropriately the mask $\mathbf{y}$ determined by intensity thresholding (see Fig. 2). There are a lot of good circle configurations $\mathbf{x}$ whose coverage of binary mask $\mathbf{y}$ are equivalent. Therefore, unknown configuration cannot be determined with certainty but rather described probabilistically by marked point process [7,8]. We need to find such a marked point process that will promote configurations coherent with the binary mask of objects and will allow to control the number of overlapping circles. So the crucial element necessary to reconstruct the silhouette of binary mask $\mathbf{y}$ is the knowledge of conditional probability mass function (pmf) $p(\mathbf{x}|\mathbf{y})$ which governs such process:

$$p(\mathbf{x}|\mathbf{y}) \propto f(\mathbf{y}|\mathbf{x})p(\mathbf{x}), \tag{1}$$

where likelihood term $f(\mathbf{y}|\mathbf{x})$ evaluates the consistency of circle configuration $\mathbf{x}$ respect to binary mask $\mathbf{y}$ and a prior term $p(\mathbf{x})$ reflects constraints on pairwise interactions between circles within configuration $\mathbf{x}$ [8]:

$$p(\mathbf{x}) = \alpha\beta^{n(\mathbf{x})} \prod_{x_i \sim x_j} h(x_i, x_j), \tag{2}$$

where $\alpha, \beta > 0$ are constants, $n(\mathbf{x})$ is the number of circles in configuration $\mathbf{x}$, h is the interaction function and $\sim$ is a symmetric and reflexive relation describing circle overlaps. If we assume that variables representing mask values $y_t \in \{0, 1\}$ are conditionally independent given configuration $\mathbf{x}$ then $f(\mathbf{y}|\mathbf{x})$ takes the following form:

$$f(\mathbf{y}|\mathbf{x}) = \prod_{t \in S(x)} b(y_t; p_N) \prod_{t \in S \setminus S(x)} b(y_t; p_B), \tag{3}$$

where $b(y_t; p_N)$ and $b(y_t; p_B)$ are Bernoulli pmf's:

$$b(y_t; p_N) = \begin{cases} 1 - p_N & \text{if } y_t = 0 \\ p_N & \text{if } y_t = 1, \end{cases} \tag{4}$$

$$b(y_t; p_B) = \begin{cases} 1 - p_B & \text{if } y_t = 1 \\ p_B & \text{if } y_t = 0. \end{cases} \tag{5}$$

They are used to evaluate the likelihood of pixels on binary mask $\mathbf{y}$ within nuclei region $S(x)$:

$$S(x) = \bigcup_{i=1}^{n} S(x_i), \tag{6}$$

and background region $S \setminus S(x)$ respectively, where S is a pixel lattice of binary mask $\mathbf{y}$ and $S(x_i)$ is the silhouette of the circle x_i. Parameter p_N describe a probability of occurring actual nuclei pixel within nuclei region $S(x)$ on binary mask $\mathbf{y}$, and p_B is a probability of occurring actual background pixel within background $S \setminus S(x)$. Both parameters were chosen arbitrarily based on results of image thresholding and data from manually annotated nuclei.

Finally, Strauss process is used to implement interaction model [1,15]:

$$p(\mathbf{x}) = \alpha \beta^{m(\mathbf{x})} \gamma^{r(\mathbf{x})}, \tag{7}$$

where $\alpha, \beta, \gamma > 0$ are constants, $m(x)$ is the number of circles in configuration and $r(\mathbf{x})$ is the number of pairwise overlaps in configuration $\mathbf{x}$. For $0 < \gamma < 1$, model exhibits repulsive forces between circles and this prevent an excessive number of overlaps in circle configurations. Finding proper configuration of circles boils down to optimization problem where Ω is a set of all possible configurations $\mathbf{x}$. To solve the problem of nuclei segmentation, we must find in Ω a configuration $\mathbf{x}$ that fits the image best without contravene a prior interaction constraints. In Bayesian framework this problem can be viewed as a maximum a posterior estimation problem [7,8]:

$$\hat{\mathbf{x}} = \arg\max_{\mathbf{x}} f(\mathbf{y}|\mathbf{x}) p(\mathbf{x}). \tag{8}$$

Unfortunately, direct sampling from $f(\mathbf{y}|\mathbf{x})$ and $p(\mathbf{x})$ is not straightforward. But, the problem becomes much more tractable if we deal with the following proportion [8]:

$$w = \ln\left(\frac{f(\mathbf{y}|\mathbf{x}_{k+1})p(\mathbf{x}_{k+1})}{f(\mathbf{y}|\mathbf{x}_k)p(\mathbf{x}_k)}\right)$$

$$= \sum_{t \in S_N}\Big(\ln\big(b(y_t; p_N)\big) - \ln\big(b(y_t; p_B)\big)\Big) \tag{9}$$

$$+ \ln\big(\gamma\big)\big(r(\mathbf{x}_{k+1}) - r(\mathbf{x}_k)\big) + \ln\big(\beta\big),$$

where $\mathbf{x}_k$ is the current configuration, $\mathbf{x}_{k+1}$ is the new prospective configuration and $S_N = \big(S(\mathbf{x}_{k+1}) \cup S(\mathbf{x}_k)\big) \setminus \big(S(\mathbf{x}_{k+1}) \cap S(\mathbf{x}_k)\big)$. If we limit the ways the new configurations $\mathbf{x}_{k+1}$ can emerge by allowing only to add single circle u or delete single circle u from the current configuration $\mathbf{x}_k$ then it becomes possible to apply steepest ascent procedure to find the local maximum. Algorithm is always choosing new configuration $\mathbf{x}_{k+1}$ to maximize proportion w. Therefore, probability never decreases at any stage and eventual convergence is guaranteed. However, algorithm usually stuck in nearest local maxima. The pseudocode of this procedure is presented as Algorithm 1.

Initialization: $\mathbf{x}_0 = \emptyset$;
for $i = 0, 1, \ldots$ **do**
  for *All* u **do**
    if $u \notin \mathbf{x}_k$ **then**
      $\mathbf{x}_{k+1} = \mathbf{x}_k \cup u$;
      $w(u) = \ln\left(\frac{f(\mathbf{y}|\mathbf{x}_{k+1})p(\mathbf{x}_{k+1})}{f(\mathbf{y}|\mathbf{x}_k)p(\mathbf{x}_k)}\right)$;
    else if $u \in \mathbf{x}_k$ **then**
      $\mathbf{x}_{k+1} = \mathbf{x}_k \setminus u$;
      $w(u) = \ln\left(\frac{f(\mathbf{y}|\mathbf{x}_{k+1})p(\mathbf{x}_{k+1})}{f(\mathbf{y}|\mathbf{x}_k)p(\mathbf{x}_k)}\right)$;
  end
  find circle u_{max} which maximizes $w(u)$;
  if $w(u) > 0$ **then**
    if $u_{max} \notin \mathbf{x}_k$ **then**
      $\mathbf{x}_{k+1} = \mathbf{x}_k \cup u_{max}$;
    else if $u_{max} \in \mathbf{x}_k$ **then**
      $\mathbf{x}_{k+1} = \mathbf{x}_k \setminus u_{max}$;
  else
    Return $\mathbf{x}_k$;
end

Algorithm 1. Steepest Ascent circle detection algorithm

3.3 Marker-Controlled Watershed

The classical watershed transform treats the image to be segmented as topographic surface I_{TM}. It segments image by flooding basins from the seeds until basins attributed to different seeds meet on watershed lines. The input of the algorithm is usually a binary mask of the image. It is transformed by the Euclidean distance transform and local maxima from this transform are used as seeds of watershed transform. Unfortunately, algorithm in this form tend to create many micro-segments [19]. To deal with this problem we used modified version of watershed that uses nuclei seeds generated by Bayesian object recognition algorithm to revise topographic map I_{TM}.

The prototype of topographic map is determined by Euclidean distance transform applied to binary mask $\mathbf{y}$ obtained after preprocessing (see Sect. 3.1). Objects determined by classical watershed are classified to be nuclei or not based on known distributions of area, roundness, and ellipticity of nuclei. Objects assessed as not-nuclei are usually clumps of nuclei. To separate them, we are using marker-controlled watershed. Necessary markers take the form of circles generated by procedure described in Sect. 3.2. Topographic map I_{TM} is modified by discovered circles to prevent over-segmentation and to allow to separate clumped nuclei.

Two different strategies of generating modified topographic map are proposed. The first method generates markers based on circle centers. It places small disks of radius 5 pixels in circle centers. Resulting markers J_1 are combined with the original topographic map I_{TM} by morphological reconstruction $\rho_{I_{TM}}(J_1)$ [17]. The algorithm is based on repeated dilations of a marker mask J_1 until the contour of the marker mask fits under a topographic map determined by the Euclidean distance transform:

$$I'_{TM} = \rho_{I_{TM}}(J_1) = \bigcup_{n \geq 1} \delta^{(n)}_{I_{TM}}(J_1). \tag{10}$$

The grayscale geodesic dilation of size n is then given by:

$$\delta^{(n)}_{I_{TM}}(J_1) = \underbrace{\delta_{I_{TM}}(\ldots \delta_{I_{TM}}(\delta_{I_{TM}}(J_1)))}_{n}, \tag{11}$$

and the elementary geodesic dilation is described by the following relationship:

$$\delta_{I_{TM}}(J_1) = (J_1 \oplus B) \cap I_{TM}, \tag{12}$$

where $(J_1 \oplus B)$ is a standard dilation of size one followed by an intersection (pointwise minimum $\cap$) and B is 4-connected neighborhood structural element with pair of horizontal and vertical connected pixels.

The second method uses whole circles as nuclei markers J_2. It applies a Euclidean distance transform for each circle. As a result we get a set of topographic maps $\{I^1_{TMC}, \ldots, I^n_{TMC}\}$. They are merged into single map by summing all maps: $I_{TMC} = I^1_{TMC} + \ldots + I^n_{TMC}$. Final topographic map used by watershed is given by $I'_{TM} = I_{TM} + I_{TMC}$.

Nuclei properly pre-segmented by classical watershed are not processed by marker-controlled watershed but are stored to include them in the final segmentation. Thus, we need initially to classify segmented objects into two classes, nuclei, and objects that do not resemble nuclei (i.e. clumped nuclei). We did this based on the area, roundness and ellipticity of segmented objects [11, 13]:

$$Roundness = \frac{4A}{\pi d^2_{max}}, \quad Ellipticity = \frac{A}{\pi \frac{d_{max}}{2} \frac{d_{min}}{2}}, \tag{13}$$

where A is the area of the object, d_{max} is the longest diagonal of the object and d_{min} is the shortest diagonal of the object. Object was recognized as single nucleus if its area was within 500 to 4000 pixels, roundness was over 0.7 and ellipticity was over 0.95. All thresholds were determined experimentally based on the set of manually segmented nuclei. All objects that meet these criteria are immediately classified as nuclei and they do not require further processing (see Fig. 2). The rest of the objects that do not meet the requirements of being single nucleus is subjected to a separation procedure by marker-controlled watershed. The final segmentation is obtained by combining results generated during both procedures (see Fig. 2).

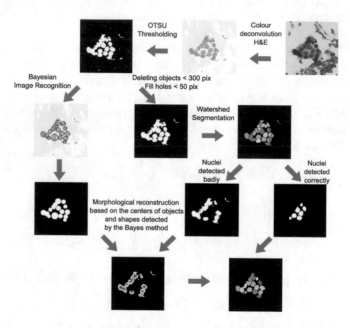

Fig. 2. Segmentation scheme – proposed method

4   Results

In order to verify the accuracy of the proposed nuclei segmentation procedure, it was applied to segment circular objects in artificially generated test images and to segment nuclei in real cytological images of breast cancer.

Preliminary experiments were conducted using artificially generated image of overlapping or touching disks. Image contains 9 different configurations of disks and have the size of 500×500 pixels. All disks have the same size determined by radii equal to 30 pixels. The intensities of background and foreground pixels were generated randomly using normal distributions: $\mathcal{N}(0.40, 0.05)$ and $\mathcal{N}(0.70, 0.05)$ respectively. The image was segmented using 3 methods: classical watershed, marker-controlled watershed with markers as circle centers and marker-controlled watershed with markers as whole circles. Each circle is described by its position and radii $r \in [15, \ldots, 35]$. The other parameters that must be defined for the Bayesian object recognition method are β and γ. As a result of the experiments, it was found that the highest accuracy was obtained for $\ln(\beta) = -600$, and $\ln(\gamma) = -700$.

In order to compare the segmentation results obtained for artificially generated test image please see Fig. 3.

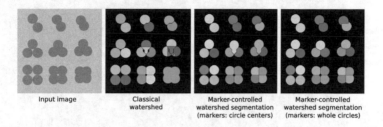

| Input image | Classical watershed | Marker-controlled watershed segmentation (markers: circle centers) | Marker-controlled watershed segmentation (markers: whole circles) |

Fig. 3. Segmentation results for a synthetic image

We can observe that the segmentation of configurations with two disks is satisfactory for all methods. They were able to segment correctly even strongly overlapping disks. In the case of 3 disks, classical watershed get correct segmentation only for the configuration with touching disks. For configurations with overlapping disks, it failed to segment them correctly. Both marker-controlled watershed methods segmented configurations with 3 disks correctly, however the method based on markers defined as the circle centers suffered from some problems with region leaks. Thus the best result was obtained by the marker-controlled watershed based on markers defined as circles. In the case of 4 disks, all methods generated correct results for touching disks and for slightly overlapping disks. For the configuration with strongly overlapping disks, classical watershed utterly failed to separate disks. Marker-controlled watershed methods had no problem even with a strongly overlapping scenario.

Satisfactory results of experiments carried out on artificially generated image allowed us to proceed to the second stage of experiment. This time, the task was to segment real nuclei. Experiment was repeated for 10 images. The results are presented in Fig. 4. Visual inspection of results allows us to state that the obtained results are satisfactory. Moreover, we can observe that marker-controlled watershed with markers as circles usually outperforms the segmentation with markers as circle centers.

The segmentation results obtained in the experiment were compared with manually annotated nuclei. In order to evaluate the results of the experiment quantitatively, two metrics were used: Jaccard distance and Hausdorff distance. Two distance matrices were determined using chosen metrics. They were storing distances between manually segmented nuclei and nuclei segmented automatically. For each manually segmented nucleus, the closest automatically

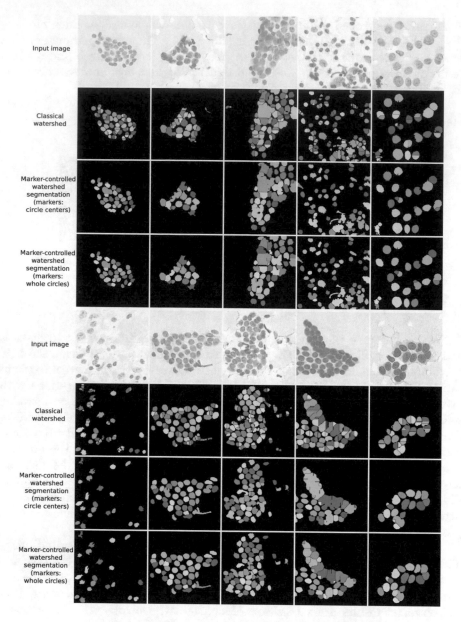

Fig. 4. Segmentation results for a cytology images

segmented object is determined and as a result we get a list of reference nuclei paired with automatically segmented nuclei. Having a set of these distances, we can compute for each image the mean distance (Jaccard and Hausdorff) and standard deviation of distances. Summary results and detailed results of individual

Table 1. The accuracy of nuclei segmentation

No	Hausdorff distance						Jaccard distance					
	Classical	Markers					Classical	Markers				
	Watershed	Circle centers		Whole circles			Watershed	Circle centers		Whole circles		
	Mean	Std	Mean	Std	Mean	Std	Mean	Std	Mean	Std	Mean	Std
1	16	9	7	6	**6**	**4**	0.51	0.27	0.24	0.12	**0.23**	**0.11**
2	29	27	16	12	**13**	**9**	0.61	0.28	0.37	0.24	**0.34**	**0.18**
3	26	**18**	21	23	**19**	19	0.62	0.28	**0.39**	0.26	0.40	**0.24**
4	30	27	**14**	24	14	**23**	0.65	0.28	**0.30**	**0.22**	0.32	0.23
5	28	24	13	14	**11**	**12**	0.51	0.32	0.26	0.27	**0.22**	**0.22**
6	22	15	**8**	**7**	8	7	0.64	0.31	**0.30**	**0.20**	0.30	0.20
7	23	27	8	14	**8**	**12**	0.49	0.32	**0.19**	0.13	**0.19**	**0.12**
8	21	17	11	10	**11**	**9**	0.54	0.29	**0.27**	0.17	**0.27**	**0.16**
9	26	**18**	25	27	**23**	24	0.62	**0.28**	0.51	0.34	**0.43**	0.31
10	32	19	14	14	**12**	**11**	0.60	0.27	0.24	0.26	**0.20**	**0.18**
All	25	20	14	15	**12**	**13**	0.58	0.29	0.31	0.22	**0.29**	**0.19**

images are presented in Table 1. They indicate that the method based on markers defined as circles is the most accurate.

5 Conclusions

The novelty of the proposed approach is the application of the stochastic geometry as a tool to generate markers for the marker-controlled watershed method. The results indicate that proposed approach eliminates over-segmentation generated by the classical watershed method. Bayesian object recognition was employed to approximate the location and size of nuclei using circles. Finally the application of the watershed transform allows to determine precise edges of nuclei. Both methods complement each other creating a very good tool for segmentation of cytological images. The experiments carried out have shown that the method performs well even for overlapped nuclei. In the future work, we plan to expand the number of examined cytological images and check the diagnostic effectiveness of the method in the malignancy classification.

Acknowledgement. The research was supported by National Science Centre, Poland (2015/17/B/ST7/03704).

References

1. Baddeley, A.J., van Lieshout, M.N.M.: Stochastic geometry models in high-level vision. In: Mardia, K.V., Kanji, G.K. (eds.) Advances in Applied Statistics, Statistics and Images: 1, pp. 231–256. Carfax Publishing, Abingdon (1993)
2. Bembenik, R., Jóźwicki, W., Protaziuk, G.: Methods for mining co-location patterns with extended spatial objects. Int. J. Appl. Math. Comput. Sci. **27**(4), 681–695 (2017)
3. Gdawiec, K.: Procedural generation of aesthetic patterns from dynamics and iteration processes. Int. J. Appl. Math. Comput. Sci. **27**(4), 827–837 (2017)
4. Kłeczek, P., Dyduch, G., Jaworek-Korjakowska, J., Tadeusiewicz, R.: Automated epidermis segmentation in histopathological images of human skin stained with hematoxylin and eosin. Proc. SPIE **10140**, 10,140:1–10,140:19 (2017)
5. Kowal, M., Filipczuk, P.: Nuclei segmentation for computer-aided diagnosis of breast cancer. Int. J. Appl. Math. Comput. Sci. **24**(1), 19–31 (2014)
6. Kowal, M., Korbicz, J.: Marked Point Process for Nuclei Detection in Breast Cancer Microscopic Images, pp. 230–241. Springer, Cham (2018)
7. van Lieshout, M.C.: A Bayesian approach to object recognition, pp. 185–190 (1991)
8. van Lieshout, M.N.M.: Markov point processes and their applications in high-level imaging. Bull. Int. Stat. Inst. **56**, 559–576 (1995)
9. Otsu, N.: A threshold selection method from gray-level histograms. IEEE Trans. Syst. Man Cybern. **9**(1), 62–66 (1979)
10. Paramanandam, M., O'Byrne, M., Ghosh, B., Mammen, J.J., Manipadam, M.T., Thamburaj, R., Pakrashi, V.: Automated segmentation of nuclei in breast cancer histopathology images. PLOS ONE **11**(9), 1–15 (2016)
11. Pentland, A.: A method of measuring the angularity of sands. Proc. Trans. R. Soc. Can. **21**(3), 43 (1927)
12. Piorkowski, A.: A statistical dominance algorithm for edge detection and segmentation of medical images. In: Information Technologies in Medicine. Advances in Intelligent Systems and Computing, vol. 471, pp. 3–14. Springer (2016)
13. Ritter, N., Cooper, J.: New resolution independent measures of circularity. J. Math. Imaging Vis. **35**(2), 117–127 (2009)
14. Ruifrok, A.C., Johnston, D.A.: Quantification of histochemical staining by color deconvolution. Anal. Quant. Cytol. Histol. **23**(4), 291–299 (2001)
15. Strauss, D.J.: A model for clustering. Biometrika **62**(2), 467–475 (1975)
16. Veta, M., Huisman, A., Viergever, M.A., van Diest, P.J., Pluim, J.P.W.: Marker-controlled watershed segmentation of nuclei in H&E stained breast cancer biopsy images. In: 2011 IEEE International Symposium on Biomedical Imaging: From Nano to Macro, pp. 618–621 (2011)
17. Vincent, L.: Morphological grayscale reconstruction in image analysis: applications and efficient algorithms. IEEE Trans. Image Process. **2**(2), 176–201 (1993)
18. Więcławek, W., Piętka, E.: Watershed based intelligent scissors. Comput. Med. Imaging Graph. **43**, 122–129 (2015)
19. Yang, X., Li, H., Zhou, X.: Nuclei segmentation using marker-controlled watershed, tracking using mean-shift, and Kalman filter in time-lapse microscopy. IEEE Trans. Circuits Syst. I Regular Papers **53**(11), 2405–2414 (2006)

Bioinformatic Tools for Genotyping of Klebsiella pneumoniae Isolates

Marketa Nykrynova[1(✉)], Denisa Maderankova[1], Matej Bezdicek[2], Martina Lengerova[2], and Helena Skutkova[1]

[1] Department of Biomedical Engineering, Brno University of Technology, Technicka 12, 616 00 Brno, Czech Republic
m.nykrynova@gmail.com
[2] Department of Internal Medicine – Hematology and Oncology, University Hospital Brno, Brno, Czech Republic

Abstract. Nowadays we use multiple molecular typing methods capable of distinguishing bacteria strains. However, a majority of these methods are time-consuming, and associated costs are not negligible. Also, reproducibility of typing results is questionable. Therefore, we propose new typing methodology based on bioinformatics. In this paper, we present an algorithm that is at the core of the new method. It consists of multiple steps, such as measuring the quality of input data, identification of genes having high diversity and analysis of results employing clustering and phylogenetic trees. Obtained results are then compared with results from the mini-MLST method.

Keywords: Genotyping · *Klebsiella pneumoniae* · Genes
Bacterial strains · Mini-MLST

1 Introduction

Typing of bacteria is important in the process of identifying relationships between microbial isolates. Finding the relation between different bacteria strains is crucial to understand outbreaks, and it helps us to track infection source and its routes [1]. It is also necessary for detection of the cross-transmission of nosocomial pathogens, its diagnosis, and treatment [2].

In the past bacteria typing was based on phenotypic and genotypic methods, but nowadays the genotypic methods are used more often because phenotypic methods cannot discriminate between closely related strains. So genotypic methods come to the fore due to their high-resolution [3]. Current typing methods can be divided into three groups: the first one are DNA methods which are based on banding patterns obtained from electrophoresis, which means that they can distinguish between different bacteria strains according to the size of DNA bands. The second group are methods based on sequencing that are able to determine strains from polymorphisms in DNA, and the last one are methods based on hybridization which rely on DNA hybridization with probes of known sequences [4].

© Springer International Publishing AG, part of Springer Nature 2019
E. Pietka et al. (Eds.): ITIB 2018, AISC 762, pp. 419–428, 2019.
https://doi.org/10.1007/978-3-319-91211-0_37

The typing methods should meet some basic requirements. They should be usable for all organisms within a species. They must have high discriminatory power and be able to distinguish between different bacterial strains. At last, they should have high reproducibility [1].

All typing methods have their strength and weaknesses, so the method selection depends on the goals of our analysis. The wet-lab typing methods are quite expensive, time-consuming and often they lack reproducibility. We propose a new typing methodology based on bioinformatic tools.

1.1 *Klebsiella pneumoniae*

Klebsiella pneumoniae is gram-negative bacteria with polysaccharide capsule which encases the whole cell and provides resistance against many host defense mechanisms [5]. This bacterium can be found in soil, water and on the surface of plants. Some strains cause hospital-acquired infections especially to patients with weakened immune system and they can spread very fast and lead to nosocomial outbreaks. It can cause pneumoniae, urinary tract infection or even sepsis when it enters the bloodstream, so it can lead to life-threatening infection [6]. In *Klebsiella's* genome, we can find many antibiotic resistance genes which protect the bacteria from antibiotic use [7].

1.2 Molecular Typing Methods

Pulsed-field electrophoresis is considered as a gold standard in molecular typing methods [1]. It has high discriminatory power, it is relatively cheap and reproducible [8]. A DNA molecule is cut with restriction enzymes and obtained fragments are separated on agarose gel by electrophoresis. During the electrophoresis, the orientation of electric field is changed in predefined time slots. After that, the gel is dyed with fluorescent pigment and is then projected with ultraviolet light. Next, we proceed to the analysis of obtained data [9]. Main disadvantages of pulsed-field electrophoresis are technical complexity, time demands as well as low discriminatory power for bands with almost same length [8].

Another typing method is the random amplification of polymorphic DNA (RAPD), and it is based on using random primers (about 10 bases) which hybridize with DNA while the annealing temperature is quite low. Primers are used to amplify selected parts of DNA. Fragments are then separated by agarose-electrophoresis, and obtained banding patterns are used to identify particular bacteria strains [2,8]. Because the method can be performed relatively quickly and due to the low price of RAPD analysis we see it often used during outbreaks. Unfortunately, it has low reproducibility [8].

Restriction fragment length polymorphism analysis is one of the first typing methods in widespread use. DNA is cleaved by often used restriction enzymes, so it produces a huge number of fragments which are then separated by electrophoresis and transferred by Southern blotting to a nylon membrane. DNA is attached to the membrane and hybridized with labeled probes which are homologous to gene we want to determine. Then we visualize and process our data [2].

The main advantage of this method is a good resolution capability, low price, quick turnaround time and it can be used for unknown samples. Same as previous method, low reproducibility is an issue [10].

Among typing methods, we also find repetitive PCR which uses primers that hybridize to noncoding intergenic repetitive sequences. DNA which lies between two repetitive elements is then amplified by PCR. Obtained fragments are separated by electrophoresis and banding patterns are then analyzed. The method is quick, easy to perform, it has high discriminatory power and can be used for a large or small number of isolates. The main disadvantage is low reproducibility [8]. To counter problems with reproducibility semiautomated rep-PCR commercial system was developed which use microfluid chip for fragments separation instead of electrophoresis [2].

Amplified fragment length polymorphism (AFLP) method is based on amplification of fragments which result from digestive DNA by restriction enzymes [1]. There are two variants of AFLP. In the first one we use two restriction enzymes and two primers, and in the second one, we use only one primer and restriction enzyme [3]. After DNA is cut with restriction enzymes, then the ends of cut parts are ligated with adaptors. Fragments with adaptors are amplified by PCR using primers which are complementary to adaptors. If we use primers which are dye by fluorescent color, then after separation we can use a sequencer to analyze samples [8]. AFLP has high discriminatory power and reproducibility [1] but it's also expensive and we need DNA samples of high-quality [2].

Variable-number tandem repeat typing is based on PCR where we amplify fragments which include short tandem repeat sequence. Fragments are then separated by electrophoresis and number of repetitive elements in amplicon is determined. The difference in number of repetitive copies on a specific spot is used to distinguish between bacterial strains [2]. The method is cheap and fast but obtained data can't be compared between labs because of low reproducibility [8].

Multilocus sequence typing (MLST) is based on amplification of mainly seven housekeeping genes. For chosen genes, the sequence about 450–500 bp is identified and sequenced [4]. To unique alleles are randomly assigned numbers. So, to each strain is assigned a seven-number allelic profile which is called sequence type [8]. The sequence type is comparable between each other to determine a relation between observed isolates [11]. The main advantage is that obtained data are unambiguous because of standardized nomenclature [8]. To disadvantages belong high prize, time demands and low discriminatory power for some pathogens [4].

Mini-MLST is derived from multilocus sequence typing and it consists of two parts. The first part is the same as in MLST, so chosen genes are also amplified by PCR, but in the second part the sequencing is replaced by high-resolution melt (HRM) analysis. Genes with high diversity are chosen for MLST, and suitable primers are then designed. After amplification of genes, the HRM analysis takes part [12]. DNA is dye with fluorescent color. During analysis, we raise the temperature so that DNA melts, and the color is loosening from DNA. As a consequence, there is a decrease in fluorescent that we measure.

We obtain melting curves and when 50% of DNA is denatured, we get melting temperature [13]. Then we use conversion key to translate Minim data into MelT profiles and also to compare data with MLST database. An advantage of the method is its price which is approximately 10–20% of MLST [14].

2 Materials and Methods

2.1 Data Validation

As a first step, the data from DNA sequencer need to be validated. Genomes were sequenced by Illumina sequencer, and we obtained paired-end reads as a result of sequencing. FastQC was used for quality controls of sequence data. Then MultiQC [15] was applied to gather obtained results into a single report. Using these two pieces of software all 12 genomes of *Klebsiella pneumoniae* were examined.

2.2 Genome Assembly

The next step after data verification is genome assembly. Burrows-Wheeler Aligner (BWA) [16] was used to assemble each genome. Reads were mapped against reference genome which is *Klebsiella pneumoniae subsp. pneumoniae HS11286*. Reference genome was acquired from NCBI database. As a first step in the assembly process, our reference sequence was set. Then paired-end reads were separately aligned. We gathered BWA output in SAM format.

In the next step samtools [17] was used to create BAM file and also to remove unmapped reads. Then our data were sorted, and an index of the BAM file was created. Now it is possible to visualize gathered data, e.g. Tablet software can be used to do a quick visual check of the assembly.

From our assembled data consensus sequence was created using samtools, bcftools and vcfutils, and this process was repeated for every genome. After that, we have 12 sequences for all genomes in FASTA format.

2.3 BLAST

We searched five allele templates (http://bigsdb.pasteur.fr/klebsiella/primers_used.html) of genes *infB, mdh, phoE, rpoB tonB*. These genes were founded in our 12 genomes using BLAST software. Then found genes are aligned.

2.4 Phylogenetic Analysis

For each genome a sequence that contains aforementioned genes one after the other was created. Obtained sequences are aligned, and for each couple of sequences, the proportional distance is calculated. A distance matrix is created from that data.

Evolution distances were calculated using Kimura model of evolution, where distances d are calculated as

$$d = -\frac{1}{2}\ln\left(1 - 2P - Q\right) - \frac{1}{4}\ln\left(1 - 2Q\right), \tag{1}$$

where P is number of nucleotides which change as a result of transition and Q as a result of transversion.

From obtained matrix which contains biological distances between pairs of sequences was constructed the phylogenetic tree using neighbor-joining method.

2.5   Cluster Analysis

For each gene and every genome, the melting temperature was calculated using website www.endmemo.com/bio/tm.php. DNA concentration was set at 200 nM, salt concentration was set at 0 mM and Mg^{2+} concentration was set at 2.5 mM.

For each pair of genomes, the distance d_{st} was calculated using Euclidean metric as:

$$d_{st}^2 = (x_s - x_t)(x_s - x_t), \tag{2}$$

where x_s and x_t are two different melting temperatures.

Then the average distance d between all pairs of objects in any two clusters was calculated as

$$d(r, s) = \frac{1}{n_r n_s} \sum_{i=1}^{n_r} \sum_{j=1}^{n_s} dist(x_{ri}, x_{sj}), \tag{3}$$

where r and s are clusters, n_r and n_s are the numbers of objects in clusters r and s and $x_r l$ or $x_s j$ is ith or jth object in cluster r or in cluster s. We used the unweighted average distance (UPGMA) to distinguish between the clusters.

As a result, we got agglomerative hierarchical cluster tree.

3   Results

We worked with 12 genomes of *Klebsiella pneumoniae* and for each one of them, the melt type was determined by mini-MLST. Genomes S13–S18 were established as one melt type and genomes S19–S24 were determined as a second melt type as we can see in Table 1.

Genotyping methods are used as distinguishing between bacterial strains using phenotypes is almost impossible due to similarities and also profiles of antibiotic resistance are identical.

For typing, 5 genes were used: *infB, mdh, phoE, rpoB* and *tonB*. Their lengths and gene products are shown in Table 2.

In the Fig. 1 we can see the comparison of 12 genomes using 5 genes. Each gene is bounded by black lines. Genes are compared to allele templates, where percentage shows match to the reference sequence. Next to the percentage value

Table 1. Genomes and their melt types

Genome	Melt type 6MelT	Genome	Melt type 6MelT
S13	23	S19	61
S14	23	S20	61
S15	23	S21	61
S16	23	S22	61
S17	23	S23	61
S18	23	S24	61

Table 2. Genes used for typing

Gene	Length [bp]	Protein
infB	318	Translation initiation factor IF-2
mdh	477	Malate dehydrogenase
phoE	420	Outer membrane pore protein E
rpoB	501	DNA-directed RNA polymerase subunit beta
tonB	414	Protein TonB

in the bracket is a number of nucleotides changes against allele templates. Graph was created by BRIG application [18].

As is depicted only one nucleotide of gene *infB* is changed in first melt type. If we examine gene *mdh* we can find out that genomes S13–S18 have only one nucleotide change and on the other hand remaining genomes have two changes. For example, *phoE* has a lot of mutations in first melt type while second melt is almost same as allele templates. First melt type has the same number of nucleotide changes in gene *tonB* and *rpoB* as a second melt type.

Founded genes were aligned using multiple sequence alignment. Example of alignment of the part of gene *phoE* is depicted in Fig. 2.

In the picture, we can see single nucleotide variations which are used for bacterial typing. For example, there are two different nucleotides on position 354, thymine for genomes S13–S18 which belong to one melt type and cytosine for genomes S19–S24 which are known as a second melt type.

Phylogenetic tree was obtained from phylogenetic analysis and is depicted in Fig. 3.

As we can see, there are two main branches, which correspond to the different melt types. Genomes S13–S18 are part of one type, and genomes S19–S24 are part of a second type.

Using aforementioned web application melting temperatures were calculated for every gene in every genome and they are shown in Table 3.

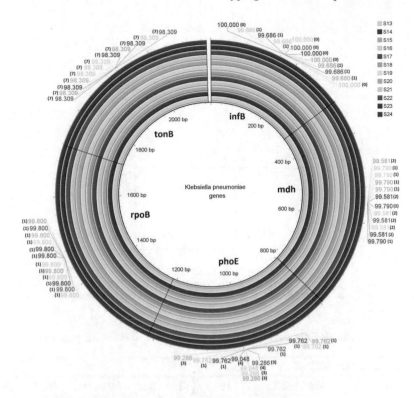

Fig. 1. Graph of selected five genes of *Klebsiella pneumoniae*

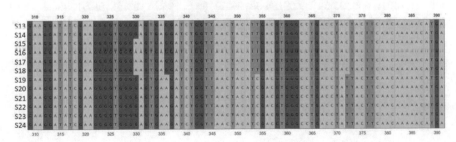

Fig. 2. A section of multialignment of gene *phoE* for 12 genomes of *Klebsiella pneumoniae*

Calculate melting temperatures were then processed by cluster analysis. The result of it is depicted in Fig. 4, where on the X axis are individual genomes and on the Y axis are Euclidean distances.

Here we can also see two well-separated clusters which belong to different melt types.

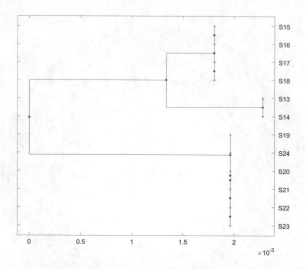

Fig. 3. Phylogenetic tree for five genes and for all genomes

Table 3. Melting temperatures for each gene and for all genomes

Melting temperatures [°C]

Genes	S13	S14	S15	S16	S17	S18	S19	S20	S21	S22	S23	S24
infB	97.03	97.03	97.03	97.03	97.03	97.03	97.13	97.13	97.13	97.13	97.13	97.13
mdh	95.59	95.59	95.59	95.59	95.59	95.59	95.51	95.51	95.51	95.51	95.51	95.51
phoE	94.92	94.92	94.89	94.89	94.89	94.89	94.88	94.88	94.88	94.88	94.88	94.88
rpoB	94.90	94.90	94.90	94.90	94.90	94.90	94.90	94.90	94.90	94.90	94.90	94.90
tonB	98.89	98.89	98.89	98.89	98.89	98.89	98.85	98.85	98.85	98.85	98.85	98.85

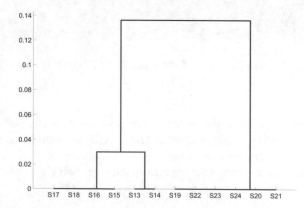

Fig. 4. Cluster analysis for melting temperatures for five genes and for all genomes

As we can see on Fig. 3 and on Fig. 4 we were also capable to distinguish between two melt types of *Klebsiella pneumoniae* using phylogenetic analysis and cluster analysis, where one group corresponds to one melt type and second group to another.

4 Conclusion

In this paper, we present a novel methodology for genotyping bacteria *Klebsiella pneumoniae* using bioinformatics methods which can distinguish among different strains of this bacteria. Because our approach is based entirely in software so the method is inexpensive to perform and fast. The only expensive part of the proposed methodology is DNA sequencing. However, the data from sequencer are usually obtained and used for more than one type of analysis, so we can use it for our purposes as well.

In contrast, contemporary methods for bacteria typing are expensive, time-consuming and they often lack reproducibility. Hence, choosing right typing method is more often than not a hard job for researchers, e.g. epidemiologist.

The results of the proposed methodology were compared to the mini-MLST-based typing method. Our software-based approach produced the results comparable to results obtained in the lab. We were also able to distinguish between two different melt types of *Klebsiella pneumoniae*. In addition, our method does not rely only on melting temperatures, but it also calculates evolution distance for phylogenetic analyses, so it is more trustworthy. Main drawback of the proposed methodology is the need to have high-quality sequence data.

Our methodology is primarily designed for genotyping *Klebsiella pneumoniae*, but in theory it can be use for genotyping *Staphylococcus aureus*, *Streptococcus pyogenes* and *Enterococcus faecium* as well as mini-MLST.

In the future our methodology can be used for genotyping during outbreaks because it can quickly deliver results of high quality.

Acknowledgement. This work was supported by grant project of the Czech Science Foundation [GACR 17-01821S].

References

1. Olive, D.M., Bean, P.: Principles and applications of methods for DNA-based typing of microbial organisms. J. Clin. Microbiol. **37**(6), 1661–1669 (1999)
2. Ranjbar, R., Karami, A., Farshad S., Giammanco G.M., Mammina C.: Typing methods used in the molecular epidemiology of microbial pathogens: a how-to guide. New Microbiologica **37**, 1–15 (2014)
3. Castro-Escarpulli, G., Alonso-Aguilar, N.M., Sanchez, G.R., et al.: Identification and typing methods for the study of bacterial infections: a brief review and mycobacterial as case of study. Arch. Clin. Microbiol. Euro Surveill. **7**, 3 (2015)
4. Li, W., Raoult, D., Fournier, P.E.: Bacterial strain typing in the genomic era. FEMS Microbiol. Rev. **33**(5), 892–916 (2009). https://doi.org/10.1111/j.1574-6976.2009.00182.x

5. Klebsiella Infections: Background, Pathophysiology. Epidemiology of Klebsiellae, Medscape (2017)
6. Klebsiella pneumoniae (ID 815) - Genome - NCBI. National Center for Biotechnology Information
7. Li, B., Zhao, Y., Liu, C., Chen, Z., Zhou, D.: Molecular pathogenesis of Klebsiella pneumoniae. Future Microbiol. **9**(9), 1071–1081 (2014). https://doi.org/10.2217/fmb.14.48
8. Sabat, A.J., Budimir, A., Nashev, D., et al.: Overview of molecular typing methods for outbreak detection and epidemiological surveillance. Eurosurveill. **18**(4), 20380 (2013)
9. He, Y., Xie, Y., Reed, S.: Pulsed-field gel electrophoresis typing of staphylococcus aureus isolates. In: Ji, Y. (ed.) Methicillin-Resistant Staphylococcus Aureus (MRSA) Protocols. Methods in Molecular Biology (Methods and Protocols), vol. 1085, pp. 103–111. Humana Press, Totowa. https://doi.org/10.1007/978-1-62703-664-1sps6
10. Tabit, F.T.: Advantages and limitations of potential methods for the analysis of bacteria in milk: a review. J. Food Sci. Technol. **53**(1), 42–49 (2016). https://doi.org/10.1007/s13197-015-1993-y
11. Maiden, M.C.J., Bygraves, J.A., Feil, E., et al.: Multilocus sequence typing: a portable approach to the identification of clones within populations of pathogenic microorganisms. Proc. Natl. Acad. Sci. USA **95**(6), 3140–3145 (1998)
12. Brhelova, E., Kocmanova, I., Racil, Z., Hanslianova, M., Antonova, M., Mayer, J., Lengerova, M.: Validation of Minim typing for fast and accurate discrimination of extended-spectrum, beta-lactamase-producing Klebsiella pneumoniae isolates in tertiary care hospital. Diagn. Microbiol. Infect. Dis. **86**(1), 44–49 (2016). https://doi.org/10.1016/j.diagmicrobio.2016.03.010
13. Tong, S.Y.C., Giffard, P.M.: Microbiological applications of high-resolution melting analysis. J. Clin. Microbiol. **50**(11), 3418–3421 (2012). https://doi.org/10.1128/JCM.01709-12
14. Andersson, P., Tong, S.Y.C., Bell, J.M., Turnidge, J.D., Giffard, P.M., Mokrousov I.: Minim typing – a rapid and low cost MLST based typing tool for Klebsiella pneumoniae. PLoS One **7**(3), e33530 (2012). https://doi.org/10.1371/journal.pone.0033530
15. Ewels, P., Magnusson, M., Lundin, S., Kaller, M.: MultiQC: summarize analysis results for multiple tools and samples in a single report. Bioinformatics **32**(19), 3047–3048 (2016). https://doi.org/10.1093/bioinformatics/btw354
16. Li, H., Durbin, R.: Fast and accurate long-read alignment with Burrows-Wheeler Transform. Bioinformatics **26**, 589–595 (2010)
17. Li, H., Handsaker, B., Wysoker, A., et al.: The sequence alignment/map format and SAMtools. Bioinformatics **25**(16), 2078–2079 (2009). https://doi.org/10.1093/bioinformatics/btp352
18. Alikhan, N., Petty, N.K., Zakour, N.L.B., Beatson, S.A.: BLAST ring image generator (BRIG): simple prokaryote genome comparisons. BMC Genom. **12**(1), 1–10 (2011). https://doi.org/10.1186/1471-2164-12-402

Modelling and Simulation

Application of Reverse Engineering in the Therapy of Lower Limb Defects

Szymon Sikorski[1(✉)], Joanna Wiśniowska[1], and Adam Konik[2]

[1] Department of Biomedical Computer Systems, University of Silesia in Katowice, ul. Będzińska 39, 41-200 Sosnowiec, Poland
szymon.sikorski@us.edu.pl

[2] City Hospitals Complex in Chorzów, ul. Strzelców Bytomskich 11, 41-500 Chorzów, Poland

Abstract. In the article, the authors describe the use of reverse engineering technology (3D scanners) and image analysis methods that allow a very accurate reflection of the curvature of the foot, making it possible to choose an orthopedic insert that provides correct support points and proper distribution of loads in the foot, thereby improving the axis of the entire lower limb. The experiment was carried out on 4 patients, which underwent the following tests: computer suboscopy, X-ray (performed on 3 patients) and a 3D footprint scan process for each patient. For each case, a spatial model was generated, reflecting the foot geometry, which became a key element in determining the therapy and conservative treatment of lower limb defects (flatfoot, calcaneal spur, hallux valgus, calluses).

Keywords: X-ray imaging · Reverse engineering · 3D scan
Surface models · 3D prototyping · Surface reconstruction

1 Introduction

Disadvantages of the lower limbs are quite common. The disadvantage of hallux valgus affects approximately 2–4% of the population [10], flat feet are widespread among children and adolescents as well as people struggling with obesity. Treatment of lower limb defects, especially foot defects, are quite complicated and difficult to diagnose medical attention. Both conservative and postoperative treatment consists in the correction of the pressure distribution and all forces acting on the foot during running and walking, as well as the creation of the correct axis of the limb. One of the commonly used solutions is the use of an orthopedic insole. The assessment of the correctness of foot construction now uses a suboscopic examination and a radiological examination. The methods used give a view on the assessment of the shape of the foot and its internal structure, but do not depict its spatial view. The physician using only subcutaneous examination and X-ray examination receives only the flat state of the foot. In many orthopedic patients, the defects of the lower limb develop at various stages

© Springer International Publishing AG, part of Springer Nature 2019
E. Pietka et al. (Eds.): ITIB 2018, AISC 762, pp. 431–441, 2019.
https://doi.org/10.1007/978-3-319-91211-0_38

of pathological changes. Often, several defects occur simultaneously in various stages of development. The answer to the problems related to the lack of personalization in orthopedics is the technology of obtaining geometry of the spatial foot in the form of 3D scanning, otherwise known as reverse engineering. Using the 3D scanning potential, it is possible to almost perfectly reflect the curvature of the foot and the selection of the insert so that it provides correct support points and proper distribution of loads in the foot, while correcting the axis of the entire lower limb. The main objective of the presented article is the use of reverse engineering methods in orthopedics as a tool supporting diagnosis and the use of spatial foot model, in order to select the correct treatment and the use of appropriate therapy in the form of conservative treatment [8,9].

2   Anatomy of the Foot

The anatomical and functional division of the foot distinguishes between the following foot parts: the rear part (the hindfoot), which directly transmits static pressure; the middle part (the midfoot), which transmits the propulsive forces and forces of stabilization on the ground; and the front part (the forefoot), which significantly supports the push-off (Fig. 1) [1].

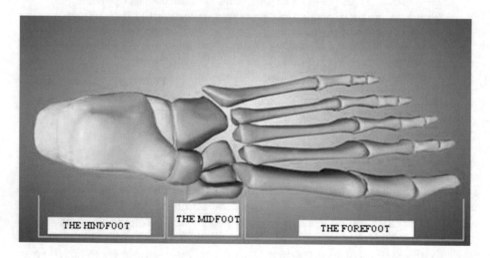

Fig. 1. The anatomical and functional division of the foot [2]

The adopted division distinguishes between three foot arches, which facilitate foot activities [2]:

– The lateral longitudinal arch of the foot increases its springiness. Its proximal supporting point is the plantar surface of the calcaneal tuberosity and the distal supporting point consists of metatarsal bone heads.

- The transverse arch is present only in a non-load-bearing foot and disappears when the foot is loaded with body weight.
- The medial longitudinal arch is called dynamic. It sits between the metatarsal bone heads and the pulps of relevant toes. Its task is to increase the foot push-off force.

3 Foot Deformation

Foot deformations stem from [3]:

- personal tendencies (weakening of the muscle-ligament system, excessive body weight, inappropriate footwear),
- acquired defects (e.g. flat foot, club foot, adducted forefoot),
- acquired defects (hallux valgus, calcaneal spur, platypodia).

4 Conservative and Operative Treatment

Conservative Treatment. Conservative treatment aims at slowing down the progression of hallux valgus and alleviating the pain. The management includes appropriately oriented physiotherapy, application of individually selected orthopedic inserts and comfortable footwear adjusted to the deformation degree [4]. The physiotherapeutic activities include, among other things, the following:

- activation of the muscles supporting the foot arches;
- strengthening of the muscles stabilizing the ankle joint;
- liquidation of Achilles tendon contracture (if present) [1].

Another type of conservative treatment is application of orthopedic inserts, which are aimed at the following:

- correction of accompanying foot defects;
- ensuring comfort by relieving the transverse arch of the foot;
- improving the functioning of the great toe during the push-off phase [1].

Operative Treatment. The only effective method of hallux valgus treatment is operative treatment. The main aim of hallux valgus classification is to facilitate the decision on the treatment method. One generally distinguishes between mild, moderate and advanced hallux valgus. No classification is perfect and the angular parameter values assessed in radiographic images are somewhat divergent. Deformations are usually classified according to the hallux valgus angle (HVA) and the intermetatarsal angle (IMA) (Table 1) [1, 2].

The basic and most important diagnostic examination in hallux valgus assessment is X-ray imaging (Fig. 2) in an A-P projection (that is, with the rays running from the top to the bottom) in the standing position. One uses the image to calculate the hallux valgus angle as well as the intermetatarsal angle between the first and second metatarsal bone.

Table 1. The relationship between hallux valgus development stages and the HVA and IMA angles

Development stage	HVA value [°]	IMA value [°]
Mild	<25	<11
Moderate	25–40	12–15
Advanced	>40	16–19
Severe	>50	>20

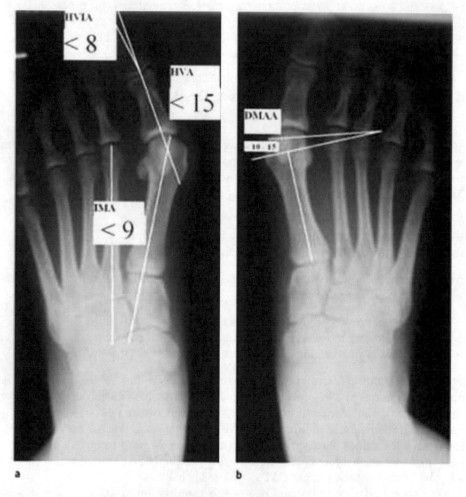

Fig. 2. Radiographic parameters plotted on radiographs in the standing position during qualifying the patient for operative treatment: (a) hallux valgus interphalangeus angle (HVIA), hallux valgus angle (HVA), intermetatarsal angle (IMA), (b) distal metatarsal articular angle (DMAA) [6]

5   Podoscopy and Radiology

Podoscopy: A Computerized Examination of the Feet. Computerized podoscopy is a fast way of diagnosing foot defects because even a cursory analysis of the image itself allows one to notice the differences between the feet (symmetry or asymmetry, hollow or flat feet etc.). The examination allows one to assess the foot shape and determine the indicators which describe its geometry and therefore provide a lot of information necessary for a correct diagnosis and appropriate treatment. This constitutes a reliable assessment of the longitudinal arch status, the hallux valgus angle (the α angle) and the fifth toe varus deformity (the β angle) [4].

During the podoscopic examination, the patient stands on the podoscope (Fig. 3). The image of their feet is recorded, scanned, automatically processed and transmitted to the computer. The examination results reveal the patients defect. The computerized examination of the foot facilitates determination of unfavorable overload of various foot parts. The podoscopic examination allows one to assess the distribution of forces in the foot and diagnose possible deformations (Fig. 4) [7].

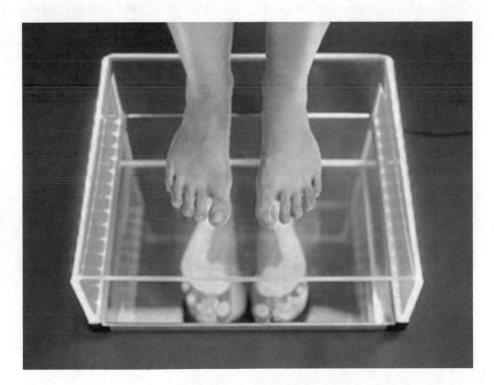

Fig. 3. A patient during the podoscopic examination [4]

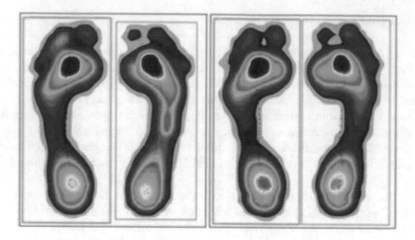

Fig. 4. A result of the computerized examination of the feet (podoscopy) [4]

Radiological Examination (X-rays). During a radiological examination, controlled doses of X-rays pass through a selected body part of the examined person and are projected onto a perpendicular plane equipped with a detector of those rays. This method is based on the differences in X-ray absorption ability between various tissues. Bones demonstrate the highest X-ray absorption (Figs. 5 and 6) of all the body tissues because they contain much more inorganic compounds (mineral salts) than other tissues [11].

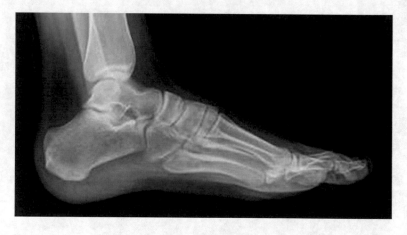

Fig. 5. An X-ray image of a flat foot

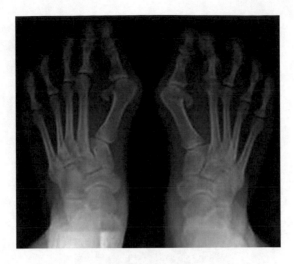

Fig. 6. An X-ray image of the feet with bilateral hallux valgus

6   Own Research

To ensure the full diagnostics of the limb defects, each patient underwent a podoscopic examination and an X-ray examination. To obtain spatial models of the feet, we collected the patients footprints in a mold filled with dental compound. We selected dental compound as the material for capturing foot geometry due to its short solidification time (approx. 1 min), relatively low price and minimal risk of an allergic reaction in the patients during casting.

During the next stage of the research, we utilized a 10 Mpix scanner by SMARTTECH SURFACE (Fig. 7) with white structured light. The scanned object was placed on a turning table to ensure the best possible scanning result. The accuracy of the scanner was 60 microns and a single measurement lasted 8 seconds [5].

The scanning produced point clouds. The technical elaboration of the obtained data consisted in correcting local discontinuities as well as removal of noise and disturbances. Then, we generated the triangle mesh representing the spatial model of the foot (Fig. 8) [6].

With computerized podoscope results, X-ray images and 3D visualization of the foot as the triangle mesh, we performed the full diagnostics of the foot to determine the foot defect. The performed examinations had three participants, who were female patients with diagnosed orthopedic defects. By combining the computerized podoscopy results, X-ray images and spatial models of the feet, we suggested solutions improving foot stability and alleviating the pain.

Patient 1. Patient 1 was a 55-year-old woman with a height of 160 cm and a weight of 80 kg. The conducted examinations (Fig. 9) and the medical history revealed calcaneal spurs in both feet and incorrect pressure distribution. The pain is present in both feet, but it becomes more intense in the left one. To correct the abnormalities in the foot and provide the patient with greater comfort, one

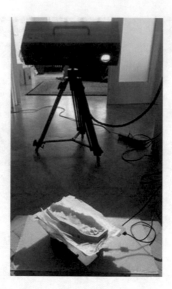

Fig. 7. 3D scanning of the foot cast

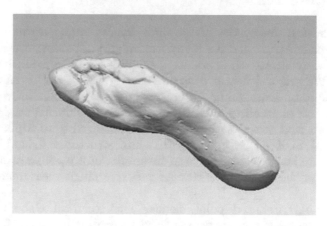

Fig. 8. The generated triangle mesh

has to relieve the longitudinal arch. Foot relief is possible by using orthopedic inserts or selecting appropriate foot-stabilizing footwear. Analyzing the spatial model, one can precisely assess the height to which the longitudinal arch has to be elevated as well as indicate the area with the biggest pressure, which is a key factor for the selection of orthopedic inserts.

Patient 2. Patient 2 was a 60-year-old woman with a height of 158 cm and a weight of 58 kg. The patient was diagnosed with hallux valgus, transverse platypodia and pain becoming more intense in the left foot. To improve foot stability and increase the patient's comfort in her everyday life, one has to elevate the transverse arch of the foot by applying conservative treatment in the form of an

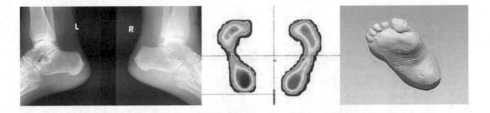

Fig. 9. Combined results of the examinations

appropriate orthopedic insert and rehabilitation. The X-ray image revealed the hallux valgus and transverse platypodia, while computerized podoscopy showed incorrect pressure distribution in the foot as well as the area with the maximal pressure. The 3D model allowed one to indicate the exact location where the treatment should be applied (Fig. 10).

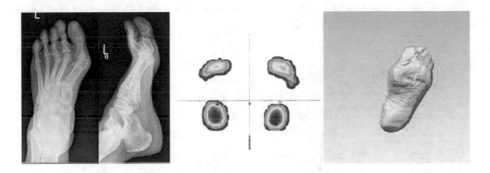

Fig. 10. Combined results of the examinations

Patient 3. Patient 3 was a 64-year-old woman with a height of 152 cm and a weight of 70 kg. The conducted examinations revealed flattening of the transverse arch, transverse platypodia, increased pressure on the heels, calluses above the head of the second metatarsal bone in the right foot, hallux valgus in the left foot as well as pain becoming more intense in the right foot (Fig. 11). The spatial visualization of the foot arches allows one to locate precisely the correction of the transverse arch, which has to be relieved. In order to alleviate the heel pain, one has to apply an elevating insert, which will restore the correct pressure distribution in the foot.

Patient 4. Patient number 4 is a woman aged 47, weighing 50 kg and height 150 cm. On the basis of the obtained tests, halux valgus and flat feet were diagnosed (Fig. 12). There are pain complaints in the left foot and the lateral ankle. The results of computer podoscopy showed increased pressure on the left foot. On the basis of the spatial model, it was proposed to raise the transverse arch using the insert with the elevation located between the first and the third

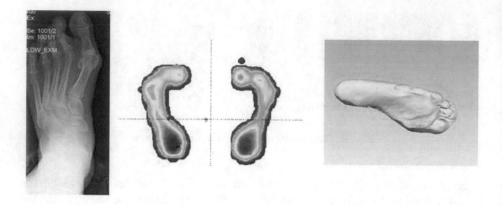

Fig. 11. Combined results of the examinations

metatarsal bone. The proposed model of the orthopedic insole will ensure proper distribution of loads in the foot, will give the correct axis of the entire limb and also reduce pain associated with complaints.

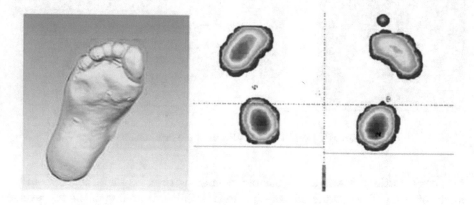

Fig. 12. Combined results of the examinations

7   Summary

Diagnosis of the defects of the lower limbs (feet) is a complex issue. Based on the examination of the podoscope and the radiological image, the doctor assesses the patient's state of health and defines the disadvantage of the patient. The conservative or postoperative treatment comes down to choosing an appropriate orthopedic insole, ensuring the correct distribution of the loads in the foot and giving the correct axis of the limb. In order to choose the right orthopedic insole to correct the defect, the geometry of the foot should be analyzed, which was obtained by reverse engineering methods. By using 3D scan of the footprint, the surface generated in the form of triangle meshes was obtained. Having a three-dimensional model of foot geometry, an orthopedic surgeon has the ability to accurately indicate the correction site and define a specific treatment area. The previous diagnostic methods showed the foot in flat space, reverse engineering methods gave a new look at orthopedic diagnosis. Spatial visualization of foot geometry is a response to the lack of personalization in orthopedics. Orthopedic defects manifest themselves in various degrees of severity, often causing deformation, which makes it difficult to locate the characteristic support points of the foot, which is problematic during the course of the diagnosis. The spatial 3D model generated by reverse engineering methods gives the opportunity to visualize atypical curvatures of the foot and thereby accurately indicate the places requiring rehabilitation or other forms of treatment.

References

1. Słonka, K., Hyla-Klekot, L.: Prophylaxis and therapy of flat feet, Opole (2012)
2. Gądek, A., Liszka, H., Łoboda, K.: Modern methods of surgical treatment of hallux valgus deformity. Clinical Department of Orthopedics and Rehabilitation of the University Hospital in Krakow (2013)
3. Napiątek, M.: Halux Valgus - from etiology to treatment, practical remarks.Chair and Department of Orthopedics and Traumatology of the Children's Medical Academy Karol Marcinkowski in Poznan (2006)
4. Mosór, K., Kromka-Szydek, M.: Influence of selected factors on foot parameters based on suboscopic examination. Current Problems of Biomechanics nr 6/2012 (2012)
5. Sikorski, S., Duda, P., Służałek, G., Majewski, Ł.: The use of 3D scanners and 3D printers in the process of product modification. In: Materials of the 21th KomPlas-Tech Conference on: Information Technology in Metal Technology, Wisla Malinka, 19–22 January (2014)
6. Sikorski, S., Duda, P., Duleba, K., Wróbel, Z.: The use of reverse engineering in the modeling of joint prostheses. Mechanik Nr 12/2016, s. 1912–1913 (2016). https://doi.org/10.17814/mechanik.2016.12.549. ISSN 0025-6552
7. Napiątek, M., Walczak, M.: Treatment of the adolescent hallux valgus (AHV) by double osteotomy of the first metatarsal. 25th Meeting of European Paediatric Orthopaedic Society, Dresden, 5–8 April 5–8 (2006)
8. Spinczyk, D., Pietka, E.: Automatic generation of 3D lung model. In: Computer Recognition Systems 2. Advances in Intelligent and Soft Computing, vol. 45, pp. 671–678 (2007)
9. Digiovanni, C.W., Greisberg, J.: Foot and Ankle and Shin Joint: Core Knowledge in Ortopaedics. Elsevier Urban & Partner, Wroclaw (2010)
10. Napiątek, M.: Crooked palis - from etiology to treatment, practical remarks. Chair and Department of Orthopedics and Traumatology of the Children's Medical Academy Karol Marcinkowski in Poznan (2006)
11. Durandet, A., Ricci, P., Hossein, A., Vanat, Q., Wang, B., Esat, I., Chizari, M.: Radiographic analysis of lower limb axial alignments. In: Proceedings of the World Congress on Engineering, WCE 2013, vol. II (2013)

3D Modeling of Leg Muscle Using Mechanochemical Representations of Muscular Tissue and Solid Fibers

Adrianna Bielak$^{(\boxtimes)}$, Radosław Bednarski, and Adam Wojciechowski

Institute of Information Technology, Lodz University of Technology,
ul. Wólczańska 215, 90-924 Lodz, Poland
adrianna.bielak.lodz@gmail.com
http://it.p.lodz.pl

Abstract. This paper presents a new 3D model of the skeletal gastrocnemius muscle. The model was created by combining the muscle fiber representation as a B-spline solid with a continual mechanochemical Usik's model, which, due to its assumptions, accounts for thermomechanochemical changes in the muscle. The use of Usik's model in the context of 3D modeling of skeletal muscle has not been met so far. As part of the experiment, an application was developed to generate a 3D muscle. Comparison of real volumes with volumes of the virtual muscles during deformations showed the same results.

Keywords: 3D musculature geometry · Gastrocnemius muscle
Continual mechanochemical model

1 Introduction

Computer modeling of the musculoskeletal system has become an indispensable part of the modern approach in the studied biomechanics of human movement. Virtual models are eagerly used in medical fields [13,14]. This gives more effective help to patients e.g. in biomechanics, including: physiotherapy, rehabilitation, orthopedics [1]. The use of modern technology allows for precise indication of all the irregularities that are difficult to observe by the human eye [2,3]. 3D muscle modeling falls into these areas.

In mechanical muscle behaviors, the following constitutive models are known: cross-bridge models, three-dimensional continual models and one-dimensional Hill-type three-component models [12]. The one-dimensional nature and the lack of consideration of the microstructural muscle characteristics of the cross-bridge and Hill-type models limit their applicability to realistic three-dimensional muscle systems [12]. In addition, Hill's model does not take into account the thermomechanical or mechanochemical reactions taking place in the muscle structures, which also affect its contraction, and thus the deformation. An alternative approach to capturing interactions between muscle structures is to represent muscles

© Springer International Publishing AG, part of Springer Nature 2019
E. Pietka et al. (Eds.): ITIB 2018, AISC 762, pp. 442–454, 2019.
https://doi.org/10.1007/978-3-319-91211-0_39

using a 3D continual approach [4] which is described in the next Section. 3D muscle models allow us to understand the form and function of skeletal muscle in ways that would be unachievable through experimental investigations alone and to a level of detail that is not possible with Hill-type lumped parameter models of muscle [11], given that there are over 300 skeletal muscles in the human body [11], which include the gastrocnemius muscle, and each of them has a differentiated course of the same structures relative to other muscles. Research studies on modeling 3D skeletal muscles with their behavior cannot complement each other [11]. The gastrocnemius muscle (in Fig. 1) was chosen because no paper was found that would examine that muscle only. It is an important muscle because it pulls the foot downwards, away from the lower leg with plantaris, soleus and fibularis longus. It can also flex the lower leg at the knee [7]. Creating 3D models for knees is important because knee joint injuries are called the 21st century epidemic [1]. Better solutions of 3D muscles models associated with the knee joint can improve research and rehabilitation in this area. The creation of such a muscle model based on the actual parameters of the patient may allow to study the behavior of the internal structures of this muscle without interfering with the patient's calf. This is especially important if we are dealing with structures that have been seriously injured or operated.

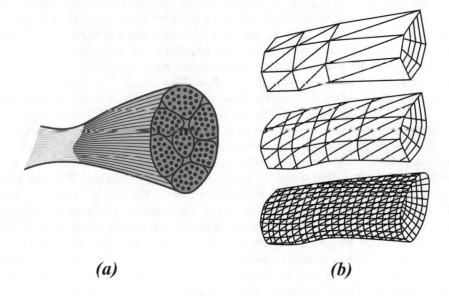

(a)   *(b)*

Fig. 1. (a) Muscle fiber [5], (b) Created visualization of a muscle fiber implemented as a volumetric B-spline solid in the developed application

This paper presents the proposal of a new 3D model of skeletal muscle and its behavior in the context of contraction and extension. Using the missing aspects in [9], namely the thermomechanical reactions in the muscle, is a new contribution to this solution. The thermomechanical Usik's model [15] was used to account for these reactions in the proposed model. No existing solution was found that would use the Usik's model in 3D skeletal muscle modeling. This representation resembles the shape of the muscle fiber structure shown in Fig. 1(a). The higher levels of tessellation are shown from the top of the Fig. 1(b).

2 Related Work

An important work related to the strain modeling of selected calf muscle was published in 1998 by Bro-Nielsen et al. [9]. They presented a mathematical primitive of the B-spline solid. The properties of B-spline basis functions allowed local deformations in shape. A continuous solid domain could be defined with inherent smoothness properties as well as an internal coordinate system that allowed parameterization of vector and scalar properties within the entire solid as well as on its boundary surface [9]. Bro-Nielsen et al. have shown that B-spline solids can be a useful primitive for developing deformable models of skeletal muscle. Their work focused on the interpretation of the muscle itself (its shape and volume), its visualization and deformation without taking into account the thermomechanical and mechanochemical properties of the muscle. Chemical reactions in the muscle cause deformation after manipulation such as bending the leg, strike, removing shoes with high heels, which implies sudden muscle stretching. The chemical reactions occurring in the muscles include the arrival of reagents at the myofibril, like the bundling of myosin and actin proteins run through the length of the muscle fiber. On the other hand, in 2005, Teran et al. [13] created a model with a high-resolution musculoskeletal geometry where B-spline solids were also used as a representation of the muscle fiber. They added Piola-Kirchhoff stress and the FVM method to compute muscle and skin deformation [13]. However, Teran et al.'s constitutive muscle model did not include the time-dependent elasticity changes, which would provide even more realistic muscle behavior.

In 2011, Spyrou et al. [12] created a 3D constitutive model for muscle and tendon tissues. They were considered as composite materials that consist of fibers and the connective tissues and biofluids surrounding the fibers. The model was non-linear, rate-dependent and anisotropic due to the presence of the fibers. The muscle fiber stress depends on the strain (length), strain-rate (velocity), and the activation level of the muscle, whereas the tendon fiber exhibits only passive behavior and the stress depends only on the strain. A methodology for the numerical implementation was based on the FVM [12]. This work presented a continuum model of muscle tissue, but it did not include thermomechanical and mechanochemical reactions in each phase of behavior, which is important and can change the values of the results forecasted in their work. Although the model was created on the basis of real data, it did not involve chemical reactions in the muscle, and thereby diffusion simulation, which could occur despite the end of the muscle-deforming force.

In 2012, Cardiff [4] developed a finite volume structural solver, implemented in the open-source software OpenFOAM which was capable of accurately predicting large displacements, large rotations and small strains for a human hip.

He developed Hill-type muscle models and implemented a novel mapped muscle attachment approach capable of accurately capturing the muscle fiber force directions. He used hexahedral, tetrahedral, polyhedral and voxel based meshes, and a comprehensive 3D mesh analysis, to create volumetric meshes of the bones, thus obtaining a model based on the FVM [4]. However, in the case of the model used for determination of muscle behavior, Cardiff used Hill's model, which does not include thermomechanical or mechanochemical reactions.

Summarizing the modern 3D model of skeletal muscle, it consists of a graphic model and a mechanical or mechanochemical model of the muscle to set its behavior. The output value of the behavior model must impact the first one to visualize shape changes in the muscle. The proposed model in [9] was supposed to show that B-spline solids could be a useful primitive for developing deformable models of skeletal muscle. The work focused on mapping the muscle with B-spline without taking into account the use of viscoelastic networks in combination with volume-preserving constraints [9]. None of the methods cited in Introduction – namely the cross-bridge model, the one-dimensional Hill-type three-component model, or the three-dimensional continual model – has been used in conjunction with the virtual representation of the muscle through B-spline. Therefore, in this work, it was decided to use this way of interpreting muscle fibers by B-spline solids, while enriching it with a continual mechanochemical model of muscular tissue by using Usik's model. The constitutive muscle model from [13] did not include the time-dependent elasticity changes, which would provide even more realistic muscle behavior. Usik's model used in this paper contains a time dependency that is not found in [13]. In [12], the FVM was used assuming that it was a geometrically intuitive and simple way of integrating the equations of motion with an interpretation compared to the simplicity of mass-spring systems. This was justified by the fact that the constitutive model could be incorporated into the FVM in contrast to models using the masses and springs system. The constitutive model for muscles in [12] included deviatoric isotropic invariants of the strain, a strain invariant associated with transverse isotropy, the fiber direction, activation in the tissue, the Mooney-Rivlin model for representing the isotropic tissues in muscle that embed the fascicles and fibers, incompressibility, active and passive muscle fiber response, the deviatoric stretch in the along-fiber direction and changes in time. These properties relate to the mechanical behavior of the muscle in the context of stress/relaxation. There are no thermomechanical aspects in this approach, such as temperature, which resolves the application of Usik's model. Referring to [4] the individual fiber distances could be employed to obtain varying forces, however, the Hill muscle parameters apply to whole muscles and obtaining parameters for individual fibers may not be possible. It was difficult to postulate the distribution of force magnitude on an attachment site without invasive in vivo measurement. For this reason, it was suggested that continuum muscle models, as opposed to discrete muscle models, might offer a greater insight with further investigation concerning modeling human muscles [4]. On the other hand, the model used does not include mechanochemical or thermomechanical reactions. Hill's type model has no explicit connection with the chemical or other internal processes taking place within the muscle, and their variation with respect to time is defined differently for the muscle in the active and passive state. These models are based on an empirical relation connecting the velocity of the contraction of the shortening element with the stress [15]. Usik's model serves as an analog of such relation. The velocity of contraction corresponds to the plastic deformation and the stress developed in it to the tension. Usik's model depends on the character of the contraction process (e.g. whether the contraction takes place at a constant strain or at a constant stress), and the mentioned relation will be different for different processes [15], also including the thermomechanical process. The approach of the proposed model could check the deformation of the muscle structure even after a direct event in the form of force. This is due to the inclusion of mechanochemical activities in Usik's model.

The contribution lies in the previously unconnected combination of the selected 3D representation of muscle tissues with a rarely used thermomechanical model. B-spline solids were applied volumetrically to the 3D representation of muscle structures. Such a solution was proposed in [9], but their work focused on the interpretation of the muscle itself, precisely its visualization and deformation without taking into account the chemical and mechanical properties of the muscle. The justification for choosing the volumetric B-spline solid as a representation of muscle structures is as follows. The volumetric shape of the B-spline solid gives the possibility to generate 3D structures real to the actual structures that make up the muscle, as seen in Fig. 1. On the other hand, Usik's model is used in a completely new context, namely 3D modeling of muscle contraction/extension, which has not been done before.

3   Gastrocnemius Muscle Model

The whole model elaboration process can be divided into 4 stages: choosing a modeled muscle, creating a muscle fiber representation using a B-spline solid, generating a volumetric muscle model with created muscle fibers, enriching the volumetric model with a graphic representation by using Usik's model as a constitutive model.

3.1   3D Fiber Representation

The gastrocnemius muscle was chosen because it is one of the major muscles in the lower legs with a relatively simple structure (two-headed). Its course and location are shown in Fig. 2.

For the muscle fiber, and therefore the most basic element of the proposed model, the volumetric B-spline solid was chosen. B-spline solids are straightforward extensions of B-spline curves and surfaces into the volumetric domain. A third parameter is added to the function to allow enumeration of points throughout a volume in addition to an iso-surface (one-parameter constant) or a streamline curve (two-parameter constant). It is represented by the following equation:

$$V(u, w, z) = \sum_{i=0}^{l} \sum_{j=0}^{m} \sum_{k=0}^{n} B_i^u(u) B_j^w(w) B_k^z(z) C_{ijk}. \qquad (1)$$

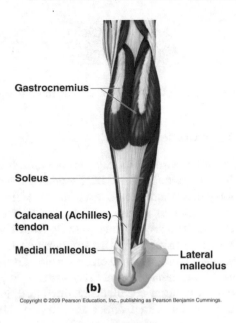

Gastrocnemius

Soleus

Calcaneal (Achilles) tendon

Medial malleolus

Lateral malleolus

(b)

Copyright © 2009 Pearson Education, Inc., publishing as Pearson Benjamin Cummings.

Fig. 2. Calf muscles [6]

Here: $C_{ijk} \in R^3$, C_{ijk} – the set of points form a control point lattice which will influence the shape of the B-spline solid, V – a parametric solid given by the tritensor product of these B-spline basis functions (in this case, the polynomials $B_i^u(u)B_j^w(w)B_k^z(z)$) with the control points in C_{ijk}.

The control points C_{ijk} can be substituted with other vector or scalar values to define other continuous fields or functions within the solid, such as continuous internal forces. The basis functions for each parameter need not all have the same order and each basis function family is indexed depending on the size of its associated knot vector, u, w or z. The knot vectors form a sequence of points that partitions the parameter domain space, determining the local region of influence for each basis function. As each control point is weighted with B-spline basis functions, moving a point will deform a region of the solid as dictated by the shape of the B-spline basis functions which are in turn determined by the knot vectors [9].

One volume of the muscle fiber was created (Fig. 3). Similarly, in [9], a natural cylindrical was chosen according to similarity cylindrical topology of muscle-like bundles after shape deformation. The use of multiple knots in the u and z parameter domains, the external control points are solely responsible for the shape of the solid boundary since the internal basis functions evaluate to zero at the boundaries. Consequently, the outer surface of a B-spline solid is equivalent to a standard B-spline surface, so it is possible to apply standard acceleration techniques to interactively update and display B-spline solids.

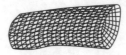

Fig. 3. A tesselated B-spline solid for a fiber muscle representation

3.2   Behavior of the Muscle

To determine the value of the force that deforms the muscle structure at a given point the Usik's model was used. In the Usik's model the muscle is treated as a multi-component homogeneous material continuum in which two phases can be distinguished, where the first one is passive, constructed from the environment of contractile proteins, and the second one is built from these contractile proteins. The passive phase is elastic, while the active phase is viscoelastic [10,15]. The center is transversal-isotropic and incompressible. The activity of the muscular tissue is governed by mechanochemical processes taking place in the tissue, within the specific ordered structures called myofibril and, in the final count, by the mechanochemical reactions which affect the form or the relative distribution of the protein molecules. Outside the myofibril there are various auxiliary systems, the connecting tissue and other muscle structures, including capillary blood vessels which serve as the source of initial chemical compounds [15]. The onset of active muscular contraction is connected with the arrival of specific reagents at the myofibril, like the bundling of myosin and actin proteins run through the length of the muscle fiber [7]. Associated with these reactions is entropy, free energy and temperature, all contained within Usik's model. Chemical reactions occur only in the active phase and the reagents can selectively pass through the cell membrane and between phases and the energy released during the reaction is directly converted into action [15]. We assume that component speeds are unmatched and insignificantly small [10].

The viscous properties depend mainly on the myofibril, while the elastic properties are governed by the connecting tissue and other structures, with each phase containing n components. Phase 1 consists of the myofibril, and Phase 2 – of all the remaining structures. The phases, in principle, differ from each other by the fact that mechanochemical reactions can only take place in one of them (in Phase 2) [15]. The elementary volume v of the continuous medium is equal to the sum of the volumes v^1 (volume of Phase 1) and v^2 (volume of Phase 2) occupied by the first and second phase, respectively. In this paper, v was represented by a B-spline solid (Fig. 4), and thus the muscle fiber.

The system describing motion of the continuous medium under consideration, possessing mechanochemical reactions, contains the following equations:

– equation of continuity having displacement vector,
– equation of conservation of momentum which accounts for stress tensor, chemical potential, the second rank tensor, mass density, the affinity of the chemical reaction, deviator of the stress tensor, time,

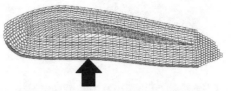

one v volume = B-spline solid muscle fibre

Fig. 4. A generated muscle created from muscle fibers represented by B-spline solids; the orange B-spline solid presents a v volume in the Usik's model; the generated muscle was cut off at its insertions to show B-spline solids inside the virtual muscle

- equation of conservation of mass of the components with deviator of the stress tensor, velocity of the influx, scalar of the rate formation, chemical potential, time,
- equation of heat influx containing tensor parameter (biofactor), one control point from the B-spline v solid, mass density, thermodynamic free energy, scalars of the rate formation, absolute temperature, deformation, source density, deviator of the stress tensor, concentration, mass, time.

After taking into account the assumptions of that model (two-phase continuum model and their properties), Usik's derived mentioned equations for each one v volume (in the case of that paper this is a one B-spline solid). These equations create a set of equations for each v volume, which is one B-spline solid from the generated muscle (Fig. 4). The system is closed by specifying the free energy of the medium on the whole (v volume which is a one B-spline solid). It gives a force for deformation in each k-th control point from one B-spline solid.

4   Experiments and Results

First, the muscle fiber was created as a volumetric B-spline solid. Vulkan API was used to visualize an effect and to optimize calculations by integrating this environment with the capabilities of modern graphic cards, namely the possibility of multithreaded calculations performed on the GPU. At this stage it was not necessary to use multithreaded calculations because generating one fiber was not an expensive procedure, albeit that step was made with the subsequent steps in mind (parallel calculations during discretization and performing these activities on the GPU). The control point lattice determines the shape of the B-spline object. Each B-spline solid has a start point in Insertion 1 (Fig. 5) and the end point in Insertion 2 (Fig. 5). It was determined by the two insertions of the gastrocnemius muscle (Fig. 2).

The control points were located in labels in the 'gastrocnemius3D.xml' XML file created for this experiment. Values for parameters were chosen from the real-life parameters of the gastrocnemius muscle [8]. Some of the real-life selected data was presented in Table 1.

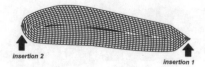

insertion 2   insertion 1

Fig. 5. Insertions of the B-spline solids from the output data of the developed application

Table 1. In vivo joint moment and architectural characteristics of the lateral gastrocnemius muscle of boys and men; a more detailed description can be found in [8]

	Men	Boys
Net PF MVC, $N \cdot m$	175.6 ± 31.7	77.4 ± 21.4†
DF MVC, $N \cdot m$	24.5 ± 8.8	13.1 ± 3.9†
DF coactivation, %	13.5 ± 5.9	11.8 ± 6.7
PF PT, $N \cdot m$	179.0 ± 33.6	79.2 ± 21.5†
Achilles tendon force, N	3865 ± 525	2268 ± 507†
GL fascicle force, N	416.2 ± 56.0	242.5 ± 51.6†
θ (rest), °	11.5 ± 2.3	10.8 ± 2.5
θ (MVC), °	18.0 ± 3.5	16.6 ± 4.6
L_f (rest), cm	8.80 ± 2.18	7.01 ± 0.79*
L_f (MVC), cm	5.5 ± 1.1	4.2 ± 0.8†
$L_f{:}L_m$	0.37 ± 0.08	0.35 ± 0.04
GL ACSA, cm^2	12.1 ± 1.9	5.6 ± 1.6†
GL Vol, cm^3	178.9 ± 178.9	64.5 ± 18.9†
GL PCSA, cm^2	32.2 ± 5.8	15.5 ± 3.2†
Moment arm length, cm	4.61 ± 0.32	3.46 ± 0.20†
Specific force, N/cm_2	13.1 ± 2.0	15.9 ± 2.7*-

*P < 0.05, †P < 0.01 [8].

```
<?xml version="1.0"?>
<gastrocnemius>
    <fiber id="0">
        <ctrlPoint>0.01, 0.002, 0.0022</ctrlPoint>
        ...
        <ctrlPoint>0.9, 0.871, 0.1</ctrlPoint>
    </fiber>
    ...
</gastrocnemius>
```
(a)

```
<?xml version="1.0"?>
<parameters>
        <massdensity>8.8</massdensity>
        <tension>5.3</tension>
        <chemicalpotential>1.244</chemicalpotential>
        <entropy>44.95</entropy>
        ...
</parameters>
```
(b)

Fig. 6. (a) The fragment from the 'gastrocnemius3D.xml' file with parameters and labels; (b) The fragment from 'gastrocnemiusDeformations.xml' file with parameters and labels

The fragment of the file and the representation of control points are given in Fig. 6(a). Each fiber label, with a special ID, has control points as a 3D point.

The final step was the set of selected muscle properties data and the substitution of Usik's muscle model into each separate volume v. The input data was located in 'gastrocnemiusDeformations.xml' XML file and all values were experimental. The labels of the XML data were adequate to Usik's equations from the 'Gastrocnemius muscle model' Section (Fig. 6(b)). The output data was a virtual, volumetrically generated muscle with deformation that was occurred in every third second. Figure 7 shows the deformation process.

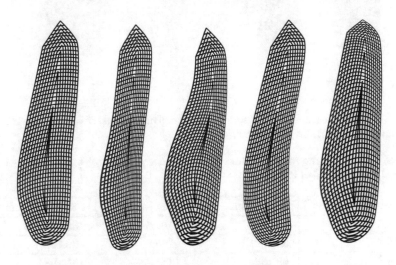

Fig. 7. The mesh of the gastrocnemius muscle; the first mesh from the left is before deformation; the other one is after deformation; each subsequent model was generated three seconds later than the previous one.

The obtained shape of the muscle was shown in Fig. 8 with the approaches discussed in the Section 'Related works'. The soleus was created by using B-spline solids but without mechanical, thermomechanical and mechanochemical properties. The semitendinosus and gluteus medius was generated using the methods described earlier. The generated gastrocnemius gives a streamlined shape characteristic for human skeletal muscles in the leg. New visualization of the same muscle was being generated every third second to check if the muscle behavior is proper, i.e. if it has smooth deformations. These actions were repeated twenty times with twenty instances of the file gastrocnemius 'Deformations.xml', with different values of the same parameters from the previous Section.

Volumes of all muscles were selected to check the accuracy of the muscle model and the potential use in biomechanical experiments. The values of real gastrocnemius muscles were taken from Table 1 from [8]. Those values were used as prerequisite parameters in the methods of muscle generation. The results were compared with the real values in Table 2.

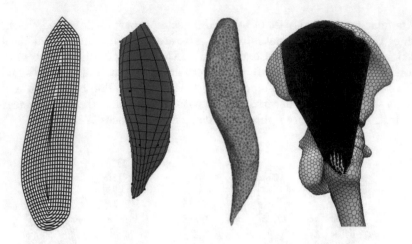

Fig. 8. From the left there is the generated gastrocnemius from this work, the soleus [9], the semitendinosus [12], the gluteus medius [4]

Table 2. The table presents real volumes of gastrocnemius muscles and obtained values of virtual gastrocnemius muscles

Real volumes [cm³]	Model volumes [cm³]	Real vol. [cm³]	Model vol. [cm³]
55.5	55.511	160.5	160.444
56.7	55.689	160.8	160.792
58.3	58.298	161.2	161.298
60.1	60.918	164.1	164.156
64.5	65.538	168.6	168.589
68.2	68.255	169.9	170.001
71.2	71.179	170.1	169.992
73.3	73.333	171.1	171.189
173.3	173.397	175.0	175.083
178.9	178.931	179.9	180.021

5   Conclusions and Discussion

The assumption was to generate a muscle with different values of the same parameters described in the previous section to check if it would assume a realistic shape. At the same time, the shape was not supposed to go beyond the physically impossible forms, such as the displacement of the lower muscle attachment into the upper one, the displacement of the fibers from the front side of the muscle to the rear wall. The 3D gastrocnemius model was created as a combination of 3D representation through B-spline solids and the continuum Usik's model, and it was successful. The work focused on combining these two solutions so that the proposed model would depend on mechanochemical reactions. Such combination using Usik's model in the context of 3D muscle modeling has not been met so far. It is close to the actual muscle structure, which affects the better relevance of results in the case of Usik's model, which, although focusing on thermomechanical phenomena occurring in the muscle, takes into account the actual muscle structure, i.e. it does not interpret it as blocks and springs, or as a continuum material composed of several layers with specific properties. Although the thermomechanical data was not based on real-life data, the comparison of real volumes with volumes of the virtual muscles, which were created based on real parameters, showed the same results (with a slight deviation in some cases). Values of those volumes did not change over time during deformations. This indicates the real volume and shape of the muscle obtained during the deformations.

References

1. Bednarski, R., Bielak, A.: Use of motion capture in assisted of knee ligament injury diagnosis. J. Appl. Comput. Sci. **26**(1) (2018, Accepted for printing)
2. Binkowski, M., Guzek, K., Napieralski, P.: Markerless assisted rehabilitation system. J. Appl. Comput. Sci. **21**(2), 7–19 (2013)
3. Nakonechny, A., Veres, Z.: The wavelet based trained filter for image interpolation. In: IEEE 1st International Conference on DSMP, pp. 218–221 (2016)
4. Cardiff, P.: Development of the finite volume method for hip joint stress analysis. A thesis submitted for the degree of Doctor of Philosophy of the National University of Ireland. University College Dublin, School of Mechanical and Materials Engineering, Dublin (2012)
5. Elitefts. https://www.elitefts.com/news/do-strength-gains-equal-size-gains/
6. Humananatomyly.com. https://humananatomyly.com/gastrocnemius-muscle/
7. Lumen. Boundless Anatomy and Physiology. Muscular System. https://courses.lumenlearning.com/boundless-ap/chapter/overview-of-the-muscular-system/
8. Morse, C.I., Tolfrey, K., Thom, J.M., Vassilopoulos, V., Maganaris, C.N., Narici, M.V.: Gastrocnemius muscle specific force in boys and men. J. Appl. Physiol. **104**(2), 469–474 (2008)
9. Ng-Thow-Hing, V., Agur, A., Ballc, K., Fiumea, E., McKeed, N.: Shape reconstruction and subsequent deformation of soleus muscle models using B-spline solid primitives. Department of Computer Science, Department of Anatomy and Cell Biology, School of Physical and Health Education, Department of Surgery, University of Toronto, Canada, May 1998
10. Oracz, M.: Usik model and classical models of muscular tissue. Zakład Mechaniki, Instytut Techniki Lotniczej i Mechaniki Stosowanej, Politechnika Warszawska, Warszawa. In: Current Problems of Biomechanics, vol. 7(1), pp. 159–164 (2007)
11. Blemker, S.S.: Three-dimensional modeling of active muscle tissue: the why, the how, the future. In: Biomechanics of Living Organs, Hyperelastic Constitutive Laws for Finite Element Modeling, University of Virginia, Charlottesville, VA, United States, vol. 7(1), pp. 361–375, June 2017
12. Spyrou, L.A., Aravas, N.: Muscle and tendon tissues: constitutive modeling and computational issues. J. Appl. Mech. **78**(4), 041015 (2011)
13. Teran, J., Sifakis, E., Blemker, S., Ng Thow Hing, V., Lau, C., Fedkiw, R.: Creating and simulating skeletal muscle from the visible human data set. IEEE Trans. Visual. Comput. Graph. **11**(3), 317–328 (2005)

14. Glinka, K., Wosiak, A., Zakrzewska, D.: Improving children diagnostics by efficient multi-label classification method. In: Pietka, E., Badura, P., Kawa, J. et al. (eds.) Information Technologies in Medicine. Advances in Intelligent Systems and Computing, vol. 471, pp. 253–266 (2016)
15. Usik, P., I.: Continual mechanochemical model of muscular tissue. In: PMM, Moscow, vol. 37, no. 3, pp. 448–458 (1973)

Sensitivity Analysis of the Insulin-Glucose Mathematical Model

Dariusz Radomski$^{(\boxtimes)}$ and Jagoda Głowacka

Institute of Radioelectronics and Multimedia Technology,
Warsaw University of Technology, Nowowiejska 15/19, 00-665 Warsaw, Poland
D.Radomski@ire.pw.edu.pl

Abstract. In this paper detailed analysis of the Hovorka model has been provided. The model describes the dynamics of glucose concentration in case of patients with type 1 diabetes mellitus. The Hovorka model is widely used as a virtual environment and also as a part of controller (so-called an internal model). Due to the popularity of the Hovorka model, its detailed analysis can be helpful in choosing the control algorithm or in simplifying the implementation. The aim was to assess how changes from their base value will affect the glucose output. Results for 3 parameters of the model: rate of an insulin elimination from a patient plasma, endogenous glucose production and total glucose fluctuations independent of insulin were compared. Another purpose of the research was to assess the model nonlinearity intensity. The study was performed on 6 patients who represent the virtual population of type 1 diabetic patients.

The performed analysis indicated that an insulin-glucose system described by the Hovorka model was weakly nonlinear. The values of the nonlinear coefficient were inter-patients varied and depended on an insulin dose. These values ranged: 0.06–10.84. The measured glucose concentration became sensitive to all studied parameters of the Hovorka model. The most sensibilized parameter were glucose fluctuations independent of insulin.

These results of the analysis may be used to develop new control algorithms based on the internal patient model. They will be able to adapt their parameters to the individual patient by updating specific value in each step of the algorithms.

Keywords: Insulin control algorithms · Sensitivity analysis
Nonlinearity analysis · Hovorka model

1 Introduction

Diabetes mellitus is a group of metabolic diseases characterized by hyperglycemia stemmed from disturbances of an insulin secretion or its biological activity. There are four types of diabetes: type 1, type 2, pregnancy diabetes and senile diabetes [1]. In 2012 approximately 422 million people suffered from diabetes. The prevalence of diabetes is 6% in a general population and 8.5% among adults [2].

© Springer International Publishing AG, part of Springer Nature 2019
E. Pietka et al. (Eds.): ITIB 2018, AISC 762, pp. 455–468, 2019.
https://doi.org/10.1007/978-3-319-91211-0_40

WHO, as well as worldwide politicians, admitted that diabetes mellitus is one of the four noncommunicable diseases which should be monitored and prevented.

Physiologically, a glucose concentration in a plasma of diabetic patients varies more deeply than in healthy humans. Depending on a glucose concentration, three glycemic states might be distinguished: normoglycemia occurs in glucose concentration between 80–140 mg/dl, hypoglycemia in a glucose concentration below 70 mg/dl and hyperglycemia above 140 mg/dl. The hypoglycemic states occur suddenly and might lead to death. They might be manifested by seizures or diabetic coma. On the other hand hyperglycemic states have usually a chronic form as a result of improper glucose controlling. Moreover, the ausemany health complications are increasing the total costs of national health care systems. The most frequent complications are: nephropathy leading to dialyzes or kidney transplantations (40% of diabetic patients), neuropathy leading to sense disorders (50% of patients have a diabetic foot syndrome after 25 years suffering from this disease), retinopathy (100% patients after 20 years) or an ischemic disease (40% patients) [3].

Type 1 is called insulin dependent diabetes and is diagnosed in 10% of diabetic patients. 85–90% constitute children or adolescents. Taking the above into account diabetes type 1 seems to be the most hazardous for patients health and simultaneously it becomes a real threat to public health systems funds due to long patients lifetime expectancy.

Type 1 is an autoimmunological disease leading to destruction of β cells of a pancreas insula and in result to discontinuation of insulin production. Therefore insulin must be administrated externally.

There are a few clinical strategies of insulin delivery in case of patients with type 1 diabetes. The most popular method are the multiple daily injections. In this method 12 h active insulin is injected using special pens two times per day. Additional short-acting insulin doses are injected around meal time to cover carbohydrate consumptions.

The second method uses low doses of short-acting insulin that is subcutaneously administrated by an infusion pump in the predetermined regular moments of a day. Also, an insulin bolus can be injected depending on a size of meal.

However, the methods mentioned above have some serious disadvantages. They work in the open loop mode so they require computing meal corrected insulin dose which is especially difficult to apply in case of child patients. The drawbacks can be overcome by using a closed loop method with a control algorithm computing an optimal insulin dose. This idea is called 'an artificial pancreas'. An implemented control algorithm mimics natural pancreas. Such an idea is presented on Fig. 1a.

The system working in a closed loop mode consists of a sensor that continuously measures glucose concentration in patient plasma, an infusion pump and a control algorithm. The measured value of the glucose concentration is transmitted to the pump processor. Then the control algorithm computes a new insulin dose ensuring normoglycemia. This cycle is repeated every 15 min. The above

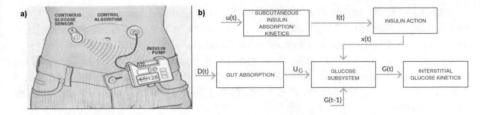

Fig. 1. (a) An idea of a closed loop system for diabetes management (https://www.thediabetescouncil.com/wp-content/uploads/2017/08/foto_no_exif.jpg) (b) The compartmental structure of the studied model elaborated by the Hovorka team. The parameter $G(t-1)$ represents subcutaneously measured glucose level

method allows to adapt better an administrated insulin dose at each time on varying conditions which stem from differences in meals, physical activities or even phases of a menstrual cycle. There are two types of closed loop system. The first one is called *hybrid closed loop system* and requires manual meal input, i.e. the amount of consumed carbohydrates. The other one, called *fully closed loop system*, estimates a meal correction based on the internal patient model.

The pivotal part of a closed loop system is a control algorithm. The most elaborated algorithms were: different version of the PID algorithm, Model Predictive Control system or Fuzzy Logic Controller [4]. A new approach uses machine learning methods, for example Reinforcement Learning [5].

The performed review of publications suggests that the control algorithms are selected almost randomly without *a prori* knowledge about a character of insulin-glucose dynamic relation. The authors apply their version of a controller and report the obtained results in the papers.

Methodologically, this approach is similar to an explorative data analysis where control algorithms are the analyzed objects. This way may cause that the proposed algorithms are too complicated in comparison to the controlled physiological process, e.g. an application of a nonlinear control algorithm for a linear process. On the contrary, a confirmatory methodology may be used. Then, a proposed control algorithm is selected on the base of *a prori* knowledge about a controlled process. In this situation a mathematical model of the process dynamics and properties of this model must be known. In our opinion the second approach is more appropriate due to existing limits and computational complexity of the algorithms.

Mathematical modeling of an insulin-glucose relation has a long history. The first model was proposed by Bergman in 1984. It is called a *minimal model* because it consists of three differential equations and four parameters [6].

At present there are two most frequently used models. The current version of the Cobelli's model was proposed in 2007. It contains 12 ordinal differential equations, 18 algebraic equations and 35 parameters. This model is approved by FDA to simulate a virtual patient with type 1 diabetes [7].

Another often exploited model is the Hovorka model that consists of 11 differential equations and 18 parameters. The values of the model parameters have been estimated individually in case of 18 patients with type-1 diabetes [8].

Moreover, there is also a model proposed by Sorensen in his PhD thesis. This model is represented by 19 differential equations and 44 parameters. It is not used in control algorithms studies because of the problems with its parameter identification and complexity [9].

Although the Cobeli's and the Hovorka models were extensively studied mainly by assessment of their prediction errors, there are several studies analyzing a character of an insulin-glucose relation based on these models. Especially there is no knowledge about a rate of the process nonlinearity. Moreover, we have poorly cognizance about influence of the model parameters on the dynamical relationship between an insulin and a glucose concentration. The last dimension is important in constructing of adaptive control algorithms which should estimate on-line values of the most sensitive parameters of the assumed model.

Therefore, the aim of this paper is to present the sensitivity analysis of the selected model studying its nonlinearity and effects of the main parameters variability on an insulin-glucose relation. The cognizance of these effects is mainly important for construction of adaptive algorithms which should estimate on-line the most sensitive model parameters. The Hovorka model has been chosen for this purpose due to its frequent application in the studies.

2   The Hovorka Model of the Insulin-Glucose Dynamic

The Hovorka model is a compartmental model. It means that the model describes a time-dependent dynamic of an insulin and glucose concentrations in biological spaces of a human organism called a compartment wherein their spatial distributions in a given space are uniforms. This model consisted of 5 compartments is depicted by 11 ordinal 1st order differential equations. A part of them is nonlinear. A virtual patient with type-1 diabetes is represented by the set of individual values of 18 model parameters [8].

The Hovorka model enables to simulate an intra-subject variability assuming oscillatory time-varied values of some model parameters. Moreover, an inter-subjects variability is modeled by setting individual-specific values of the parameters. This procedure allows to obtain a population of the simulated patients.

There are two model inputs: an administrated insulin dose computed by a control algorithm and consumed carbohydrate amount denoted by $u(t)$ and $D(t)$ respectively. The model output is a glucose concentration in a patient plasma expressed by $G(t)$. The compartmental structure of the Hovorka model is shown in the Fig. 1b.

The mathematical equations that represent a given compartment are presented below. The model variables and parameters are listed in the Table 1.

Subcutaneous Insulin Absorption and Kinetics Model. Insulin is administrated into a patient organism subcutaneously. The kinetics of this process is

Table 1. Variables and parameters of the Hovorka's model

Table 1. Variables and parameters of the Hovorka's model

Variable/ /Parameter	Unit	Description	Parameters Character (I)dentified/ (P)*riori*	Variability (O)sciltotory/(S)tationary
Q_1, Q_2	mmol	Glucose mass in accessible and non-accesible space	—	—
k_{12}	1/min	Rate of a glucose transfer from a accessible to non-accessible space	I	O
V_G	L	Glucose volume in accessiblespace	P	S
G	mmol/L	Measured glucose concentration	—	—
EGP	mmol/min	Endogenous glucose production	I	O
U_G	mmol/min	Rate of a glucose absorption in a intestine	—	—
F_{01}^C	mmol/min	Total glucose fluctuations independent of insulin	I (*based on* (17))	O
F_R	mmol/L per min	Renal clearance	—	—
I	mU/L	Insulin concentration in patient's plasma	—	—
x_1, x_2, x_3		State variables representing insulin-glucose relations	—	—
$k_{ai,i=1,2,3}$	1/min	Rates of insulin absorption	I (*based on* (7))	O
$k_{bi,i=1,2}$	1/min^2 per mU/L	Activation rate of remote insulin	I (*based on* (7))	O
k_{b3}	1/min per mU/L	Deactivation rate of remote insulin on endogenous glucose	I	O
V_I	L	Insulin volume in a patient's plasma	—	—
U_I	mU	Insulin mass in a patient's plasma	—	—
k_e	1/min	Rate of an insulin elimination from a patient's plasma	P	O
k_a	1/min	Rate of an insulin absorption	P	O
R_{thr}	mmol/L	Glucose threshold for a renal clearance	P	S
S_1, S_2	mU	Insulin masses in accessible and non-accesible space	—	—
u	U	Administered rapid-active insulin	—	—
G_1, G_2	mmol	Glucose masses in a available and non-available space	—	—
$D(t)$	mmol/min	Amounts of carbohydrates consumed at the moment t	—	—
R_{cl}	1/min	Renal clearance rate	P	S
t_{max}	min	Time to a maximal glucose concentration	P	S
Bio	–	Meal carbohydraates availability	P	S
C	mmol/L	Glucose concentration in a subcutaneous compartment	—	—
k_{a_int}	1/min	Glucose transfer rate between an interstitial and a plasma	P	O

described as follows:

$$\frac{dS_1(t)}{dt} = u(t) - k_a S_1(t) \tag{1}$$

$$\frac{dS_2(t)}{dt} = k_a S_1(t) - k_a S_2(t) \tag{2}$$

The absorbed insulin is transferred into a patient plasma according to the formula:

$$\frac{dI}{dt} = \frac{k_u S_2(t)}{V_I} - k_e I(t) \tag{3}$$

Insulin Action Compartment. This following state equations describe the biological effect of an insulin on a glucose concentration in a patient organism:

$$\frac{dx_1}{dt} = -k_{b1} x_1(t) + S_{IT} k_{b1} I(t) \tag{4}$$

$$\frac{dx_2}{dt} = -k_{b2} x_2(t) + S_{ID} k_{b2} I(t) \tag{5}$$

$$\frac{dx_3}{dt} = -k_{b3} x_3(t) + S_{IE} k_{b3} I(t) \tag{6}$$

The coefficients S_{IT}, S_{ID}, S_{IE} are called the sensitivity coefficients and represent the following relations between the activation and deactivation rates:

$$S_{IT} = \frac{k_{a1}}{k_{b1}}; \quad S_{ID} = \frac{k_{a2}}{k_{b2}}; \quad S_{IE} = \frac{k_{a3}}{k_{b3}} \tag{7}$$

Model of a Gut Absorption. The kinetic of the carbohydrate consumption form a meal is given by the equations formed by Worthington in the paper [10]:

$$\frac{dG_1(t)}{dt} = -\frac{G_1(t)}{t_{max}} + Bio \cdot D(t) \tag{8}$$

$$\frac{dG_2(t)}{dt} = \frac{G_1(t)}{t_{max}} - \frac{G_2(t)}{t_{max}} \tag{9}$$

Glucose fluctuations after a meal depend on a velocity of a glucose absorption of the intestine. The glucose absorption coefficient is denoted by U_G and has the form:

$$U_G = \frac{G_2}{t_{max}} \tag{10}$$

This gut model is also used in the simulator of virtual patients with Type-1 diabetes [11].

Glucose Subsystem. This compartment is characterized by two state variables. The Q_1 variable expresses a glucose amount in an accessible space, i.e. in a plasma while the Q_2 denotes its amount in a non-accessible space, i.e. in peripheral tissues. After a meal consumption, carbohydrates are decomposed into simple sugars so a glucose concentration is elevates and transferred into tissues. The kinetics of these processes are given in the following formulas:

$$\frac{dQ_1(t)}{dt} = -\left[\frac{F_{01}^c}{V_G G(t)} + x_1(t)\right] Q_1(t) + k_{12} Q_2(t) - F_R + EGP + U_G(t) \tag{11}$$

$$\frac{dQ_2(t)}{dt} = x_1(t) Q_1(t) - [k_{12} + x_2(t)] Q_2(t) \tag{12}$$

The model output being a glucose concentration in a plasma is computed in a classical output equation:

$$y(t) = G(t) = Q_1(t) / V_G \tag{13}$$

Model of Interstitial Glucose Kinetics. A sensor used for continuous glucose monitoring *de facto* measures a glucose concentrated in an interstitial space which is a liner correlated with a plasma concentration of this substance. Thus, the below equation quantifies the kinetic of glucose transporting into an interstitial fluid:

$$\frac{dC(t)}{dt} = k_{a\_int} [G(t) - C(t)], \tag{14}$$

where k_{a_int} is a rate of glucose transport between a plasma and an interstitial space.

Additionally, the Hovorka model considers the nonlinear constrains resulted from the following physiologically significant processes:

– production of an endogenous glucose defined by the function:

$$EGP = \begin{cases} EGP_0 \left[1 - x_3(t)\right] \text{ if } EGP \geq 0 \\ 0 \text{ else} \end{cases} \quad (15)$$

– renal clearance of a glucose when its concentration exceeds the threshold R_{thr} given by:

$$F_R = \begin{cases} R_{cl}\left(G - R_{thr}\right)V_G \text{ if } G \geq R_{thr} \\ 0 \text{ else} \end{cases} \quad (16)$$

– total glucose fluctioations independent on a glucose described as:

$$F_{01}^c = \frac{F_{01}^s G}{(G + 1.0)}, \text{ where } F_{01}^s = \frac{F_{01}}{0.85} \quad (17)$$

– time till achieving a maximal glucose concentration is computed in that way:

$$t_{max} = \begin{cases} t_{max\_ceil}, \text{ if } U_G > U_{G\_ceil} \\ t_{max}, \text{ else} \end{cases}, \text{ where } t_{max\_ceil} = \frac{G_2}{U_{G\_ceil}} \quad (18)$$

For simulation of an intra-variability values of some model parameters were assumed oscillatory time varied. The oscillatory amplitudes were equal to 5% of the nominal parameter values, the oscillatory periods were 3 hours and the oscillatory phases and some of the others were drawn from *a priori* uniform distribution defined on the interval [0; 1].

Although the Hovorka model seems to be at least globally identifiable, it is not a clinically identifiable model. The definition of clinical identification was proposed by Radomski in [12] and it means that all models parameters can be identified based on data accessible in a routine clinical examination of a patient. The set of these data can be strongly limited because of bioethical regulations or health risky invasive measurements. Therefore, only eight out of 18 parameters were individually estimated based on clinical measurements. Other ones were randomly drawn from normal or lognormal distributions according to [8]. The characterizations of the model parameters are given in the Table 1.

The Hovorka model was implemented in the Matlab environment and solved using the Runge-Kutta formula.

The Fig. 2 presents the results of the model simulation performed on a random patient. It shows the outcomes of all compartments. A meal is delivered at the 1st minute. The simulation of the inter-individual variability for 6 patients being a studied virtual group is illustrated in the Fig. 3. These patients showed significant inter-individual variability. Administration of the same insulin doses together with the same meal amounts and the same initial glucose concentration caused the different glycemic curves for the 10 h prediction. For example, despite of the daily insulin applications of two patients no. 2 and no. 4 were similar their dynamics were of glucose concentrations were different. It also justifies a need of sensitivity analysis.

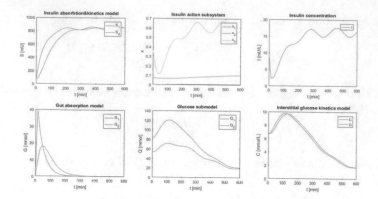

Fig. 2. Results of the Hovorka model simulation of all compartments. A simulated meal was delivered at 1st minute. Due to discrepancies in scales, insulin kinetics compartment has been presented on two figures, called 'Insulin absorption & kinetics model' and 'Insulin concentration'

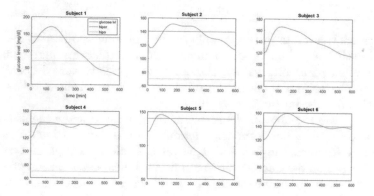

Fig. 3. Simulated inter-patients differences in a glucose response on the same insulin doses

3   Methods of the Nonlinearity and Sensitivity Analysis

The first step of the performed model sensitivity analysis was to determine an intensity of a model nonlinearity. This feature is important while projecting the control algorithm. A strong nonlinear control process surely requires a nonlinear controller. However, nonlinear control algorithms are computationally complex so they require much time to calculate insulin doses. Also, the problem with numerous local minimas appears, so the computed insulin dose may not be optimal in a given state of patient health.

On the other hand, weakly nonlinear controlled process enables to use a linearized controller where the number of linearization steps depends also on nonlinear intensity of the controlled object. Small number of these steps significantly accelerates computation. Finally, a nearly linear process can be successively controlled by a linear controller, for example PID. Currently, a PID controllers were used in commercial versions of the insulin delivered systems. According to our best knowledge, nonlinearity of the Hovorka model has not been studied.

Despite the most of mathematical equations are linear but some of them use variables with nonlinear constrains. For example the (11) equation uses the variable F_R with the piece linear constrain given by the (16) formula. Therefore it is difficult to perform a theoretical analysis of the Hovorka model nonlinearity. We studied it in simulation environment, applying the method described in [13]. Let y_o will be an output on the studied model (i.e. a simulated glucose concentration) without any control signals, i.e. without the externally administrated insulin. y_1 denotes a model response on the step of an insulin dose u_1. Respectively, y_2 will be a simulated glucose concentration in response to the step of the insulin dose equaled to $u_2 = \gamma u_1$ for $\gamma > 0$. Then, the following coefficient has been introduced:

$$\eta = \max_t \frac{|\delta(t) - \gamma|}{|\gamma|}, \text{where } \delta(t) = \frac{y_2(t) - y_0}{y_1(t) - y_0} \tag{19}$$

The coefficient η describes an intensity of a model nonlinearity. It is equaled to 0 for a linear model and tends to infinity as a model nonlinearity increases. This coefficient was used for an estimation of the nonlinear intensity for the Hovorka model.

In general, physiological processes are always nonstationary because biological properties of the organism and external factors that activates them are time-dependent. Therefore, adaptive control algorithms are recommended for the considered issue. Such algorithms on-line estimate some parameters which represent the mentioned source of nonstationarity. There is an important question - which model parameters should be estimated on-line? They must meet two conditions. The adaptive model parameters ought to be clinically identifiable and have significant influence on the insulin-glucose interaction. Thus, a parameters sensitive analysis was performed to find out the most sensitive parameters.

Generally, any mathematical model of a system can be represented by the expression $y = M(u, \mathbf{P})$, where M is a function mapping an input signal u on an output signal y and $\mathbf{P}$ is a vector of its parameters. Thus, a parameter sensitivity index is defined as:

$$S_\theta \overset{def}{=} \frac{\partial y}{\partial \mathbf{P}} \tag{20}$$

For simple models, particularly when M is a linear function the index can be analytically computed. This approach is called a direct sensitivity analysis.

For complex models two indirect manners of sensitivity analysis are used. The objective of local sensitivity analysis is to analyze the influence of a local perturbation of a parameter around its chosen value on the model output. While global sensitivity analysis studies an influence of all possible parameter values on the model output.

Typically, local sensitivity analysis is performed using a finite difference approximation of the derivative (18). Global sensitivity analysis employs Monte Carlo methods to sample the whole range of the parameter values assuming a probability distribution function defined on this range. Then, the variance based forms of (18) are used computing the variance of the model output conditioned on the studied parameter [14].

In this paper local sensitivity analysis with the 2nd order finite difference approximation due to the following reasons. From the controller point of view it is important to find how the assumed deviation from the patient-specific (nominal) values of the studied parameters affect the glucose concentrations. Moreover, population probability distribution functions of these parameters are not known and they did not have an uniform or Gaussian form.

Thus, let $q\left(y(t\,|P_o + \Delta P)\right)$ denotes a value of a model output in a response to replacing the parameter value P_o with the value $P_o + \Delta P$. We used the time-dependent sensitivity index defined as:

$$SI_{PQ}(t) = \left[G(t\,|P_o + \Delta P) - G(t\,|P_o - \Delta P)\right]/2\Delta\mathrm{P} \qquad (21)$$

Moreover, the time-dependent robustness coefficient was applied to normalize the sensitivity index relatively to the parameter changing:

$$EI_{PQ}(t) = \left[\frac{P_0}{G(t\,|P_o)}\right] SI_{PQ}(t) \qquad (22)$$

Additionally, the time-dependent relative sensitivity was computed to assess a model output residuum caused by the change in model parameter values:

$$\delta_{PQ}(t) = \frac{|G(t\,|P_0 \pm \Delta P) - G(t\,|P_0)|}{|G(t\,|P_0)|} \cdot 100\% \qquad (23)$$

Next the time median and time maximal values of the coefficients (19)–(23) were calculated.

The sensitivity analysis was performed in the 'one-at-time' methodology which means that all other model parameters were maintained constant. According to the Chassin et al. suggestions expressed in [15], a sensitivity of the studied parameter was analyzed assuming two conditions: first, when the parameter deviation was equal to 5% of the basic parameter value identified for a given patient and second, when this disturbance was equal to 30%.

Selection of the model parameters assigned for a sensitivity analysis is a difficult problem because of its arbitral character. The forms of the model equations suggest that a nonlinearity is directly associated with the glucose compartments. So, the performed sensitivity analysis obeys the following parameters: EPG_o, F_{01} and k_e. An influence of an insulin dose and inter-patients variability on the sensitivity were also studied.

4   Results

The results of the nonlinear intensity of the Hovorka model obtained for the six patients are presented in the Table 2. They are obtained for the different insulin doses and different γ values. The test insulin doses were 0.5, 0.75 or 1 U/h for $\gamma = 2$ and 0.5 and 1.5 U/h for $\gamma = 3$. These results seem to show relation between the Hovorka model nonlinearity and the inter-patients variability. Moreover, the insulin-doses dependence exists too. It is illustrated in the Fig. 4. The most 'nonlinear patient' is the patient no. 4. He/she is characterized by the 10-fold greater value of the renal clearance in comparison to the other patients. A renal glucose elimination is described by the nonlinear Eq. (16).

The results of the performed sensitivity analysis is summarized in the Table 3.

The analysis shows that the parameters EGP_0 and F_{01} are more influential on glucose concentrations than the k_e parameter. Probably it stems from the formula of the model Eqs. (15) and (17). Particularly the F_{01} variability may decrease a robustness of a non-adaptive control algorithm. The Fig. 5 shows the courses of the glucose concentrations depending on the studied disturbances of these parameters for the same insulin profile.

Table 2. The values of η coefficient obtained for different test situations

Ins. dose	Patient						Mean	Std. Dev.
u(t) [U/h]	1	2	3	4	5	6		
0.5 & 1	0.06	0.08	0.09	4.38	0.25	0.42	0.88	1.57
0.5 & 1.5	0.27	0.33	0.30	10.84	0.35	2.73	2.47	3.85
1 & 2	0.95	0.67	0.73	1.36	0.85	1.50	1.01	0.31
0.75 & 1	0.84	0.62	0.66	9.86	0.71	1.40	2.35	3.37

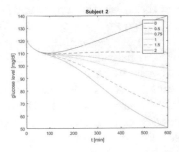

Fig. 4. Courses of glucose concentrations depending on the insulin doses obtained for the simulated patient no. 2

Table 3. The patients-averaged values of sensitivity indexes for the studied Hovorka model parameters in the different tests

Param	k_e		EGP_0		F_{01}	
	Mean	Std. dev.	Mean	Std. dev.	Mean	Std. dev.
$SI_{5\%}$	326.44	210.31	11518.44	6522.57	11968.46	5921.11
$EI_{5\%}$	0.17	0.12	0.91	0.44	0.93	0.47
$SI_{30\%}$	342.96	212.19	11021.45	4429.68	11289.92	3766.49
$EI_{30\%}$	0.17	0.12	0.89	0.34	0.89	0.38
$\delta_{-5\%}$	0.85	0.59	4.75	1.96	4.48	2.63
$\delta_{+5\%}$	0.80	0.58	4.38	2.47	4.78	2.15
$\delta_{-30\%}$	6.11	4.01	31.37	9.86	22.86	14.18
$\delta_{+30\%}$	4.18	3.11	22.10	13.03	30.38	10.71

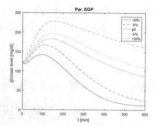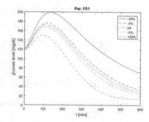

Fig. 5. Influence of the studied parameters on glucose profiles for the exemplary patient with the same insulin doses

5   Conclusion

The problem of persisting normoglycemia in patients suffering from type-1 diabetes is still unsolved. It seems that the adaptive closed loop systems are inevitable future of diabetic therapies. In this context, developing more detailed models, as well as providing broad analysis of the existing models of the physiological mechanism maintaining normoglycemia, is necessary. The results of such analyses can be very useful for construction of new algorithms enable to compute an optimal dose of administrated insulin.

According to the best authors' knowledge, there is the first paper presenting the effect of detailed sensitivity analysis of the Hovorka model. The obtained results of a model nonlinearity can be the useful indicator to select a proper model into a 'model based' controller. Low degrees of the nonlinearity enables to use simpler control algorithms which require less computational resources. It also supports and explains well approximation of the Hovorka model by the linear ARX and Box-Jenking models ($R^2 > 50\%$) presented in [16]. However, we firstly note that this approximation may be worse when the controlled patient has the higher renal clearance (the case of the fourth simulated patients).

Sensitivity analysis of the selected model parameters gives theoretical fundaments to confirm the clinical Hovorka's propositions. On the base of clinical experiences Hovorka *et al.* the nonlinear model based controller with Bayesian estimation and adaption of the five parameters: $S_{IT}, S_{ID}, S_{IE}, F_{01}$ and EGP_o. All these parameters are time-varying (Table 2) [8].

In the next studies fluctuations of the endogenous glucose and carbohydrate bioavailability were adapted [18,19].

The above presented original result shows the significant influence of k_e on the glucose concentration. It is important advice to elaborate an estimation method for this parameter and incorporate its adaptation in control algorithms. It is a possible direction for control algorithm improvement.

Moreover, further sensitivity analyses of the remained model parameters are necessary to design more flexible control algorithms.

However, based on obtained results, at least locally linearized algorithms might be postulated. This conclusion is coherent with the concept to approximate The Hovorka model by the successively linearized neural or fuzzy models which are computationally more efficient and can be used as an 'internal model' in an adaptive regulator [19].

Acknowledgement. The authors thank Dr. Malgorzata Wilinska and Prof. Roman Hovorka from Wellcome Trust-MRC Institute of Metabolic Science, University of Cambridge for their kind and advices during model implementation.

References

1. Clinical recommendations for the management of patients with diabetes 2016. Guideline of the Polish Diabetes Association
2. World Health Organization, Global Report on Diabetes (2016)
3. Kapica-Topczewska, K., Snarska, K., Bachórzcwska-Gajewska, H., Drozdowski, W.: Powikłania neurologiczne cukrzycy. Terapia **3**(236), 56–61 (2010). (in Polish)
4. Trevitt, S., Simpson, S., Wood, A.: Artificial pancreas device systems for the closed-loop control of type 1 diabetes: what systems are in development? J. Diab. Sci. Technol. **10**(3), 714 723 (2016)
5. Daskalaki, E., Diem, P., Mougiakakou, S.G.: Model-free machine learning in biomedicine: feasibility study in type 1 diabetes. PLoS ONE **11**(7), e0158722 (2016)
6. Chee, F., Fernando, T.: Closed-Loop Control of Blood Glucose, vol. 368. Springer Science & Business Media, Heidelberg (2007)
7. Dalla Man, C., Rizza, R.A., Cobelli, C.: Meal simulation model of the glucose-insulin system. IEEE Trans. Biomed. Eng. **54**(10), 1740–1749 (2007)
8. Hovorka, R., Canonico, V., Chassin, L.J., Haueter, U., Massi-Benedetti, M., Federici, M.O., Wilinska, M.E.: Nonlinear model predictive control of glucose concentration in subjects with type 1 diabetes. Physiol. Meas. **25**(4), 905 (2004)
9. Sorensen, J.T. A physiologic model of glucose metabolism in man and its use to design and assess improved insulin therapies for diabetes (Doctoral dissertation, Massachusetts Institute of Technology) (1985)
10. Worthington, D.R.L.: Minimal model of food absorption in the gut. Med. Inform. **22**(1), 35–45 (1997)

11. Hovorka, R.: Artificial pancreas project at Cambridge 2013. Diabet. Med. **32**(8), 987–992 (2015)
12. Tadeusiewicz, R., Augustyniak, P. (eds.): Podstawy inżynierii biomedycznej. Wydawnictwa AGH (2009). (in Polish)
13. Söderström, T.D., Stoica, P.G.: Identyfikacja systemów. Wydawnictwo Naukowe PWN (1997). (in Polish)
14. Cacuci, D. G.: Sensitivity and Uncertainty Analysis, Volume I: Theory. CRC Press, Boca Raton (2003)
15. Chassin, L.J., Wilinska, M.E., Hovorka, R.: Evaluation of glucose controllers in virtual environment: methodology and sample application. Artif. Intell. Med. **32**(3), 171–181 (2004)
16. Finan, D.A., Zisser, H., Jovanovic, L., Bevier, W.C., Seborg, D.E.: Identification of linear dynamic models for type 1 diabetes: a simulation study. IFAC Proc. Vol. **39**(2), 503–508 (2006)
17. Elleri, D., Allen, J.M., Kumareswaran, K., Leelarathna, L., Nodale, M., Caldwell, K., et al.: Closed-loop basal insulin delivery over 36 hours in adolescents with type 1 diabetes: randomized clinical trial. Diab. Care **36**(4), 838–844 (2013)
18. Elleri, D., Allen, J.M., Nodale, M., Wilinska, M.E., Mangat, J.S., Larsen, A.M.F., et al.: Automated overnight closed-loop glucose control in young children with type 1 diabetes. Diab. Technol. Ther. **13**(4), 419–424 (2011)
19. Radomski, D., Lawrynczuk, M., Marusak, P., Tatjewski, P.: Modeling of glucose concentration dynamics for predictive control of insulin administration. Biocybernet. Biomed. Eng. **30**(1), 41–53 (2010)

Limitations of Corneal Deformation Modelling During IOP Measurement – A Review

Magdalena Jędzierowska[(✉)], Robert Koprowski, and Zygmunt Wróbel

Faculty of Computer Science and Material Science, Institute of Computer Science, Department of Biomedical Computer Systems, University of Silesia, ul. Będzińska 39, 41-200 Sosnowiec, Poland
magdalena.jedzierowska@us.edu.pl

Abstract. This paper examines practical constraints and problems related to modelling of the human cornea during intraocular pressure measurement using Corvis ST. It highlights the essential role of corneal deformation image processing and analysis in the field of numerical modelling. By combining these two disciplines: biomechanics, which deals with modelling the behaviour of biological structures, and image processing methods, it is possible to verify and compare the values obtained for the tested models in numerical experiments with those obtained through image analysis. In the case of a biomechanical model of the eyeball, for which no 'gold standard' has yet been developed, the possibility of such a comparison is particularly important and valuable.

Keywords: Corneal deformation · Biomechanics · Dynamic numerical simulations · Corvis ST · Image processing

1 Introduction

Thanks to the dynamic development of anterior segment modern imaging techniques, there have appeared new possibilities for analysis and processing of the acquired images [1,2]. Especially in this area images derived from anterior segment optical coherence tomography (AS-OCT) [3] and non-contact Corvis ST tonometer, are now very often subject to quantitative and qualitative analysis [4–8]. The reason for their growing popularity in the field of image processing is undoubtedly the fact that both devices have the potential of corneal deformation imaging during intraocular pressure (IOP) measurement. The undisputed leader in corneal deformation imaging during IOP measurement is the Corvis ST tonometer. This device has the ultra-fast Scheimpflug camera that records 4,330 corneal images per second during its dynamic deformation resulting from an air puff (Fig. 1). So far, in the literature, there have been numerous proposals for image processing and analysis dedicated to this technology. The use of the Corvis ST tonometer to measure intraocular pressure (IOP) and to evaluate

© Springer International Publishing AG, part of Springer Nature 2019
E. Pietka et al. (Eds.): ITIB 2018, AISC 762, pp. 469–480, 2019.
https://doi.org/10.1007/978-3-319-91211-0_41

the biomechanical properties of the cornea, which are directly linked with its dynamic deformation, was the subject of several studies [9–15]. However, this device provides many more options for measurement of corneal properties after the application of additional tools and procedures available in the field of image processing.

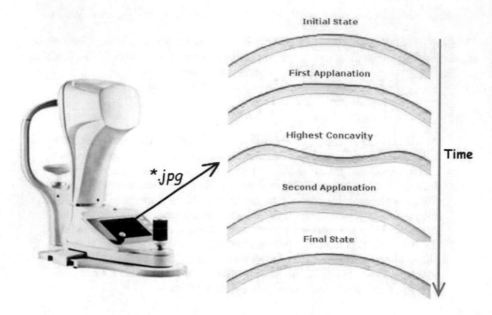

Fig. 1. Schematic diagram of the corneal deformation measurements using the Corvis ST tonomet

The human eye when measured with a non-contact tonometer such as Corvis ST is subjected to external forces. Such an examination enables analysis of biomechanics of the eyeball, and more specifically the cornea, which directly responds to an external stimulus [16,17]. By combining two disciplines, namely biomechanics, which deals with modelling the behaviour of biological structures, and image processing methods, it is possible to verify and compare the values obtained for the tested models in numerical experiments with those obtained through image analysis. In the case of a biomechanical model of the eyeball, for which no 'gold standard' has yet been developed the possibility of such a comparison is particularly important and valuable. An example would be the problem of modelling corneal geometry, which may vary between individuals and change as a result of disease (e.g. keratoconus). Therefore, the possibility of obtaining the actual parameters describing corneal geometry, such as the curvature, enables correction and individual adjustment of the parameters and assumptions defined during the construction of a numerical model.

The aim of this study was to present and comment the limitations and problems of modelling the cornea in dynamic conditions that occur during tonometry tests. The essential role of corneal deformation imaging with Corvis ST in the field of numerical modelling is also highlighted.

2   Modelling of the Eyeball

Image processing of dynamic corneal deformation allows for direct analysis of the phenomena occurring during tonometry tests. Despite undeniable advantages of this approach, qualitative and quantitative evaluations of the acquired images in isolation from the biology and biomechanics of the depicted structures can lead to incomplete and misleading conclusions, detached from actual conditions. Therefore, it is necessary to know the environment in which specific imaging tests are performed. Explanation of some of the facts observed using advanced image processing algorithms may be easier if there is a verification with biomechanical models. The role of biomechanics and modelling is extremely vital, and development of a commonly accepted model, which would perfectly reflect the physical parameters, is an important yet difficult task.

The first attempts at modelling the human cornea were made at the end of the nineteenth century. These models had a simplified form and the cornea was reduced to a spherical membrane of the same material properties and linear-elastic behaviour. With the development of computer technology, there appeared solutions of numerical models of the entire eyeball based on the finite element method (FEM). Since then, no one has managed to develop a model of the eyeball or the model of the cornea itself, which would fully reflect the physical properties of this organ.

3   Numerical Models of Dynamic Corneal Deformation

A review of the current literature on modelling the cornea during IOP measurement indicates a variety of proposals addressing the evaluation of the selection and measurement of corneal biomechanical parameters.

Some authors suggest inverse modelling using the FEM. This approach takes into account correction of the material properties of the modelled structures. Bekesi et al. [18] used imaging of corneal deformation resulting from an air puff (using Corvis ST), which was combined with the technique of inverse modelling using the FEM. The purpose was to obtain proper mechanical parameters of the studied hydrogel polymer model of cornea and porcine corneas. Simulations carried out after the correction of material properties allowed for the reconstruction of the corneal profile deformation curves obtained experimentally using Corvis ST. For the experiment, three model corneas with different thicknesses were used: 350 μm, 450 μm and 550 μm and two porcine corneas. IOP was constant, set to 15 mmHg. The authors believe that in view of the above the presented approach can be successfully used in modelling the human cornea.

Another work [19] developed a model, which estimate cornea linear elastic and viscous properties. Similar to [20], Kling et al. applied the inverse modelling approach to match the results obtained for the proposed model with the dynamic response of the cornea under experimental conditions. The aim of the model was to recreate the mechanism of corneal deformation under the influence of a collimated air pulse. The model was verified using data obtained experimentally – imaging of deformation of the porcine and human cornea using Corvis ST. The authors also examined the effect of different factors, including IOP (values from 15 to 35 mmHg), on the process of corneal deformation in the model. The assumptions adopted in [19] describe the model as two-dimensional and symmetrical. Only half of the eyeball including the cornea, sclera and limbus was under consideration (structures are shown in Fig. 2). The geometry of the sclera was taken from works of literature, and the limbus was defined as the interface between the cornea and the sclera. The shape of the cornea was modelled on the basis of images from the Scheimpflug camera (Corvis ST). The issue of fluid in the eye was approximated to a single fluid compartment model. The limbus and sclera were defined as purely elastic materials, noting at the same time that such an approach presents only the macroscopic scale of the behaviour of both structures during dynamic deformation. Reported results have shown that the mean corneal Young's modulus was 0.71 MPa for the virgin human cornea and 13.2 MPa for the cross-linked porcine cornea. One of the key elements was describing the corneal material as linear viscoelastic. The approach to this problem presented by Kling et al. has been contradicted by the recent publications [21, 22] which support the hypothesis that during the dynamic tonometry test any viscous property of the cornea cannot be activated as the duration of the air pulse is too short. Consequently, the influence of viscosity in the biomechanical response to the air-puff deformation has limited relevance.

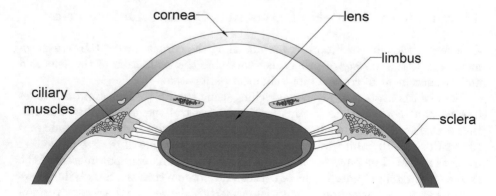

Fig. 2. Schematic diagram of the anterior segment of the eye. Structures shown include the cornea, limbus, sclera, ciliary muscles and lens

One of the works presenting the above theory is the paper of Roy et al. that aimed to develop a three-dimensional finite element model of the whole eyeball and improve the method of inverse modelling [21]. The designed model contained elements that had not been previously included, namely: transversely isotropic structure of the cornea resulting from intersection of lamellae, which constitute a single layer of collagen fibres. Also in this publication, the authors used the possibility of imaging two-dimensional cross-sections of the cornea in the course of its deformation using Corvis ST. The measurements performed on one eye on each of 10 patients. During the tests, displacement of the outer edge of the cornea in relation to its original position was determined in real time. These measurements of corneal deformation were used in inverse modelling. It is also worth noting that in their work, they took into account the impact of the entire eyeball and the resistance of fatty tissues and muscles on the amplitude of corneal deformation. What is more, the influence of IOP (13, 15 and 17 mmHg) on the estimated biomechanical parameters was also examined.

When studying diverse approaches to dynamic corneal deformation modelling, attention should also be paid to publications [23–25], which discuss corneal vibrations during its deformation resulting from external pressure. Han et al. [23] proposed a simple one degree-of-freedom biomechanical model describing corneal deformation caused by an air pulse. The model assumed a viscoelastic material structure of the cornea with a specific weight (affecting corneal displacement). Numerical results for the model were compared with measurements made using two non-contact tonometers, namely Ocular Response Analyzer (ORA) and Corvis ST. The numerical simulations made it possible to obtain curves depicting corneal displacement over time. These waveforms proved to be very similar to those obtained from ORA. However, significant differences were introduced by some changes in the model parameters: corneal mass, elasticity modulus (ranging from 38 to 50) and damping coefficient (set values: 0 and 0.0003). Analysis of various configurations of the presented parameters enabled Han et al. to conclude that corneal vibrations appearing after applying dynamic external force are mainly affected by the corneal mass and elasticity modulus. However, the simulated results are different from those observed on images from the Corvis ST tonometer. Vibrations on these images are observed during maximum corneal deflection (the largest concave) and definitely do not last throughout the entire measurement process. The above is in contrast to the model data where vibrations persist until the moment when cornea moves back to its initial state. Given present constraints on the model, it can only partially represent characteristics of corneal dynamics. An important observation is the supposition that the resulting vibrations can reflect the characteristics of the natural frequencies of the cornea.

In [25], the authors present another approach to modelling the cornea in dynamic conditions. The main element of assumptions was treating the eyeball as a perfectly spherical membrane of uniform thickness and material from which the membrane was made as uniform (both cornea and iris were classified in the same class of materials and it was assumed that the eyeball is filled completely with water). When considering this model, the authors suggested, that natural vibrations of the eyeball are mainly dominated by the fluid in its interior and not by the properties of the membrane itself.

Some selected elements considered as significant during cornea deformation modelling were listed in Table 1.

Table 1. Summary of selected model elements referred from other studies

	Kling et al. [19]	Roy et al. [21]	Han et al. [23]	Shih et al. [25]
Dynamic conditions	Yes	Yes	Yes	Yes
Model verification with Corvis ST	Yes	Yes	Yes	Yes
Model geometry	2D axis-symmetric cornea model defined based on Scheimpflug images	3D cornea model constructed using the tomographic data from a Pentacam	Nonlinear corneal model constructed in one dimension (mass- spring-damper model)	Spherical diaphragm model of an eyeball
Material	Corneal modeled as a linear viscoelastic material	Cornea modeled as a hyperelastic, fiber dependent elastic material	Cornea modeled as viscoleastic material	Diaphragm material represented only by corneal properties
Consideration of ocular fluid	Yes	No	No	Yes
Simulation of corneal vibrations	No	No	Theoretical simulations indicate the presence of corneal vibration during air puff test	Model considered the oscillation of the entire eyeball
Separation of eyeball reaction	No	No	No	No
Consideration of ocular muscles	Yes	Yes	No	No

4   Image Analysis – Selected Aspects Influencing Cornea Modelling

Analysis of images from the Corvis ST tonometer enables extraction of new information and parameters relating to, for example, vibrations of the cornea, or to change in geometry when measuring intraocular pressure.

The nature of corneal deformation changes studied in works [26,27] was associated with the occurring lesions – keratoconus. In [26] the proposed analysis of the different stages of corneal deformation is aimed at extracting characteristic parameters associated with corneal vibrations during its deformation. However, the problem of the occurrence of corneal vibrations and their frequency due to external stimuli has been previously described [28], the presented data did not provide information on the analysis of corneal vibrations during its deformation in a tonometry test. In an attempt to examine this phenomenon corneal oscillations occurring during Corvis ST measurements were identified [26]. Changes associated with high frequencies of corneal vibrations – above 100 Hz and low frequencies – below 100 Hz were distinguished. Moreover, on the basis of the frequency analysis, the authors proposed a number of new parameters directly related to corneal vibrations at its characteristic points. By combining these new parameters with the characteristics of patients with keratoconus (the length of the first applanation, corneal thickness and IOP), the quality of the classification of this disease has been improved. The results described in the work of Koprowski et al. shed new light on the biomechanical aspects of corneal deformation. Furthermore they open, previously described to a lesser extent, a new issue of corneal vibrations induced by an air stream, which in numerical models are still simplified or completely omitted.

The dynamics of corneal deformation and intraocular pressure measurement are also affected by corneal thickness and ocular anatomy. The measurement of central corneal thickness (CCT) in static conditions is widely recognized as extremely important, if not essential for the diagnosis of diseases of the eye and observation of patients after refractive surgery [29,30]. A group of scientists in work [31], addressed the issue of correction of dynamic corneal thickness. They referred to their previous work [32] where corneal thickness was measured on the basis of a series of images acquired from Corvis ST. Upon completion of the measurements, it turned out that the cornea at the point of its maximum deflection is thinner than when measured under static conditions. However, this fact without correction of distortions resulting from the method of imaging with the Scheimpflug camera did not fully reflect reality. Therefore, the main aim of the study of Li et al. [31] was to evaluate the effect of Scheimpflug distortions and to develop a method of their correction in the measurement of central corneal thickness during its dynamic deformation. After applying a new, proprietary method for correcting these distortions, there was an increase in the value of CCT at the time of greatest deflection by 66 ± 34 μm, which is 2.5% of its original value. The authors have expressed some objections to the observed changes and pointed out that further studies on the presented problem are necessary. However, variations in corneal thickness caused by external forces (air puff) may reflect the biomechanical properties of the cornea. Perhaps the confusion regarding the origin of this phenomenon can be explained by advanced biomechanical analysis of the dynamic model of the cornea.

5   Discussion

The issue of modelling the eyeball and cornea in static conditions has been presented repeatedly [33–36]. With the development of anterior segment imaging methods, in particular, the technologies for capturing the structures of visual organs during their dynamic responses to external stimuli, the need to simulate the occurring processes has emerged. Although it would seem that all the necessary tools are already available, the problem turns out to still be a difficult task. This is due to the need to describe many factors influencing the nature of a dynamic response.

The main problems met in modelling dynamic corneal deformation include: description of the shape and geometry of the cornea, determination of its material properties, consideration of the presence of liquid between the cornea and the sclera, acceptance of boundary conditions related to the effect of the limbus and accommodative system on the dynamics of deformation [22]. In addition, there is also the problem of modelling the force causing deformation, which is the air stream.

By using the experimental studies performed with, for example, the Corvis ST tonometer, it is possible to accurately model the shape and geometry of the cornea using the inverse modelling method [19–21,37]. It should be noted that images from the Corvis ST device show only sections of the cornea at a specified point. This approach introduces a number of limitations since corneal geometry is strongly affected by inter-individual factors, which vary depending on the point of the section. Moreover, the construction of the cornea may be asymmetrical, particularly in the case of degenerative diseases, such as keratoconus. Unfortunately, at the moment there is no imaging technique which would allow for three-dimensional imaging of corneal deformation during intraocular pressure measurement. However, given the technological advances of anterior segment imaging methods, it is believed that in the near future these limitations will be overcome.

A description of the corneal material poses more difficulties. Currently, it is known that the cornea is composed of six layers [38], of which stroma has the largest area. Accordingly, researchers often simplify the structure of the corneal material only to this 'thickest' layer. In spite of strict guidelines and insightful considerations of the structure of lamellae, forming a system of collagen fibres, according to the authors' knowledge, none of the developed cornea models fully takes into account the remaining structures of the cornea. The big unknown in this regard is the recently discovered Dua's layer, whose impact on the biomechanics of the human eye has not yet been investigated.

Another aspect is the lack of uniform boundary conditions defining the attachment of the eyeball. Some authors ignore the undoubted influence of the limbus and external muscles of the eyeball on the dynamics of the deformation process [39], 'fixing' the cornea in a rigid manner. Moreover, a description of the limbus material, which together with the ciliary muscle form a structure capable of changing its tensile stiffness, is very simplified. The assumptions describing this structure with material parameters of the cornea or sclera may not be appropriate. However, there are only unconfirmed hypotheses on this subject.

The important issue, which is the distinction between modelling the response of the cornea itself and modelling the response of the entire eyeball, cannot be ignored. In the first of these cases, during model development, it should be remembered that the response of the entire eyeball to an air pulse must be subtracted from the response (reaction) of the cornea itself. The effect of the eyeball reaction on the dynamic response of the cornea and its importance has been documented in [40].

Today, according to the authors' knowledge, there is no model that would allow for the simulation of corneal vibrations during IOP measurements using non-contact Corvis ST. The key issue is to explain the phenomenon of vibration. The shape of cornea vibrations occurring during its deformation is known thanks to the analysis of images from the Corvis ST tonometer [26]. They can be observed mainly in the phase of maximum deflection when the cornea 'ripples' and begins to return to its original shape. However, despite stringent assumptions, the models known from the literature ignore many aspects that prevent the correct presentation of this phenomenon. Among other things, internal reflections of the wave of air at the border of two centres, the cornea and the sclera, are omitted. There is also no modelling of high-frequency corneal vibrations – above 400 Hz.

To conclude, the main limitations in the corneal deformation modelling during IOP measurement are: 3D modelling of the corneal shape and geometry (currently there is no corneal imaging technique capable of presenting the dynamic corneal deformation in 3D); description of corneal material that will include all of the six cornea layers; defining the boundary conditions that will consider the impact of limbus and the external eyeball muscles; including in the model the corneal vibrations which occur during the tonometry test.

6   Summary

Nowadays, analysis and processing of medical images is a widely used tool to support the work of doctors of various disciplines and among other areas of science [41–43]. Thanks to advanced technologies, devices such as Corvis ST, dedicated to medical measurements, provide additional information, in this case in the form of two-dimensional images. The relationships and characteristics of the structures observed through the use of appropriate imaging tools often require a physical explanation. Therefore, the combination of biomechanics dealing with modelling of structures and organs of the human body, with advanced image analysis are complementary. This is also relevant to the issue of corneal deformation resulting from an air puff during non-contact tonometry tests. Although this topic is still being developed, there is no 'gold standard' for the model of the eyeball. The models presented in this paper include a number of restrictions that require reconsideration and verification with the information derived from corneal image analysis.

References

1. Rio-Cristobal, A., Martin, R.: Corneal assessment technologies: current status. Surv. Ophthalmol. **59**, 599–614 (2014)
2. Konstantopoulos, A., Hossain, P., Anderson, D.F.: Recent advances in ophthalmic anterior segment imaging: a new era for ophthalmic diagnosis? Br. J. Ophthalmol. **91**, 551–557 (2007)
3. See, J.L.S.: Imaging of the anterior segment in glaucoma. Clin. Experiment. Ophthalmol. **37**, 506–513 (2009)
4. Koprowski, R., Rzendkowski, M., Wróbel, Z.: Automatic method of analysis of OCT images in assessing the severity degree of glaucoma and the visual field loss. Biomed. Eng. Online **13**, 16 (2014)
5. Koprowski, R., Siedlecki, D., Kasprzak, H., Wróbel, Z.: Rapid dynamic changes of the geometry of the anterior segment of the eye: a method of automatic spatial correction of a temporal sequence of OCT images. Comput. Biol. Med. **72**, 132–137 (2016)
6. Gao, Z., Bu, W., Zheng, Y., Wu, X.: Automated layer segmentation of macular OCT images via graph-based SLIC superpixels and manifold ranking approach. Comput. Med. Imaging Graph. **55**, 42–53 (2016)
7. Kasprzak, H., Boszczyk, A.: Numerical analysis of corneal curvature dynamics based on Corvis tonometer images. J. Biophotonics **9**, 436–444 (2016)
8. Ji, C., Yu, J., Li, T., Tian, L., Huang, Y., Wang, Y., Zheng, Y.: Dynamic curvature topography for evaluating the anterior corneal surface change with Corvis ST. Biomed. Eng. Online **14**, 53 (2015)
9. Hong, J., Xu, J., Wei, A., Deng, S.X., Cui, X., Yu, X., Sun, X.: A new tonometer-the Corvis ST tonometer: clinical comparison with noncontact and Goldmann applanation tonometers. Invest. Ophthalmol. Vis. Sci. **54**, 659–665 (2013)
10. Valbon, B.F., Ambrosio Jr., R., Fontes, B.M., Alves, M.R.: Effects of age on corneal deformation by non-contact tonometry integrated with an ultra-high-speed (UHS) Scheimpflug camera. Arq. Bras. Oftalmol. **76**, 229–232 (2013)
11. Nemeth, G., Hassan, Z., Csutak, A., Szalai, E., Berta, A., Modis, L.: Repeatability of ocular biomechanical data measurements with a Scheimpflug-based noncontact device on normal corneas. J. Refract. Surg. **29**, 558–563 (2013)
12. Ambrosio Jr., R., Ramos, I., Luz, A., Faria, F.C., Steinmueller, A., Krug, M., Belin, M.W., Roberts, C.J.: Dynamic ultra high speed Scheimpflug imaging for assessing corneal biomechanical properties. Rev. Bras. Oftalmol. **72**, 99–102 (2013)
13. Smedowski, A., Weglarz, B., Tarnawska, D., Kaarniranta, K., Wylegala, E.: Comparison of three intraocular pressure measurement methods including biomechanical properties of the cornea. Investig. Ophthalmol. Vis. Sci. **55**, 666–673 (2014)
14. Koprowski, R.: Automatic method of analysis and measurement of additional parameters of corneal deformation in the Corvis tonometer. Biomed. Eng. Online **13**, 150 (2014)
15. Tian, L., Wang, D., Wu, Y., Meng, X., Chen, B., Ge, M., Huang, Y.: Corneal biomechanical characteristics measured by the CorVis Scheimpflug technology in eyes with primary open-angle glaucoma and normal eyes. Acta Ophthalmol. **94**, e317–e324 (2016)
16. Kling, S., Hafezi, F.: Corneal biomechanics – a review. Ophthal. Physiol. Opt. **37**, 1–13 (2017)
17. Jedzierowska, M., Koprowski, R., Wrobel, Z.: Overview of the ocular biomechanical properties measured by the ocular response analyzer and the corvis ST. Inf. Technol. Biomed. **4**, 377–386 (2014)

18. Bekesi, N., Dorronsoro, C., De La Hoz, A., Marcos, S.: Material properties from air puff corneal deformation by numerical simulations on model corneas. PLoS One **11**, e0165669 (2016)
19. Kling, S., Bekesi, N., Dorronsoro, C., Pascual, D., Marcos, S.: Corneal viscoelastic properties from finite-element analysis of in vivo air-puff deformation. PLoS One **9**, e104904 (2014)
20. Nguyen, T.D., Boyce, B.L.: An inverse finite element method for determining the anisotropic properties of the cornea. Biomech. Model. Mechanobiol. **10**, 323–337 (2011)
21. Sinha Roy, A., Kurian, M., Matalia, H., Shetty, R.: Air-puff associated quantification of non-linear biomechanical properties of the human cornea in vivo. J. Mech. Behav. Biomed. Mater. **48**, 173–182 (2015)
22. Simonini, I., Angelillo, M., Pandolfi, A.: Theoretical and numerical analysis of the corneal air puff test. J. Mech. Phys. Solids. **93**, 118–134 (2016)
23. Han, Z., Tao, C., Zhou, D., Sun, Y., Zhou, C., Ren, Q., Roberts, C.J.: Air puff induced corneal vibrations: theoretical simulations and clinical observations. J. Refract. Surg. **30**, 208–213 (2014)
24. Kling, S., Akca, I.B., Chang, E.W., Scarcelli, G., Bekesi, N., Yun, S.-H., Marcos, S.: Numerical model of optical coherence tomographic vibrography imaging to estimate corneal biomechanical properties. J. R. Soc. Interface **11**, 20140920 (2014)
25. Shih, P.-J., Cao, H.-J., Huang, C.-J., Wang, I.-J., Shih, W.-P., Yen, J.-Y.: A corneal elastic dynamic model derived from Scheimpflug imaging technology. Ophthal. Physiol. Opt. **35**, 663–672 (2015)
26. Koprowski, R., Ambrosio, R.: Quantitative assessment of corneal vibrations during intraocular pressure measurement with the air-puff method in patients with keratoconus. Comput. Biol. Med. **66**, 170–178 (2015)
27. Koprowski, R., Ambrosio, R., Reisdorf, S.: Scheimpflug camera in the quantitative assessment of reproducibility of high-speed corneal deformation during intraocular pressure measurement. J. Biophotonics **8**, 968–978 (2015)
28. Kling, S.: Corneal Biomechanical Properties: Measurement. Modification and Simulation. Institutio de Oftalmobiologia Aplicada, Spain (2014)
29. Antonios, R., Fattah, M.A., Maalouf, F., Abiad, B., Awwad, S.T.: Central corneal thickness after cross-linking using high-definition optical coherence tomography, ultrasound, and dual Scheimpflug tomography: a comparative study over one year. Am. J. Ophthalmol. **167**, 38–47 (2016)
30. Huseynova, T., Waring, G.O., Roberts, C., Krueger, R.R., Tomita, M.: Corneal biomechanics as a function of intraocular pressure and pachymetry by dynamic infrared signal and Scheimpflug imaging analysis in normal eyes. Am. J. Ophthalmol. **157**, 885–893 (2014)
31. Li, T., Tian, L., Wang, L., Hon, Y., Lam, A.K.C., Huang, Y., Wang, Y., Zheng, Y.: Correction on the distortion of Scheimpflug imaging for dynamic central corneal thickness. J. Biomed. Opt. **20**, 56006 (2015)
32. Hon, Y., Li, T., Zheng, Y., Lam, A.K.C.: Corneal thinning during air puff indentation. Invest. Ophthalmol. Vis. Sci. **55**, 3707 (2014)
33. Pandolfi, A., Manganiello, F.: A model for the human cornea: constitutive formulation. Biomechan. Model. **5**, 237–246 (2006)
34. Cavas-Martinez, F., Fernandez-Pacheco, D.G., De la Cruz-Sanchez, E., Nieto Martinez, J., Fernandez Canavate, F.J., Vega-Estrada, A., Plaza-Puche, A.B., Alio, J.L.: Geometrical custom modeling of human cornea in vivo and its use for the diagnosis of corneal ectasia. PLoS One **9**, e110249 (2014)

35. Simonini, I., Pandolfi, A.: Customized finite element modelling of the human cornea. PLoS One **10**(6), e0130426 (2015)
36. Nejad, T.M., Foster, C., Gongal, D.: Finite element modelling of cornea mechanics: a review. Arq. Bras. Oftalmol. **77**, 60–65 (2014)
37. Bekesi, N., Kochevar, I.E., Marcos, S.: Corneal biomechanical response following collagen cross-linking with Rose Bengal-green light and riboflavin-UVA. Investig. Ophthalmol. Vis. Sci. **57**, 992–1001 (2016)
38. Dua, H.S., Faraj, L. a, Branch, M.J., Yeung, A.M., Elalfy, M.S., Said, D.G., Gray, T., Lowe, J.: The collagen matrix of the human trabecular meshwork is an extension of the novel pre-descemet's layer (Dua's layer). Br. J. Ophthalmol. **98**, 691–697 (2014)
39. Ali, N.Q., Patel, D.V., McGhee, C.N.: Biomechanical responses of healthy and keratoconic corneas measured using a noncontact Scheimpflug-based tonometer. Invest. Ophthalmol. Vis. Sci. **55**, 3651–3659 (2014)
40. Koprowski, R., Lyssek-Boron, A., Nowinska, A., Wylegala, E., Kasprzak, H., Wrobel, Z.: Selected parameters of the corneal deformation in the Corvis tonometer. Biomed. Eng. Online **13**, 55 (2014)
41. Wójcicka, A., Jędrusik, P., Stolarz, M., Kubina, R., Wróbel, Z.: Using analysis algorithms and image processing for quantitative description of colon cancer cells. In: Pietka, E., Kawa, J., Wieclawek, W. (eds.) Information Technologies in Biomedicine, vol. 3, pp. 385–395. Springer, Cham (2014)
42. Popielski, P., Koprowski, R., Wróbel, Z., Wilczyński, S., Doroz, R., Wróbel, K., Porwik, P.: The matching method for rectified stereo images based on minimal element distance and RGB component analysis. In: Nguyen, N.T., Iliadis, L., Manolopoulos, Y., Trawiński, B. (eds.) Computational Collective Intelligence: 8th International Conference, ICCCI 2016, Halkidiki, Greece, 28–30 September 2016, Proceedings, Part II, pp. 482–493. Springer, Cham (2016)
43. Walczak, M.: 3D measurement of geometrical distortion of synchrotron-based perforated polymer with Matlab algorithm. In: Pieketka, E., Badura, P., Kawa, J., Wieclawek, W. (eds.) Information Technologies in Medicine: 5th International Conference, vol. 1, pp. 245–252. Springer, Cham (2016)

Sensitivity Analysis of Biomedical Models Using Green's Function

Krzysztof Łakomiec[(✉)], Karolina Kurasz, and Krzysztof Fujarewicz

Institute of Automatic Control, Silesian University of Technology,
Akademicka 16, 44-100 Gliwice, Poland
krzysztof.lakomiec@polsl.pl

Abstract. One of the important steps of analysis of any mathematical model is the sensitivity analysis. The most frequently used type of sensitivity analysis is the local parametric sensitivity analysis that answers the question how changes of model's parameters influence the solution of the model. It is routinely used but it can be applied only for constant parameters. It cannot be applied for non-stationary parameters nor for varying in time external input signals. The full information about the sensitivity in such a case can be given by the sensitivity analysis using Green's function. This work describes a toolbox written in MATLAB environment, which can be useful in sensitivity analysis of biomedical models described by system of ordinary differential equations. To illustrate this type of sensitivity analysis, we use the created tool to analyze a model of cell signaling pathway of p53 protein, which plays crucial role in the response of tumor and healthy cells to radiotherapy.

Keywords: Sensitivity analysis · Ordinary differential equations
Green's function

1 Introduction

Ordinary differential equations (ODE) are most often used to model real dynamical systems. Especially in biomedicine and systems biology the ODE models are usually used to describe the complex phenomena in living cells. Due to complexity of biomedical systems the models usually contain very large number of equations and parameters. To analyze these complex models (for example to simplify them) we can utilize the sensitivity analysis.

Sensitivity analysis of mathematical models is the study of how the change of input arguments of the model (parameters or input signals) affects the change of particular output of the model. This information can be used to better understand the system representing by particular mathematical model, therefore the methods of sensitivity analysis are often used in many fields of science and technology. Overview of different methods of sensitivity analysis can be found in work [8]. The general classification of methods of sensitivity analysis may be done by dividing them into two main groups:

© Springer International Publishing AG, part of Springer Nature 2019
E. Pietka et al. (Eds.): ITIB 2018, AISC 762, pp. 481–492, 2019.
https://doi.org/10.1007/978-3-319-91211-0_42

– Local sensitivity analysis — in which there is a local (nominal) point of analysis. Usually, in these methods the particular partial derivatives are calculated.
– Global sensitivity analysis — in which the entire available space of possible values is taken into account. In this type of sensitivity analysis different Monte-Carlo methods are often used [18].

This work is focused on first-order local sensitivity analysis. The term order in local sensitivity analysis indicates the order of derivatives which are calculated. This type of sensitivity analysis has been used in our previous works to compute gradients of minimized objective functions and utilized during gradient-based parameter estimation of mathematical models of different types [1–5,9,11–13], or during gradient-based control optimization [6].

Usually the local sensitivity analysis is used in a so-called parametric way. It means that the value of a given parameter is perturbed but it takes the same perturbed value through whole time horizon.

Another work [15] describes a dynamical method of sensitivity analysis for ODE systems by calculation of the so-called Green's function. The Green's function can give a dynamical insight how a change (in different perturbation times) of a signal/parameter propagates through the system. Unfortunately, the authors of [15] only describe the approach but do not share any computational tool. One of the aims of the present work is to fill this gap. We develop in Matlab environment a convenient tool that can be used for dynamical sensitivity analysis of any non-linear ODE model by using Green's function.

There are many tools written in MATLAB environment especially designed for sensitivity analysis of systems described by ordinary differential equations. A well-known tool to sensitivity analysis of ODE systems is a set of functions called SENS_SYS and SENS_IND [7]. These functions are written as an extension to the original MATLAB ODE15s function. Another tool widely used for sensitivity analysis of ODE systems is MATLAB SimBiology^{TM} [14] toolbox which uses the complex-step method to approximate the requested derivatives. Mentioned tools have one common disadvantage — they are only capable to calculation the parametric sensitivity and they cannot calculate the sensitivity for different perturbation times of particular variable.

In this article as an example of biomedical model for which we analyze sensitivity using the Green's function is p53-MDM2 model [16], which plays crucial role of in the cell's response to ionizing radiation. Radiotherapy is a part of cancer treatment to control or kill tumor cells and it may be curative in a number of types of cancer if they are localized to one area of the body. The p53 pathway controls hundreds of genes and their products, that respond to a large variety of stress signals among others, the one caused by radiotherapy.

There are studies describing the sensitivity analysis for the p53 model eg. simple p53-MDM2 regulatory module [17] or more complex model of ATM/p53/NF-κB pathways [10] where the authors focus on parametric sensitivity analysis. In those studies the authors did not use the approach that is utilized in this article.

2 Local Sensitivity Analysis

In this section we present the basics of the classical local parametric sensitivity for dynamical systems. Then the sensitivity analysis by using Green's function will be introduced and compared to the previous one.

2.1 Parametric Sensitivity Analysis

Let us consider that the analysed system is given as a following state-space representation:

$$\begin{cases} \dot{x}(t) = f(x(t), u(t)) \\ y(t) = g(x(t)) \end{cases} \tag{1}$$

where $x(t) \in R^n$, $y(t) \in R^m$ are vectors of state variables and output variables of the system respectively. $u(t) \in R^q$ is a vector of external inputs (stimulations) or non-stationary parameters. $f(\cdot)$ and $g(\cdot)$ are non-linear functions of appropriate dimensions that are differentiable w.r.t. their arguments.

To keep the mathematical description simple we do not introduce additional vector of parameters. Instead of this we assume that parameters are elements of vector $u(t)$ and they are constant for stationary parameters and may vary in time for non-stationary parameters.

The sensitivity model for (1) can be described by following equations:

$$\begin{cases} \dot{\overline{x}}(t) = A(t)\overline{x}(t) + B(t)\overline{u}(t) \\ \overline{y}(t) = C(t)\overline{x}(t) \end{cases} \tag{2}$$

where $\overline{x}(t), \overline{u}(t), \overline{y}(t)$ are variations of state, input and output of the original system (1). Matrices $A(t)$, $B(t)$ and $C(t)$ are constructed by linearisation of the functions $f(\cdot)$ and $g(\cdot)$ along nominal trajectories:

$$A(t) = \left.\frac{\partial f(\cdot)}{\partial x(t)}\right|_{nom}, \qquad B(t) = \left.\frac{\partial f(\cdot)}{\partial u(t)}\right|_{nom}, \qquad C(t) = \left.\frac{\partial g(\cdot)}{\partial x(t)}\right|_{nom}. \tag{3}$$

The classical parametric sensitivity of the ith output with respect to jth stationary parameter u_j

$$s_{ij}(t) = \frac{\partial y_i(t)}{\partial u_j} \tag{4}$$

is a solution (function of time) of the sensitivity model (2) under a single non-zero step-wise input signal $\overline{u}_j(t) = 1$, $t \geq 0$ and initial conditions $\overline{x}(0) = \frac{\partial x(0)}{\partial u_j}$.

This way of sensitivity analysis is the most popular way of local sensitivity analysis. Unfortunately, it can be applied only for constant parameters. In this way we cannot discover the influence of non-stationary parameters or external input signals varying in time that affect the system.

2.2 Sensitivity Analysis by Using Green's Function

The sensitivity model (2) under zero initial condition can be also described by following integral operator:

$$\overline{y}(t) = \int\limits_0^t K(t,\tau)\overline{u}(\tau)d\tau \tag{5}$$

where $K(t,\tau)$ is a kernel of the integral operator and is called *Green's function*.

The Green's function has two arguments t and τ. $K(t,\tau)$ can be interpreted as a sensitivity of instantaneous value of the output $y(t)$ with respect to instantaneous value of input/parameter $u(\tau)$. It allows existence of variation of the parameter at any time and, as consequence, allows the sensitivity analysis with respect to non-stationary parameters and other inputs varying in time.

A cross-section of $K(t,\tau)$ for fixed $\tau = \tau_0$ is an impulse response $\overline{y}(t)$, $t \geq \tau_0$ of the sensitivity model (2) caused by the Dirac impulse applied at time τ_0.

On the other hand a cross-section of $K(t,\tau)$ for fixed $t = t_0$ can be interpreted as a sensitivity of the instantaneous value $\overline{y}(t_0)$ on previous stimulation $\overline{u}(\tau)$, $\tau \leq t_0$ — see integral operator (5).

For linear time-invariant (LTI) systems both cross-sections are symmetric and are equal to the classical impulse response. For linear time-variant systems (LTV) these two cross-sections may have in general different shape.

3 Mathematical Model of p53-MDM2 Cell Regulatory Module

As an exemplary biomedical model, for which we apply the sensitivity analysis using Green's function, we use a deterministic model of the p53-MDM2 protein complex [16]. The p53-MDM2 protein complex is responsible for various task in the cell. The most important task for p53-MDM2 pathway are:

- detection of DNA damage,
- arrest the cell cycle during repair (not included in analyzed model),
- in the case that if particular DNA damage cannot be repaired then lead the cell to apoptosis.

The analyzed model describes changes over time the amounts of various agents involved in p53-MDM2 signaling pathway and is defined by following system of ordinary differential equations:

$$\frac{d}{dt}PTEN(t) = t_1 PTEN_t(t) - d_2 PTEN(t) \tag{6}$$

$$\frac{d}{dt}PIP_p(t) = a_2(PIP_{tot} - PIP_p(t)) - c_0 PTEN(t)PIP_p(t) \tag{7}$$

$$\frac{d}{dt}AKT_p(t) = a_3(AKT_{tot} - AKT_p(t))PIP_p(t) - c_1 AKT_p(t) \tag{8}$$

$$\frac{d}{dt}MDM(t) = t_0 MDM_t(t) + c_2 MDM_p(t) - a_4 MDM(t)AKT_p(t) + \quad (9)$$

$$- \left(d_0 + d_1 \frac{N^2(t)}{h_0^2 + N^2(t)} \right) MDM(t)$$

$$\frac{d}{dt}MDM_p(t) = a_4 MDM(t)AKT_p(t) - c_2 MDM_p(t) + \quad (10)$$

$$+ e_0 MDM_{pn}(t) - \left(d_0 + d_1 \frac{N^2(t)}{h_0^2 + N^2(t)} \right) MDM_p(t) - i_0 MDM_p(t)$$

$$\frac{d}{dt}MDM_{pn}(t) = i_0 MDM_p(t) - e_0 MDM_{pn}(t) + \quad (11)$$

$$- \left(d_0 + d_1 \frac{N^2(t)}{h_0^2 + N^2(t)} \right) MDM_{pn}(t)$$

$$\frac{d}{dt}P53_n(t) = p_0 - \left(a_0 + a_1 \frac{N^2(t)}{h_0^2 + N^2(t)} \right) P53_n(t) + c_3 P53_{pn}(t) + \quad (12)$$

$$- (d_3 + d_4 MDM_{pn}^2(t))P53_n(t)$$

$$\frac{d}{dt}P53_{pn}(t) = \left(a_0 + a_1 \frac{N^2(t)}{h_0^2 + N^2(t)} \right) P53_n(t) - c_3 P53_{pn}(t) + \quad (13)$$

$$- (d_5 + d_6 MDM_{pn}^2(t))P53_{pn}(t)$$

$$\frac{d}{dt}MDM_t(t) = 2s_0 P_A(t) - d_7 MDM_t(t) \quad (14)$$

$$\frac{d}{dt}PTEN_t(t) = 2s_1 P_A(t) - d_8 PTEN_t(t) \quad (15)$$

$$\frac{d}{dt}N(t) = d_{DAM} R(t) - \frac{N(t)d_{REP}P_A(t)}{N(t) + N_{SAT}P_A(t)} + a_6 \left(\frac{A(t)}{A_{max}} \right)^4 \quad (16)$$

$$\frac{d}{dt}A(t) = p_1 \frac{q_3 P53_{pn}^2(t)}{q_4 + q_3 P53_{pn}^2(t)} - d_9 A(t) \quad (17)$$

where:
AKT_p — active form of AKT,
MDM_t — MDM2 transcript,
MDM — cytoplasmic MDM2,
MDM_p — phosphorylated cytoplasmic MDM2,
MDM_{pn} — phosphorylated nuclear MDM2,
$P53_n$ — inactive form of nuclear p53 dimers,
$P53_{pn}$ — active form of nuclear p53 dimers,
$PTEN_t$ — PTEN transcript,
$PTEN$ — cytoplasmic PTEN,
PIP_p — active form of PIP3,
N — number of double strand breaks (DSBs) in DNA,
R — irradiation signal,
A — level of apoptotic factors.

486   K. Łakomiec et al.

The reader interested in details can find full description of the model and values of the parameters in [16].

Simulation of the model and the sensitivity analysis have been done two times: for initial conditions taken from [16] which are different than the steady state and initial conditions that are equal to the stable steady state (Table 1).

Table 1. Initial conditions of the model

Initial condition	Non-steady state value	Steady state value
$PIP_p(0)$	1.00E+05	1.08E−05
$AKT_p(0)$	1.00E+05	4.04E+03
$MDM(0)$	8.64E+03	2.90E−03
$MDM_p(0)$	1.37E+04	4.99E+04
$PTEN(0)$	0	1.48E+05
$MDM_{pn}(0)$	2.28E+05	1.66E+05
$P53_n(0)$	3.68E+04	1.03E+05
$P53_{pn}(0)$	5.90E+03	6.94E+04
$MDM_t(0)$	15	1.30E+02
$PTEN_t(0)$	0	7.41E+01
$N(0)$	0	5.03E−02
$A(0)$	0	4.06E+04

The final time for analysis is set to 90 h. Simulations of the model for two variables: $P53_{pn}$ and MDM_{pn} are presented in Fig. 1.

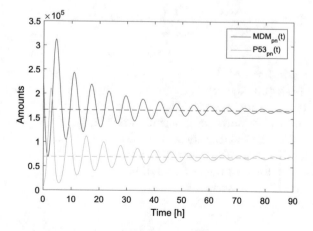

Fig. 1. Simulation of the model, dashed lines: steady state initial conditions, solid lines: non-steady state initial conditions

4   MATLAB Tool

In order to automate the calculation the sensitivity for different perturbation times a tool in MATLAB environment called GFODES was created. GFODES can be downloaded from MathWorks File Exchange site[1]. The user only need to provide a model in a symbolic form and names of variables which perturbation should be analyzed. The sensitivity system (2) is created from symbolic form of the model by using MATLAB Symbolic Toolbox. The user can use this tool in two ways: by creating the input file for the tool, or by use the provided graphical user interface.

5   Results

Now let us consider that we want to know how a perturbation of irradiation signal R in different times (from 0 to the final time 90 h) affects the number of $P53_{pn}$, MDM_{pn} molecules and the number of DNA damage N. To achieve that we need to calculate three different Green's functions. They are presented in Figs. 2, 3 and 4 respectively.

All three figures present also impulse responses of the sensitivity model (cross-sections of the Green's function) caused by impulsive stimulation applied at different times.

It is interesting to observe that for initial conditions that are different than the steady state (left panels) the impulse responses for the $P53_{pn}$ and MDM_{pn} are very different and depends strongly on the time τ of the impulsive stimulation. For example the sensitivity of both $P53_{pn}$ and MDM_{pn} are much higher on radiation at time 6 [h] than radiation applied at times 0 or 9 [h].

For initial conditions that are equal to the steady state (right panels) the shape of the impulse responses are similar and do not depend on the time of the stimulation.

The general conclusion that can come from this example is that for any non-linear dynamical model that does not work in steady state (i.e. there is a transition state caused by specific initial condition and/or external stimulation) the sensitivity analysis by using Green's function gives us much more information about classical parametric sensitivity analysis. Using this approach we can obtain impulsive responses on perturbation of parameter/signal at any time and this responses can be very different. Moreover, the non-stationary behavior of the system may be caused by another stimulation of different type, e.g. chemotherapy, which may be utilized in combined therapy.

The results of how irradiation in different times can change the levels of particular proteins can be also interesting from medical point of view. For example, in radiotherapy it is important to know which time of irradiation is the best for patients. A helpful tip to answer this question can be the results obtained from dynamic sensitivity analysis of various mathematical models describing the process of cellular response to irradiation.

---

[1] https://www.mathworks.com/matlabcentral/fileexchange/66028-gfodes.

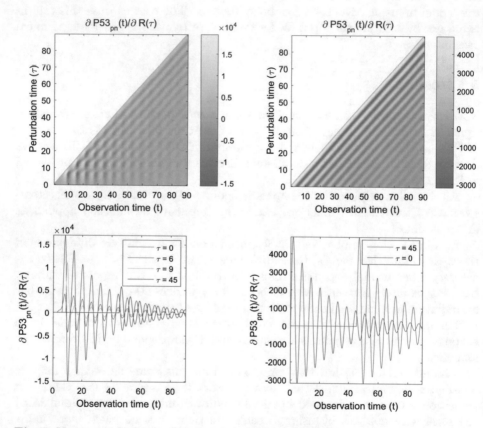

Fig. 2. Upper panels: The calculated Green's functions for the model depicting how a perturbation of R in different times τ affects the change of number of $P53_{pn}$ molecules at time t. Lower panels: cross-sections of particular Green's function in different perturbation times. Right panels: steady state initial conditions, left panels: non-steady state initial conditions

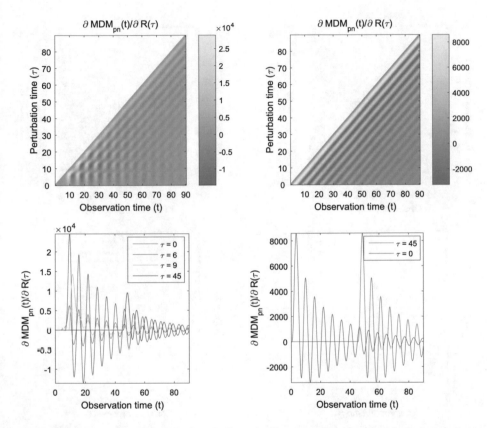

Fig. 3. Upper panels: the calculated Green's functions for the model depicting how a perturbation of R in different times τ affects the change of number of MDM_{pn} molecules at time t. Lower panels: cross-sections of particular Green's function in different perturbation times. Right panels: steady state initial conditions, left panels: non-steady state initial conditions

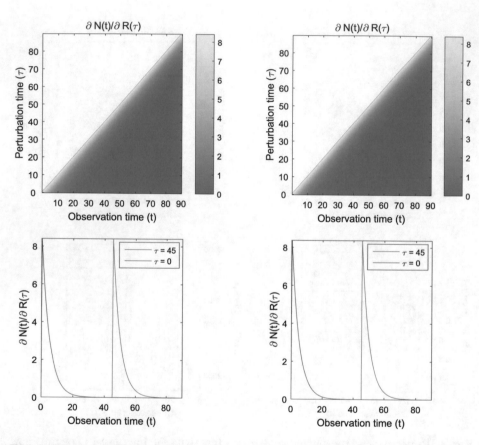

Fig. 4. Upper panel: The calculated Green's function for the model depicting how a perturbation of R in different times τ affects the change of number of DNA damage N at time t. Lower panels: cross-sections of particular Green's function in different perturbation times. Right panels: steady state initial conditions, left panels: non-steady state initial conditions

6   Conclusions

In this work we analyzed how changes of irradiation in different perturbation times affect the change of three crucial variables in the p53–MDM2 model by using the concept of Green's function. Results show that in sensitivity analysis of complex biomedical models the big importance have the dynamic methods, in which the particular parameter/signal is perturbed in different times.

Additionally, a tool in MATLAB environment which utilize the concept of Green's function to sensitivity analysis of system described by differential equations was created. The sensitivity system which is needed to calculate the Green's function is created by using the MATLAB Symbolic Toolbox from symbolic form of the model. The model and the sensitivity system are solved by using built-in MATLAB ODE solvers. The user should only provide the model in a symbolic form and names of state variable/parameter which should be analysed. The initial version of the tool can be downloaded from MathWorks File Exchange site. The tool will be constantly updated to provide a very reliable and useful software for sensitivity analysis.

Acknowledgement. This work was supported by the Polish National Science Centre under grant DEC-2016/21/B/ST7/02241 (K.F.) and by the Silesian University of Technology under grants BKM-508/RAU1/2017/12 (K.K.), BK-204/RAU1/2017/3 (K.Ł.). Calculations were performed using the infrastructure supported by the computer cluster Ziemowit (www.ziemowit.hpc.polsl.pl) funded by the Silesian BIO-FARMA project No. POIG.02.01.00-00-166/08 and expanded in the POIG.02.03.01-00-040/13 in the Computational Biology and Bioinformatics Laboratory of the Biotechnology Centre at the Silesian University of Technology.

References

1. Fujarewicz, K.: Estimation of initial functions for systems with delays from discrete measurements. Math. Biosci. Eng. **14**(1), 165–178 (2017). https://doi.org/10.3934/mbe.2017011
2. Fujarewicz, K., Galuszka, A.: Generalized backpropagation through time for continuous time neural networks and discrete time measurements. In: Rutkowski, L., Siekmann, J., Tadeusiewicz, R., Zadeh, L.A. (eds.) Artificial Intelligence and Soft Computing - ICAISC 2004. Lecture Notes in Computer Science, vol. 3070, pp. 190–196 (2004). https://doi.org/10.1007/978-3-540-24844-6_24
3. Fujarewicz, K., Kimmel, M., Lipniacki, T., Swierniak, A.: Adjoint systems for models of cell signaling pathways and their application to parameter fitting. IEEE ACM Trans. Comput. Biol. Bioinform. **4**(3), 322–335 (2007). https://doi.org/10.1109/tcbb.2007.1016
4. Fujarewicz, K., Kimmel, M., Swierniak, A.: On fitting of mathematical models of cell signaling pathways using adjoint systems. Math. Biosci. Eng. **2**(3), 527–534 (2005). https://doi.org/10.3934/mbe.2005.2.527
5. Fujarewicz, K., Łakomiec, K.: Parameter estimation of systems with delays via structural sensitivity analysis. Discr. Continuous Dyn. Syst. Ser. B **19**(8), 2521–2533 (2014). https://doi.org/10.3934/dcdsb.2014.19.2521

6. Fujarewicz, K., Łakomiec, K.: Adjoint sensitivity analysis of a tumor growth model and its application to spatiotemporal radiotherapy optimization. Math. Biosci. Eng. **13**(6), 1131–1142 (2016). https://doi.org/10.3934/mbe.2016034

7. Garcia, V.: Sensitivity analysis for ODEs and DAEs, MATLAB central file exchange. https://www.mathworks.com/matlabcentral/fileexchange/1480-sensitivity-analysis-for-odes-and-daes. Accessed 25 Mar 2016

8. Hendrickson, R.: A Survey of Sensitivity Analysis Methodology. National Bureau of Standards, NBSIR 84-28114, Washington DC (1984)

9. Jakubczak, M., Fujarewicz, K.: Application of adjoint sensitivity analysis to parameter estimation of age-structured model of cell cycle. In: Pietka, E., Badura, P., Kawa, J., Wieclawek, W. (eds.) Advances in Intelligent Systems and Computing, vol. 472, pp. 123–131. Springer (2016). https://doi.org/10.1007/978-3-319-39904-1_11

10. Jonak, K., Kurpas, M., Szoltysek, K., Janus, P., Abramowicz, A., Puszynski, K.: A novel mathematical model of ATM/p53/NF-κb pathways points to the importance of the DDR switch-off mechanisms. BMC Syst. Biol. **10**(1), 75 (2016). https://doi.org/10.1186/s12918-016-0293-0

11. Kumala, S., Fujarewicz, K., Jayaraju, D., Rzeszowska-Wolny, J., Hancock, R.: Repair of DNA strand breaks in a minichromosome in vivo: kinetics, modeling, and effects of inhibitors. Plos One **8**(1), 1–12 (2013). https://doi.org/10.1371/journal.pone.0052966

12. Łakomiec, K., Fujarewicz, K.: Parameter estimation of non-linear models using adjoint sensitivity analysis. In: Advanced Approaches to Intelligent Information and Database Systems, Studies in Computational Intelligence, vol. 551, pp. 59–68. Springer (2014). https://doi.org/10.1007/978-3-319-05503-9_6

13. Łakomiec, K., Kumala, S., Hancock, R., Rzeszowska-Wolny, J., Fujarewicz, K.: Modeling the repair of DNA strand breaks caused by γ-radiation in a minichromosome. Phys. Biol. **11**(4), 045003 (2014). https://doi.org/10.1088/1478-3975/11/4/045003

14. MathWorks MATLAB SimBiology release 2015b, Natick, Massachusetts, United States (2015)

15. Perumal, T.M., Wu, Y., Gunawan, R.: Dynamical analysis of cellular networks based on the Green's function matrix. J. Theor. Biol. **261**(2), 248–259 (2009). https://doi.org/10.1016/j.jtbi.2009.07.037

16. Puszynski, K., Hat, B., Lipniacki, T.: Oscillations and bistability in the stochastic model of p53 regulation. J. Theor. Biol. **254**(2), 452–465 (2008). https://doi.org/10.1016/j.jtbi.2008.05.039

17. Puszynski, K., Lachor, P., Kardynska, M., Smieja, J.: Sensitivity analysis of deterministic signaling pathways models. Bull. Pol. Acad. Sci. Tech. Sci. **60**(3), 471–479 (2012)

18. Saltelli, A., Ratto, M., Andres, T., Campolongo, F., Cariboni, J., Gatelli, D., Saisana, M., Tarantola, S.: Global Sensitivity Analysis: The Primer. Wiley, New York (2008)

Analytics in Action on SAS Platform

Automatic Classification of Text Documents Presenting Radiology Examinations

Monika Kłos[1], Jarosław Żyłkowski[2], and Dominik Spinczyk[1(✉)]

[1] Faculty of Biomedical Engineering, Silesian University of Technology,
Roosevelta 40, 41-800 Zabrze, Poland
dspinczyk@polsl.pl
[2] Second Department of Clinical Radiology, Medical University of Warsaw,
Banacha 1a, 02-097 Warszawa, Poland
http://ib.polsl.pl

Abstract. The paper presents the classification of text documents presenting radiology examinations, taking into consideration two groups: cases with aneurysms and those without it. A database containing descriptions of 1284 cases was classified using the maximum entropy algorithm and frequent phrase extraction. It was revealed that the best method was the classifier using the maximum entropy algorithm based on nouns. The best result obtained was 90% of sensitivity and 70% of specificity. The worse diagnostic capacity demonstrates frequent phrase extraction algorithm. The other classifiers turned out to be less effective, than the random ones.

Keywords: Medical records · Text mining · Text classifiers
Maximum entropy classifiers · Frequent phrase extraction classifiers

1 Introduction

The development of IT has increased the popularity of using computers and mobile devices. The amount of data is growing and finding the information needed is becoming more difficult. The expansion of technology conducts also to creating Hospital Information Systems. There are two types of data in hospitals: text data and image data, but the first type is more common.

Classifying, tagging and clustering of the data increases their utility. If the existing groups of topics in the data are completely unknown then clustering is useful [1]. In presented work we focused on classification of the text documents, which contained descriptions of computed tomography examinations.

The documents were segregated into two classes: (1) cases with aneurysms and (2) those without it. The aneurysms are blood-filled balloon-like bulge in the wall of a blood vessels. These most common diseases of blood vessels localized in brain, often do not show any symptoms, but their rupture can cause a spontaneous subarachnoid hemorrhage. There is a 30% risk of death or permanent

© Springer International Publishing AG, part of Springer Nature 2019
E. Pietka et al. (Eds.): ITIB 2018, AISC 762, pp. 495–505, 2019.
https://doi.org/10.1007/978-3-319-91211-0_43

neurological deficits causing the disablement. In order to find the best treatment, knowledge of morphology, size and location of aneurysms is very important. The treatment of uncontrolled aneurysms is especially controversial. On one hand the surgery can prevent apoplexy, but on the other hand, it can cause post surgery complications. Frequently the risk of preventive treatment exceeds the risk of natural course of the disease.

The aim of this paper is to develop an automatic method of the classification of short text documents containing descriptions of head computer tomography examinations.

This paper proceeds as follows. Section 2 presents five general stages of our work: creation of taxonomy, division of the document into teaching and learning set, classifier selection, quality of assessment of classification and classification of text documents related to aneurysms.

Experimental results are presented in Sect. 3. Finally, Sect. 4 contains discussion and plans for future work.

2   Materials and Methods

To achieve the goal of this paper, the work was divided into several stages. At the beginning, the descriptions of computer tomography examinations were selected from a database. Subsequently, the taxonomy was created. After dividing the cases into training and testing sets, the classifier was selected. These steps are described in more detail in Subsects. 2.1–2.3.

2.1   Creation of Taxonomy

To classify text documents, the term taxonomy should be defined. This is a set of methods and classification rules. Depending on the complexity of the classes, there exist: flat taxonomy, where each of the classes is on the same level and they do not divide further into subcategories and hierarchical taxonomy, where at least one class has subcategories.

It is important to choose class names, so that the document can be uniquely identified. Another important aspect is the creation of classes, that cover all cases.

In this paper we have selected flat taxonomy with two classes: Aneurysms and Without aneurysms. Our taxonomy is presented on the diagram (Fig. 1).

2.2   Division of the Documentation Into: Teaching Set and Testing Set

The next step is generating a metadata, that is structuring facts used to describe information resources. In order to do this, we need to separate the data into:

– testing data set – which best represents each category. These collections are used for each classification method;

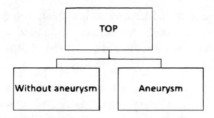

Fig. 1. Flat taxonomy

– training data set – which should be similar to the test sets. They are only used in statistical classification and in rule-based classification methods.

The analyzed data was divided into three sets:

1. training set for class Aneurysms – consisting of 50% of documents in the examined category;
2. training set for class Without Aneurysms – consisting of 50% of cases in considered class;
3. testing set – consisting of documents that did not occur in previous collections.

2.3   Classifier Selection

The classification of text documents concerns a wide range of topics. It can, for example, deal with recognition of the language of the analyzed documents or identification the author of the text. An important issue is also data structurization.

On the basis of the learner set, the classifier creates rules, so that it is possible to verify which class the document belongs to. The general diagram of the classifier work is shown in Fig. 2.

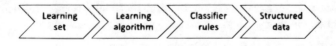

Fig. 2. Stages of the classifier

Regardless of the algorithm used, text documents are classified into matching classes based on the string of characters that holds the information. Depending on how the document is assigned to a class, we can distinguished:

1. Rule systems – in which categories are assigned by rules and heuristics;
2. Systems with supervised learning – where, relying on learning set, the features are used to train classifier;

3. Systems with unsupervised learning – in which the algorithm without the knowledge of the output labels, finds the rule that determines the output on its own. For example, when data set is not divided into classes, clustering can be used to group the most similar documents.

It was decided to choose rule-based classifiers. In this approach, user of the system can manually define a list of terms, that will create a classification rule. It is also possible to use automatic rules generator. The ability to modify automatic classification rules facilitates the work and accelerates the creation of classifiers.

We can distinguish two types of rules: (1) linguistic and (2) logic (called also boolean). In taxonomy, one class can use either boolean or linguistic rules. However, it is not possible to apply a rule that incorporates both types of rules to the same class.

Linguistic rules are based on the percentage of the accuracy of the document with a given principle of classification. The rule contains terms in which each has a weight. The sum of the weights of the words in the analyzed document determines its level of hit. Depending on the threshold, the document will either be classified or not.

Logic rules combine terms with boolean operators. If the document meets the assumptions, it is included in a class. Application of boolean rules takes more time than linguistic, but they are more precise.

Regardless of the type of rule, in order to create one, it is necessary to know the unique terms of each class. To detect unique words SAS Enterprise Miner is used to find uncommon words. There were created dictionaries for every group, first few terms of each category were presented in the Table 1. The dictionaries have been translated into English, which caused a repetition of some of these words, due to seven grammatical cases in Polish language. Ending of nouns change depending on the gender, number and case of that noun. After comparison of dictionaries it was found that unique terms are very rare. Because in this stage it was revealed that it was impossible to find specific terms for each class, in such manner it was preferred to work on automatic rules generators.

Automatic rules generators allow to identify ideals, terms and other relevant features of each category. Most commonly used classifiers are:

- Frequent Phrase Extraction – this algorithm uses the most common terms in the corpus of documents. The created list does not include weight of terms. This approach combines the advantages of statistical and rule-based methods;
- Support vector machine (SVM) – it is one of the most popular algotirhms, especially used for specyfic texts. It is succesfully used to classify such diseases as cancer and diabetes. The classifier treats the document as point in space, mapped in such a way, that the document classes are separated by a possibly wide gap. The category assignment for the parsed document follows when you map a document to this space and assign it the appropriate category, depending on which side of the gap is the case in question [2,5];
- K nearest neighbours (KNN) – this simple method classifies independent data, based on their similarity to the examples in the training data set.

Table 1. Dictionaries for each classes

Without aneurysms				Aneurysms			
Term	Role	Number of lectures in class	Number of documents	Term	Role	Number of lectures in class	Number of documents
permeable	Adjective	506	157	aneurysm	Noun	2178	790
a.	Noun	462	147	a.	Noun	1206	548
cervical	Adjective	429	150	aneurysm	Noun	1004	636
narrowing	Noun	395	118	aneurysm	Noun	840	504
artery	Noun	309	194	right	Adjective	784	532
segment	Noun	273	124	artery	Noun	737	383
stenoses	Noun	252	93	left	Adjective	717	480
permeable	Adjective	243	61	brain	Noun	716	453
spinal	Adjective	211	126	brain	Noun	715	453
intracranial	Adjective	210	171	right	Adjective	701	506
internal	Adjective	206	123	left	Adjective	675	472
neck	Adjective	205	75	research	Noun	614	430
left	Adjective	190	126	mm	Abbr.	612	289
preamble	Adjective	185	117	neck	Noun	513	366
research	Noun	177	133	about	Adverb	469	251
right	Adjective	168	111	this	Own name	454	411
important	Adjective	165	70	neck	Adjective	452	307
segment	Noun	163	84	front	Adjective	432	324
side	Noun	154	85	segment	Noun	424	277
tt	Noun	153	96	this	Own name	412	387
left	Adjective	148	106	direct	Adjective	386	302
common	Adjective	142	78	artery	Noun	373	228
istotnych	Adjective	140	54	neck	Adjective	371	266
change	Noun	140	102	intracranial	Adjective	368	321

The algorithm compares the analyzed document with the examples memorized while learning process of the classifier and finds the nearest neighbors for the given case (according to the previously mentioned proximity criterion). The main disadvantage of this algorithm is the speed with large data sets [2,5];

- Naive Bayes classifier (NB) – this probabilistic classifier assumes, that the probability of occurrence of a word is independent of its position in the document and the length of the analyzed document. The estimated probability of classifying a word into a class is expressed by the ratio of the number of words appearances in the training data for the class in question to the total number of word expressions in the training data for that class. The probabilities of all words in the class must sum up to 1 [7];

- Maximum entropy classifiers (MaxEnt) – this is probabilistic classifier belonging to the exponential model class. It does not assume, like Bayes Classifier, that functions are conditionally independent of each other. It is used to solve a variety of such problems [3,8].

There are many articles using SVM and KNN classifiers to text classification, for example System for Natural Language Processing presented in the publication [5]. The autors of the article [3] have found, that text mining can successfully support the Vaccine Adverse Event Reporting System, and the most commonly used classifiers are the rule-based, Naive Bayes and SVM classifiers.

Out of the known classifiers we decided to apply MaxEnt Classifier and Frequent Phrase Extraction. The method using Maximum Entropy is widely used for a variety of tasks. For example it is applied to tagging part of speech, language modeling or text segmentation. Authors of the article [6] emphasize that this approach is promising technique for text classification. We decided to use algorithm based on frequency of the phrase, because of its simplicity.

Comparison of results obtained from both methods can show, if less frequently used methods work in text classification.

2.4   Quality Assessment of Classification

It is worth mentioning, that the performance of the classifier might be faulty. We distinguish two types of correct decisions: true positive TP – proper indication of the class being analyzed and true negative TN – appropriate rejection case from the considered class.

There are two types of mistakes: false positive FP – incorrect choosing of inspected class and false negative FN – faulty passing by the examined class.

A good classifier should have minimum FP and TN values. However, in case of diagnosing the disease in another way, the case will be considered, when the classically classified person is at risk and otherwise, when the person is labeled as a healthy person.

To compare the results obtained by different algorithms, the statistical measures of the performance of a binary classification test were calculated. The first one is sensitivity, also called true positive rate (TPR), which can be calculated from the formula:

$$TPR = \frac{TP}{TP + FN}. \tag{1}$$

Maximum value of TPR (equal to 1) informs us that all cases considered as ill have been diagnosed.

The second often used quality assessment of classification is specificity (SPC), defined as:

$$SPC = \frac{TN}{TN + FP}. \tag{2}$$

SPC equal to 1 means that all healthy cases have been marked as healthy.

The most commonly used parameter is FPR (false positive rate), which value can be determined using the formula:

$$FPR = \frac{FP}{FP + TN} = 1 - \frac{TN}{TN + FP} = 1 - SPC. \tag{3}$$

After calculating those values, the analyzed classifier can be placed in ROC space (receiver operating characteristic).

There are other measures of the quality assessment of classification:

- positive predictive value (PPV), according to the procedure:

$$PPV = \frac{TP}{TP + FP}.$$

(4)

- negative predictive value (NPV), applying the formula:

$$NPV = \frac{TN}{TN + FN}.$$

(5)

- prevalence (PV), defined as:

$$PV = \frac{TP + FN}{TP + TN + FN + FP}.$$

(6)

- accuracy (ACC), calculated from the formula:

$$\begin{aligned} ACC &= \frac{TP + TN}{TP + TN + FN + FP} \\ &= \frac{TP}{TP + FN} \cdot PV + \frac{TN}{TN + FP} \cdot (1 - PV) \\ &= TPR \cdot PV + SPC \cdot (1 - PV) \end{aligned}$$

(7)

2.5 Classification of Text Documents Related to Aneurysms

Data set consists of 1284 radiological reports of head studies. For each class, the number of words in the study have been analyzed. The results were collected and presented in the Table 2. The average length of document is of about 50 words.

Table 2. Analysis of text documents of each class

Class	Quantity of documents	Number of words			
		Minimum	Maximum	Average	Median
Without aneurysms	378	0	148	47	38
Aneurysms	906	0	162	51	46

Experiment consists of the following steps:

- Text import – save each record in database as separate text file;
- Text parsing – find terms in the document and transform them into frequency matrix. This stage creates dictionaries for each class;
- Text classification – apply two algorithms of classification: Frequent Phrase Extraction and MaxEnt with different settings;
- Analysis – calculate several quality measures of decision rules for each classifier and show them in ROC space.

The calculations were made using SAS Text Analytics in Enterprise Text Miner Application and SAS Content Categorization Studio. The analysis concerned short textual documents in Polish, which contain about 50 words.

3   Results and Conclusions

Using two classification algorithms: MaxEnt and classifier based on frequent phrase extraction and available program parameters, 8 cases were generated:

1. Frequent phrase extraction: best speed or best quality,
2. Maximum entropy classifiers (MaxEnt):
   (a) weighted linguistic rules based on word,
   (b) weighted linguistic rules based on noun phrase,
   (c) weighted linguistic rules based on words or noun phrase,
   (d) boolean rules based on words,
   (e) boolean rules based on noun phrase,
   (f) boolean rules based on words or noun phrase.

Summing up the results obtained by the classifiers created in SAS Content Categorization Studio, the Table 3 which collected the results of the work of all classifiers was created.

Table 3. Results of classification

Algorithm	TP	FN	FP	TN	TPR	SPC	FPR	PPV	PV	ACC
B freq quality	7	182	452	1	0.037	0.002	0.998	0.015	0.294	0.012
T freq quality	68	385	187	2	0.150	0.011	0.989	0.267	0.706	0.109
B freq speed	9	180	450	3	0.048	0.007	0.993	0.020	0.294	0.019
T freq speed	12	441	188	1	0.026	0.005	0.995	0.060	0.706	0.020
B ent-wl W	100	88	287	167	0.532	0.368	0.632	0.258	0.293	0.416
T ent-wl W	55	399	88	100	0.121	0.532	0.468	0.385	0.707	0.241
B ent-wl N	130	59	164	289	0.688	0.638	0.362	0.441	0.294	0.653
T ent-wl N	410	43	64	125	0.905	0.661	0.339	0.865	0.706	0.833
B ent-wl WN	146	43	118	335	0.772	0.740	0.260	0.553	0.294	0.749
T ent-wl WN	413	40	68	121	0.912	0.640	0.360	0.859	0.706	0.832
B ent-bool W	105	84	442	31	0.556	0.066	0.934	0.192	0.285	0.205
T ent-bool W	361	92	134	55	0.797	0.291	0.709	0.729	0.706	0.648
B ent-bool N	66	134	373	80	0.330	0.177	0.823	0.150	0.306	0.224
T ent-bool N	235	218	165	24	0.519	0.127	0.873	0.588	0.706	0.403
B ent-bool WN	107	81	418	35	0.569	0.077	0.923	0.204	0.293	0.222
T ent-bool WN	396	57	141	48	0.874	0.254	0.746	0.737	0.706	0.692

First column of the Table 3 contains abbreviation of the adopted algorithm and it parameters. First letter of the shortcut means classes: 'B' defines Without Aneurysms and 'T' – Aneurysms. Consecutive characters of abbreviation interpret used algorithm: Frequent Phrase Extraction (freq) and Maximum Enthropy (ent). The remaining symbols of an alphabet symbolize parameters of each method.

These algorithms are described in the Sect. 2.3.

As shown in the analysis of individual parameters allowing for evaluation of diagnostic rules, the worst diagnostic ability had the algorithm based on the frequency of expression. And the best method was the Maximum Entropy classifier, which generated weighted linguistic rules.

For better visualization of the results, the classifiers are marked on the ROC space (Fig. 3).

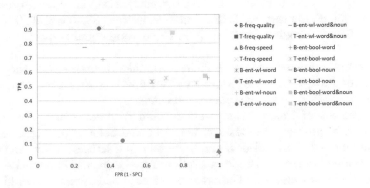

Fig. 3. ROC space with the used classifiers

Three groups of classifiers can be observed on the chart. First of them contains the worst methods, that used frequent phrase extraction. Next part include classifiers worse, than the random ones. These all classifiers using the maximum entropy algorithm, that creates the logical rules. Last fraction is composed from maximum entropy approaches, that construct the weighted linguistic rules.

4   Discussion

Interdisciplinary projects combining medicine and technical science, like biomedical engineering, enable supporting doctors. The work done has allowed to find the algorithm, which made classification of data into two groups possible.

Text documents are made from descriptions of radiological examinations that in Poland are often recorded by the doctor on the dictaphone and prescribed by a medical secretary. It is worth mentioning, that the purpose of the description is to provide information about the condition of the patient, rather than maintaining all the correct of Polish grammar and stylistic rules. Some of the descriptions have copied fragments of text from other studies, because in such diseases time is very crucial.

Descriptions of radiological examinations, stored in the Radiology Information System database, are short text documents consisting about 50 words. The database contains 1284 described cases. It was revealed that the most successful method was based on classifier using the maximum entropy algorithm based on nouns. It was shown, that the linguistic rules were more effective than boolean rules. The best result obtained was 90% of sensitivity and 70% of specificity. The worse diagnostic capacity demonstrates frequent phrase extraction algorithm. The other classifiers turned out to be less effective, than the random ones.

Comparable results where obtained by rule-based classifier, presented in the article [4], where the method obtained about 79.05% sensitivity and 94.80% of specificity. Another results also worthy of comparison have been presented in publication [5]. SVM classifier TPR is equal to average 87.43% and PPV is equal to about 76.94%. Results obtained by KNN method equal respectively 78.50% and 65.38%.

The results obtained are not sufficient to make diagnosis, but they may be the basis for further analysis. Maximum entropy classifier based on weighted linguistic rules allow to get satisfactory effects.

Improvement of classification results could include better preparation of descriptions, before they can be classified. As noted before, these texts consist of a great number of abbreviations, scribbled text and letters. A detailed analysis of all the abbreviations used and translation from Latin should be made, and the synonym dictionary created. The creation of such a dictionary should be consulted with the radiologist, in order to correct and complement the synonyms. In addition, it will be useful to create a list of strict terms, indicating the presence of tetracycline or a healthy case. The study can also be enlarged, by discovering more types of aneurysms.

Acknowledgement. This research was supported by the Polish Ministry of Science and Silesian University of Technology statutory financial support partially by grant No. BK-200/RIB1/2016 and grant No. BK-200/RIB1/2017.

References

1. Spinczyk, D., Dzieciatko, M.: Similarity search for the content of the medical records. In: Information Technologies in Medicine. Advances in Intelligent Systems and Computing, vol. 471, pp. 489–501 (2016)
2. Ahmad, M.: Machine learning approach to text mining: a review. J. Adv. Res. Comput. Sci. Softw. Eng. **4**, 1125–1131 (2014)
3. Berger, A., Pietra, V., Pietra, S.: A maximum entropy approach to natural language processing. Comput. Linguist. **22**, 39–71 (1996)
4. Botist, T., Nguyen, M., Woo, E., Markatou, M., Ball, R.: Text mining for the vaccine adverse event reporting system: medical text classifiaction using informative feature selection. J. Am. Med. Inform. Assoc. **18**, 631–638 (2011)
5. Khachidze, M., Tsintsadze, M., Archuadze, M.: Natural language processing based instrument for classification of free text medical records. BioMed. Res. Int. **2016**, 10 (2016)
6. Ningam, K., Lafferty, J., McCallum A.: Using maximum entropy for text classification (1999)

7. Ningam, K., McCallum, A., Thrun, A., Mitchell, T.: Text classification from labeled and unlabeled documents using EM. Mach. Learn. **39**, 103–134 (2000)
8. Pang, B., Lee, L., Vaithyanathan, S.: Thumbs up? Sentiment classification using machine learning techniques. In: Association for Computational Linguistics, vol. 22 (2002)

Similarity Search for the Content of Medical Records Using Unstructured Data

Sylwia Wilczek[1], Kinga Gawrysiak[2], and Dominik Spinczyk[1(✉)]

[1] Faculty of Biomedical Engineering, Silesian University of Technology,
Roosevelta 40, 41-800 Zabrze, Poland
dspinczyk@polsl.pl
[2] Warsaw School of Economy, Aleja Niepodległości 162, 00-001 Warsaw, Poland
http://ib.polsl.pl

Abstract. Clustering large amounts of unstructured data is an important challenge in contemporary medicine and biology. This article presents an automatic clustering method for unstructured medical data. The presented method consists of the following main steps: transformation of the document corpus to a frequency matrix of terms; dimensionality reduction of the frequency matrix of terms using principal component analysis (PCA); the direct comparison of pairs of documents similarity measures using the cosine and correlation distances; and finding the optimal number of groups for expertly labelled data sets by treating the clustering problem as an optimization problem in which the objective function is an F measure to be optimized via the selection of parameter values such as PCA resolution and the similarity threshold of the pairs of documents. The usefulness of the proposed methodology was demonstrated by performing calculations on three data sets: short sentences divided into three themes, radiological reports of aneurysms, and radiological reports of abdomen studies. A common barrier in clustering unstructured data is difficulty in results interpretation. To overcome this limitation, the utility of presentation methods, including group histograms, similarity matrices, plots of document assignment to founding clusters, F-measure interpolation and alphabetical- and term-frequency dictionaries, are presented. Excluding the labelling step, the presented method is completely automated and can be used as a preliminary data analysis method for large bodies of text to discover potential groups of interesting topics.

Keywords: Medical records · Direct comparison of medical text
Similarity search · Clustering of medical data
Clustering of unstructured data · SAS Text Miner

1 Introduction

Clustering unstructured data is currently an important task. The four existing groups of text-clustering methods, namely dictionary-based approaches, rule-based approaches, machine learning approaches and manual annotation, have

© Springer International Publishing AG, part of Springer Nature 2019
E. Pietka et al. (Eds.): ITIB 2018, AISC 762, pp. 506–517, 2019.
https://doi.org/10.1007/978-3-319-91211-0_44

disadvantages [1,2]. First, all of these methods require high user engagement. Dictionary-based learning approaches tend to miss undefined terms that are not present in the dictionary [3], while rule-based approaches require rules that identify terms from text, and the resulting rules are often not effective in all cases [3]. Machine learning approaches generally require standard annotated training data sets that are typically laborious to build [4]. The main motivation of this work is to propose a completely automatic text-clustering method. A similar approach can be found in different reports. Amine et al. studied and compared three-text clustering methods, namely, an ascending hierarchical clustering method, a self-organizing map (SOM)-based clustering method and an ant-based clustering method, using three similarity measurements, namely, the cosine distance, the Euclidean distance and the Manhattan distance. Evaluation based on the F-measure showed the best results for the SOM-based clustering method using the cosine distance [5]. Safeer et al. discussed a k-means clustering algorithm for clustering unstructured text documents that we also implemented, beginning with the representation of unstructured text and reaching the resulting set of clusters. Based on the analysis of the resulting clusters for a sample set of documents, they also proposed a technique to represent documents that could further improve the clustering results [6].

The goal of the study is to directly compare the contents of text documents to find the clusters. The method described here is a further development of a previously presented method [7]. This report is organized as follows. In the Materials and methods section, the main decisions in the processing steps are presented, namely, the representation of information in the text-document corpus, the dimensionality reduction of the frequency matrix of terms, the similarity measures for text documents and the organization of the calculation to find the best solution. The Results section presents the outcomes that were obtained, and the Discussion and Conclussion section summarizes the presented approach.

2   Methods

The main idea of the present work is to directly compare the contents of text documents. The steps of the proposed method are:

- representation of information in the text-document corpus,
- dimensionality reduction of the frequency matrix of terms,
- similarity measures for text documents,
- finding the optimal number of groups,
- visual interpretation of results.

They are presented in the Sects. 2.1–2.5.

2.1   Representation of Information in the Text-Document Corpus

In the presented method, we applied the bag-of-words approach in SAS Text Miner. This approach collects the frequency list of word occurrences in each document in a single column. The columns are then combined into a single frequency matrix:

$$a = \begin{bmatrix} a_{11} & \cdots & a_{1n} \\ \cdots & a_{ij} & \cdots \\ a_{m1} & \cdots & a_{mn} \end{bmatrix}$$

where a_{ij} represents the element of the frequency matrix; m represents the number of rows of the frequency matrix, which corresponds to the number of terms included in the frequency matrix, and n represents the number of columns in the frequency array, which corresponds to the number of documents in the corpus. The column number represents the index of the input document, and the row number represents each term's index. The value of each matrix element corresponds to the number of occurrences of a specific term in the document. The details, advantages and disadvantages of this approach have been previously described [7].

2.2   Dimensionality Reduction of the Frequency Matrix of Terms

In text mining, the issue 'length of query' indicates that every term existing in the document is treated as a separate feature, resulting in a large frequency-matrix size. Consequently, it becomes difficult to prepare an efficient list of words that can find a specific document precisely; a second challenge is the large size of the feature space. Because of these difficulties, dimensionality reduction is necessary. In our approach, the principal component analysis (PCA) method is used. The reduction of the dimensionality is based on a singular value decomposition method for a frequency matrix of terms that decomposes the input matrix into independent linear components. The details of this method can be found in the references describing the algebraic calculations [8–10].

2.3   Similarity Measures for Text Documents

In the present method, the cosine distance and correlation metric are used to directly compare the contents of the text documents. The details, advantages and disadvantages of this approach have been previously described [7]. The cosine distance is defined as:

$$dys_{cos}(doc_1, doc_2) = \frac{term(doc_1) \cdot term(doc_2)}{|term(doc_1)||term(doc_2)|},$$

where: $term(doc_i)$ – vector representing a set of terms used in the i-th document.

When the vectors are normalized, the cosine distance is defined as the scalar product of document vectors: $dys_{cos}(doc_1, doc_2) = \sum_{i=1}^{m} doc_1^i doc_2^i$. The correlation distance is based on the sample correlation between points (treated as sequences of values). It is calculated as:

$$dys_{Jacc}(doc_1, doc_2) = \frac{|term(doc_1) \cap term(doc_2)|}{|term(doc_1) \cup term(doc_2)|},$$

where: $term(doc_i)$ – vector representing a set of terms used in the i-th document.

2.4 Finding the Optimal Number of Groups

The main parameters of the proposed method are the resolution of the dimensionality reduction method, the similarity measure and the selection of the similarity measure threshold value. The four criteria most commonly used to evaluate an unsupervised classification of text documents are as follows [5].

- Very large volumes of unstructured data should be able to be processed. In our case, critical calculations are parallelized using a graphical processing unit to improve calculation times.
- The results must be easy to read. The system must offer various visualization modes for the results. In our case, to improve results interpretation, the following two types of dictionaries are created for each selected group:
  - an alphabetical dictionary that presents the included terms in alphabetical order, and
  - a term frequency dictionary that presents the included terms according to their frequency.
  The dictionaries for each group are created based on the corresponding columns in the frequency matrix.
- The data must be as homogeneous as possible within each group, and the groups as distinct as possible; to assess homogeneity within groups and differentiation among groups, the F measure was used.

The clustering results for different parameters are evaluated using the F-measure:

$$F = \sum_{i=1}^{l} \frac{Nci}{N} \sum_{k=1}^{K} \frac{2Recall(i,k) \cdot Precision(i,k)}{Recall(i,k) + Precision(i,k)}$$

where i represents the number of the predefined class, K represents the number of clusters in the unsupervised classification, Nci represents the number of documents of class i and N represents the total number of documents in the text corpus. Additionally,

$$Precision(i,k) = \frac{Nik}{Nk}$$

where Nik represents the number of documents of the i-th class in the cluster Ck, and Nk represents the number of documents in cluster Ck. Additionally,

$$Recall(i,k) = \frac{Nik}{Nci}$$

The parameters of the proposed method change in the following sets of values,

- PCA resolution $low = 0.3$, $medium = 0.5$, $high = 0.9$,
- similarity measure = $cosine$, $Jaccard$,
- selected similarity measure threshold value = $0.5 - 1$,

and clustering is performed. The selection of the best case is based on the F-measure. For the best case, the dictionaries of the included terms for existing clusters are created to emphasize the criterion of the result interpretation.

2.5   Visual Interpretation of Results

One common challenge in working with unstructured data clustering results is their interpretation. The 'length of query' issue was mentioned above because it causes objective difficulties in embracing the results. Currently, a visual analytics paradigm has been proposed to solve this problem [11]. Such an approach is possible because of a significant increase in computing performance and in the size of the address space of computers. Visual interpretation includes two important factors. First, an increase in the transparency of information presentation is one of the main goals of creating and developing the current information system. Second, visualization takes advantage of the great cognitive abilities of the human vision system and combines in a synergistic way with the increasing capabilities of modern computer systems. The ideal tool for data visualization is characterized by the following features: conciseness, or the ability to present a large amount of information; relativity and proximity, or the ability to present clusters, their differences and outliers; focus with context, or the ability to interactively present selected features in their wider context; zoomability, or the ability to quickly change the presented scope; and 'right brain' stimulation, or the ability to support the human cognitive process [11]. Given these criteria and the types of charts used for the presentation of unstructured data, the following visual presentation elements are proposed: a set of groups, dictionaries of groups, a histogram of the number of groups, a similarity matrix of document pairs (valid values are presented only in the lower part of the matrix below the diagonal, because of the symmetry of the matrix), the F-measure for labelled data sets according to calculation parameters and the similarity of individual groups according to specific terms.

3   Materials

The usefulness of the proposed methodology was demonstrated by performing calculations on three data sets:

- The first data set consists of dozens of short sentences divided into three themes; the data set is labelled, and the number of groups is known and is equal to three.
- The second data set consists of 100 radiological reports of aneurysms; the data set is labelled, and the number of the group is known and is equal to two.
- The third data set consists of 100 radiological reports of abdominal studies. The average length is approximately 200 words. The style of the language includes conventional radiological terminology; the data sets that are unlabelled, and the number of groups is unknown.

4   Results

The obtained results for first, second and third data set are presented in Figs. 1–2, Figs. 3–4 and Figs. 5–6, respectively.

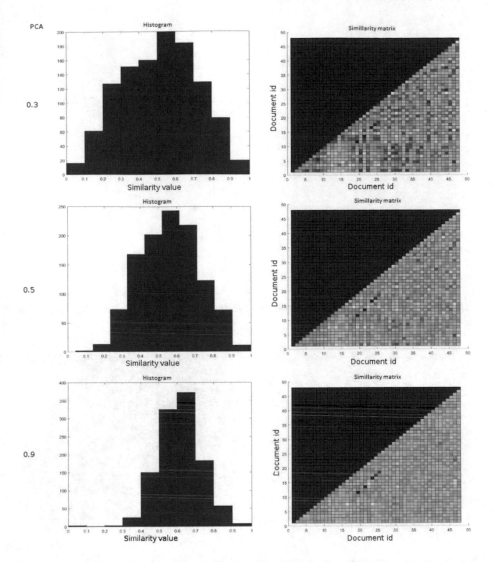

Fig. 1. Group histograms and similarity matrices for the first data set using the cosine distance as a similarity measure

The heat map presents the similarity of documents in pairs. In heat maps, identical documents are marked in blue, while the ones most distant from each other are in yellow. Because the similarity matrix is symmetrical, one part under the diagonal is presented.

The histograms presents the number of documents pair that presents the value of similarity metrics at the specific level.

In heat maps with the increasing value of the clustering parameter, which is the PCA cut-off threshold, the number of pairs of documents with low similarity decreases, between 0.5 and 0.7 increase, and above decrease. At the same time

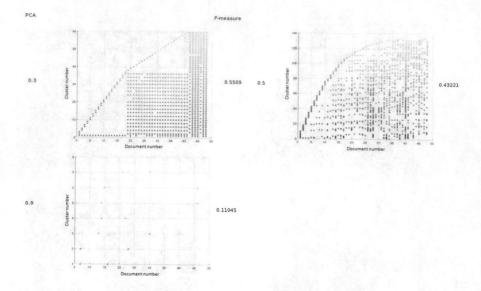

Fig. 2. Assignment of documents to clusters found for the first data set using the cosine distance as a similarity measure

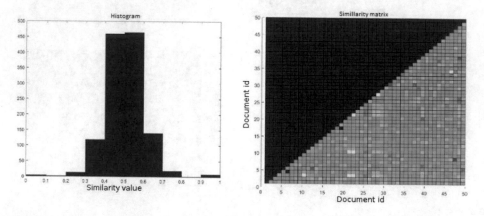

Fig. 3. Group histograms and similarity matrix for the second data set using the cosine distance as a similarity measure

increasing the threshold of the similarity measure, the number of couples fulfilling the condition decreases, which causes a smaller number of elements in the found clusters.

The analysis of the results from the first data set indicates that PCA resolution determines the number of clusters found for a given similarity threshold (left column in Fig. 1). The reader might also notice the impact on the length of the vector representing the document characteristics in the corpus, and thus the value of the similarity matrix (right column in Fig. 1). In the case in which

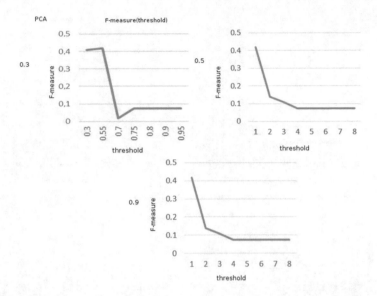

Fig. 4. F-measure values corresponding to similarity measure threshold values for the second data set using the cosine distance as a similarity measure

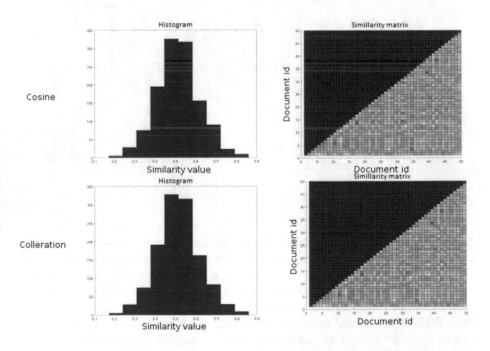

Fig. 5. Group histograms and similarity matrices for the third data set

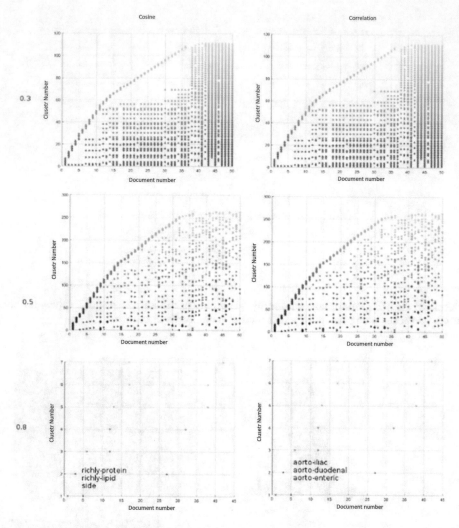

Fig. 6. Assignment of documents to clusters found for the third data set

documents belonging to the class indicated by an expert are known, it is possible to calculate the value of a numerical measure of F, indicating the quality of the clustering (Fig. 2). Continuing with this theme, one can treat the problem of clustering as an optimization problem, where the objective function is an F measure that is to be optimized through the selection of parameter values such as PCA resolution and similarity threshold. This approach is presented in the analysis of the second data set, consisting of 100 radiological reports of aneurysms that are labelled; the number of groups is known and equals two. The similarity matrix and number of identified clusters are presented in Fig. 3. The interpolation of the F-measure as a function of the PCA resolution and similarity measure

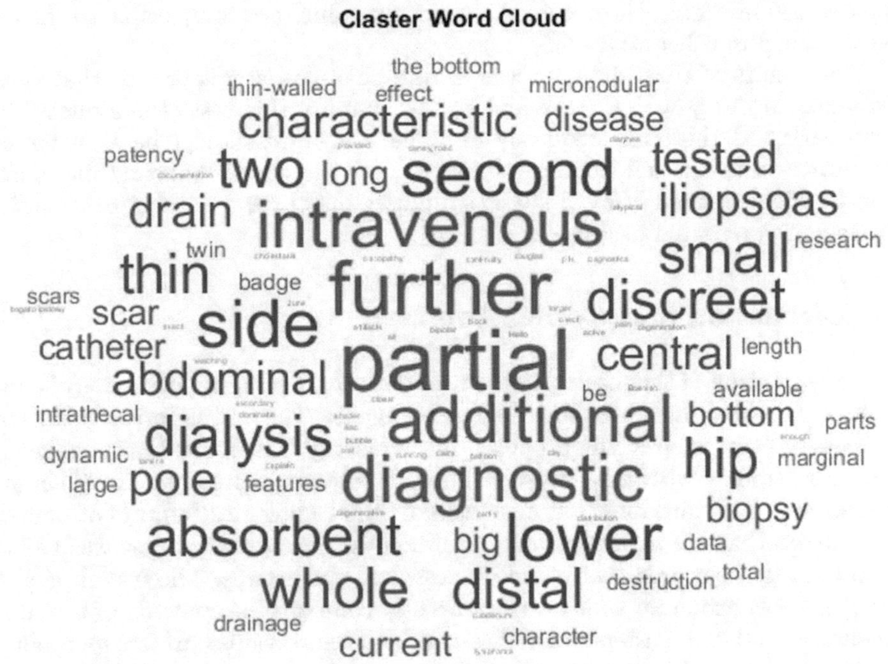

Claster Word Cloud

Fig. 7. Example of Word cloud using cosine distance

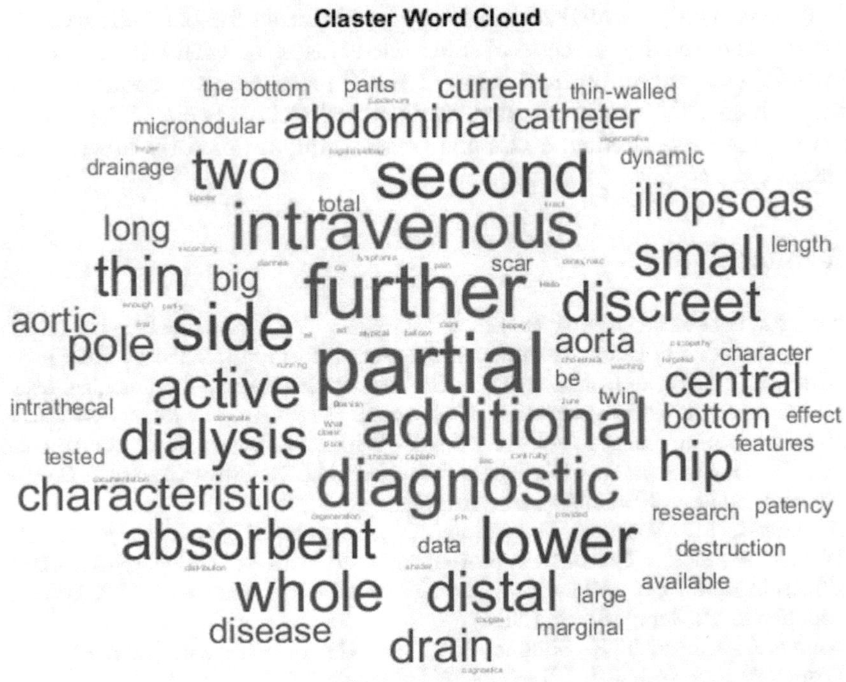

Claster Word Cloud

Fig. 8. Example of Word cloud using correlation distance

is presented in Fig. 4. The obtained F-measure values are comparable to the values obtained in other studies [5].

The results of third data set was to find characteristic keywords that could differentiate the groups (Figs. 7 and 8). To simplify this task, the alphabetical dictionary and the term frequency dictionary are presented (the alphabetical dictionary is in the left column of Fig. 6, and the term frequency dictionary is in the right column of Fig. 6). The similarity matrix and number of identified clusters are presented in Fig. 5.

5   Discussion and Conclusion

The presentation of the results for the first data set, consisting of dozens of short sentences divided into three themes, has two goals. The first is to verify the correctness of every step of the proposed methodology. The second is to make the end user familiar with the proposed form of the result presentation. The goal of analysing the third data set, consisting of 100 radiological reports of abdominal studies that are unlabelled and an unknown number of groups, was to find characteristic keywords that could differentiate the groups. The overall goal of the study was achieved, which was to directly compare the contents of text documents to find the clusters. The obtained F-measure values are comparable to the values obtained in other studies [5].

In this paper, a method to find similarities among medical record documents is presented using SAS Text Miner for data processing, which allows process Polish language. The presented methodology can be used for both supervised and unsupervised clustering. In cases of supervised clustering with labelled data sets, it is possible to find an optimal value of the F measure by selecting parameter values such as PCA resolution and similarity threshold value. This optimization step may be treated as a training phase using an expertly labelled subset of a large data corpus.

References

1. Zhu, F., Patumcharoenpol, P., Zhang, C., Yang, Y.: Biomedical text mining and its applications in cancer research. J. Biomed. Inform. **46**, 200–211 (2013)
2. Kawa, J., Juszczyk, J., Pyciński, B., Badura, P., Piętka, E.: Radiological atlas for patient specific model generation. Adv. Intell. Syst. Comput. **84**, 69–84 (2014)
3. Rebholz-Schuhmann, D., Jepes, A., Li, C., Kafkas, S., Lewin, I., et al.: Assessment of NER solutions against the first and second CALBC Silver Standard Corpus. J. Biomed. Seman. **2**(Suppl. 5), S11 (2011)
4. Krallinger, M., Vasquez, M., Leitner, F., Salgado, D., Chatr-Aryamontri, A., Winter, A., et al.: The protein-protein interaction tasks of BioCreative III: classification ranking of articles and linking bio-ontology concepts to full text. BMC Bioinform. **12**(Suppl. 8), S3 (2011)
5. Amine, A., Elberrichi, Z., Simonet, M.: Evaluation of text clustering methods using WordNet. Int. Arab J. Inf. Technol. **7**(4), 349–357 (2010)

6. Safeer, Y., Mustafa, A., Noor, A.A.: Clustering unstructured data. Int. J. Comput. Sci. Inf. Secur. **8**(2), 174–180 (2010)
7. Spinczyk, D., Dziecitko, M.: Similarity search for the content of medial records. In: Information Technologies in Medicine. Advances in Intelligent Systems and Computing, vol. 471, pp. 489–501 (2016)
8. Albright, R.: Taming Text with the SVD. SAS Institute White Paper (2004)
9. Meyer, C.: Matrix Analysis and Applied Linear Algebra. SIAM, Philadelphia (2000)
10. Vandenberghe, L.: Applied Numerical Computing (lecture) (2011)
11. Keim, D., Kohlhammer, J., Ellis, G., Mansmann, F.: Mastering the Information Age Solving Problems with Visual Analytics. Eurographics Association, Goslar (2013)

New Challenges for Information Technologies in Medicine: Big Data Analysis?

Zdzisław S. Hippe[✉] and Rafał Niemiec

University of Information Technology and Management (UITM),
35-225 Rzeszow, Poland
zhippe@wsiz.rzeszow.pl

Abstract. The first aim of the paper is to investigate whether the very promising method of data analysis (the Big Data Analysis, further called BDA) – used now across various domains – can serve for information technologies in medicine, in the area of planning pathways of organic syntheses. The eventual usage of BDA in the field stated is meant within a speculation – synthesis of new drugs. Therefore characteristic features of BDA are here briefly discussed; they are commonly marked by (five) letters V, coming from the following concepts: Volume, Velocity, Variety, Veracity, Value. In the research performed it was found that BDA unfortunately seems to have rather restricted applicability in planning of chemical compounds; rather we have to focus in details of a single, chosen reaction. Therefore in a second part of the paper – in its core – the Achmatowicz reaction is selected to expose the required ingenuity in organic synthesis. As a pattern for discussion, the structure of Bao Gong Tung A molecule, a novel natural product showing strong antiglaucoma properties, was fixed.

Keywords: Volume · Velocity · Variety · Veracity · Value
Spatial structures · Achmatowicz reaction · Bao Gong Teng A

1 Introduction

Problems discussed here are related to specific area of knowledge: synthesis of organic compounds, within a speculation – synthesis of new drugs. Operational research programs of European Union (EU) are for years focusing giant intellectual and financial potential on these questions [8]. It seems, however, that this potential does not keep pace with new challenges: increasing number of growing old population (specific drugs are required), unknown illnesses (new pharmaceuticals are requested) and formation of mutant bacteria (usually resistant to standard antibiotics). Thus it is obvious that automation of methods used for planning of chemical syntheses is extremely important as well for individuals (health of individual citizens), as for society (health of a nation) [2].

© Springer International Publishing AG, part of Springer Nature 2019
E. Pietka et al. (Eds.): ITIB 2018, AISC 762, pp. 518–524, 2019.
https://doi.org/10.1007/978-3-319-91211-0_45

2   Background Theory

The characteristic feature of the discussed logistic-analytical BDA process relies on joint analysis of various data types, publicly available in the Internet, kept in hospitals, in libraries, in museums – generally analysis of all data stored anywhere. Hence, BDA processes strict data, fuzzy data, rough data, suppressed data; it also run a collective analysis of medical data, medicine books and ebooks, tweets, posts, and even medical blogs. Recently published review of research devoted to BDA [7] suggests that machine learning may be used to enhance the restriction of multiplicity of applied procedures, and to leave out or omit excessive or false processing results.

2.1   Preliminaries of the BDA Methodology

The BDA methodology characterizes – across various domains – by specific features, named after the first letter of the word describing a given property. So, we have V for (Volume) – it stands for immense and rising number of collected and analyzed data. The next V (Velocity) is connected with speed of data creation and supplying them to the system for analysis. This term relates also to local algorithms used for data processing and computing of results gained. The next V (Variety) points out the heterogeneity and complexity of analyzed data. Somewhat later other V was added for (Veracity); this term relates to quality of processed data. The main problem here is the adherence to the truth of tweets, posts, blogs and various uncertain data created within flash mobs and other groups of interests. And the last V (Value) points out that BDA should provide a new insight into data, allowing the best (economically) decision [7].

It was found however, that within a broad BDA (to the core of different domains), discovery of confabulation about not existing situations was neglected. Substitution of facts by fantasy is typical for most folks; for example an allocation to ourselves untrue features, gifts or skills. And, what is extremely dangerous (specially for Information Technologies in Medicine), a sinister custom to propagate deliberate incorrect views and/or incorrect evaluation of phenomenon, problems or projects. So, the current BDA seems to be spoiled by fabricated data, by titles or books connected with real or fictitious authors, ghost libraries, faint TV images, or even some things seen in a delirium, hence doubly nonexistent [3].

3   Planning Syntheses of Organic Compounds

Talking about planning syntheses of organic compounds (largely built from C, H, O, and N atoms, additionally from P, S, halogens and some metals), we have to stress that the chemical route design has to pay heed to a range of difficult criteria, such as availability of commercial quantities of starting materials, chemical safety concerns and potential hazards, toxicity, environmental considerations ('green chemistry'), cost of goods, quality criteria, prior art and the intellectual situation, etc. [2]. Thus, it appears interesting to investigate whether the BDA methodology can be successfully applied in synthesis of chemical compounds (in other words: in planning pathways of organic syntheses).

Design (planning) of chemical syntheses is considered as one of the most difficult fields of research [4,5]. This situation is caused by motives mentioned below:

– multitude of the analyzed objects (over 13 million of known carbogenes),
– size of the solution space (medical diagnosis $\sim 10^{40}$, chess $\sim 10^{80}$, chemical synthesis $\sim 10^{120}$),
– level of processing complexity – rising for the following items:
  • digits and numbers,
  • regular text (is one-dimensional and unidirectional),
  • chemical structures (are three-dimensional and multidirectional).

Additionally, the situation is complicated by a phenomenon of structural isomerism. A compound $C_6H_{13}NO_2$ (quite small molecule) has over 10 000 of isomers, whereas the molecule $C_{25}H_{52}$ (also a small molecule, built from only C and H atoms) counts more than 32 million of isomers! [4].

3.1 Concluding Remarks on BDA in Planning Syntheses

Genuine article adding up the discussed field [2], unfortunately has a review-advertising essence: research results (in AstraZeneca) were obtained using known tool – hence, recommended indirectly.

Owing to a lack of global standardization of computer program systems (and also interfaces) for automatic syntheses design, even the superficial evaluation of BDA application in planning of chemical syntheses is restricted, or even not possible. It is also not known whether exist data (available elsewhere) on untrue (fabricated) chemical reactions.

To summarize the first part of the executed research, we should accept the statement that BDA has definitely restricted applicability in planning of chemical reactions; currently (say, within next 2–3 years) rather we have to focus in details on a single, chosen reaction. Following this stream, the Achmatowicz reaction [1] was selected as a next topic of article.

4   The Achmatowicz Reaction

The Achmatowicz reaction (see Fig. 1) is now frequently used in synthesis of important substances, having curing properties against many illnesses, giving occasionally a very good background for medical information systems. It was also used for the total synthesis of Bao Gong Teng A [9], a novel natural product showing strong antiglaucoma properties.

This reaction was also applied in a project devoted to automatic generation of the library of monosaccharides.

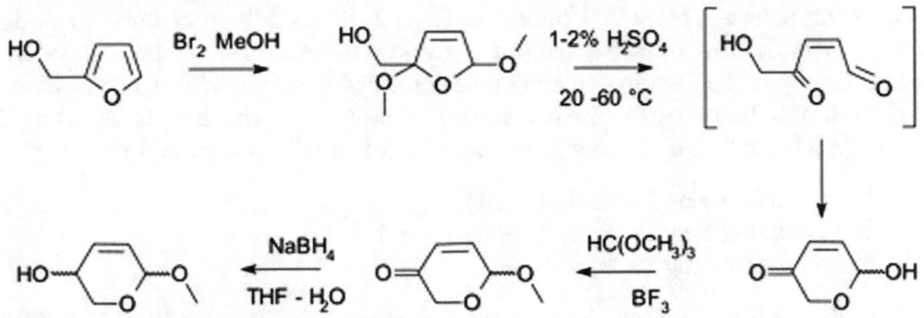

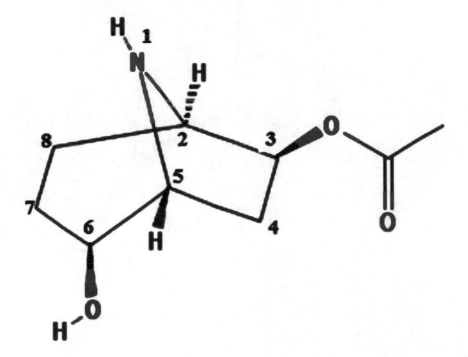

Fig. 1. General flow of Achmatowicz reaction

4.1   The Bao Gong Teng A Molecule

Let us now focus our attention on the spatial structure of the Bao Gong Teng A molecule (see Fig. 2), its proper chemical name and summaric formula.

The proper chemical name of the investigated molecule sounds as:

[(1R,4S,5R,7S)-4-hydroxy-8-aza-bicyclo[3.2.1]octan-7-yl] acetate],

whereas its summaric formula is: $C_9H_{15}NO_3$.

Fig. 2. Bao Gong Teng A

Looking at the synthesized molecule (Fig. 2) it is really very hard to understand – without deep knowledge about organic synthesis – how the scheme shown on Fig. 1, may be applied in conversion of some starting materials to complicated ensembles of substructures (mostly rings), contained in the Bao Gong Teng A. Looking attentively we see that the compound formally contains 3 rings:

– 1→5. membered ring (1, 2, 3, 4, 5, 1),
– 1→6. membered ring (1, 2, 8, 7, 6, 5, 1) and
– 1→7. membered ring (2, 3, 4, 5, 6, 7, 8, 2).

The discussion of a stepwise sequence of the synthetic transformation [9] to get the Bao Gong Teng A molecule, is beyond the scope of the article. But this example shows that currently more valid is

– the detailed analysis of a given (selected) reaction,
– analysis the architecture of particular compounds involved in the conversion,
– looking for active bonds or active items,
– analysis of steric situation,
– possible catalysts, temperature, solvent
– and required environment of the reaction (acidic, basic, neutral, or even unknown).

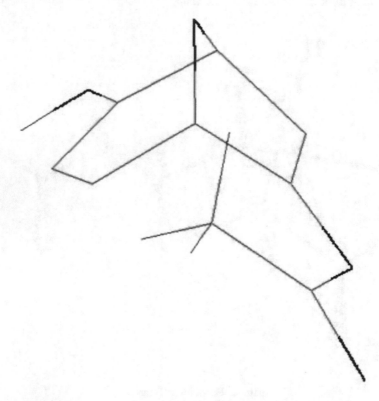

Fig. 3. Bao Gong Teng A molecue displayed in the form of sticks

These parameters can be guessed having insight into details of molecular structures, length of various bonds, rotation of some groups, etc.

This specific ('molecular') insight into chemical structures is elegantly simplified using, for example, the HyperChem molecular modelling software [6]. In Fig. 3 we have the molecule displayed in the form of sticks. Particular atoms are not shown here explicitly, but chemists easily recognize oxygens (marked in red) and nitrogen (marked in blue).

Another possibility is to show the molecule using rendering of Balls and Cylinders (Fig. 4). Both Figs. 3 and 4 are displayed in the form of zero-point energy, in other words – as fixed conformations having the lowest potential energy [6].

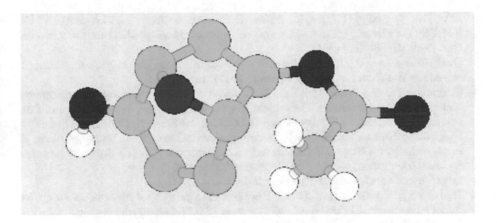

Fig. 4. Bao Gong Teng A structure shown using rendering Balls and Cylinders

4.2 Concluding Remarks

This chapter shows how enjoyable is the synthetic analysis of any reaction, organic molecule and the consideration of laboratory details. The emotional attitude of many (all?) chemists and other people involved in information technologies in medicine, supports planning of syntheses, no matter how it is done. In person or automatically, using any available design system. Even now some of these systems supplies valuable results – they create the ideas on possible pathways of synthesis of not very complex structures. Usually, the results can be classified into three categories:

1. reactions whose evaluation indicates full possibility of their laboratory implementation;
2. reactions which display a considerable level of ingenuity and lead to interesting conclusions on the strategy of synthesis of a considered compound. Frequently, these may be reactions altogether not taken into account, requiring careful evaluation referring to original literature data; and

3. reactions which seem to be unrealistic or too complicated at current level of organic synthesis.

However, for the practical application of BDA in information technology in medicine we have to wait.

References

1. Achmatowicz Jr., O., et al.: Synthesis of methyl 2,3-dideoxy-DL-alk-2-enopyranosides from furan compounds: a general approach to the total synthesis of monosaccharides. Tetrahedron **27**(10), 1973–1996 (1971). https://doi.org/10.1016/s0040-4020(01)98229-8
2. Bøgevig, A., Federsel, H.J., Huerta, F., Hutchings, M.G., Kraut, H., Langer, T., Löw, P., Oppawsky, C., Rein, T., Saller, H.: Route design in the 21st century - the IC SYNTH software tool as an idea generator for synthesis predictions. Org. Process Res. Dev. **19**, 357–368 (2015)
3. Dunin-Wąsowicz, P.: Polska biblioteka widmowa. Leksykon książek zmyślonych, Narodowe Centrum Kultury, Warszawa (2017). (in Polish)
4. Grzymała-Busse, J.W., Hippe, Z.S., Mroczek, T.: Eksploracja danych medycznych. Metody sztucznej inteligencji w projektowaniu syntez leków, Wyższa Szkoła Informatyki i Zarządzania - Wydawnictwo IVG, Rzeszów-Szczecin (2015). (in Polish)
5. Hippe Z.S.: Human interaction in planning chemical syntheses. Some problems of retrosynthesis. In: Hippe Z.S., Kulikowski J.L., Mroczek T. (eds.) Human-Computer Systems Interaction, pp. 67–1 79. Springer, Cham (2018)
6. http://hyper.com/. Accessed 18 Sept 2017
7. Japkowicz N., Stefanowski J. (eds.): Big Data Analysis - New Algorithms for a New Society. Studies in Big Data, vol. 16. Springer (2016). https://doi.org/10.1007/978-3-319-26989-4_1
8. Warren, S., Wayatt, P.: Organic Synthesis. The Disconnection Approach. Wiley, Chichester (2013)
9. Zhang, Y., Liebeskind, L.S.: Organometallic enantiomeric scaffolding: organometallic chirons. Total synthesis of (-)-Bao Gong Teng A by a molybdenum-mediated [5+2] cycloaddition. J. Am. Chem. Soc. **128**(2), 465–472 (2006)

Application of Text Analytics to Analyze Emotions in the Speeches

Mariusz Dzieciątko[✉]

SAS Institute, Gdanska 27/31, 01-633 Warszawa, Poland
mariusz.dzieciatko@sas.com
http://www.sas.com

Abstract. The paper presents the different aspects of analyzing public speeches of deputies in the Parliament (Sejm) of the Republic of Poland with use of SAS tools for text analytics. A document repository was created based on publicly available transcriptions of speeches for 7th (from Nov 2011 to Nov 2015) and 8th (from Nov 2015 to Jan 2018) term of the Parliament (Sejm). A database contains 440 pdf files with transcriptions of the full-day parliament session. This repository was cleaned and pre-processed, every file was split into a set of personal speeches. As a result, the source data table contains 350 000 records. The aim of the experiment was to check whether automatic analysis of text data is suitable for monitoring the 'temperature' of the Parliament (Sejm) debates and the main elements of the rhetoric used.

Keywords: Text mining · Text classifiers · Emotion
Affective verbal stimuli · Nencki affective word list
Frequent phrase extraction classifiers

1 Introduction

The development of the Internet has caused a revolution in the ease of access to information but also in the possibility of creating and publishing new content. Further acceleration appeared along with the existence of social media. Today's man is bombarded with a huge amount of information every day, and only a part of them is able to consume. In addition, custom search engines like Google create something like virtual reality by matching search results to the searcher's preferences.

The advantages of the Internet have also been noticed by state institutions. The Internet allows you to increase the transparency of all transactions, law-making processes, etc. Here, however, there is a problem how to find a place in this thicket of information? One day of sitting of the Sejm is on average 130 pages of the transcript. The database which was analyzed contains 350,000 Sejm statements. And that's not all. In addition, there are transcripts of committee meetings, Sejm papers with bills, resolutions, etc. The most comprehensive bill in the Sejm of the Republic of Poland has 1170 pages! It's hard to navigate in such a mass of information.

© Springer International Publishing AG, part of Springer Nature 2019
E. Pietka et al. (Eds.): ITIB 2018, AISC 762, pp. 525–536, 2019.
https://doi.org/10.1007/978-3-319-91211-0_46

And here is the place to use text mining tools to support the automatic processing of text data. The analysis of text data, which is unstructured, is carried out in two stages. The first stage consists in transforming loose text using Natural Language Processing (NLP) tools into a matrix whose columns correspond to words and records to documents. In the simplest form, this approach is called a bag of words. The second stage is the use of data mining, machine learning, and deep learning algorithms to discover knowledge. To get a picture of the work of parliament, government and MPs from these perspectives, from the perspective of cool, non-emotional analytics. Most of the work related to this study has been done with SAS Text Analytics tools that natively support the Polish language.

Data, which are the basis of this study, come from www.sejm.gov.pl.

The aim of this study is to demonstrate the suitability and capabilities of both supervised and unsupervised analysis of unstructured text data.

This paper is organized as follows:

- Section 2 presents preprocessing step and four applications: preprocessing of PDF transcript files, linguistic characteristics of parties and leaders, intensiveness of accusing by words, analysis of expressed emotions with use of NAWL, Social Network Analysis for verbal disputes between Members;
- Section 3 includes experimental results;
- Section 4 contains discussion and plans for future work.

Another example of text analysis is the analysis of Conover [15] who investigated the political alignment of Twitter users. Various aspects of unstructured data such as sentiment analysis, classification, and prediction of political orientation are currently being researched [16–18].

2 Process, Materials and Methods

The diagram Fig. 1 shows the main components of the process of processing, analyzing, modeling and visualizing unstructured data. These components are described more specifically in Sect. 2. The number in circles refer to subsections numbers.

2.1 Source Selection

Almost all analyzes of text data from the Internet begin at the site of data source selection. In the presented experiment all data needed for the analysis were collected from the domain www.sejm.gov.pl. The data concerned deputies' speeches at plenary sessions of the Sejm, basic data of deputies such as membership in parliamentary clubs, electoral districts, education, and profession.

2.2 Web Crawling

After identifying sources, the next step is downloading files from the Internet and creating a local file repository. The source documents were mainly in HTML and PDF format. A program written using the SAS 4GL programming language was used to download files.

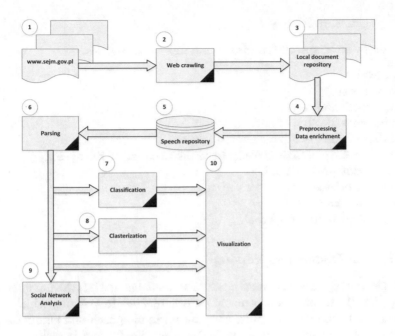

Fig. 1. Process of text analysis

2.3   Document Repository

A local document repository is a place where original versions of source files downloaded from the Internet are stored. This solution allows you to save time and minimize the load on web servers, as well as the ability to experiment freely with the transformation of source files into text documents for further analysis.

2.4   Documents Preprocessing and Data Enrichments

At this stage, the source files in HTML and PDF format are transformed into text documents with a unified code page and then loaded into tables in the SAS format. Text from documents in PDF format was extracted using the Apache Tika toolkit. In this step, documents from all-day sessions of the parliament are split into the statements of individual persons, the author of the speech and possibly the author of the inclusions to the speech are identified. Documents are cleared of unnecessary elements such as the table of contents, word splits related to moving to a new line. Then the result table is combined with other collected tables so as to obtain a single table containing all data of deputies. The source files are converted using regular expressions, rule-based classifiers, and entity extraction. This process requires a lot of attention because the source files contain many disturbances in their structure. The quality and reliability of the final results depend largely on the correctness of this step.

2.5 Speech Repository

The main table in speech repository contains data as below:

1. Speech ID,
2. Speech text,
3. Author of the speech,
4. Parliamentary club of author,
5. Author of the disturbance of the speech,
6. Parliamentary club of author of the disturbance of the speech,
7. Parliament session number,
8. Author position,
9. Source file name,
10. Considered point of debate.

2.6 Speech Documents Parsing

In the next step, text documents are processed using Natural Language Processing (NLP) techniques. Documents are subjected to parsing, which divides documents into individual words, marking parts of speech and eliminating various forms of the same word through steaming. Each term is assigned weights using the chosen method. The result of this step is text documents described in numerical form and therefore ready for further analysis using data mining and machine learning methods. For term frequencies, logarithm weighting functions

$$g(f_{ij}) = \log_2(f_{ij} + 1), \tag{1}$$

where f_{ij} – frequency of term i in document j, were chosen because it dampens the effect of terms that occur many times in a document.

The experiment for term weighting methods mainly used Entropy and Mutual Information [11] with the parliament club's name as a target variable. These methods are useful for distinguishing important terms from others. In general, the assumption is that terms that are useful are those that occur in only a few documents but many times in those few documents. Entropy term weighting:

$$w_i = 1 + \sum_j \frac{(f_{ij}/g_i) \log_2(f_{ij}/g_i)}{\log_2(n)} \tag{2}$$

where, g_i is the number of times that term i appears in the document collection, and n is the number of documents in the collection, j is a document. Weight is greater for terms that occur infrequently in the document collection by using a derivative of the entropy measure found in information theory.

Mutual Information term weighting

$$w_i = \max_{C_k} \left[\log \left(\frac{(P(t_i, C_k)}{P(t_i)P(C + k)} \right) \right] \tag{3}$$

where, $P(t_i)$ is the proportion of documents that contain term t_i. $P(C_k)$ is the proportion of documents that belong to category C_k. And $P(t_i, C_k)$ is the proportion of documents that contain term t_i and belong to category C_k.

Mutual Information weight is proportional to the similarity of the distribution of documents that contain the term to the distribution of documents that are contained in the respective category.

Effective work with text documents would be much more difficult without the possibility of eliminating various forms of words (steaming). This is a particularly important topic in the case of Polish language. SAS Text Miner uses dictionary-based stemming (also known as lemmatization), which unlike tail-chopping stemmers, produces only valid words as stems.

Table 1. Example of steaming

Language	Steam	Terms
English	baloon	baloons
French	aller	vais, vas, va, allons, allez, vont
Polish	poseł	posła, posłem, posłowi, pośle, posłowie, posłami, posłom, posłach

2.7   Text Classification

Many problems of automatic analysis of unstructured data, just like in data mining, can be reduced to the classification task. Basically, there are two approaches here.

The first one is based on a rule classifier which, based on the expanded linguistic rules, classifies the document in accordance with the prepared taxonomy. This taxonomy can be built manually by a domain expert, generated automatically on the basis of the training set or be a combination of both previous approaches. Most often it starts with the initial generation of rules and then it is done manually. This approach offers very high accuracy of classification up to 95% by the cost of a large amount of manual work.

The second approach is based on the construction of a statistical classifier using machine learning methods [9]. Based on the training set with assigned values of the target variable, a model is built using methods such as decision tree, logistic regression, neural networks, random forests or gradient boosting. Next, the above model is used for the scoring of new data. This approach is much faster, however, the achieved accuracy of the classification is at the level of 85% and therefore worse than in the first method.

An exemplary task solved using both approaches is sentiment analysis. The approach based on a rule classifier has greater possibilities to consider the context of words that are carriers of sentiment than the statistical approach. There is the possibility of partial recognition of irony, sarcasm, citation or paraphrases.

Nencki Affective Word List (NAWL)[2] is a database of 2902 Polish words and their ratings connected to different aspects of expressing emotions that are freely accessible to the scientific community for non-commercial use. The database is a Polish adaptation of the Berlin Affective Word List-Reloaded (BAWL-R), commonly used to investigate the affective properties of German words. Affective normative ratings were collected from 266 Polish participants (136 women and 130 men). In order to analyze the emotions that accompany speakers in parliament, the flat taxonomy of five basic emotions such as **Happiness**, **Anger**, **Sadness**, **Fear** and **Disgust** was used built on the basis of Nencki Affective Word List (NAWL). The taxonomy is presented in the diagram (Fig. 2). This work uses several rule-based classifiers and based on a statistic model proposed by Ningham et al. [7].

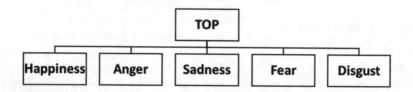

Fig. 2. Flat emotion taxonomy

2.8   Text Clustering

Clustering [10] is a technique used to group similar documents, but it differs from categorization in that documents are clustered without predefined topics. To determine clusters in text documents, unsupervised methods are used. The most widespread algorithms are:

- Support vector machine (SVM)[4,5] – classifier, which aims to determine the hyperplanar separating with the maximum margin examples belonging to different classes. The classifier treats a document as a point in a multidimensional space.
- K nearest neighbors (KNN)[4,5] – one of the non-parametric regression algorithms. The definition of 'closest neighbors' comes down to minimizing a certain metric that measures the distance between vectors of explanatory variables of two observations. Usually, Euclidean metrics or Mahalanobis metrics are used here. The k nearest neighbors algorithm is especially useful when the relationship between variables is complex or atypical, i.e. difficult to model in the classic way.

In the case of cluster analysis of text documents, in addition to selecting the algorithm, it is important to select the features that represent the documents. Possible representations are:

- all words after steaming – an ineffective approach due to the very large size of the analyzed matrix;

- a number of the most common words – a method that gives satisfactory results, it is difficult to choose the number of representatives. It may happen that documents will appear without any representation;
- SVD coefficients – Latent Semantic Analysis (LSA)[13] method, analyzing relationships between a set of documents and the terms they contain by producing a set of concepts related to the documents and terms. LSA assumes that words that are close in meaning will occur in similar pieces of text. A singular value decomposition (SVD) is used to reduce the number of columns while preserving the similarity structure among rows. Columns represent documents, rows represent terms.

2.9   Social Network Analysis [12] for Textual Data

Based on the extraction of entities from text documents, it is possible to create graphs representing various dependencies. Such entities may be people, addresses, ideas, used terms, nouns defining the subject of statements and many more. The graph created on the basis of the entity can then be analyzed using social network analysis methods. Depending on the selection of the entity and the distance between them (direct neighborhood, sentence, paragraph, document), this method can be used to analyze collocation or coexistence.

As an example in this study, a graph was built based on the interaction between the deputy appearing on the rostrum and the person speaking from the plenary hall.

2.10   Results Visualization

The final stage of the analysis of text data is the presentation of results. For this purpose, tools from the business intelligence group are most often used. Depending on the chosen visualization method, it may be necessary to prepare input data through aggregation or transposition. Most of the visualizations in this study were made with the use of the SAS Output Delivery System [14] which offers very large possibilities of adapting graph elements to the user's needs.

3   Results and Conclusions

At the stage of parsing, the part of speech is marked, which were used to compare a linguistic characteristic of the parliamentary clubs of the Sejm of the 7th and 8th term Fig. 3. It can be noticed that opposition parties have a higher share of verbs in relation to the other parts of speech than in the situation of these parties in the government (e.g. k01 (16.1% to 18.5%), k06 (16.8% to 17.1%) – government during the 7th term, k02 (17.3% to 16.2%) – government during the 8th term).

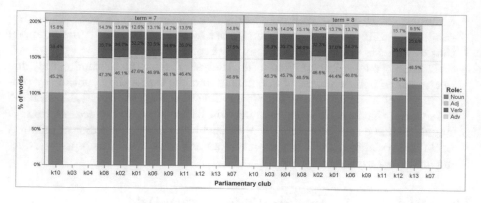

Fig. 3. Part of speech by parliamentary club

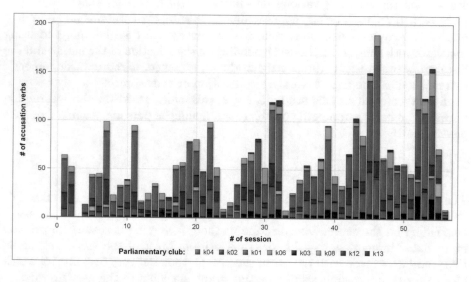

Fig. 4. Intensity of using accusation verbs by session (the 8th term)

The next figure Fig. 4 details the observations from the previous analysis for the Sejm of the 8th term. As a dictionary, 213 verbs have been chosen here, which are commonly perceived as an accusation, attack. Here you can clearly see a significant advantage of the participation of opposition clubs (k01, k04, k06, k12).

Based on the verbs dictionary used in the previous step, one can follow the changes in the rhetoric of statements in the next dozen sessions of the parliament Fig. 5. The most frequently appearing terms in subsequent periods are shown in Table 2.

Table 2. The most frequently appearing terms in subsequent periods

Session	Most frequent terms
1–10	you liquidate, you have forgotten
11–20	you can not, you have forgotten
21–30	break, promised
31–40	you destroy, you take away
41–50	you lie, you cheat
51–56	you lie, you do not know

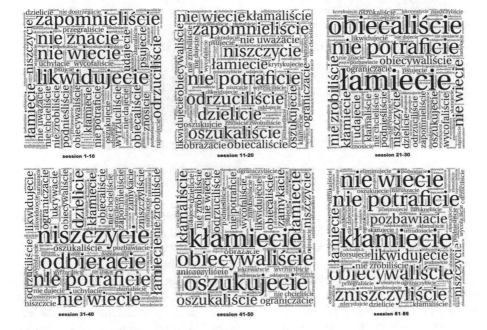

Fig. 5. Changes in the rhetoric of speeches – accusing verbs (the 8th term)

Sentiment analysis [8] is the frequently appearing in the literature and recently also in business applications, which is usually limited to assigning one of three emotional polarizations at the document level – negative, neutral or positive. In this work, a step further was presented and an analysis of the basic five emotions raised by the statements of MPs from the Sejm rostrum. In order to define the emotions more precisely, each of the words of the NAWL [2] database was assigned the weight as a standardized distance of a given word from the dominant emotion

$$d_i = \frac{\max(distance_i) - distance_i}{\max(distance_i) - \min(distance_i)} \tag{4}$$

where i is dominant emotion, d is a weight of a term. At the document level, the emotion most strongly represented is assigned. In order to obtain percentage shares of particular emotions at the level of parliamentary clubs, aggregation was made from the level of documents and percentages were calculated. The results are shown in Fig. 6. The dominating emotion is a joy (above 54%). However, there is a significant increase in the share of anger and sadness among opposition parties in the 8th term of the Sejm in relation to the 7th term, e.g. for k01: anger from 9.8% to 12.5%, sadness from 2.7% to 4.9%.

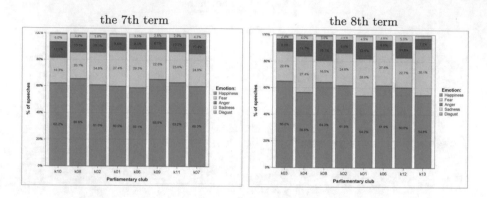

Fig. 6. Emotions expressed by MPs for Sejm of the Republic of Poland

Very promising results are brought together by methods of text mining and social networks analysis. It gives the possibility of an easy analysis of links between various objects extracted from documents. An example of such an analysis is the extraction of the names of authors of speeches and names of interfering persons from texts. The network shown in Fig. 7 is visualized using the Walshaw [3] algorithm, which is responsible for the distribution of network nodes on the plane. The green color of the node means the person at the rostrum, the red color of the person from the parliament room, the intermediate color the person who appears in both roles. Edge colors mean the aggressor's parliamentary club and the thickness of the line's intensity of interaction. Due to the significant level of complexity of the full graph, only people with more than 20 interactions were selected.

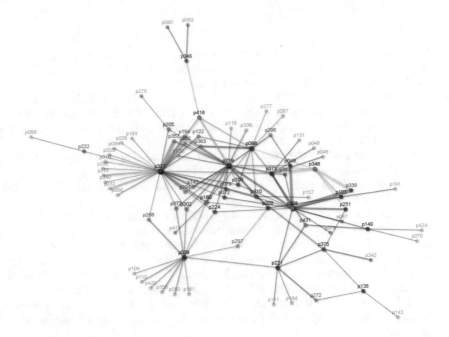

Fig. 7. Social Network Analysis for verbal disputes between Members (the 8th term)

4 Discussion

The development of text analysis tools opens up completely new possibilities for exploring unstructured data. The ability to mark parts of speech, extraction of selected entities, supervised and unsupervised grouping of documents to content, combining qualitative and quantitative data, the use of collocation capabilities using graphs presents new challenges for scientists to discover unknown areas of social behavior.

The presented results of the experiment prove the usefulness of text analytics tools for automatic monitoring of the quality of parliamentary debate as well as a precise analysis of the topics discussed and the rhetoric used. The use of social network analysis and graph visualization tools significantly improves the process of analyzing connections between various objects, allowing a deeper understanding of the existing relationships.

Analysis of sentiment or emotions may still be burdened with errors due to the problems of automatic dealing with irony, sarcasm, etc. However, even with today's accuracy of algorithms reaching up to 90% of this type of analysis can be helpful in the work of sociologists.

References

1. Spinczyk, D., Dzieciatko, M.: Similarity search for the content of the medical records. In: Information Technologies in Medicine. Advances in Intelligent Systems and Computing, vol. 471, pp. 489–501 (2016)
2. Riegel, M., Wierzba, M., Wypych, M., Żurawski, Ł., Jednoróg, K., Grabowska, A., Marchewka, A.: Nencki Affective Word List (NAWL): the cultural adaptation of the Berlin Affective Word List-Reloaded (BAWL-R) for Polish. Behav. Res. Methods **47**(4), 1222–1236 (2015)
3. Walshaw, C.: A multilevel algorithm for force-directed graph drawing. In: International Symposium on Graph Drawing, pp. 171–182 (2000)
4. Ahmad, M.: Machine learning approach to text mining: a review. J. Adv. Res. Comput. Sci. Softw. Eng. **4**, 1125–1131 (2014)
5. Khachidze, M., Tsintsadze, M., Archuadze, M.: Natural language processing based instrument for classification of free text medical records. BioMed Res. Int. (2016)
6. Berger, A., Pietra, V., Pietra, S.: A maximum entropy approach to natural language processing. Comput. Linguist. **22**, 39–71 (1996)
7. Ningam, K., McCallum, A., Thrun, A., Mitchell, T.: Text classification from labeled and unlabeled documents using EM. Mach. Learn. **39**, 103–134 (2000)
8. Pang, B., Lee, L., Vaithyanathan, S.: Thumbs up? Sentiment classification using machine learning techniques. In: Association for Computational Linguistics, vol. 22 (2002)
9. Sebastiani, F.: Machine learning in automated text categorization. ACM Comput. Surv. **34**(1), 1–47 (2002)
10. Liritano, S., Ruffolo, M.: Managing the Knowledge Contained in Electronic Documents: a Clustering Method for Text Mining, pp. 454–458. IEEE (2001)
11. Yang, Y., Pedersen, J.O.: A comparative study on feature selection in text categorization. In Machine Learning: Proceedings of the Fourteenth International Conference (ICML 1997), pp. 412–420 (1997)
12. Scott, J.: Social Network Analysis, SAGE Publication Ltd. (2017)
13. Landauer, T.K., Dumais, S.: Latent semantic analysis. Scholarpedia **3**(11), 4356 (2008)
14. SAS 9.4 Output Delivery System: User's Guide, Fifth Edition. http://documentation.sas.com
15. Conover, M.D., Goncalves, B., Ratkiewicz, J., Flammini, A., Menczer, F.: Predicting the Political Alignment of Twitter Users. In: 2011 IEEE Third International Conference on Privacy, Security, Risk and Trust and 2011 IEEE Third International Conference on Social Computing, Boston, MA, pp. 192–199 (2011)
16. Spinczyk, D., Nabrdalik, K., Rojewska, K.: Computer aided sentiment analysis of anorexia nervosa patient's vocabulary BioMedical Engineering OnLine 201817:19. https://doi.org/10.1186/s12938-018-0451-2
17. Kaya, M., Fidan, G., Toroslu, I.: Sentiment analysis of Turkish Political News. In: 2012 IEEE/WIC/ACM International Conferences on Web Intelligence and Intelligent Agent Technology (2012)
18. Acharya, A., Crawford, N., Maduabum, M.: 'A Nation Divided': Classifying Presidential Speeches. http://cs229.stanford.edu/proj2016/report/AcharyaCrawfordMaduabum-ClassifyingPresidentialSpeeches-report.pdf

Assistive Technologies and Affective Computing (ATAC)

Sensor Headband for Emotion Recognition in a Virtual Reality Environment

David Krönert[1]([⊠]), Armin Grünewald[1], Frédéric Li[2],
Marcin Grzegorzek[2], and Rainer Brück[1]

[1] Medical Informatics and Microsystems Engineering,
University of Siegen, 57076 Siegen, Germany
david.kroenert@uni-siegen.de
[2] Research Group for Pattern Recognition, University of Siegen,
57076 Siegen, Germany
http://www.eti.uni-siegen.de/mim/

Abstract. Due to global digitalisation, teaching in virtual reality is becoming a growing market. Compared to learning in class, individual learning scenarios are possible. To find out, if a person is currently stressed or overstrained and the training course thus should be adapted, it is necessary to detect the emotional state of the person. Therefore in this paper a sensor headband is introduced, which is able to measure certain physiological values such as galvanic skin conductance, blood volume pulse or body temperature. With the help of feature extraction it is then possible to determine, which emotional state relevant in learning scenarios is predominate.

Keywords: Emotion recognition · Virtual reality · Sensors · GSR
BVP

1   Introduction and Motivation

Global digitalisation, in all areas of everyday life, forces companies to rethink and adapt to the new circumstances and requirements of new business models through individual courses. More and more companies plan to train their workforce in virtual reality (VR), especially when new equipment and operations should be part of the training content. Germany's national train system company Deutsche Bahn will train all employees working on their new express train by the end of 2018 in VR, and comparable approaches exist e.g. at Wal-Mart and UPS [4]. Additional examples are in the field of medical education, where the placement of an external ventricular drain (neurosurgical procedure) or vascular interventional surgery is trained using VR [5,11].

One way to increase the efficiency of such a training system is to automatically adapt the learning scenarios to each individual user. To achieve this, it is necessary to obtain information of the current emotional state of the user.

© Springer International Publishing AG, part of Springer Nature 2019
E. Pietka et al. (Eds.): ITIB 2018, AISC 762, pp. 539–548, 2019.
https://doi.org/10.1007/978-3-319-91211-0_47

As shown later, different approaches exist in current research to perform emotion recognition. To address this topic the collaborative research project 'ELISE' [3] has been launched in 2016 in order to develop an interactive and emotionally sensitive learning systems for the preservation of competences in business process management. These courses in VR make it possible to go through three-dimensional and multimedia visualized business processes (so-called 'Process Walkthroughs'). The learning content and the business process management game are customized to learners' emotions and moods such as happiness, boredom or frustration based on biomedical data in order to increase the individual success of the subject (see Fig. 1).

Due to digitized progression of sensor technology in wearables, new various biosensors have been developed to detect, collect and analyze signals from the human body. To improve the quality of these sensors, filters and amplifiers are used to eliminate noises and to extract critical physiological signals with high accuracy. The detection of emotions can then be performed by applying machine learning and pattern recognition algorithms on large amounts of data acquired by the sensors.

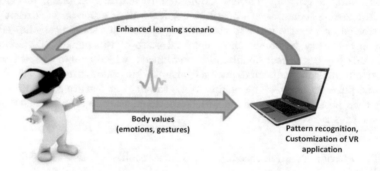

Fig. 1. Entire emotion recognition system in ELISE

In this paper, a hardware system for emotion recognition in VR will be presented along with first experimental results. To obtain the physiological data required for the pattern recognition analysis, an experimental emotion induction setup was designed and then employed on different test subjects. The remaining part of this paper is structured as follows: at first, the current state-of-the-art in the research field of emotion recognition is presented. After that, the design and implementation of the hardware system for emotion recognition and the emotion induction experimental setup are described. Preliminary results of a first data acquisition session are then presented, and an outlook on future works finally concludes the paper.

2   State of the Art

Different approaches exist to achieve emotion recognition. Due to increased computing power, more efficient GPUs and new algorithms, the analysis of facial images has become one of the most promising solutions. In [9] a system is proposed, which uses facial landmarks to detect negative, positive and blank emotions in real time. In [1], the authors present a mobile solution using the camera of a smartphone and an app to recognize facial expressions. However, these solutions cannot be deployed in a virtual reality setting, since the VR headset covers important parts of the face. The same applies for speech recognition, which has been successfully shown to be effective for emotion recognition in [13]. Instead, the measurement of body parameters should be used to determine the emotional state of a person. This has been done in [10], where the heart rate, skin conductance and skin temperature have been monitored. The sensors are placed on a finger and the system aims at detecting the emotions happiness, sadness, anger and a neutral attitude. In [12], Electroencephalogram (EEG), Electrooculogram (EOG) and Electromyogram (EMG) are recorded in addition of the Skin Conductance to monitor the levels of valence and arousal of the subject. Thereby arousal indicates the level/amount of a physical response and valence if it is perceived rather positive or negative. Several other approaches exist, e.g. as shown in [2,14]. However, all approaches vary in their precision and have in common the fact that they focus on basic emotions instead of emotional states relevant for learning such as boredom or frustration. Furthermore the sensors are placed on different locations on the body, including some which might not be suitable for applications using Virtual Reality.

3   Design and Implementation

Taking into account the requirements of the ELISE project, our whole system for emotion recognition is laid out to be compatible with a virtual reality headset, whereas other parts of the body like hands for instance should not be involved. The following sensors were selected to record the physiological signals used to recognize emotions and moods:

- Blood Volume Pulse (BVP),
- Photoplethysmogram – Oxygen saturation in blood (PPG),
- Galvanic skin response (GSR),
- Skin temperature,
- Electroencephalography (EEG), not evaluated in this paper,
- Electrooculography (EOG), not evaluated in this paper.

Unlike EEG and EOG, the placement of the BVP and GSR sensors is usually not done on the head. The solution we are proposing for the BVP and GSR measurements is therefore novel.

3.1   Concept

The architectural concept of the entire system for emotion recognition is shown in Fig. 2. The microcontroller, as the central element, connects and controls the individual sensors and preprocesses the digital measurement signals. For further processing and evaluation the sensor data are sent to any powerful station via bluetooth. To attach the different sensors and electrodes to the head, an elastic headband (Fig. 3) was used. In a subsequent version this headband could be directly fixed on a virtual reality headset.

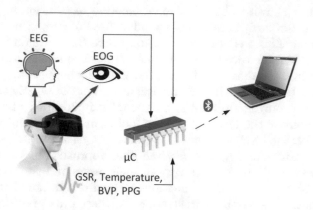

Fig. 2. Architectural concept

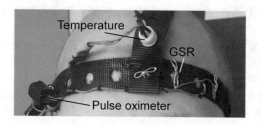

Fig. 3. Headband with sensors

3.2   Hardware Architecture

The basic structure of the emotion recognition system is presented schematically in Fig. 4. The two subsystems for EEG and EOG and the GSR sensor are connected via integrated analogue/digital converter. The pulse oximeter sensor and infrared temperature sensor operate digitally via the 'Inter-Integrated Circuit' bus (I^2C bus).

GSR

Strong impulsive emotions can stimulate the sympathetic nervous system, which produces more sweat on skin. Fluctuations are caused by changes in electrical conductivity. The GSR sensor is a voltage divider and is shown in Fig. 5. The electrodes are attached directly to the body. The human body works like a large resistor (defined as resistor R2 in Eq. 1), so that the output V_{out} (P02) of the circuit depends on the voltage divider equation.

$$V_{out} = P02 = V_{cc} \cdot \frac{R_1}{R_1 + R_2} \tag{1}$$

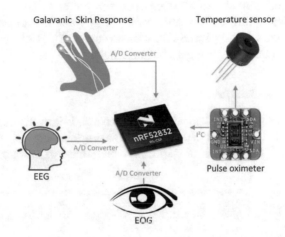

Fig. 4. Schematic structure

If the resistance of the skin decreases, the voltage rises in relation to the output of the circuit. In order to reduce the total voltage on the skin, an additional resistor R6 of 68 kΩ is added into the circuit.

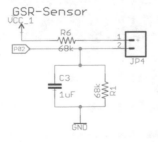

Fig. 5. Schematic diagram of GSR

544   D. Krönert et al.

Temperature

The infrared sensor MLX90614 from *Melexis – Microelectronic Integrated Systems* is a highly sensitive digital 16-bit sensor. Its accuracy is ±0.5° and its working range lies between −40 to +125 Celsius for temperature measurements [8].

BVP

The basic function of a pulse oximeter is based on measurement of light absorption or light reflection and is used to measure the arterial oxygen saturation of haemoglobin and the heart rate. The MAX30102 sensor from *Maxim Integrated* uses daylight suppression and works with an analog/digital converter up to 18-bits. The converter operates with a sampling rate from 50 Hz to 3.2 kHz. Discrete time filters remove disturbing interferences of 50/60 Hz and low-frequency ambient frequencies. An integrated on-chip temperature sensor calibrates the entire system depending on the measured temperature and compensates for faulty measurements during the SpO2 measurement [7]. Both modules communicate via the standard I^2C-compatible interface.

3.3 Data Transmission

Except for smaller partial calculations, the recorded data are not processed on the microcontroller. For analysing and evaluating the signals, they are transferred to external computers or laptops which have more potent hardware.

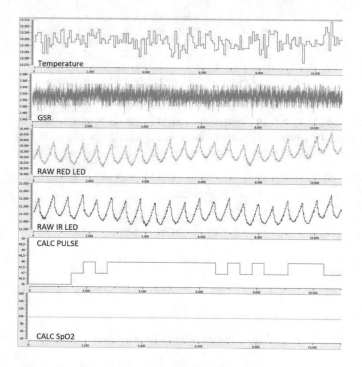

Fig. 6. Example values in Serialplot [6]

The transmission is carried out in 8-bit data packets, which are serially trans-ferred using the UART interface. Two 8-bit data packets are combined to form a data record.

A total of 9 data records are transmitted and visualized using the Serialplot software [6], which is in particular suitable for the interpretation of different binary formats (like integers or floating point numbers) and ASCII characters. In addition, several channels can be plotted simultaneously and commands can be returned to the source system. The data records can then be saved by the software as a CSV (Coma Seperated Values) file for later analysis. Figure 6 shows an example of processed and transmitted data record, visualized in the Serialplot software.

4   Experimental Setup

4.1   Emotion Induction

To find out whether emotion recognition is possible with the selected sensors, extensive data acquisition sessions with several test subjects are necessary. Emo-tion induction experiments were carried out in the second half of 2017 in a labora-tory of University of Siegen at the Chair of Medical Informatics and Microsystem Engineering. In order to induce the mentioned emotions, test subjects were asked to perform different games or tasks. These tests were divided into the following three experiments, each being 5-min long:

1. Listening to the song 'Delibes (1870): Mazurka aus Coppelia' while reading vignettes of cheerful sentences at predefined intervals.
2. Flash-based game 'Frusta Bit', which can only be controlled by a computer mouse, where the test subject has to navigate through a labyrinth and col-lect balls while avoiding walls and obstacles. After each level, the difficulty increases. If the subjects complete the first eight levels under a certain time of 5 min, they are promised to get a reward. The experiment is rigged due a second wireless mouse of the supervisor, so the subject can never reach the objective.
3. A four-minute long boring video 'The Most Boring Video Ever | DELETED SCENES' [15] shows two men hanging clothes on a clothesline and talking to each other only occasionally.

Before and after each experiment, the test subjects were asked to fill out a questionnaire about their current emotional state in order to verify the feasibilty of the emotion induction. Each data record obtained after each experiment was then associated with a label corresponding to the dominant emotion reported in the post-experiment questionnaires.

4.2   Preliminary Data Exploration

In order to carry out a basic preliminary study of the data, we used physio-logical data from three subjects who reported feeling happy/bored/frustrated

after taking the experimental setup described in Sect. 4.1. We then analysed the
potential efficiency of some very simple features (i.e. attributes of the data which
are relevant for the recognition problem) for a potential classification of those
three emotions. A sliding time window segmentation approach (see Fig. 7) was
firstly employed to divide the data acquired from the sensors into smaller segments, and limit the quantity of data on which features are computed. A time
window of a fixed size was slid on the sensor data records (with a fixed stride)
to yield data frames.

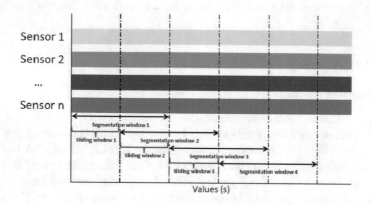

Fig. 7. Sliding window algorithm

Simple statistical features (e.g. mean, standard-deviation, max, min, amplitude) were then computed on the frames obtained this way, and for each sensor
channel separately. For a basic qualitative study, we plotted histograms of the
values of features we extracted from the frames of the whole dataset. Two examples are shown in Figs. 8 and 9. The histograms for the mean of Heart Rate
(displayed in Fig. 8) show that even simple statistical features might have a use
for the distinction of the emotions considered in our study: feature values for
'boredom' are skewed toward low values and is indicative of a lower pulse during
the boredom induction experiment. The histogram also shows us that high values of the mean of the pulse could be used to distinguish 'frustration' from the
two other emotions. However, plotting the histograms of other features (such as
the mean of RED_raw in Fig. 9) also highlighted potential difficulties to obtain
an user-independent emotion recognition system, related to the high intra-class
variability of the classification problem: the three distributions of features visible
in Fig. 9 correspond to the three subjects of the dataset, and show that different
subjects in the same emotional state can provide sensor values very different
from each other. Further studies to find more elaborated features able to bypass
this issue (e.g. based on the Fourier transform or deep-learning) will be carried
out on a dataset including more subjects and all sensors in the future.

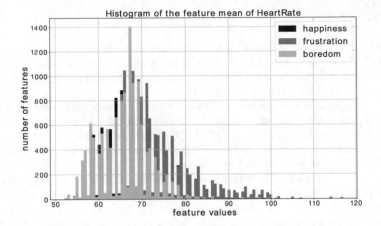

Fig. 8. Arithmetic mean of calculated heart rate

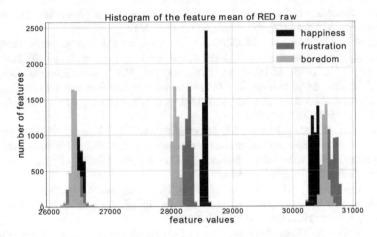

Fig. 9. Arithmetic mean of raw data from the red LED of the pulse oximeter

5   Conclusion and Future Work

The presented compact microcontroller-supported system for emotion recognition was developed at the Chair of Medical Informatics and Microsystems Engineering for application in a virtual reality environment. First experimental results have shown that the system delivers reliable biomedical data and further gives positive indication for the recognition of emotions relevant in learning scenarios. Future steps will include data acquisition runs on a higher number of subjects, with the inclusion of all sensors. Once the full dataset is acquired, studies to find more relevant features for an user-independent emotion recognition (e.g. Fourier or deep-learning based) will be carried out. The efficiency of the features found will be evaluated in a standard supervised learning framework using a SVM classifier.

References

1. Alshamsi, H., Meng, H., Li, M.: Real time facial expression recognition app development on mobile phones. In: 12th International Conference on Natural Computation, Fuzzy Systems and Knowledge Discovery (ICNC-FSKD) (2016). https://doi.org/10.1109/FSKD.2016.7603442
2. Das, P., Khasnobish, A., Tibarewala, D.: Emotion recognition employing ECG and GSR signals as markers of ANS. In: Conference on Advances in Signal Processing (CASP) (2016). https://doi.org/10.1109/CASP.2016.7746134
3. ELISE: Elise-förderprojekt - lebenslanges lernen mit gefühl, spaß und technik (2016). http://elise-lernen.de/. (in German)
4. Fink, C.: VR Training Next Generation of Workers (2017). https://www.forbes.com/sites/charliefink/2017/10/30/vr-training-next-generation-of-workers
5. Guo, S., Cai, X., Gao, B., Yuhua, J.: An improved VR training system for vascular interventional surgery. In: IEEE International Conference on Robotics and Biomimetics (2016). https://doi.org/10.1109/ROBIO.2016.7866567
6. hackaday.io: Serialplot - Realtime Plotting Software (2017). https://hackaday.io/project/5334-serialplot-realtime-plotting-software
7. Maxim Integrated: Datenblatt: Max30102. https://datasheets.maximintegrated.com/en/ds/MAX30102.pdf. Accessed 05 Dec 2017
8. Melexis: Datasheet: Mlx90614. https://www.melexis.com/-/media/files/documents/datasheets/mlx90614-datasheet-melexis.pdf. Accessed 05 Dec 2017
9. Nguyen, B.T., Trinh, M.H., Phan, T.V., Nguyen, H.D.: An efficient real-time emotion detection using camera and facial landmarks. In: Seventh International Conference on Information Science and Technology (ICIST) (2017). https://doi.org/10.1109/ICIST.2017.7926765
10. Quazi, M.T., Mukhopadhyay, S.C., Suryadevara, N.K., Huang, Y.M.: Towards the smart sensors based human emotion recognition. In: IEEE International Instrumentation and Measurement Technology Conference (I2MTC) (2012). https://doi.org/10.1109/I2MTC.2012.6229646
11. de Ribaupierre, S., Armstrong, R., Noltie, D., Kramers, M., Eagleson, R.: VR and AR simulator for neurosurgical training. In: IEEE Virtual Reality (VR) (2015). https://doi.org/10.1109/VR.2015.7223338
12. Torres-Valencia, C.A., Alvarez, M.A., Orozco-Gutierrez, A.A.: Multiple-output support vector machine regression with feature selection for arousal/valence space emotion assessment. In: 36th Annual International Conference of the IEEE Engineering in Medicine and Biology Society (EMBC) (2014). https://doi.org/10.1109/EMBC.2014.6943754
13. Vinay, G.S., Mehra, A.: Gender specific emotion recognition through speech signals. In: International Conference on Signal Processing and Integrated Networks (SPIN) (2014). https://doi.org/10.1109/SPIN.2014.6777050
14. Wiem, M.B.H., Lachiri, Z.: Emotion recognition system based on physiological signals with raspberry pi III implementation. In: 3rd International Conference on Frontiers of Signal Processing (ICFSP) (2017). https://doi.org/10.1109/ICFSP.2017.8097053
15. youtube.com: The Most Boring Video Ever | Deleted Scenes (2016). https://www.youtube.com/watch?v=s34zGmq3rXQ

EEG-Based Mental Task Classification with Convolutional Neural Networks – Parallel vs 2D Data Representation

Bartłomiej Stasiak$^{(\boxtimes)}$, Sławomir Opałka, Dominik Szajerman,
and Adam Wojciechowski

Institute of Information Technology, Łódź University of Technology,
ul. Wólczańska 215, 93-005 Łódź, Poland
bartlomiej.stasiak@p.lodz.pl

Abstract. In this paper a convolutional neural network, CNN, is trained
to perform mental task recognition on the basis of the EEG signal. We
address the problem of EEG data representation and processing, comparing two different approaches to the construction of the convolutional
layers of the CNN. We demonstrate that splitting the input EEG data
into individual channels and frequency bands is beneficial in terms of the
generalization error, although the training process is faster and more stable if complete, unsplit two-dimensional spectrograms of the EEG signal
are processed.

Keywords: Convolutional neural network CNN
Brain-computer interface · Electroencephalography

1 Introduction

Electroencephalography (EEG) is a well-known diagnostic tool routinely used
by neurologists in many medical conditions affecting the central nervous system.
Apart from its clinical significance, non-invasive measurement of electrical brain
activity is one of the most studied technologies applied for the construction of
brain-computer interfaces (BCI). This type of a communication channel between
the user's brain and the external devices has significant advantages, including
real-time operating with low latency, as well as portability, ease of use and low
cost of the associated equipment. On the other hand, the EEG signal is recorded
by the electrodes placed on the scalp surface of the user which results in poor
signal-to-noise ratio and low selectivity, as compared to more invasive techniques,
such as electrocorticography. Each electrode produces its output averaged over
a relatively large area of the brain cortex which imposes the need of sophisticated post-processing and advanced analytical methods to extract the useful
information.

© Springer International Publishing AG, part of Springer Nature 2019
E. Pietka et al. (Eds.): ITIB 2018, AISC 762, pp. 549–560, 2019.
https://doi.org/10.1007/978-3-319-91211-0_48

In this paper we present machine-learning approach to classify three types of tasks imagined by the user, on the basis of the EEG recording. For this purpose, we explore the potential of the convolutional neural networks (CNN), comparing two different neural architectures associated with two different methods of EEG data presentation and processing.

2   Previous Work

The complexity of the brain activity patterns and the very coarse information available from the standard EEG signal entails the need for robust data-processing methods. Machine learning approach has been demonstrated to yield satisfactory results both in clinical cases, including i.a. stroke rehabilitation [3] or epilepsy treatment [2] and in more general applications, such as sleep stages classification [4], event-related potentials (ERP) analysis [5] and controlling the movement of a robot [1] in the unknown environment. Artificial neural networks (ANN) are typically applied here as trainable classification tools, with *convolutional neural networks* (CNN) being one of the most prominent examples studied recently.

Convolutional neural networks are primarily designed to analyze visual information in a way resembling the hierarchical processing of images performed by the human brain. The hidden layers (*convolutional layers*) perform linear filtering of the input image with adaptable convolution kernels. Their outputs are called *feature maps* [6,10], since they actually describe locations of certain features of the image on different levels of abstraction. The neural architecture and the functional principles of the CNNs are biologically inspired and the analogies to some elements of the human visual system allowed to significantly reduce the connections between layers and to share neural weights between individual neurons [8,11,15]. In this way, raw input images may be directly processed (without any preceding feature-extraction step), which had been always considered too computationally complex for classical neural architectures, such as multi-layer perceptrons (MLP) or radial-basis function networks (RBF).

Another factor, that allowed for the successful CNN applications in image recognition tasks (ImageNet Large Scale Visual Recognition Challenge, ILSVRC [7,9,12,13]) is the computational potential of modern graphics processing units (GPUs) facilitating efficient training of 'deep' neural architectures with many hidden layers, so that they can model complex dependencies inherent to real-world problems [6,9,14].

In typical image classification tasks, the CNN significantly reduces the dimensionality of the input data in each consecutive hidden layer, by reducing the size of its output feature map w.r.t. its input. This reduced data representation is then fed to a general-purpose classifier, such as a multi-layer perceptron. This is advantageous, because the MLP itself is also a neural network, so it can be implemented just as a set of additional, densely connected neural layers (*inner-product layers*) appended to the CNN and trained jointly (CNN+MLP network as a whole) with a gradient optimization technique [6,14].

Apart from image analysis, convolutional neural networks have been successfully applied in many other areas, including speech recognition [16,17] and music information retrieval [18–21]. They have also been used for brain signal analysis and decoding, as evidenced by the most recent research, including i.a. seizure prediction [23,24], EEG-based rhythm stimuli recognition [25], event related potential detection [26] and driver's cognitive performance prediction [27]. A particular application area is motor imagery classification in which the user mentally simulates certain actions [28–30], which may be detected in the EEG signal and used as the information source for BCI interface, e.g. to control the movements of a prosthesis or other external devices. A comprehensive survey of current research on CNN-based EEG signal analysis and classification may be found in [22].

Despite the reported successful applications, there is still much room for improvement and research, concerning i.a. the choice of EEG data representation and the design of the neural architecture of the CNN. It should be stressed that in the case of the EEG analysis, the input data characteristics is significantly different from what the convolutional networks have been specifically designed for, i.e. from typical images. The choice of the right data representation and the processing scheme is therefore not obvious and indeed, several different approaches have been proposed hitherto.

The initial convolutional layers of the network are often constructed so that they process the data along one dimension only (along the time axis) [22,28, 29]. It means that all EEG signals (from the individual electrodes) are first processed separately by parallel sections of the CNN and only then are they merged and processed jointly by the intermediate hidden convolutional layers and finally by the densely connected output layers (the MLP section). Some authors however start from processing the input data across frequency channels, postponing the filtration along time axis to the next convolutional layer [30]. The number of convolutional layers is typically limited to 2 [28,30] although some authors tested also much 'deeper' architectures (e.g. shallow, deep and residual networks considered in [22] have 2, 5, and 31 layers, respectively). Also, the kernel sizes and the number of MLP units in the classifier part is much varied and different data reduction methods are applied (e.g. max-pooling in [22,29] and average pooling in [28]).

In the present work we compare two different architectures of the convolutional neural network in the task of mental imagery classification. The typical parallel layout (one-dimensional processing of the input data) is contrasted with two-dimensional approach in which both time and frequency dimensions are processed simultaneously from the very first layer of the network. The strengths and the shortcomings of both approaches are discussed and the potential areas of application are indicated. The dataset used for training and testing the proposed CNNs is described in the next section and in the following section the details of the two CNN architectures are explained. The results obtained in experimental evaluation are presented and discussed in Sect. 5.

3 Dataset

The dataset used in our experiments (BCI Competition III, dataset V [31]) is composed of 12 sessions in which a user ('subject'), while being monitored by the EEG device, was performing mental actions of one of the three possible kinds (classes):

1. Imagined repetitive left hand movement,
2. Imagined repetitive right hand movement,
3. Generation of words beginning with the same (random) letter.

Each session lasted 4 min during which the user was consecutively performing the actions in random order. Each action lasted ca 15 s and the user switched to another one without any break (the data was recorded continuously). The raw EEG signal was post-processed in the following way. First, it was spatially filtered by means of a surface Laplacian computed globally with a spherical spline of the 2nd order [31] and then the power spectral density (PSD) was computed with the window size of 1000 ms and the hop-size of 62.5 ms. The resulting data represent the frequency spectra of individual EEG channels limited to the band of 8–30 Hz (alpha and beta waves) with the frequency resolution of 2 Hz. Each second of the recording of one EEG channel is therefore represented by 12×16 spectrogram matrix (12 frequency components $\times$ 16 'hops' i.e. time-shifts per second). Eight centro-parietal channels: C3, Cz, C4, CP1, CP2, P3, Pz, and P4 are monitored, which yields $12 \times 16 \times 8 = 1536$ values per second in total. This data is accompanied by the expected target labels of the mental action being currently taken by the user (one label per time shift, i.e. 16 labels per second, correspondingly), as demonstrated in Fig. 1.

Three users took part in the data collection process (exactly 4 sessions for each user). For each user, three sessions are treated as the training data source, while the fourth session is used for testing. In our tests, both training and testing of the CNN is done independently for every user, so the whole available database is in fact considered to be composed of three independent datasets (one dataset per user), each containing three training sessions and one test session. This is consistent with the approach presented in other works [29,31] and it reflects the very individual, user-specific characteristics of the EEG data, which generally makes the construction and training of universal classifiers a very difficult task.

The input data is split into 1s-long fragments (16 consecutive columns of the spectrogram matrix) by the sliding window technique with original hop-size of 62.5 ms. The set of 8 such fragments (one fragment for one channel) is a single input to the CNN network for which we expect to obtain the class label prediction at the network output.

4 CNN Architecture

Two different architectures of the CNN are analyzed and compared, as mentioned in Sect. 2. In opposition to many proposed approaches based on one-dimensional

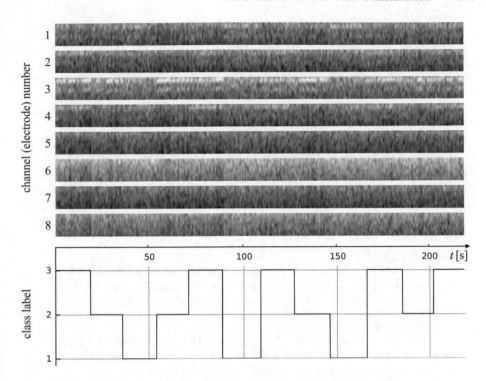

Fig. 1. The spectrograms of the 8 EEG channels (top) and the corresponding mental task labels (bottom). The plots are time-aligned, the ordinate of the spectrograms represents frequency (8–30 Hz) and the gray-scale intensity level is the PSD value

convolution in the first neural layer, we decided to process the input data in two dimensions immediately at the first convolutional layer (Fig. 2).

This solution is similar to the method of sound signal representation for CNN-based music information retrieval tasks [18, 21] in which the short-time Fourier transform (STFT) is used to obtain the sound spectrograms. These spectrograms are then treated as images (optionally cut into consecutive fragments along time with the sliding window technique), which makes the CNN directly applicable. We further make use of the possibility of multi-channel image analysis – which in typical applications is used to feed RGB images directly to the CNN – to mix

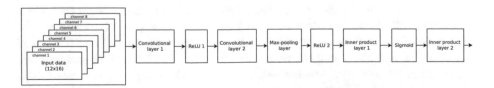

Fig. 2. The 2D architecture of the convolutional neural network

together the input data from all 8 EEG channels. The input data may therefore be seen as an 8-channel 'image', where a single channel is represented by one of the 8 spectrograms shown at the top of Fig. 1. Such 'image' is naturally cut into fragments of the width corresponding to 1 s of the EEG data recording (16 columns in our case), as explained in the previous section.

The proposed architecture contains two convolutional layers with non-linear activation function (parametric rectified linear unit, PReLU). After the second convolutional layer we use a max-pooling layer. Two final layers are inner-product (dense) layers, as they play the role of the classifier (the MLP). The first one has a sigmoidal activation function and the last one contains three linear neurons associated with the three expected output class labels, respectively. In the search of the appropriate complexity of our network, we have used various number of neurons in the individual layers. Three representative examples are as follows:

1. 'Big' network (2D-big):
   – Conv. layer 1 : 96 kernels (7×3, stride: 1) – output size: 10×10,
   – Conv. layer 2 : 50 kernels (3×3, stride: 1) – output size: 8×8,
   – Max-pool layer : (2×2, stride: 2) – output size: 4×4,
   – Inner product layer: 96 neurons.
2. 'Medium-sized' network (2D-med):
   – Conv. layer 1 : 30 kernels (7×3, stride: 1) – output size: 10×10,
   – Conv. layer 2 : 15 kernels (3×3, stride: 1) – output size: 8×8,
   – Max-pool layer : (2×2, stride: 2) – output size: 4×4,
   – Inner product layer: 96 neurons.
3. 'Small' network (2D-small):
   – Conv. layer 1 : 10 kernels (7×3, stride: 1) – output size: 10×10,
   – Conv. layer 2 : 10 kernels (3×3, stride: 1) – output size: 8×8,
   – Max-pool layer : (2×2, stride: 2) – output size: 4×4,
   – Inner product layer: 10 neurons.

Note that, the input size is 12×16 ($\times 8$ channels), and also the kernel dimensions in the convolutional layers are the same in all three cases. Several other configurations have also been tested but they either introduced no significant changes or they were remarkably inferior.

The second architecture (Fig. 3) is based on a layout more typically used for EEG data processing, in which the convolution is done in one dimension only (in time). The input data is divided into $12 \times 8 = 96$ vectors (each vector represents a single frequency band from a single channel) where each of these vectors contains 16 values (representing 16 consecutive points in time). Every vector is processed by its own convolutional network with one-dimensional kernels. In other words, we use 96 one-dimensional CNNs in parallel, where every such CNN is defined similarly to the convolutional part of our first (i.e. 2D) architecture. More precisely, it has two convolutional layers with 50 kernels of size 5×1, and 20 kernels of size 3×1, respectively, as well as the PReLU activation function and the max-pooling layer (also one-dimensional). The data from all these CNNs are concatenated and further processed by the MLP part, which is identical to the MLP part used in the 2D architecture (two dense layers with 96/3 neurons and sigmoidal/linear activation functions, respectively).

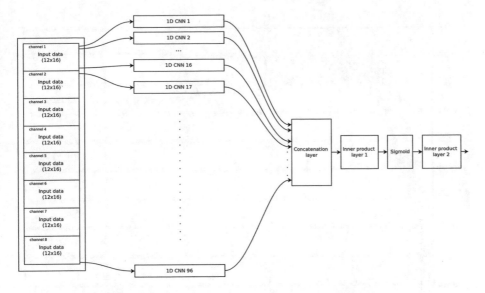

Fig. 3. The parallel architecture of the convolutional neural network

5   Experimental Evaluation

All the experiments were done with Caffe deep learning framework [32] on a machine with Tesla K80 GPU accelerator. Each neural network was trained on the same data composed of three independent datasets (one dataset from one user). Our main goal was to compare the capabilities and learning dynamics of the two different neural architectures presented in the previous section. We have therefore used uniform training parameters and stopping criterion for all the networks. The fixed number of 150 000 iterations was used with training batch size of 1000 input spectrogram fragments ($12 \times 16 \times 8$). We used AdaGrad optimization algorithm which has already proved to yield good results for the same task and dataset [29].

In order to evaluate the quality of the obtained results, we periodically performed classification of both the training and the testing sets, during the training process (every 300 training iterations). Unsurprisingly, the classification accuracy on the training dataset was continuously improving, while on the testing set some generalization error could be observed in the late phase of the training.

The generalization error is known to be dependent on the relation between the network complexity and the dataset size and characteristics. For the fixed dataset, we could expect that the parallel architecture, having ca 4 times more neural weights than the 2D-big network, would be more prone to over-fitting, but it appeared that it is just the opposite. The parallel network had very low generalization error and in some cases its classification accuracy on the *testing dataset* kept enhancing even at the end of the training process, as demonstrated in Fig. 4.

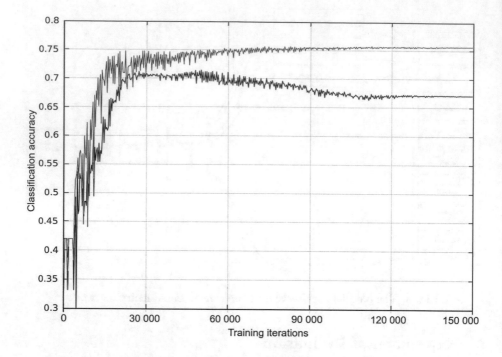

Fig. 4. Example (for 'user 2' dataset) of the evolution of the classification accuracy on the testing set during the training process for the 2D-big architecture (black plot) and for the parallel architecture (gray plot)

On the other hand, the analysis of the classification results on the *training set* revealed that the 2D architecture learns much better, in some cases achieving accuracy over 90% for the more 'rich' variants (2D-big, 2D-med). The results for all the investigated networks are displayed in Table 1.

For each user and each network three values are presented:

1. Train – the classification accuracy on the *training set* at the end of training,
2. Test Max – the best classification accuracy on the *testing set* obtained anytime during the training process,
3. Test Final – the classification accuracy on the *testing set* at the end of training.

The first value shows the learning potential of the network, the second value indicates the best result that would theoretically be achieved on the testing set if the optimal stopping condition was applied (e.g. by using a separate validation set), and the third value enables to assess the generalization error increase for the over-trained network. Each value in Table 1 is the arithmetic mean of three individual repetitions of the training process for given settings (each repetition starts with random values of the initial neural weights). The results are usually quite stable among the repetitions, as demonstrated by the standard deviation (σ)

Table 1. Classification accuracy [%] with (σ) value

Net arch.	User 1			User 2			User 3		
	Train	Test max	Test final	Train	Test max	Test final	Train	Test max	Test final
2D big	99.66 (0.02)	81.38 (0.47)	78.75 (0.52)	94.30 (2.27)	71.33 (0.09)	67.95 (0.67)	63.39 (1.33)	56.15 (0.58)	51.59 (0.27)
2D med	96.88 (0.61)	81.72 (0.48)	80.03 (0.69)	90.13 (1.09)	71.12 (0.13)	66.75 (1.08)	63.07 (3.05)	55.10 (0.23)	51.15 (1.08)
2D small	89.86 (1.36)	80.51 (0.44)	79.85 (0.76)	75.91 (3.67)	69.66 (1.59)	68.10 (0.58)	53.93 (0.13)	55.24 (0.50)	50.11 (2.86)
Parall. arch.	86.82 (0.06)	83.21 (0.49)	82.99 (0.53)	72.98 (0.12)	75.89 (0.07)	75.65 (0.07)	53.13 (0.18)	54.43 (0.41)	51.83 (0.09)

values at the bottom of each cell. It should be noted that the users differ much in terms of the ability to generate consistent EEG signal for the three predefined mental tasks. The data authored by the third user seems to be definitely the least representative [31].

The presented results clearly show that, although the 2D architecture is capable of learning the training data almost perfectly, if provided with sufficiently many hidden units (accuracy of 99.63% for the 2D-big network and 'user 1' dataset), it performs significantly worse for the unseen (testing) data. Reducing the network complexity by decreasing the number of hidden units does not seem to help – only the training classification drops, as expected.

On the other hand, the parallel architecture is much more difficult to train (the training lasts several times more, and the training error usually decreases much slower than for the 2D networks), but the network is more robust and achieves better results on the unseen data than any of the investigated 2D networks, at least in the case of the first two users. The final classification accuracy obtained for user 2 on the testing set is even better than on the training set which seems counterintuitive. This probably results from relatively high oscillations of the training error for consecutive batches of the input data (the training process is generally slow and not very stable for the parallel network) and from the particular composition of the training and testing 'user 2' dataset.

In terms of general effectiveness, the presented CNN networks are on par with other solutions presented in literature [29,33,34]. For more rigorous comparison, the appropriate stopping criterion should be applied on the basis of the training set. This is especially important for the 2D architecture, where the over-fitting is likely to occur. It is interesting to note here, that the complexity (capacity) of a classification model seems to be much higher in the case of the 2D architectures, despite the radically lower number of adjustable parameters (neural weights). This seems to result from the possibility of modeling the subtle dependencies between channels and frequency bands from the very first convolutional layer of the network. Unfortunately, these dependencies do not generalize well, so limiting the initial layers to process individual channels and bands, as it is done in the parallel architecture, seems to be more relevant and suited for the EEG data processing.

Still, the capability of the 2D-big network to learn the training data almost perfectly is appealing, and some methods of limiting the generalization error, e.g. by dropout or regularization techniques, definitely seem to be worth pursuing. On the other hand, it might be valuable to search for the methods of pruning the parallel architecture to make it learn faster and more reliably, while still keeping the generalization error low. The third alternative is to merge the two considered architectures, e.g. by individually processing all EEG channels in parallel, but without splitting them into separate frequency bands, thus retaining the two-dimensional structure of the first convolution layer. These potential directions will be considered in the future research.

6   Conclusion

In this paper we have compared two architecture types of a convolutional neural network, and the associated methods of input data presentation, in the problem of EEG signal analysis and mental task classification. The experimental results show better generalization properties of the parallel approach in which all the frequency bands of all the channels (electrodes) are processed by individual one-dimensional convolutional networks. In the second approach, based on immediate processing of the input data in two dimensions, the neural network learns much easier and faster, but it does not generalize equally well. Both approaches enable to obtain classification accuracy results exceeding 80% on the testing dataset, which seems very promising in terms of practical applications and effective brain-computer interface (BCI) construction.

Acknowledgement. We would like to thank Dr. Arkadiusz Tomczyk (Institute of Information Technology, Łódź University of Technology) for kindly providing the computational resources to run the experimental evaluation of our CNN models.

References

1. Tonin, L., Carlson, T., Leeb, R., Millan, J.d.R.: Brain-controlled telepresence robot by motor-disabled people. In: IEEE EMBS 2011, pp. 4227–4230 (2011)
2. Gadhoumi, K., Lina, J.-M., Mormann, F., Gotman, J.: Seizure prediction for therapeutic devices: a review. J. Neurosci. Methods **260**, 270–282 (2016)
3. Ramos-Murguialday, A., Broetz, D., Rea, M., Läer, L., Yilmaz, O., Brasil, F.L., Liberati, G., Curado, M.R., Garcia-Cossio, E., Vyziotis, A., Cho, W., Agostini, M., Soares, E., Soekadar, S., Caria, A., Cohen, L.G., Birbaumer, N.: Brain-machine interface in chronic stroke rehabilitation: a controlled study. Ann. Neurol. **74**(1), 100–108 (2013)
4. Jain, V.P., Mytri, V.D., Shete, V.V., Shiragapur, B K.: Sleep stages classification using wavelet transform & neural network. In: BHI 2012 IEEE-EMBS, pp. 71–74 (2012)

5. Liu, M., Ji, H., Zhao, C.: Event related potentials extraction from EEG using artificial neural network. In: Congress on Image and Signal Processing, pp. 213–215 (2008)
6. Cireşan, D.C., Meier, U., Masci, J., Gambardella, L.M., Schmidhuber, J.: Flexible, high performance convolutional neural networks for image classification. In: IJCAI 2011, pp. 1237–1242 (2011)
7. Deng, J., Dong, W., Socher, R., Li, L.-J., Li, K., Fei-Fei, L.: ImageNet: a large-scale hierarchical image database. In: CVPR 2009 (2009)
8. Fukushima, K.: Neocognitron: a self-organizing neural network model for a mechanism of pattern recognition unaffected by shift in position. Biol. Cybern. **36**, 193–202 (1980)
9. Krizhevsky, A., Sutskever, I., Hinton, G.E.: Imagenet classification with deep convolutional neural networks. In: Pereira, F., Burges, C.J.C., Bottou, L., Weinberger, K.Q. (eds.) Advances in Neural Information Processing Systems 25, pp. 1097–1105. Curran Associates Inc., Red Hook (2012)
10. LeCun, Y., Bengio, Y.: Convolutional networks for images, speech, and time-series. In: Arbib, M.A. (ed.) The Handbook of Brain Theory and Neural Networks. MIT Press, Cambridge (1995)
11. LeCun, Y., Bottou, L., Bengio, Y., Haffner, P.: Gradient-based learning applied to document recognition. In: Proceedings of the IEEE, pp. 2278–2324 (1998)
12. Nguyen, T.V., Lu, C., Sepulveda, J., Yan, S.: Adaptive nonparametric image parsing. CoRR, abs/1505.01560 (2015)
13. Zeiler, M.D., Fergus, R.: Visualizing and understanding convolutional networks. CoRR, abs/1311.2901 (2013)
14. Stasiak, B., Tarasiuk, P., Michalska, I., Tomczyk, A., Szczepaniak, S.P.: Localization of Demyelinating Plaques in MRI using Convolutional Neural Networks. In: BIOSTEC 2017, pp. 55–64 (2017)
15. Tarasiuk, P., Pryczek, M.: Geometric transformations embedded into convolutional neural networks. J. Appl. Comput. Sci. **24**(3), 33–48 (2016)
16. Sainath, T.N., Kingsbury, B., Saon, G., Soltau, H., Mohamed, A. R., Dahl, G., Ramabhadran, B.: Deep convolutional neural networks for large-scale speech tasks. Neural Netw. **64**, 39–48 (2015)
17. Sercu, T., Puhrsch, C., Kingsbury, B., LeCun, Y.: Very deep multilingual convolutional neural networks for LVCSR. In: ICASSP 2016, pp. 4955–4959 (2016)
18. Mońko, J., Stasiak, B.: Note onset detection with a convolutional neural network in recordings of bowed string instruments. In: Dziech, A., Czyżewski, A. (eds.) Communications in Computer and Information Science, vol. 785, pp. 173–185 (2017)
19. Troxel, D.: Music transcription with a convolutional neural network. In: ISMIR 2016
20. Stasiak, B., Mońko, J.: Analysis of time-frequency representations for musical onset detection with convolutional neural network. Ann. Comput. Sci. Inf. Syst. **8**, 147–152 (2016)
21. Schlüter, J., Böck, S.: Improved musical onset detection with convolutional neural networks. In: ICASSP 2014, pp. 6979–6983 (2014)
22. Schirrmeister, R.T., Springenberg, J.T., Fiederer, L.D.J., Glasstetter, M., Eggensperger, K., Tangermann, M., Hutter, F., Burgard, W., Ball, T.: Deep learning with convolutional neural networks for EEG decoding and visualization. Hum. Brain Mapp. **38**, 5391–5420 (2017)
23. Page, A., Shea, C., Mohsenin, T.: Wearable seizure detection using convolutional neural networks with transfer learning. In: ISCAS 2016, pp. 1086–1089 (2016)

24. Liang, J., Lu, R., Zhang, C., Wang, F.: Predicting seizures from electroencephalography recordings: a knowledge transfer strategy. In: ICHI 2016, pp. 184–191 (2016)
25. Stober, S.: Learning discriminative features from electroencephalography recordings by encoding similarity constraints. In: Bernstein Conference (2016)
26. Cecotti, H., Graser, A.: Convolutional neural networks for P300 detection with application to brain-computer interfaces. IEEE Trans. Pattern Anal. Mach. Intell. **33**(3), 433–445 (2011)
27. Hajinoroozi, M., Mao, Z., Jung, T.-P., Lin, C.-T., Huang, Y.: EEG-based prediction of driver's cognitive performance by deep convolutional neural network. Sig. Process. Image Commun. **47**, 549–555 (2016)
28. Sakhavi, S., Guan, C., Yan, S.: Parallel convolutional-linear neural network for motor imagery classification. In: EUSIPCO 2015, pp. 2736–2740 (2015)
29. Szajerman, D., Smagur, A., Opałka, S., Wojciechowski, A.: Effective BCI mental tasks classification with adaptively solved convolutional neural networks. In: 18th International Symposium on Electromagnetic Fields in Mechatronics, Electrical and Electronic Engineering (ISEF) Book of Abstracts, pp. 1–2 (2017)
30. Tang, Z., Li, C., Sun, S.: Single-trial EEG classification of motor imagery using deep convolutional neural networks. Optik Int. J. Light Electron Opt. **130**, 11–18 (2017)
31. Millán, J.d.R.: On the need for on-line learning in brain-computer interfaces. In: Proceedings of IEEE International Joint Conference on Neural Networks, pp. 2877–2882 (2004)
32. Jia, Y., Shelhamer, E., Donahue, J., Karayev, S., Long, J., Girshick, R., Guadarrama, S., Darrell, T.: Caffe: Convolutional Architecture for Fast Feature Embedding. In: ACM MM 2014, pp. 675–678 (2014)
33. Lin, C.-J., Hsieh, M.-H.: Classification of mental task from EEG data using neural networks based on particle swarm optimization. Neurocomputing **72**(4–6), 1121–1130 (2009)
34. Agarwal, S.K., Shah, S., Kumar, R.: Classification of mental tasks from EEG data using backtracking search optimization based neural classifier. Neurocomputing **166**, 397–403 (2015)

Computer Aided Feature Extraction in the Paper Version of Luria's Alternating Series Test in Progressive Supranuclear Palsy

Paula Stępień[1]($\boxtimes$), Jacek Kawa[1], Dariusz Wieczorek[2], Magda Dąbrowska[3], Jarosław Sławek[3,4], and Emilia J. Sitek[3,4]

[1] Faculty of Biomedical Engineering, Silesian University of Technology, Roosevelta 40, 41-800 Zabrze, Poland
paula.stepien@polsl.pl
[2] Department of Rehabilitation, Medical University of Gdansk, Gdańsk, Poland
[3] Neurology Department, St. Adalbert Hospital, Copernicus PL Ltd., Gdańsk, Poland
[4] Department of Neurological and Psychiatric Nursing, Medical University of Gdansk, Gdańsk, Poland

Abstract. Luria's Alternating Series Test (AST) is a popular bedside graphomotor task used to assess set-shifting both in patients with focal brain damage and with neurodegenerative disease. Several approaches to automate its assessment are available, yet they require digitizers or other electronic devices. However, archived data from the past 60 years are stored only on paper. This pilot study concerns the extraction of the features from the paper version of AST using image processing algorithms.

In this study, AST data from twenty two cases with progressive supranuclear palsy are processed. Each case contains reference data (a pattern sequence drawn by the examiner) and diagnostic data (continuation of the pattern drawn by the patient). Spatial-based features as well as (novel) erosion bar charts (EBC) are extracted from the initial characters of the examiner and patient sequence. The results are evaluated to find parameters that are statistically different between the groups. The results indicate that patients typically write larger characters than examiners, yet their pen-paper pressure is smaller.

Keywords: Neurodegeneration · Writing assessment · Dementia
Luria's test · Movement disorders · Progressive supranuclear palsy

1 Introduction

Modern neuropsychological assessment approach to the differential diagnosis of neurodegenerative diseases affecting basal ganglia has to address the patient's cognitive profile in the context of his/her motor function. In dementia syndromes

© Springer International Publishing AG, part of Springer Nature 2019
E. Pietka et al. (Eds.): ITIB 2018, AISC 762, pp. 561–570, 2019.
https://doi.org/10.1007/978-3-319-91211-0_49

associated with movement disorders, e.g. progressive supranuclear palsy (PSP), it is sometimes difficult to disentangle motor and cognitive components of deficient performance on executive tasks. However, executive tasks requiring motor reactions such as go/no go or conflicting reactions are very sensitive in PSP [15]. A simple clinical battery was published in the 1966 by Alexander Romanovich Luria (often referred to as the 'father of modern neuropsychological assessment' [11]), in the book *Higher cortical functions in man* based on 25 years of observations [5]. In his work, Luria described twelve methods to investigate the cortical functions in local brain lesions. The main goal of his research was to gather information that would help scientists design a tool to identify the locus of brain damage, as at the time of development of those tasks (during the II World War) neuroimaging techniques were not available. The investigation of motor functions concerned, among other things, the hand movements.

The techniques introduced by Luria are the cornerstone of the Luria-Nebraska neuropsychological battery (LNNB), which incorporates the mentioned test as well as the traditional American psychometric procedures. The evaluation provided by the battery is often described as 'brief but comprehensive'. However, the whole procedure takes about three hours. Frequently, only specific tasks are performed in the specialist's office [3]. One of these tasks is Luria's alternating series test (AST), in which the subject is asked to continue a pattern given by the specialist. The pattern consists of alternating squares and triangles, therefore it is universal and can be easily used worldwide, regardless of the subject's mother tongue. This makes it popular among researchers.

The AST is a clinical test administered both by behavioral neurologists and neuropsychologists. Due to its simplicity and brevity it may be used at various stages of dementia. The visuographic task of AST, engages both cognitive processing and motor activity and also assesses set-shifting and inhibitory control [1]. The assessment is usually quantitative, yet sometimes the percentage of perseverative shapes in reference to all shapes drawn by the patient in a line is computed [13]. Apart from executive components of the task (set-shifting and inhibitory control), which are important for examining patients with dementia affecting mainly the frontal lobe, the task may be used to assess graphomotor parameters. In patients with hypokinesia, it may show the progressive reduction of drawings in a line. In patients with hyperkinesia, it may show size irregularity or a tendency to increase the size of the shapes, etc. Thus, it may reveal both micrographia and macrographia.

The technological advances are usually applied in computerized neuropsychological test batteries [8] that can be used with patients with mild cognitive impairment or mild dementia. Computerized executive tasks are very complex and their use is not feasible at bedside or with patients with moderate dementia. On the contrary, writing and drawing assessments [16] are widely used in the clinical practice but usually those tasks are assessed only qualitatively. Graphomotor set-shifting tasks may allow the analysis of both executive and motor features when qualitative analysis is supplemented with quantitative approach.

The availability of modern devices such as tablets, digitizers, and touch-screens made the measurement of additional writing features, such as pressure or acceleration of the pen, possible. Research using electronic devices was conducted on groups with Parkinson's [2,6,9], Huntington's [10], and Alzheimer's diseases [12] as well as mild cognitive impairment [4].

In their work [7], Nõmm et al. extracted features such as velocity, acceleration, jerk, number of strokes, pressure, horizontal and vertical components from the AST. They designed a method consisting of four tasks: (1) continuing, (2) copying and (3) tracing the pattern, and (4) copying a sinusoidal line on a tablet using a stylus. Interestingly, only kinematic features were taken into account.

Despite all the recent work on AST, one must not forget, that dynamic approach can only be applied to the contemporary data, whereas over the past 60 years the Luria test data were collected using a sheet of paper and a pencil. The archived cases combined with patient's record may contain vital data for the understanding of the processes standing behind neurological diseases. Moreover, the paper version is still in use, as not all psychologists own digitizers or are even familiar with such equipment.

This study is concerned with the paper version of AST. The long-term goal is to automatically process the test and extract features for analysis. The aim of presented step is to select features to differentiate between the characters drawn by the examiner and the patient part of the sequence (transition between the given pattern and the patient continuation).

During the presented processing, test sheets are first digitized and manually cropped to the region of interests. Then, the sequence of rectangles and triangles is manually separated into individual characters and attributed either to examiner (usually four or five initial characters) or patient (following characters). Finally, every character is subjected to the features extraction process, including spatial features as well as novel erosion bar charts (EBC) features. Extracted data are then statistically analyzed in the examiner and patient groups.

2 Materials and Methods

Luria's alternating sequences test was administered in the context of comprehensive neuropsychological assessment. During AST administration, the patient was seated at the desk with the elbow of the dominant hand positioned comfortably on the desk surface. If vision correction was necessary, the examinee was asked to wear eyeglasses. Then, the patient was presented a short sequence of alternating connected shapes, open triangles and squares, all drawn by the examiner. Next, the examinee was asked to continue the pattern until the end of the page, if possible without lifting the pen.

The task was administered to 22 patients (13 men and 9 women, mean age 67 ± 8 years), with clinical diagnoses of probable or possible progressive supranuclear palsy (PSP), as established by an experienced movement disorder specialist.

A4 paper and a Grip 2001 HB Faber-Castell pencil were used. Cases were digitized using HP Deskjet Ink Advantage K209a scanner at 600 dpi (Fig. 1) and stored as grayscale, uncompressed TIFF (Tagged Image File Format) files.

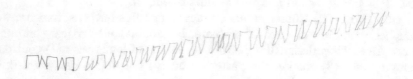

Fig. 1. An example of the Luria's alternating series test

At the next step (Fig. 2) the data were transferred into the MATLAB 2017b environment. Each correctly placed character was manually labeled as rectangle or the triangle. Misplaced characters and artifacts (e.g. additional lines between characters) were tagged accordingly and excluded from further analysis. Additionally, each triangle and rectangle was marked as drawn by either the expert (usually initial three pairs of rectangles and triangles) or the patient (continuation of the sequence).

Finally, the characters were thresholded and subjected to feature extraction. As the goal of the study was to detect the moment in which the drawing person changes (transition between pattern and continuation) and not how the characters alter in time (which may be considered at later time), only the first two available rectangles and triangles drawn by expert and patient were processed. Both character groups were regarded separately.

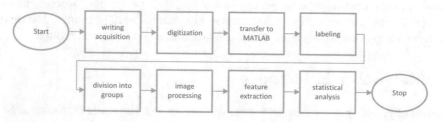

Fig. 2. Workflow of the presented approach

2.1   Extracted Features

The feature extraction was carried out automatically (Fig. 3). First, each character was fitted into a separate rectangle (bounding box). Height and width of the bounding box defined the basic dimensions. However, the characters may have been skewed or rotated, so at the next step the characters were straightened and the dimensions were estimated once again. During straightening procedure, an ellipse was first defined such that is has the same normalized second central moment as the character (Eq. 1).

$$m_{pq} = \int\limits_{-\infty}^{\infty} \int\limits_{-\infty}^{\infty} (\mathbf{x} - \overline{\mathbf{x}})^p (\mathbf{y} - \overline{\mathbf{y}})^q f(\mathbf{x},\mathbf{y}) \mathrm{d}x \mathrm{d}y \qquad (1)$$

The inclination of the longer axis of the ellipse determines the angle of the rotation and the character was straightened. The bounding box of the processed character defined a second set of dimensions.

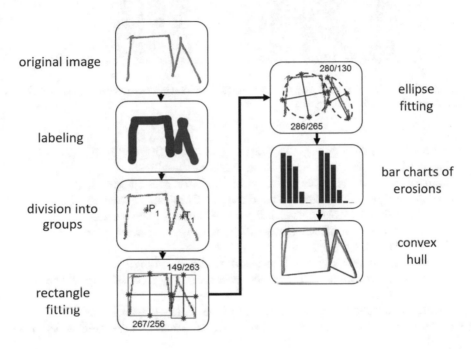

Fig. 3. Labeling and image processing

At the following step a set of novel features, the erosion bar charts (EBC), were calculated. The binary image was subjected to iterative erosion using a 1-by-1 structuring element: at the each iteration, the drawn lines were 'peeled off' by one pixel from both sides (Fig. 4a). After the completion of each step, the percentage of character's removed pixels was calculated (Fig. 4b). This procedure was carried out as long, as there were object pixels remaining.

Finally, a convex hull of the character was defined. The ratio of the number of character (object) pixels to the area of convex hull defined its opacity.

The feature vector for each character contains:

- width – the width of the rectangle in which the character was fitted (mm),
- height – the height of the rectangle,

a)

b)

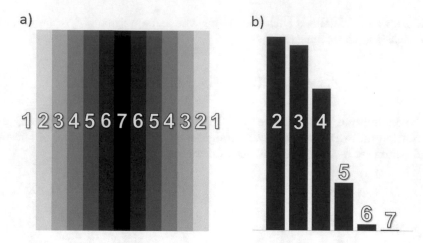

Fig. 4. The erosion steps (a) and the bar chart representing the percentage of the pixels being eresed in each of them (b)

- minor ellipse axis length – the shorter axis of the fitted ellipse,
- major ellipse axis length – the longer axis of the ellipse,
- inclination – the inclination of the longer ellipse axis (degrees),
- eccentricity of the ellipse – the distance from the center to the focus of the ellipse dived by the distance from the center to the vertex,
- width' – the width of the rectangle in which the character was fitted after the straightening procedure,
- height' – the height of the rectangle after straightening,
- convex hull – the area of the smallest convex polygon containing all the points of the character,
- opacity – the percentage of character pixels in the convex hull,
- mean thickness of bold lines – the mean thickness of lines thicker than one pixel,
- erosion bar charts (EBC) – the percentage of erased pixels in each 'peeling off' procedure.

2.2   Statistics

In the statistical analysis for the continuous data, the normality of the distribution was first verified using the Shapiro-Wilk W test. Depending on the outcome of the Shapiro-Wilk W test ($\alpha = 0.95$), the data was analyzed using either t-test ($p > 0.05$, null hypothesis not rejected, distribution presumably normal) or the Mann-Whitney U test. Depending on distribution variance, Welch's t-test or Student's t-test was employed. For discrete data, the Mann-Whitney U test was always used.

3   Results

The results of the feature extraction are presented in the Tables 1, 2, 3, 4 and 5.

In the case of spatial parameters, the height and width of the bounding box before and after the straightening procedure, the ellipse axes lengths and the area of the convex hull differ significantly between examiner and patient groups for rectangles and triangles. In both groups the size of the characters drawn by the patients is bigger than drawn by examiner. The interquartile range (IQR) of all features is distinctly bigger in the patient cases (Tables 1 and 2). A similar tendency can be seen in the features analyzed using the Welch's t-test (Table 3). The standard deviation (std) in the patient group is twice as big as in the expert group. For triangles the Student's/Welch's t-test results are not included, as none of the discriminant features is normally distributed.

Table 1. Mann-Whitney U test summary for triangles (only parameters with p-value < 0.05 are included)

Feature	Expert				Patient				p-value
	Median	IQR	Min	Max	Median	IQR	Min	Max	
Width [mm]	6.31	1.31	4.36	10.37	7.83	4.34	3.98	15.58	0.0006
Height [mm]	10.33	1.33	7.75	13.21	11.49	4.34	5.33	18.37	0.0012
Width' [mm]	10.73	1.84	8.17	13.12	12.30	4.64	6.05	19.86	0.0005
Height' [mm]	6.03	1.52	3.81	11.43	7.35	4.00	3.85	15.50	0.0009
Minor ellipse axis length [mm]	11.26	2.04	8.80	14.72	12.82	4.97	5.49	21.52	0.0012
Convex hull [mm^2]	39.95	11.42	23.40	64.91	50.54	39.44	14.89	130.90	0.0001

Table 2. Mann-Whitney U test summary for squares (only parameters with p-value < 0.05 are included)

Feature	Expert				Patient				p-value
	Median	IQR	Min	Max	Median	IQR	Min	Max	
Height [mm]	10.52	2.07	8.59	13.21	12.93	3.09	7.45	19.05	<0.0001
Height' [mm]	11.26	1.97	4.49	15.50	12.45	3.51	7.41	22.18	0.0002
Minor ellipse axis length [mm]	16.42	3.09	11.33	21.50	17.30	6.01	11.59	39.93	0.0005
Major ellipse axis length [mm]	12.12	2.29	3.99	14.61	13.69	3.81	8.00	24.37	<0.0001
Convex hull [mm^2]	99.36	26.80	27.70	167.19	113.69	69.30	62.09	426.21	<0.0001

Expert and patient triangles (Table 4) and squares (Table 5) differ also with respect to the novel EBC (erosion bar charts) feature in its first (EBC1), third (EBC3) and fourth (EBC4) step. In the first step of the iterative erosion, almost the half of the character written by patients is erased, while it is only one third in case of expert's characters. The percentage of erased patient's lines between steps changes also in a more dynamic way. Yet the std and IQR are bigger in the expert group for the first and fourth step.

Table 3. Welch's t-test summary for squares (only parameters with p-value < 0.05 are included)

Feature	Expert				Patient				p-value
	Mean	Std	Min	Max	Mean	Std	Min	Max	
Width [mm]	10.19	1.84	4.74	13.89	12.01	3.61	7.28	25.36	0.0001
Width' [mm]	12.25	1.80	9.53	16.09	14.98	3.70	8.64	28.54	<0.0001

Table 4. Mann-Whitney U test summary for erosion steps for triangles

Step	Expert				Patient				p-value
	Median	IQR	Min	Max	Median	IQR	Min	Max	
EBC1	0.32	0.20	0.25	0.66	0.46	0.12	0.30	0.61	0.0002
EBC3	0.23	0.06	0.08	0.26	0.16	0.03	0.10	0.21	<0.0001
EBC4	0.14	0.12	0.00	0.20	0.08	0.05	0.00	0.16	0.0084

Table 5. Mann-Whitney U test (EBC1, EBC4)/Welch's t-test (normally distributed EBC3) summary for erosion steps for squares.

Step	Expert				Patient				p-value
	Median	IQR	Min	Max	Median	IQR	Min	Max	
EBC1	0.31	0.18	0.25	0.68	0.47	0.11	0.31	0.67	<0.0001
EBC4	0.16	0.11	0.00	0.21	0.08	0.06	0.00	0.14	<0.0001
Feature	Expert				Patient				p-value
	Mean	Std	Min	Max	Mean	Std	Min	Max	
EBC3	0.20	0.04	0.06	0.26	0.15	0.03	0.05	0.20	<0.0001

4   Discussion and Summary

The dimension of the characters drawn by patients are distinctively bigger than the dimensions of the expert's characters despite the fact, that only initial patient characters were considered. These findings are consistent for both character groups: the triangles and the squares.

Moreover, almost half of the lines written by PSP patients would be erased by the first erosion step (EBC1 feature). Yet only one-third of the lines drawn by the doctor would be erased in this step. Given the shape of the character was similar, this indicates that the lines written by PSP patients were more frequently thin. One possible explanation for this observation is a smaller pencil-paper pressure, which resulted in thinner lines in the patient group. This relation should become a subject of further examination. Interestingly, the time-averaged pressure was one of the features investigated by Nõmm [7], yet it was not discussed in the paper.

The EBC features look promising from the perspective of distinguishing the examiner and patient characters in automated processing. An ensemble, bagged-trees classifier build upon the EBC1–EBC4 features for squares shows 84.1% accuracy (5-fold validation) in the examined dataset. Similar classifier build upon all differentiating features shows 87.5% validation (5-fold validation). For the triangles it is 85.2% and 87.5%, respectively.

However, there are several limitations of the study. The writing samples examined in the study were collected by only one examiner. Distinguishing the examiner and patient based on the EBC features alone may not be possible when multiple examiners are involved. However, the identity of the expert should not affect the observed patient's inclination to macrographia. As impulsivity, disinhibition or perseveration are among cognitive symptoms of PSP included in the current Movement Disorder Society clinical criteria of PSP (and they may manifest in behavior, language or motor performance [18]), it remains to be established in further studies if macrographia, observed in PSP can help in distinguishing patients with PSP from patients with Parkinson's disease, who have a tendency to micrographia. Macrographia could be a potential marker of disinhibition.

Additionally, the patient cohort consisted only of patients diagnosed with progressive supranuclear palsy. Distinguishing the patient/examiner characters might be difficult or impossible in more heterogeneous group. However, this limitation does not affect our current research where only preselected archive cases are considered. Moreover, this study focused only on the quantitative analysis of graphomotor characteristics of AST and did not address its executive components directly, that was analyzed elsewhere [17].

The performances of the AST are usually not flawless. Some patient add unwanted additional lines or characters. It this study, each character was labeled manually by an expert. Such an approach allowed to avoid the artifacts resulting form the erroneous character segmentation. The next step in the research will be the automatic segmentation and recognition of the drawn characters replacing the cumbersome and time-consuming manual segmentation.

Acknowledgement. We would like to thank Andre Woloshuk for his English language corrections.

References

1. Diesfeldt, H.F.A.: Visuographic tests of set shifting and inhibitory control. The contribution of constructional impairments. J. Neuropsychol. **3**(1), 93–105 (2009)
2. Drotár, P., Mekyska, J., Rektorová, I., Masarová, L., Smékal, Z., Faundez-Zanuy, M.: Analysis of in-air movement in handwriting: a novel marker for Parkinson's disease. Comput. Methods Program Biomed. **117**(3), 405–411 (2014). https://doi.org/10.1016/j.cmpb.2014.08.007. ISSN 0169-2607
3. Golden, C.J., Freshwater, S.M.: Luria-Nebraska neuropsychological battery. In: Understanding Psychological Assessment, pp. 59–75. Springer, Boston, MA (2001)

4. Kawa, J., Bednorz, A., Stępień, P., Derejczyk, J., Bugdol, M.: Spatial and dynamical handwriting analysis in mild cognitive impairment. Comput. Biol. Med. **82**, 21–28 (2017). https://doi.org/10.1016/j.compbiomed.2017.01.004. ISSN 0010-4825
5. Luria, A.R.: Higher Cortical Functions in Man. Springer Science & Business Media, Heidelberg (2012)
6. Nackaerts, E., Nieuwboer, A., Farella, E.: Technology-assisted rehabilitation of writing skills in Parkinson's disease: visual cueing versus intelligent feedback. Parkinson's Dis. **2017**, 1–7 (2017). https://doi.org/10.1155/2017/9198037
7. Nõmm, S., Toomela, A., Kozhenkina, J., Toomsoo, T.: Quantitative analysis in the digital Luria's alternating series tests. In: 2016 14th International Conference on Control, Automation, Robotics and Vision (ICARCV), Phuket, pp. 1–6 (2016). https://doi.org/10.1109/ICARCV.2016.7838746
8. Parsons, T.D.: Neuropsychological assessment 2.0: computer-automated assessments. In: Clinical Neuropsychology and Technology, pp. 47–63. Springer International Publishing (2016). https://doi.org/10.1007/978-3-319-31075-6_4
9. Phillips, J.G., Stelmach, G.E., Teasdale, N.: What can indices of handwriting quality tell us about Parkinsonian handwriting? Hum. Mov. Sci. **10**(2–3), 301–314 (1991). https://doi.org/10.1016/0167-9457(91)90009-M. ISSN 0167-9457
10. Phillips, J.G., Bradshaw, J.L., Chiu, E., Bradshaw, J.A.: Characteristics of handwriting of patients with Huntington's disease. Mov. Disord. **9**, 521–530 (1994). https://doi.org/10.1002/mds.870090504
11. Proctor, H.: Revolutionary thinking: a theoretical history of Alexander Luria's Romantic science (Doctoral dissertation, Birkbeck, University of London) (2016)
12. Schröter, A., Mergl, R., Bürger, K., Hampel, H., Möller, H.J., Hegerl, U.: Kinematic analysis of handwriting movements in patients with Alzheimer's disease, mild cognitive impairment, depression and healthy subjects. Dement. Geriatr. Cogn. Disord. **15**, 132–142 (2003)
13. Sitek, E.J., Kawa, J., Stępień, P., Brockhuis, B., Kluj-Kozłowska, K., et al.: Makrografia jako jeden z objawów agrafii wykonawczej u pacjenta z wariantem behawioralnym otępienia czołowo-skroniowego. Pol. Przegl. Neurol. t. **13**(Supl. A), s. A100 (2017). ISSN: 1734-5251
14. Weiner, M., Hynan, L., Rossetti, H., Falkowski, J.: Luria's three-step test: what is it and what does it tell us? Int. Psychogeriatr. **23**(10), 1602–1606 (2011). https://doi.org/10.1017/S1041610211000767
15. Sitek, E.J., Konkel, A., Dąbrowska, M., Sławek, J.: Utility of Frontal Assessment Battery in detection of neuropsychological dysfunction in Richardson variant of progressive supranuclear palsy. Neurol. Neurochir. Pol. **49**(1), 36–40 (2015). https://doi.org/10.1016/j.pjnns.2014.12.002. Epub Dec 9, 2014
16. Sitek, E.J., Narożańska, E., Konieczna, S., Brockhuis, B., Wieczorek, D., Wszolek, Z.K., Sławek, J.: Drawing analysis in the assessment of patients with neurodegenerative diseases. Neurology **88**(2), 218–219 (2017). https://doi.org/10.1212/WNL.0000000000003496
17. Sitek, E.J., Wieczorek, D., Konkel, A., Dąbrowska, M., Sławek, J.: The pattern of verbal, visuospatial and procedural learning in Richardson variant of progressive supranuclear palsy in comparison to Parkinson's disease. Psychiatr. Pol. **51**(4), 647–659 (2017). https://doi.org/10.12740/PP/OnlineFirst/62804. Epub Aug 29, 2017
18. Höglinger, G.U., Respondek, G., Stamelou, M., Kurz, C., Josephs, K.A., Lang, A.E., et al.: Clinical diagnosis of progressive supranuclear palsy: the movement disorder society criteria. Mov. Disord. **32**(6), 853–864 (2017)

Video-Based Automatic Evaluation
of the 360 Degree Turn Test

Patrycja Romaniszyn[1], Paula Stępień[2(✉)], Agnieszka Nawrat-Szołtysik[3],
and Jacek Kawa[1]

[1] Faculty of Biomedical Engineering, Silesian University of Technology,
Roosevelta 40, 41-800 Zabrze, Poland
[2] Faculty of Automatic Control, Electronics and Computer Science,
Silesian University of Technology, Akademicka 16, 44-100 Gliwice, Poland
paula.stepien@polsl.pl
[3] The Jerzy Kukuczka Academy of Physical Education in Katowice,
Mikolowska 72b, 40-065 Katowice, Poland

Abstract. In this paper, an automatic, offline evaluation method of
the 360 Degree Turn Test based on a video recording is presented. The
provided approach is used to measure the time the patient needs to:
(1) rotate $360°$ in a given direction, (2) pause and (3) repeat the first
part of the test in the opposite direction without losing balance.

The method is evaluated using 30 samples registered in a group of
13 residents of a Social Assistance Center resulting in a $2.42\,\text{s} \pm 5\,\text{s}$ mean
absolute error and $19.85\% \pm 30.52\text{pp}$ mean of the absolute values of the
relative error. The results are promising in terms of the automatic assessment of the balance.

Keywords: Telemedicine · Telegeriatrics · 360 Degree Turn Test
Berg balance scale

1   Introduction

According to the World Health Organization [22] in Europe, people older than
60 constitute about 20% of the total population. 15% of the population are over
80 and this number is expected to rise up to 26% by 2050 [5]. Due to these demographic changes, geriatrics is gaining importance. The goal of geriatric medicine
is primarily to provide both mental and physical fitness to the people over the
age of 65 and to protect them from social exclusion, as seniors contribute to the
proper functioning of society – either within the family, the local community or
total population [22]. In order to provide seniors with the best possible quality of
life, their physical fitness must be taken care of first. Early distinction between
the natural and the pathological aging process is vital to ensure trouble-free
access to various tests used to diagnose motor disorders. Today, mobile phones
and other mobile applications are a promising tool for improving the quality
of older people's lives [13]. Telegeriatrics was introduced to involve them in the

© Springer International Publishing AG, part of Springer Nature 2019
E. Pietka et al. (Eds.): ITIB 2018, AISC 762, pp. 571–579, 2019.
https://doi.org/10.1007/978-3-319-91211-0_50

diagnostic. Its mission is to combine traditional geriatrics with modern technology and to continuously improve existing applications and diagnostic methods.

The comfort of life depends, to a huge extent, on the state of health and the ability to exist independently. While getting older, the human organism changes and gets weaker which affects the functions of the motor system and hinders the proper maintenance of correct body posture. The worsening of vision and balance increases the risk of falls and injuries in people over 60 years of age [6]. About 40% of people over 65 fall at least once each year. Furthermore, 20–60% of older patients hospitalized after hip fractures resulting from falls require assistance for everyday tasks up to 2 years after the accident, even if they were living independently before [9]. However, in many cases, the fall could be prevented, provided that adequate intervention was introduced (e.g. introduction of a walking aid). The at-risk group might be selected using balance assessment tools.

In standard medical procedures, balance analysis is mostly based on clinical and observational methods. One of the most commonly used methods of balance evaluation in medical facilities is the Berg Balance Scare (BBS). It consists of 14 exercises that reflect the daily activities of an elderly person in both dynamic and static situations. These include: changing the position from standing to sitting or standing with closed eyes. Each of these tasks is evaluated in a five-point scale from 0 to 4, where 0 means a poorly executed exercise or the inability to complete the directions, and 4 indicates a perfect or an almost perfect realization. A patient can score a maximum of 56 points [2]. The Berg Balance Scale is considered more reliable than other stability tests [12]. Moreover, the Berg Balance Scale is not only used as a diagnostic tool for elderly persons, but also has been also used in evaluating imbalances in children with cerebral palsy [8]. Typically, the entire test takes about 20 min and requires the presence of an expert.

The existing attempts to automate the Berg Balance Scale assessment involve force platforms or inertial sensors. In one of these attempts, the balance training was evaluated on the Force Platform with Visual Feedback (FPVF) [19]. Berg Balance Tests have been also used to create games that run on Android OS. Its purpose is to analyze the movement of the user based on data collected from the sensors on the sole of the shoe during exercises compliant with BBS [3]. In our previous works we already presented applications to automate two Berg Balance Scale tasks evaluation based on video recordings: reaching forward with outstretched arm while standing (the measurement of the maximum distance a patient can lean – the 8th task of the BBS) [14] and standing on one leg (automatic one-step assessment of leg movements – the 14th test of the BBS) [7]. Our goal is to design, step by step, a system that would enable the automatic assessment of the full BBS in domestic conditions. In this paper, an approach to automate the evaluation of the 11th task of the BBS, a 360 Degree Turn Test, is presented.

Apart from being the element of the BBS, the 360 Degree Turn Test is a reliable and easily-managed clinical tool to assess the ability of subjects with chronic stroke [17] and can be performed not only by elderly people for balance diagnosis, but also as a tool to assess the progress of rehabilitation. The test is also used to examine associations between measures of static and dynamic balance and performance of mobility task in senior adults [18].

According to the BBS protocol, in the 360 Degree Turn Test, the patient should turn completely around in a full circle, then pause and turn a full circle in the other direction. The patient is assigned 4 points, if he/she is able to turn 360 degree safely in 4 seconds or less. Three points are assigned if the patient is able to turn 360 degree safely in 4 seconds or less for one side only. The patient can score two points when the entire task is performed safely in more than 4 seconds, one point when strict supervision or verbalization was needed, and no points if the patient loses balance and needs assistance [2].

The method presented in the paper automates the assessment of the 360 Degree Turn Test. It is based on our previous approach [15] in which points automatically found by the Kanade-Lucas-Tomasi (KLT) flow [10] on the patient's body were used as markers. If a point changed its position in a consecutive frame, it was assessed as moving and the maximum time of the movement of all points was treated as the time needed to perform the exercise. In this paper, this approach is referred to as 'non-face gating' (NFG). This method was prone to errors and required a separate time measurement for each turn direction. Therefore an additional step has been added to improve the time assessment based on the face visibility (method referred hereafter as 'face gating', FG). The algorithm requires the test to be recorded beforehand. Processing is performed offline. To the best of our knowledge, this is the only automated attempt to assess the 11th BBS exercise, also known as the stand-alone 360 Degree Turn Test, based on video processing.

2   Material and Method

In this section the research set-up has been presented.

2.1   Material

The research group consisted of 13 residents (12 women and 1 man) of the St. Elisabeth Social Assistance Center in Ruda Śląska. All participants were over 60 years old (min. 61, max. 92, average age 81 ± 8 years), able to walk with assistance or independently (full BBS performed at least a week prior to examination: min. 31, max. 56, avg. 46 ± 7 pts.). Before the examination, all patients were informed about the goal of the study and consent has been obtained.

The test was performed in a dedicated room serving also as a fitness room for the center's residents. A trained physiotherapist supervised the performances and provided help in the patient lost his or her balance. Loose railings were an additional protection against accidental falls. The 360 Degree Turn Test was always performed as the first of four registered exercises. Standard BBS protocol was used, yet participants were allowed up to four attempts of each test (if multiple attempts were registered, they were all analyzed).

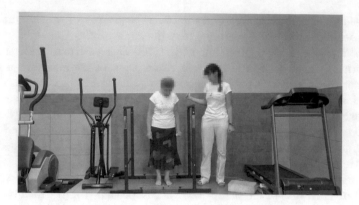

Fig. 1. Patient during exercise

Data for the analysis was acquired using the high-definition video recorder (50 fps, 1920×1080 px) fixed to a tripod and encoded using FFH264 codec. Prior to analysis, the recordings were manually clipped to the beginning/end of the whole exercise with a margin of ca. Two seconds (Fig. 1) and subsampled to the low-resolution 192×108 px.

2.2 Method

The processing algorithm consisted of two main steps: (1) preprocessing and region of interest (ROI) selection, (2) movement tracking and time estimation. Compared to the NFG algorithm (presented in [15]), the second step was extended to include the face-based movement gating (Fig. 2).

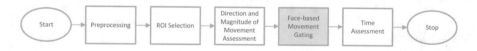

Fig. 2. Workflow of the presented method. New processing step marked gray

2.3 Preprocessing and Region of Interest Selection

During preprocessing, each frame was first converted to grayscale and subjected to the histogram equalization. Next, the Viola-Jones algorithm was applied to detect a patient face [23]. A rectangular region featuring the highest number of face detections defined the ROI enclosing whole body [4] using standard body proportions:

$$ROI = [x_{face} - width_{face}, y_{face} - height_{face}, 3 \cdot width_{face}, 9 \cdot height_{face}] \quad (1)$$

where $[x_{face}, y_{face}, height_{face}, width_{face}]$ denotes the region with the highest number of face detections.

2.4   Movement Tracking and Time of Full Turn Estimation

In the next step, the point-tracking algorithm was used to estimate the direction and magnitude of movement. Initial points for tracking were selected within the previously defined ROI in the first frame using the Shi-Tomasi [16] corner metric. The Kanade-Lucas-Tomasi algorithm [10] was then employed to estimate the new position of tracked points on the following frames and to validate it; during validation, tracking was repeated backward in order to see whether the procedure is reversible or not defining, respectively, a valid or invalid found.

In each step, if a point changed it's position substantially in consequent frames, it was considered as moving. Moving points determined the general direction of movement (left or right):

$$x_{avg}^n = \frac{1}{k} \sum_k \left(x_k^n - x_k^{n-1} \right) \qquad (2)$$

where x_k^n, x_{n-1}^k denotes the horizontal position of a tracked point k in the frame n and $n+1$, respectively.

Once the movement was processed, the face detection was employed again to time the full-turn exercise: the moment of disappearance of the patient's face during a single, mostly uninterrupted (short pauses allowed) movement left or right, determined the beginning of a turn, while its reappearance marked the end of the rotation. The face disappearance (reappearance) was considered valid if a frame was not detected (or detected) in at least half of the frames within a 2 s window (mean filter of a width of two frames per seconds-width is employed). The procedure compensated the eyeblinks or misdetections caused by the background. In cases where the face disappearance/reappearance was not detected, the beginning/end of the turn was set as the beginning/end of the point movement (as it was in NFG).

Then, the correctness of the whole exercise was assessed. The exercise was performed correctly if the following sequence of movements was detected: rotation in a given direction, pause and re-rotation. During this procedure, the number of turns was retrieved as well as the total time of the whole exercise.

3   Results

During the examination, 30 recordings of 13 volunteers were collected (Table 1). They were first processed using the method presented in [15] (timing based on magnitude of movement, without face gating; denoted NFG). Next, the same cases were processed using the method presented in the paper, with face-based timing (denoted FG). In both cases, if time estimation was not possible, it was assumed, that no turn has been completed (0 s).

In all cases, the presented FG method featuring additional face-based gating performed no worse than the previous approach featuring only movement-magnitude-based time assessment (NFG). NFG did not allow the successful processing of the whole examination recording. In the previous work [15], the recording had to be manually divided. Here the algorithm was able to calculate the longest time the points were continuously moving in one direction.

Table 1. Total time of the 360 Degree Turn Test (including all steps). FG/NFG denote 'face gating' and 'no face gating' methods, respectively. All times and absolute errors are given in seconds. 'Abs. Relative Error' stands for absolute value of the relative error. Cases marked by asterisks feature single turn (*) or triple (**) full turns

Case	Patient id	Sex	Age	Time in seconds					Abs. Relative Error (FG)
				Real	NFG	Abs.Err	FG	Abs.Err	
1	1	F	88	14.47	2.1	12.37	13.9	0.57	3.94%
2				9.5	0	9.5	10.3	0.8	8.42%
3	2	F	92	13.5	2.1	11.4	12.58	0.92	6.81%
4				19.1	2.1	17	19.7	0.6	3.14%
5	3	F	91	14	2.1	11.9	14.3	0.3	2.14%
6	4	F	77	24.3	0	24.3	0	24.3	100%
7				9.8	0	9.8	10.1	0.3	3.06%
8*	5	F	88	8.41	2.1	6.31	5.8	2.61	31.03%
9*				13.6	0	13.6	13.56	0.04	0.29%
10	6	F	83	8	0	8	9.5	1.5	18.75%
11				4.38	0	4.38	0	4.38	100%
12				9	2.2	6.8	9.42	0.42	4.67%
13				15.92	2.2	13.72	16.72	0.8	5.03%
14	7	M	80	21	2.1	18.9	14.96	6.04	28.76%
15*				10	2.1	7.9	9.52	0.48	4.80%
16				13.2	2.4	10.8	12.3	0.9	6.82%
17	8	F	87	13	0	13	12.54	0.46	3.54%
18				15	2.1	12.9	14.5	0.5	3.33%
19				17	2.8	14.2	17.04	0.04	0.24%
20	9	F	81	20	2.1	17.9	5.04	14.96	74.80%
21				21	2.1	18.9	18.38	2.62	12.48%
22	10	F	72	11	0	11	10.2	0.8	7.27%
23				11	0	11	5.4	5.6	50.91%
24	11	F	83	9.28	0	9.28	8.42	0.86	9.27%
25				7	2.1	4.9	6.6	0.4	5.71%
26*				4.5	2.5	2	4.1	0.4	8.89%
27	12	F	61	8.2	2.1	6.1	8.47	0.27	3.29%
28				8	0	8	7.88	0.12	1.50%
29	13	F	74	10.2	0	10.2	10.8	0.6	5.88%
30**				12	0	12	12.06	0.06	0.50%
Avg.						11.27		2.42	19.85%
Std.						4.76		4.99	30.52pp

In several cases (no. 2, 9, 10, 17, 23, 24, 28–30), inclusion of the additional face-gating step enabled the metrics to be calculated when they were undetectable using the NFG method (NFG method was unable to find the end of the movement and, consequently, provided no time information). In cases 6 and 11, the ROI was incorrectly selected (in subsequent steps no 360 degree turn was detected), as the patients were turning around watching their feet.

4   Discussion

The obtained results are promising in terms of automation of the balance assessment. In 22 cases (73%), the absolute error of the presented method with face-based movement gating did not exceed 1 s and would have no impact on the final grade (in each of these cases both the real time of the turn and estimated time exceeded the 4 s threshold).

Moreover, the inclusion of the face-based movement gating improved the overall accuracy of the approach. The error of the original, NFG method (without face-based time gating) has in 27 cases (90%) been substantially reduced, while in remaining cases it remained on the same level. Besides, the addition of the face-based movement gating seem to improve the overall robustness of the NFG method which proved to be almost completely useless in this study: in most cases, in the NFG method, the turn has been prematurely assessed as finished and improperly timed due to some minor downturns or pauses. Furthermore, the addition of the extra step did not increase the computational complexity; the results of the face detection performed at the Region of Interests selection step can be directly reused at the face gating step (i.e. the processing time of the FG and NFG methods is comparable).

Retrospectively, the inclusion of the face visibility condition as a determinant of the beginning or the end of the movement seems natural. It may not be a universal solution for all the troublesome cases, though. The face might not be visible (or detectable by the employed classifier). Patient may also shake the head during registration, delaying (or accelerating) the detection of the beginning/end of the exercise. Future version should improve the detection by providing a reliable, alternative option. Patients with balance issues tend to move slowly and are often gazing on their feet. This fact makes the face detection cumbersome. Still, it seems to be a better solution than markers attached to the garments or body, distracting the movement and causing unnecessary stressful situations.

The presented approach features several limitations. If a patient loses his or her balance during the exercise, the score should be lowered, regardless of the time of the 360 degree turn. The imbalance detection problem should be addressed during further research. Moreover, the registration environment can affect the overall performance of the method: light changes, presence of bystanders etc. This factor limits the possible application from technical point of view.

Another severe limitation is not specific to the presented method itself, but results from the general concept of the full automation of the balance test assessment. The subject of the examination are presumably members of the group featuring high risk of fall. Their safety should therefore be always concerned and unsupervised exercise should be avoided, which mitigates the need for full automation. However, the availability of automatic assessment may increase the objectivity even in supervised cases. Moreover, it enables the evaluation of the balance in the presence of otherwise untrained caregivers.

5   Summary

In this paper a novel method of assessment of the 360 degree turn has been presented. The approach presented in [15] has been improved by addition of the face-based movement gating: face disappearance/reappearance is used to precisely time the exercise.

The method has been tested in a group of 13 residents of a Social Assistance Center. 30 cases have been registered and analyzed. Evaluation has been performed against the manually acquired reference data. The results seem promising in terms of automatic assessment of the 360 Degree Turn Test.

Acknowledgement. This research was partially founded by: the Polish Ministry of Science and SilesianUniversity of Technology statutory financial support No. BK-200/RIB1/2017 and statutory financial support for young researchers BKM-510/RAu-3/2017.

We would like to thank Andre Woloshuk for his English language corrections.

References

1. Allert, G., Blasszauer, B., Boyd, K., Callahan, D.: The goals of medicine: setting new priorities. Hastings Center Rep. **26**(6), S1–27 (1996)
2. Berg, K.O., Wood-Dauphinee, S.L., Williams, J.I., Maki, B.: Measuring balance in the elderly: validation of an instrument. Can. J. Public Health **83**, S7–11 (1992). Revue canadienne de sante publique
3. Brassard, S., Otis, M.J.D., Poirier, A., Menelas, B.A.J.: Towards an automatic version of the berg balance scale test through a serious game. In: Proceedings of the Second ACM Workshop on Mobile Systems, Applications, and Services for Healthcare, p. 5. ACM, November 2012
4. Cai, Q., Aggarwal, J.K.: Tracking human motion using multiple cameras. In: Proceedings of the 13th International Conference on Pattern Recognition, vol. 3, pp. 68–72. IEEE, August 1996
5. Davies, E., Higginson, I.J.: Better palliative care for older people. World Health Organization (2004)
6. Granacher, U., Gollhofer, A., Hortobágyi, T., Kressig, R.W., Muehlbauer, T.: The importance of trunk muscle strength for balance, functional performance, and fall prevention in seniors: a systematic review. Sports Med. **43**(7), 627–641 (2013)
7. Kawa, J., Stępień, P., Kapko, W., Niedziela, A., Derejczyk, J.: Leg movement tracking in automatic video-based one-leg stance evaluation. Comput. Med. Imaging Graph. Official Journal of the Computerized Medical Imaging Society (2017)
8. Kembhavi, G., Darrah, J., Magill-Evans, J., Loomis, J.: Using the berg balance scale to distinguish balance abilities in children with cerebral palsy. Pediatr. Phys. Ther. **14**(2), 92–99 (2002)

9. Kłak, A., Raciborski, F., Targowski, T., Rzodkiewicz, P., Bousquet, J., Samoliński, B.: A growing problem of falls in the aging population: a case study on Poland - 2015–2050 forecast. Eur. Geriatr. Med. **8**(2), 105–110 (2017). https://doi.org/10. 1016/j.eurger.2017.02.004. ISSN 1878-7649
10. Tomasi, C., Kanade, T.: Detection and tracking of point features (1991)
11. Nascher, I.L.: Geriatrics: The Diseases of Old Age and Their Treatment, Including Physiological Old Age, Home and Institutional Care, and Medico-legal Relations. P. Blakiston's Son & Company (1914)
12. Newstead, A.H., Hinman, M.R., Tomberlin, J.A.: Reliability of the berg Balance Scale and balance master limits of stability tests for individuals with brain injury. J. Neurol. Phys. Ther. **29**(1), 18–23 (2005)
13. Plaza, I., Martín, L., Martin, S., Medrano, C.: Mobile applications in an aging society: status and trends. J. Syst. Softw. **84**(11), 1977–1988 (2011)
14. Romaniszyn, P., Buchalik, A., Bilut, B., et al.: Automatic distance calculation in the functional reach test. Adv. Biosci., 7–12 (2016)
15. Romaniszyn, P., Stępień, P., Buchalik, A.: Automatic evaluation of the 360 degrees turn test. In: 15th Students' Science Conference FULL PAPERS, pp. 267–272 (2017)
16. Shi, J., Tomasi C.: Good features to track. In: 1994 Proceedings of IEEE Conference on Computer Vision and Pattern Recognition, Seattle, WA, pp. 593–600 (1994). https://doi.org/10.1109/CVPR.1994.323794
17. Shiu, C.H., Ng, S.S., Kwong, P.W., Liu, T.W., Tam, E.W., Fong, S.S.: Timed 360 degree turn test for assessing people with chronic stroke. Arch. Phys. Med. Rehabil. **97**(4), 536–544 (2016)
18. Shubert, T.E., Schrodt, L.A., Mercer, V.S., Busby-Whitehead, J., Giuliani, C.A.: Are scores on balance screening tests associated with mobility in older adults? J. Geriatr. Phys. Ther. **29**(1), 33–39 (2006)
19. Srivastava, A., Taly, A.B., Gupta, A., Kumar, S., Murali, T.: Post-stroke balance training: role of force platform with visual feedback technique. J. Neurol. Sci. **287**(1), 89–93 (2009)
20. Steves, C.J., Spector, T.D., Jackson, S.H.: Ageing, genes, environment and epigenetics: what twin studies tell us now, and in the future. Age Ageing **41**(5), 581–586 (2012)
21. Szczerbinska, K., Pietryka, A.: Rozwój geriatrii w krajach europejskich-historia i zasoby (część 1). Gerontologia Pol. **16**(2), 61–73 (2008). (in Polish)
22. World Health Organization. World report on ageing and health (2015). Luxembourg, Luxembourg, pp. 1–260 (2016)
23. Viola, P., Jones, M.J.: Robust real-time face detection. Int. J. Comput. Vision **57**(2), 137–154 (2004)

Usability of Dynamic Thermography for Assessment of Skeletal Muscle Activity in Physiological and Pathological Conditions – Preliminary Results

Dariusz Radomski[1(✉)] and Krzysztof Kruszewski[2]

[1] Institute of Radioelectronics and Multimedia Technology,
Warsaw University of Technology, Nowowiejska 15/19, 00-665 Warsaw, Poland
d.radomski@ire.pw.edu.pl
[2] Laboratory of Thermographic and Energy Measurements, Przy Agorze 28/32,
01-930 Warsaw, Poland

Abstract. The paper presents the use of dynamic thermography in an assessment of quadriceps activity during a static load in healthy persons and patients with spastic quadriplegia. The differential thermograms relating to the muscle localisation were quantitatively described by the mean and standard deviation of pixels thermal values belonging to the ROI. The obtained trends in temperature distribution in healthy persons correspond to blood flow changes observed by other authors. These trends were opposite to the trend received for the first time in a spastic person. These results suggest that a dynamic thermography may have a potential application in the assessment of spasticity intensity.

Keywords: Dynamic thermography · Spasticity
Isometric contraction · Static load

1 Introduction

Thermography is a technique used to measure and visualize spatial distribution of object's temperature arising from thermal processes which occurs in the studied object. Historically, thermographic static photos were the only means of measurement, and thus only thermal processes being in an equilibrium could be observed. The development of thermographic cameras enabled the use of thermography to analyze thermal phenomenon in a nonequilibrium. Therefore, several new notions associated with thermography became of interest in the literature, though these are not precisely defined. Thus, we assume the following meaning of often used terms: active thermography, passive thermography and endogenic dynamic thermography. Suszynski established that active thermography measures time and spatially distributed thermal response of an object to external stimulation. On the contrary, passive thermography measures thermal processes occurring in the studied object being in its 'natural state' without

© Springer International Publishing AG, part of Springer Nature 2019
E. Pietka et al. (Eds.): ITIB 2018, AISC 762, pp. 580–588, 2019.
https://doi.org/10.1007/978-3-319-91211-0_51

any stimulation [1]. These terms are sufficient in studying technical inanimate objects. Continuing the above classification, we introduce) third type i.e. endogenic dynamic thermography that monitors object's thermal response to an internal stimulation resulted from unnatural state of the studied object. One of the possible applications of such thermography in medicine, is physiotherapy.

Currently, more and more approaches used in physiotherapy are based on scientific evidences. Therefore, physiological measurements are becoming the bases of daily clinical decisions made by physiotherapists.

The major physiotherapy treatments concern muscle functions, aiming to improve their effectiveness in athletes or to restore their activity in patients. The particular challenge for physiotherapists is rehabilitation of neurological patients. The current literature demonstrates an increase in the prevalence of neuromuscular conditions caused by strokes in particular [2].

The most popular method used in clinical assessment of muscle activity beside clinical examination is electromyography. It measures the bioelectrical activity of the examined muscle and therefore allows for diagnosis of central or systemic causes of muscle impairments. It can also be used to evaluate progress during the course of rehabilitation. However, the precise EMG parameters for clinical assessments have not been established and thus the consensus among clinicians and scientists regarding this matter is low.

Another method of assessing muscle activity is the continuous measure of the force generated by the evaluated muscle. This method however only provides a rough estimation of the muscle activity thus it is used mainly to assess training progress.

The least frequently used method of muscle evaluation is thermography. This technique enables visualization of spatial distribution of the temperature registered in the muscle projection on the skin by thermographic camera. Qualitative and post-hoc analysis is used for these distributions. Thermography was used to identify myofascial trigger points for an assessment of the upper trapezius muscle temperature in women with and without neck pain [3]. Moreover, a delayed onset muscle soreness can be detected by this method too [4]. A relationship between skin temperature and muscle activation during incremental cycle exercise was identified [5]. Interestingly, Adate et al. investigated use of the thermographic method of a compensative mechanism of postural muscles during an experimental leg difference [6]. These publications supported the use of the thermography in physiotherapy. Nevertheless, the above mentioned studies have only employed thermographic photos, so a dynamic phenomenon of a muscle activity was not observed. Moreover, none of the these studies have included patients with neuromuscular problems.

One of the most prevalent neuromuscular disorders is spasticity, most commonly caused by stroke, brain traumas, spinal cord injuries or cerebral palsy [7]. By definition, spasticity is a hyper-reflex in response to a muscle stretch because of brain injuries which suppress the hypertonic muscle tension generated by the spinal cord. The strength of the hypertension is proportional to the stretching movement's velocity [8].

Although a spastic individual is a frequent patient in the department of physiotherapy, there is no reliable method to assess the intensity of this symptom. Current literature only highlights the Modified Ashworth Scale as a suitable clinical measure. Yet, the recent meta-analysis published by Meseguer-Henarejos and colleagues indicates poor inter-rater reliability of this scale, particularly for the lower limbs (studies averaged $\kappa^+ = 0.36$)) [9]. Therefore, there is a clear need for a new clinically flexible way to quantify spastic intensity.

Our previous study [10] showed that there was a link between the temperature of a thigh surface and the force of a quadriceps muscle during a static load. Therefore, one could speculate that an isometric tension is associated with a specific pattern of temperature changes; a phenomena that has not been studied before. Additionally, we aim to test if spasticity can modify the identified population trends.

The aim of this study was to establish the trends of temperature distribution during a static load of the quadriceps muscles in healthy population (control group) and run comparative analyses against the trends observed in a spastic patient.

2   Methods

To identify the trend changes of temperature distributions measured on a surface of the thigh skin during a static load of the quadriceps muscle, experiments outlined below were performed. Figure 1 presents the scheme of the laboratory stand.

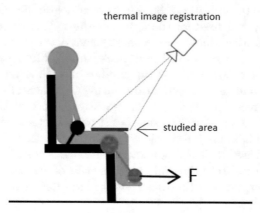

Fig. 1. The scheme of the laboratory stand used for measuring changes in temperature distributions associated with the static load of the quadriceps

The experiments were carried out in subsequent steps:

- the participant was asked to sit in the laboratory armchair, which was adjusted to their posture and size, ensuring that the desired right angles in hip and knee joints were obtained. The trunk and legs were stabilized using mechanical stabilizers.
- the thermographic camera was placed 1 m away from the studied thigh and focused individually on each thigh.
- the participant was then asked to relax for 30 s
- the participant then received the instructions to kick and keep their knee in a submaximal tone erectors for 30 s. The dynamics of temperature distribution were measured.
- the dynamics of a temperature distribution was measured again, three minutes after muscle relaxation.

This process allowed us to observe time-varying and space-varying changes of the temperature distribution on the thigh surface during a concentrative strain of the quadriceps muscle. The temperature distributions were measured by the FLIR camera, model E40 with 30 frames per a second.

Seventeen women and 16 men were studied with a mean age of 24 ($SD = 1.5$). All participants were healthy students of physiotherapy at the Józef Piłsudski University of Physical Education in Warsaw recruited volountairly. 28 participants indicated being physically active at least once a week. This group served as the control group. Additionally, a man aged 46 years with spastic quadriplegia caused by cerebral palsy was tested to verify a potential different thermal trend associated with a spasticity.

The study protocol was approved by the Bioethical Committee and conducted in accordance with the rule of Good Clinical Practice.

Finding a trend in the muscle temperatures during a static load and a rest phase requires a parameterization method of the registored thermal imagoo. For this purpose we manually marked an area of a quadriceps muscle on the thermal images for each participant.

Because we used a dynamic thermography, thermal image being a temperature distribution can be represented as $T(x, y, k)$ for $x, y \in$ ROI and in the kth frame. To intensify the observed time-varying thermal changes, the following differential images were analyzed:

$$T_D(x, y, k) = T(x, y, k) - T_{ref}(x, y, k), \tag{1}$$

where

$$T_{ref}(x, y, k) = \frac{1}{50} \sum_{k=1}^{50} T(x, y, k) \tag{2}$$

is the thermal image resulted from averaging of 50 initial frames registered in a steady state before loading. Therefore, a differential image shows changes in a thermal distribution in relation to an initial physiological state of the studied muscle. Moreover, the images registered during loading were averaging to filter noise.

Although there are many parameterization methods of images, we have chosen the classic one to ensure easy biological interpretation of the obtained results. Thus we used two parameters: the spatial mean temperature and the spatial standard deviation.

The spatial mean temperature of a differential ROI consisted of $N \times M$ pixels computed for every $k = 1, \ldots K$ frames

$$m(k) = \frac{1}{NM} \sum_{i=1}^{N} \sum_{j=1}^{M} T_\Delta (x_i, y_j, k) \tag{3}$$

The spatial standard deviation of the temperature belonging to the ROI;

$$s(k) = \sqrt{\frac{\sum_{i=1}^{N} \sum_{j=1}^{M} (T_D(x_i, y_j, k) - m(k))^2}{NM}} \tag{4}$$

The value of $s(k)$ may be interpreted as variation of myocytes activating during a static load.

Software. ROI marking and image parameters computing were done using Flir Tools 4.2 and ResearchIR max 4.30. The ROI were determined manually. In the performed study images corrections for thigh movements were not needed because the limb of each seated participant was accurately fixed in three points (see Fig. 1). Moreover, the ROI included such the area of the muscle which did not vary from a frame to a frame in the frontal plane of a thigh. We ensured that the correlation between frames containing a binary contour of the studied leg was constant and equaled approximately to 0.96. The further analysis was performed using Matlab 2016b.

3   Results

The performed experiments and images analyses led to the following results. Figure 2 represents the differential thermal ROIs obtained in different periods of quadriceps activations for a randomly chosen healthy participant. We observed that during the static load of the quadriceps, the areas where relative temperature was decreased were enlarged. At the end of the muscle contraction an increase of local temperature was observed. This trend was continued during rest when the quadriceps was relaxed.

The opposite trend was observed in the patient with spastic quadriplegia demonstrated in Fig. 3. The muscle relaxation was not associated with temperature increase.

In order to better present the above dissimilarity, the average trend for the control group was computed for the two ROIs parameters m, s. Figures 4 and 5 confirm that the spastic person has different trends in these parameters in comparison to the control group. These trends are agreed with the changes in thermographic images presented in Figs. 2 and 3. One way ANOVA was performed

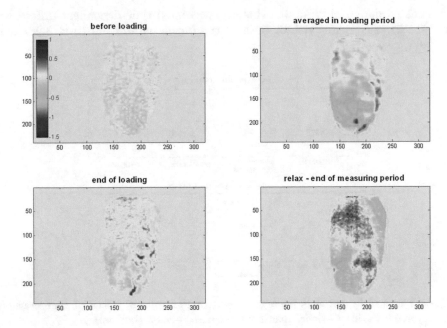

Fig. 2. The differential thermographic ROIs obtained for a random healthy person depending on the quadriceps activities

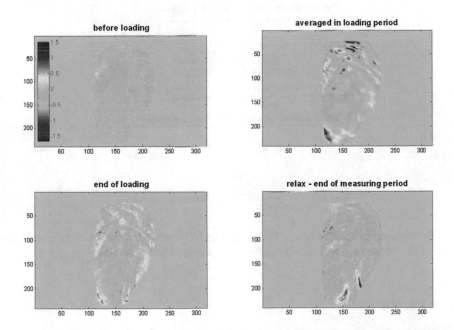

Fig. 3. The differential thermographic ROIs obtained for the spastic participant depending on the quadriceps activities

for repeated data and it showed that the presented time-dependent differences were statistically significant for both of the image parameters ($p < 0.001$ and $p < 0.05$, respectively).

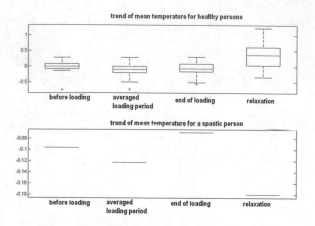

Fig. 4. The healthy subjects averaged trend of ROIs mean values of temperatures (upper) in comparing to their trend for the spastic person (bottom)

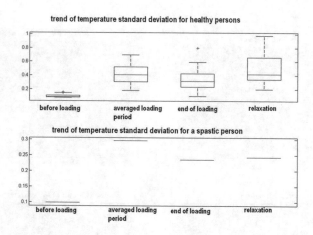

Fig. 5. The control group averaged trend of the ROIs standard values of temperatures (upper) in comparison to their trend for the spastic person (bottom)

4   Conclusions

This is the first ever study to present the time-varying trends of temperature distributions in healthy population during a static load of the quadriceps muscle. The results obtained for the control group are strongly compliant with the studies performed by McNeil et al. [11], who studied blood flow during isometric contractions in dorsiflexion of feet. During 100 percent of the maximal voluntary contraction (MVC), blood flow drops at the beginning of a contraction and it subsequently increases. Moreover, in the 30% MVC the measured blood flow by a tibial artery was initially increased too. The last phenomenon may explain the intersubject variability observed in our measurements because not everyone reached and kept the maximal voluntary contraction during a load. Stopping of blood flow during a muscle concentration disables the transfer of by convection. In this situation heat is transferred out only by conduction which is also limited by the contracted quadriceps. After muscle relaxation, turbulent blood flow appears in the arteries so convection is recovered and causes the temperature to increase rapidly.

To our best knowledge, there is no data investigating blood flow during an isometric concentration of a spastic muscle. The obtained preliminary observations suggest an opposite thermal trend in spastic patients in comparison to healthy population. It may result from significant lower percent of MVC as well as a longer duration of muscle relaxation. The increased tonus of a spastic muscle may impede blood flow restoration after contraction so convection cannot be recovered. The quadriceps may become overheated and less biomechanically efficient.

Therefore, dynamic thermography may be useful to monitor spastic intensity during the rehabilitation process.

References

1. Suszynski, Z.: Termografia aktywna. Wydawnictwo Politechniki Koszalinskiej (2013). (in Polish)
2. Icks, A., Claessen, H., Kvitkina, T., Narres, M., Weingärtner, M., Schwab, S., Kolominsky-Rabas, P.L.: Incidence and relative risk of stroke in the diabetic and the non-diabetic population between 1998 and 2014: a community-based stroke register. PLoS One **16**(12(11)) (2017)
3. Dibai-Filho, A.V., Guirro, E.C., Ferreira, V.T., Brandino, H.E.: Guirro, M.O.V.R.J.: Reliability of different methodologies of infrared image analysis of myofascial trigger points in the upper trapezius muscle. Braz. J Phys Ther. **19**(2), 122–128 (2015)
4. Dibai-Filho, A.V., Packer, A.C., Costa, A.C., Berni-Schwarzenbeck, K.C., Rodrigues-Bigaton, D.: Assessment of the upper trapezius muscle temperature in women with and without neck pain. J. Manipulative Physiol. Ther. **35**(5), 413–417 (2012)
5. Quesada, J.I.P., Carpes, F.P., Bini, R.R., Palmer, R.S., Pérez-Soriano, P., de Anda, R.M.C.O.: Relationship between skin temperature and muscle activation during incremental cycle exercise. J. Therm. Biol. **48**, 28–35 (2015)
6. Abate, M., Carlo, L.D., Romualdo, S.D., Ionta, S., Ferretti, A., Romani, G.L., Merla, A.: Postural adjustment in experimental leg length difference evaluated by means of thermal infrared imaging. Physiol Meas. **31**(1), 35–43 (2010)
7. Moharic, M.: Research on prevalence of secondary conditions in individuals with disabilities: an overview. Int. J. Rehabil Res. **40**(4), 297–302 (2017)

8. Nahm, N.J., Graham, K.H., Gormley, M.E., Georgiadis, A.G.: Management of hypertonia in cerebral palsy. Curr. Opin. Pediatr. (11) (2017)
9. Meseguer-Henarejos, A.B., Sánchez-Meca, J., López-Pina, J.A., Carles-Hernández, R.: Inter- and intra-rater reliability of the Modified Ashworth Scale: a systematic review and meta-analysis. Eur. J. Phys. Rehabil Med. (2017)
10. Radomski, D., Kruszewski, K.: Measurement automation monitoring. **63**(04), 139–142 (2017)
11. McNeil, C.J., Allen, M.D., Olympico, E., Shoemaker, K.J., Rice, C.L.: Blood flow and muscle oxygenation during low, moderate, and maximal sustained isometric contractions. Am. J. Physiol. Regul. Integr. Comp. Physiol. **309**(5), R475–81 (2015)

Three-Dimensional Children Gait Pattern – Reference Data for Healthy Children Aged Between 7 and 17

Katarzyna Jochymczyk-Woźniak[1]($\boxtimes$), Katarzyna Nowakowska[1],
Robert Michnik[1], Marek Gzik[1], Piotr Wodarski[1], Joanna Gorwa[2],
and Piotr Janoska[3]

[1] Faculty of Biomedical Engineering, Department of Biomechatronics,
Silesian University of Technology, Roosevelta 40, Zabrze, Poland
Katarzyna.Jochymczyk-Wozniak@polsl.pl

[2] Faculty of Physical Education, Sport and Rehabilitation, Department of Theory
and Methodology of Sport, Poznań University of Physical Education, Poznań, Poland

[3] The Katowice Institute of Information Technologies, Katowice, Poland

Abstract. The research aimed to determine the standards of kinematic
quantities and indices of regularity, namely the Gillette Gait Index and
the Gait Deviation Index related to children aged between 7 and 17
as well as the identification of differences concerning the above-named
quantities according to age and height. The study group consisted of
56 healthy children aged 7 to 17. The tests were performed using the
BTS Smart system. The original applications developed in the Matlab
environment for all of the children subjected to the tests enabled the
identification of the Gillette Gait Index (GGI) and the Gait Deviation
Index (GDI). Detailed analysis involved a set of sixteen variables describing gait kinematics; the above-named variables are used when creating
the GGI. The children were divided into five groups in relation to age
and six groups in relation to height. Time values of the angles of the
joints were registered and then the GGI and the GDI were calculated.
Sixteen parameters composing the GGI were determined for all of the
children constituting the test group. The confirmation or the exclusion
of differences between age-related and height-related groups was based
on statistical analysis. The identified courses of the kinematic time series
can be used as normative in relation to patients aged 7–17.

Keywords: Gait analysis · Normal pattern · Gillette Gait Index
Gait Deviation Index · Kinematics

1 Introduction

Gait analysis is currently more and more widely used in clinical evaluation,
especially when it comes to patients, who present central nervous system (CNS)
disorders. Based on experimental studies using systems, which enable three-
dimensional analysis, an enormous set of data is generated, including spatio-
temporal parameters, kinematic values and ground reaction force components

© Springer International Publishing AG, part of Springer Nature 2019
E. Pietka et al. (Eds.): ITIB 2018, AISC 762, pp. 589–601, 2019.
https://doi.org/10.1007/978-3-319-91211-0_52

[6,9,14,16]. Results obtained in the experimental tests are increasingly commonly applied when creating mathematical models of the human motor system enabling a non-invasive identification of loads of the skeletal-muscular system [14].

In clinical practice the interpretation of results from patients, who present pathological gait, relies on comparing the patient's results to the norm [3,9,22]. Up to this time studies that aimed to determine a model of gait for children have been performed by a number of authors, but most of them focused on such spatio-temporal parameters as walking speed, cadence or step length. Such studies were performed by, for example, Pierce et al. (children aged 6–14, a total of 213 subjects) [15] and Dusing et al. (children aged 1–10, a total of 405 subjects) [5]. The spatio-temporal parameters can be appointed quite easily, while they are very important when it comes to gait patterns. Steinwender et al. [22], who examined a total of 20 children, aged 7–15, apart from the spatio-temporal parameters also appointed the dynamic and kinematic values, relating them then to values obtained from children with cerebral palsy (CP). Next Stansfield et al. [21] examined a total of 16 children, aged 7–12, while analyzing the regression between walking speed and the dynamic and kinematic values. Schwartz et al. [20] checked the impact of walking speed on the dynamic and kinematic parameters performing tests on a group of 83 healthy children, aged 4–17. The differences between children's and adults' gait were studied by Ganley et al. [6], who did their research on a group of fifteen seven-year-old children and fifteen adults, analyzing their walking speed, cadence, step length, sagittal plane angles, joint moments and force values. Studied changes in the walking speed, step length, cadence and range of motion in 33 healthy children during 5 consecutive years, at the time of the initial tests the children were 7 years old, and were 11 at the end of the study. The study was performed using the Vicon system. Holm et al. [8] examined 360 children, aged 7–12, using GAITRite, focusing on the step length during walking at a speed of 1.5 m/s, spotting some significant differences based on age.

Tools for the triplanar analysis of motion provide an extensive amount of data including time-spatial parameters, kinematic quantities, dynamic quantities, including the components of ground reaction force or muscular action potentials. Although the above-named results properly depict therapeutic progress, yet on their basis it is difficult to unequivocally diagnose improvement triggered by a given therapy or compare a number of competitive methods used when treating a given condition. Quite frequently, the use of a specific therapy leads to the improvement of certain gait parameters but to the deterioration of others. In such situations it is difficult to clearly ascertain whether the stereotype of gait has improved or deteriorated. Recent years have seen the advent of several factors describing the gait of a person using one non-dimensional numerical value. The most commonly applied gait indices are the Gilette Gait Index (GGI), Gait Deviation Index (GDI), Gait Profile Score (GPS) [1,2,4,9,16,19,20].

Even though so many authors have been studying the topic of healthy children's gait patterns, none has compared the gait of children differing in age, height and sex. In view of the foregoing, this research work aimed to identify the standards of gait-related kinematic quantities and indices of regularity the Gillette Gait Index and the Gait Deviation Index related to children aged between 7 and 17.

2   Materials and Methods

The experimental tests of gait were conducted using the BTS Smart system (BTS S.p.A., Milan, Italy), which enables a three-dimensional analysis of gait. The system consisted of six opto-electronic digital cameras, which make it possible to record the location of passive markers in space. Frequency of sampling of the cameras during the test equalled 250 Hz. Placement of markers was done in compliance with Helen Hayes protocol, calculations were done on the basis of a model built in the BTS System. Ethical approval for this study was obtained from the Ethics Committee of Medical University of Silesia, Poland (no. KNW/0022/KB1/19/11).

Within the framework of this study, a total number of 80 children aged 7–17 was examined, including 56 healthy children without motor organ disorders, who made up the final test group. Healthy children, without defects or diseases affecting the motor system, participated in the study. The age of children was 11.0 ± 3.0 y.o., body mass: 41.8 ± 13.2 kg and body height: 1.47 ± 0.17 m. Before the start of the gait examination the necessary anthropometric measurements were performed and then each child walked the trial path ten times. In further analysis the average of all strides for each child was used. During the study the children walked at their natural, self-selected speed. For the needs of analysis the children were divided into five age groups and six height groups (Table 1).

The parameters recorded within the research-related tests were used to create the standards of gait-related kinematic quantities for healthy children. In addition, the use of original applications developed in the Matlab environment (The MathWorks, Inc., United States) enabled the identification of gait-related indices, i.e. Gillette Gait Index (GGI) and Gait Deviation Index (GDI), very useful tools to assess gait abnormalities, defined as a scaled distance between the subject gait and the average of gait for a control group [19,20]. A detailed analysis was performed on a set of sixteen distinctive spatio-temporal and kinematic parameters of clinical significance, as suggested by Schutte et al. [19] such as: time of toe off (1), walking speed (2), cadence (3), mean pelvic tilt (4), range of pelvic tilt (5), mean pelvic rotation (6), minimum hip flexion (7), range of hip flexion (8), peak abduction in swing (9), mean hip rotation in stance (10), knee flexion at initial contact (11), time of peak knee flexion (12), range of knee flexion (13), peak dorsiflexion in stance (14), peak dorsiflexion in swing (15), mean foot progression angle (16). The research also involved a detailed statistical analysis of the results obtained in the tests in respect of the children's age and height.

Analysis of Results. The normative courses of kinematic quantities, i.e. the courses of angles of the pelvis and in the joints of lower limbs are presented in Fig. 1. To determine the standard of children's gait, the results of kinematic

Table 1. Characteristics of the age- and height-based test group

Age groups [years]	Number of children in the study group	Height [cm]	Weight [kg]
7–8	16	128.62 ± 5.59	28.57 ± 5.26
10–11	19	141.5 ± 7.84	40.11 ± 8.28
12–13	6	156 ± 7.37	44.33 ± 9.61
14–15	6	170.26 ± 9.21	54.67 ± 7.47
16–17	9	169.66 ± 5.74	59.56 ± 7.45
Height category [cm]	Number of children in the study group	Age [years]	Weight [kg]
119–129	8	8.11 ± 1.17	26.57 ± 8.14
130–139	13	8.54 ± 1.05	32.32 ± 4.0
140–149	13	10.23 ± 0.6	41.55 ± 5.60
150–159	6	12.0 ± 1.67	44.17 ± 8.42
160–169	8	14.75 ± 1.91	56.38 ± 9.80
170–183	8	15.38 ± 0.92	59.25 ± 3.28

quantities subjected to the analysis were averaged and standardised in relation to a single cycle of gait. The gait-related indices of regularity the Gillette Gait Index and the Gait Deviation Index were determined in relation to all persons subjected to the tests. Using one numerical value, the above-named indices indicate whether the patient's gait is proper (Table 2).

Table 2. Mean, maximum and minimum values as well as the standard deviation of the GGI and GDI in relation to the group of patients with proper gait

	GGI	GDI
mean	15.71	99.23
std	5.68	8.37
max	30.00	121.07
min	7.46	78.95

Sixteen parameters (elements) composing the GGI were determined for all of the children constituting the test group. The mean values along with the standard deviation of the selected 16 parameters are presented in Table 3. The analysis of the test results was based on statistical and comparative methods. Gini coefficient (a statistical measure of the degree of variation represented in a set of values) were used to identify the degree of concentration of individual parameters in the groups. The normality of the distribution of the individual parameters of the Gillette Gait Index was verified using the Shapiro-Wilk test. For an adopted significance level of 0.05, distribution normality was not revealed only in relation to parameter P6 (mean pelvic rotation in the transverse plane). Because of the normality of the distribution of 15 analysed parameters, the statistical effect of the age and height on the above-named quantities was determined using the ANOVA single-factor analysis (a stronger parametric test) or the Kruskal-Wallis test (a weaker non-parametric test) (Table 4). The zero hypothesis (H0) signifies the lack of statistical differences in a given parameter in relation to age or height, whereas the alternative hypothesis (H1) signifies that age or height has a statistical effect on a given parameter. The Kruskal-Wallis test was performed for parameter P6, i.e. the mean pelvic rotation in the transverse plane. The above-named test provided similar results as the stronger test of the ANOVA single-factor analysis. Table 4 contains the critical values of distribution F and of the chi-squared distribution in relation to corresponding levels of significance (5% and 1%). If a value calculated in the test was higher than the appropriate critical value, the zero hypothesis (H0) was rejected, whereas the alternative hypothesis was adopted (H1).

Table 3. Mean value of 16 selected parameters necessary to determine the value of the GGI along with the standard deviation for the group of children with regular gait

No.	GGI parameters	Average value for the control group
1	Time of toe off (% gait cycle)	58.92 ± 1.5
2	Walking speed/leg length	1.56 ± 0.28
3	Cadence (step/s)	2.06 ± 0.24
4	Mean pelvic tilt (°)	7.4 ± 4.57
5	Range of pelvic tilt (°)	4.01 ± 1.07
6	Mean pelvic rotation (°)	-0.88 ± 2.13
7	Minimum hip flexion (°)	-9.75 ± 7.78
8	Range of hip flexion (°)	46.16 ± 5.84
9	Peak abduction in swing (°)	-11.58 ± 2.26
10	Mean hip rotation in stance (°)	3.68 ± 7.69
11	Knee flexion at initial contact (°)	11.51 ± 4.41
12	Time of peak flexion (% gait cycle)	70.46 ± 1.16
13	Range of knee flexion (°)	58.88 ± 3.74
14	Peak dorsiflexion in stance (°)	13.29 ± 3.64
15	Peak dorsiflexion in swing (°)	4.69 ± 3.42
16	Mean foot progression angle in stance (°)	-11.17 ± 4.68

3 Discussion

Systems for the triplanar analysis of motion enable a very detailed analysis of locomotor functions. The time-spatial parameters of gait can be identified using

Table 4. The results of ANOVA and Kruskal-Wallis (K.W.*) one-way analysis of variance for all 16 parameters in relation to age and height

Parameter	ANOVA in relation to age	ANOVA in relation to height
1	1.97	3.11
2	10.13	13.60
3	10.97	12.06
4	3.54	3.85
5	5.78	4.85
6	1.92*	9.86*
7	1.29	0.63
8	1.59	2.51
9	1.93	1.34
10	2.29	0.88
11	2.92	2.12
12	1.32	3.41
13	0.51	1.79
14	1.15	3.05
15	0.49	2.02
16	1.33	1.30
	$F = 2.56$ (5%), 3.72 (1%) *Kruskal-Wallis test chi $= 9.488$ (5%), 13.277 (1%)	$F = 2.40$ (5%), 3.41 (1%) *Kruskal-Wallis test chi $= 11.070$ (5%), 16.086 (1%)

very simple and inexpensive devices such as timers, measuring tapes, photocells etc. This might be one of the reasons for which researchers often analyse changes in the time-spatial parameters of gait in their works [5,6,8,15]. Scientific publications contain little information concerning changes in the kinematic quantities of children's gait in relation to age and height. The authors identified the courses of normative quantities in relation to children aged 7–17, constituting the basis of the clinical analysis of patients suffering from various conditions [9]. The obtained courses of the kinematic quantities were compared with the results obtained for a 31-strong group of patients (aged 6–17) with regular gait, presented in the publication by Pinzone et al. [17]. Gait-related experimental tests for the above-named test group were performed at the Royal Children's Hospital in Melbourne using the Vicon system and the AMTI force plates. Figure 1 present the courses of the mean value and of the standard deviation in relation to angles of the pelvis and angles in the joints of lower limbs obtained in individual research and in the study by Pinzone et al. [17]. The obtained course of the kinematic quantities coincide [17]. Undoubtedly, it would be highly recommendable to perform the quantitative comparison of the curves of the normative quantities presented by various research centres.

Table 5 compares the obtained values of the Gillette Gait Index and of its 16 constituent parameters with the results obtained by other authors in relation to the group of children and adults [1,4,16–19]. An average value of the GDI for the group of patients with regular gait equals 100.62 ± 10.77 in the work by Molloy et al. [12]. Minimum and maximum values of the GDI obtained in own research (max: 121.07, min: 78.95) coincide with the extreme ranges of values of this index in Molloy et al. [12]. The calculated numerical values of the GGI and GDI coincide with the results obtained by other authors [1,9,18–20].

When analysing the values of the individual GGI constituent parameters obtained in various research centres (see Table 5), it was ascertained that many of the results were similar to those obtained in the individual research. The mean values of parameters P1 and P2, i.e. the percentage of the stance phase and the rate of gait standardised in relation to height, were comparable in all of the tests involving the group of healthy children. The research publications concerning adults' gait revealed a slightly higher (approximately by 3%) mean value of the percentage of the stance phase and a greater step frequency than those in the group of healthy children. Greater result discrepancies in the research works were noticed in relation to parameter P4, i.e. the value of the mean anteversion of the pelvis. A greater difference could be ascribed to a slightly different manner used when selecting a marker sticking area on the sacral bone. However, the analysis of the alterations in pelvic inclination in the sagittal plane during gait revealed a significant coincidence of the values. In addition, the values of the mean pelvic rotation in a single gait cycle, which, when determined in the individual research amounted to $-0.88° \pm 2.13°$, proved similar as well. The individual research-related tests saw the highest values of parameters P8 and P9, i.e. the range of movement in the hip joint in the sagittal plane and the maximum abduction in the hip joint during the swing phase of gait. Significantly lower values concerning the above-named parameters in relation to the other research works were seen in the publication by Romei et al. [18], and, as regards the value of the maximum abduction in the hip joint, also in the publication by Schutte [19]. The publication by Assi et al. [1] presented a significantly higher value of parameter P10, i.e. the mean rotation in the hip joint during the stance phase of gait (different from the remaining results). The mean value of the above-named parameter obtained in the individual research amounted to $3.68° \pm 7.69°$ and was similar to the results obtained by Romei et al. and Pinzone et al. [17,18]. The mean value of flexion in the knee joint at the beginning of the gait cycle amounted to $11.51° \pm 4.41°$ and was higher by a few degrees than that presented in the publications by the other authors. The values of P12, i.e. time preceding the maximum flexion of the knee were similar in the works of all of the authors. In addition, all of the analysed children's gait-related publications presented comparable values concerning the range of movement in the knee joint in the sagittal plane, restricted within the range of $54°$–$59°$. The highest values of parameters P14 and P15 i.e. the peak dorsal flexion in the stance phase and in the swing phase of gait were presented in the publication by Assi et al. [1]. The numerical values of the above-named parameters in the individual research were similar to those obtained for children

Table 5. Values of the GGI and of its 16 constituent parameters in relation to patients with regular gait obtained in individual research and in research by other authors [1,3,16–19]

	Children					Children & Adults	Adults	
	Own research	Pinzone et al. Centre one	Pinzone et al. Centre two	Assi et al.	Schutte et al.	Romei et al.	Pietraszewski et al.	Cretual et al.
Age (years)	7÷17	4÷17	6÷17	5÷15	5÷18	7÷28	22±1	22÷57
Group number	56	81	31	56	24	25	17	25
Time of toe off (% gait cycle)	58.92±1.5	60	60	58.09±1.83	61.87±2.67	58.36±1.96	65.1	62.60
Walking, speed/leg length	1.56±0.28	1.55±0.24	1.69±0.18	1.52±0.30	1.43±0.21	1.63±0.13	1.45±0.18	1.57
Cadence (step/s)	2.06±0.24	2.05±0.27	2.13±0.25	1.88±0.23	1.94±0.11	1.91±0.31	1.84±0.14	1.87
Mean pelvic tilt (°)	7.4±4.57	11.96±5.20	12.12±5.34	8.10±4.00	9.26±4.26	9.43±5.20	–	−5.75
Range of pelvic tilt (°)	4.01±1.07	2.00±0.25	1.79±0.46	3.57±1.60	3.57±1.60	3.81±1.25	1.2	3.56
Mean pelvic rotation (°)	−0.88±2.13	0.03±4.09	−0.05±4.10	−0.04±2.52	0.15±2.51	−0.78±3.19	–	−0.12
Minimum hip flexion (°)	−9.75±7.78	−5.27±6.49	−7.23±7.03	−5.10±6.50	−11.14±6.75	−6.59±6.00	–	−11.18
Range of hip flexion (°)	46.16±5.84	42.73±6.50	44.65±6.89	43.40±4.50	45.00±5.15	38.98±4.24	45.5	44.72
Peak abduction in swing (°)	−11.58±2.26	−7.25±3.11	−7.73±3.37	−8.00±3.50	−0.30±3.27	−0.16±3.53	–	6.73
Mean hip rotation in stance (°)	3.68±7.69	−1.95±9.80	3.54±7.24	31.90±14.00	10.91±7.33	2.03±8.98	–	−0.52
Knee flexion at initial contact (°)	11.51±4.41	5.49±5.24	6.79±4.48	8.50±6.50	6.83±4.69	6.24±4.54	–	9.42
Time of peak flexion (% gait cycle)	70.46±1.16	72	72	71.70±2.30	71.40±2.70	70.06±1.85	–	72.91
Range of knee flexion (°)	58.88±3.74	56.72±b3.79	59.14±5.87	53.60±8.00	54.44±10.59	56.34±4.60	56.1	60.30
Peak dorsiflexion in stance (°)	13.29±3.64	11.37±6.06	13.34±3.37	17.00±6.80	13.31±6.45	11.68±3.76	–	15.97
Peak dorsiflexion in swing (°)	4.69±3.42	1.63±4.52	1.68±4.00	9.00±5.60	3.21±4.88	3.82±4.08	–	10.41
Mean foot progression angle in stance (°)	−11.17±4.68	−6.1±7.0	−8.6±6.6	−8.4±6.7	−9.76±6.46	−11.26±6.50	–	1.84
GGI (min ÷ max)	15.71	–	–	27	15.7	16.36	–	15.7
	(7.46÷30)			(9÷45.5)	(8.2÷26.9)	(6.85÷16.36)		(6.9÷33.8)

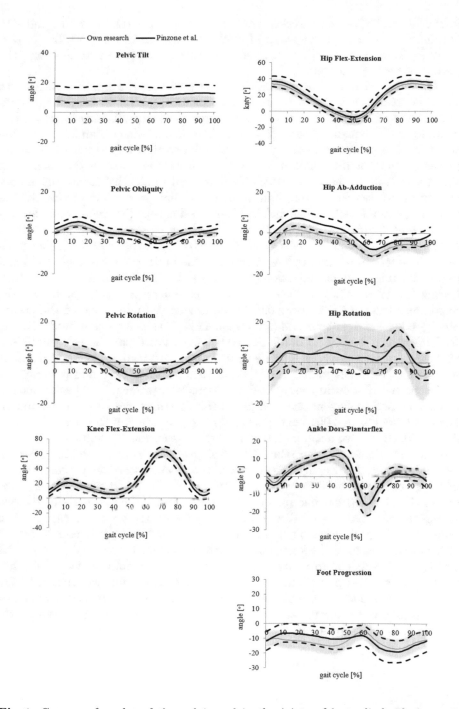

Fig. 1. Courses of angles of the pelvis and in the joints of lower limbs during gait determined in the individual research (n = 56) and by Pinzone et al. (n = 31) [17]

in the remaining research works. The mean values of parameters P14 and P15 obtained in relation to the group of adults referred to in the work by Cretual et al. [4] were by a few degrees higher than those obtained when analysing the groups of healthy children.

The range of values concerning the mean position of the foot in relation to the directional line in the stance phase amounted to $-11.17° \pm 4.68°$ in the individual research and coincided with the ranges of results obtained in relation to children in the remaining tests [1, 17–19]. The mean value obtained in relation to adults and published in the work by Cretual et al. diverged from the above-presented range and amounted to 1.84° [4]. In addition, within the confines of this research work, the Gini coefficients were used to identify the degree of concentration related to the distribution of individual parameters of the Gillette Gait Index in the defined age and height-related groups (Table 1). The parameters having the highest Gini coefficient in relation to age included parameter 6 (mean pelvic rotation in the sagittal plane)–0.5593, parameter 16 (mean position of the foot in relation to the directional line in the stance phase)–0.468 and parameter 9 (minimum abduction of the hip joint)–0.4403. In turn, parameters having the lowest Gini coefficient included parameter 12 (time preceding the maximum flexion of the knee)–0.0035, parameter 1 (percentage of the stance phase)–0.0062 and parameter 3 (step frequency)–0.0439. The parameters having the highest Gini coefficient in relation to height included parameter 9 (minimum abduction of the hip joint)–0.5302, parameter 16 (mean position of the foot in relation to the directional line in the stance phase)–0.5237 and parameter 6 (mean pelvic rotation in the sagittal plane)–0.3231, whereas parameters having the lowest Gini coefficient included parameter 12 (time preceding the maximum flexion of the knee)–0.0048 and parameter 1 (percentage of the stance phase)–0.0076. To confirm or exclude the differences between the age and height-related groups it was necessary to use the ANOVA single-factor analysis and the Kruskal-Wallis rank test. The applied tests revealed the greatest statistical differentiation of the groups (both in terms of age and height) in relation to parameter 2 (standardised gait rate) and parameter 3 (step frequency). The analysis of the age groups revealed that the smallest differences between the groups were related to parameter 15 (peak dorsal flexion in the swing phase) and parameter 13 (range of flexion-extension of the knee joint), whereas as regards the height groups the smallest differences were related to parameter 7 (minimum flexion of the hip joint in the sagittal plane) and 16 (mean position of the foot in relation to the directional line in the stance phase). The calculations were also performed differentiating between the right and left limbs, yet the results obtained were nearly identical to the mean value.

4   Summary

The experimental tests concerning the gait of children aged 7–17 enabled the development of the standards concerning the values of time-spatial parameters and standard alterations in kinematic quantities. In addition, it was possible to identify the normative ranges of the Gait Deviation Index and the Gillette Gait Index as well as of 16 parameters constituting the GGI (similar to the results obtained by other authors) [1,18–20]. However, because of the significant numbers of factors affecting the variability of measurements, each research centre should have their own standards of gait parameters. The differences of the GGI parameter values in relation to the defined age and height groups were subjected to statistical tests. Although the tests revealed the existence of statistically relevant differences concerning the parameters constituting the GGI in relation to the defined age groups (5 parameters) and height groups (6 parameters), the authors recommend that the identified courses of the kinematic quantities be used as normative in relation to patients aged 7–17. The foregoing was confirmed by the fact that the greatest differences between the groups were obtained in relation to the time-spatial parameters (parameter 2 and 3). Taking into account the fact that most of the Gillette Gait Index constituent parameters did not differ statistically in the individual age and height groups, it could be concluded that the identified normative range was appropriate for the entire range of age. The concluding remarks were confirmed by information found on reference research publications stating that the coordination of upper and lower body parts improves until the end of the sixth year of age. The locomotion and the sense of equilibrium among children above six years of age do not differ significantly from the adults' motion standards. Some alterations do occur in relation to the gait stereotype, yet they are characterised by the improvement of previously acquired skills and not by the emergence of new standards. Reference publications state that 7-year old children have fully formed and mature gait [6].

References

1. Assi, A., Ghanem, I., Lavaste, F., Skalli, W.: Gait analysis in children and uncertainty assessment for Davis protocol and Gillette Gait Index. Gait Posture **30**(1), 22–26 (2009)
2. Baker, R., McGinley, J.L., Schwartz, M.H., Beynon, S., Rozumalski, A., Graham, H.K., Tirosh, O.: The gait profile score and movement analysis profile. Gait Posture **30**(3), 265–269 (2009)
3. Cretual, A., Bervet, K., Ballaz, L.: Gillette Gait Index in adults. Gait Posture **32**(3), 307–310 (2010)
4. Bober, T., Dziuba, A., Kobel-Buys, K., Kulig, K.: Gait characteristics following Achilles tendon elongation the foot rocker perspective. Acta Bioeng. Biomech. **10**(1), 37–42 (2008)
5. Dusing, S., Thorpe, D.: A normative sample of temporal and spatial gait parameters in children using the GAITRite electronic walkay. Gait Posture **25**(1), 135–139 (2007)

6. Ganley, K.J., Powers, C.M.: Gait kinematics and kinetics of 7-year-old children: a comparison to adults using age-specific anthropometric data. Gait Posture **21**(2), 141–145 (2005)
7. Hillman, S.J., Stansfield, B.W., Richardson, A.M., Robb, J.E.: Development of temporal and distance parameters of gait in normal children. Gait Posture **29**(1), 81–85 (2009)
8. Holm, I., Teter, A.T., Fredriksen, P.M., Vollestad, N.: A normative sample of gait and hopping on one leg parameters in children 7–12 years of age. Gait Posture **29**(2), 317–321 (2009)
9. Jurkojć, J., Michnik, R., Guzik-Kopyto, A., Gzik, M., Rycerski, W.: Kinematic differences in gait obtained for people with right and left paresis. In: Piętka, E., Kawa, J. (eds.) Information Technologies in Biomedicine, Lecture Notes in Bioinformatics, vol. 7339, pp. 464–471 (2012)
10. Michnik, R., Jochymczyk-Woźniak, K., Kopyta, I. (eds.): Use of engineering methods in gait analysis of children with cerebral palsy. Wyd. Politechniki Śląskiej, 98–15 (2016). (in Polish). ISBN 978-83-7880-398-0
11. Michnik, R., Nowakowska, K., Jurkojć, J., Jochymczyk-Woźniak, K., Kopyta, I.: Motor functions assessment method based on energy changes in gait cycle. Acta Bioeng. Biomech. **19**(4), 63–75 (2017)
12. Molloy, A., McDowell, B.C., Kerr, C., Cosgrove, A.P.: Further evidence of validity of the Gait Deviation Index. Gait Posture **31**(4), 479–482 (2010)
13. Nowakowska, K., Michnik, R., Jochymczyk-Woźniak, K., Jurkojć, J., Mandera, M., Kopyta, I.: Application of gait index assessment to monitor the treatment progress in patients with cerebral palsy. In: Piętka, E., Badura, P., Kawa, J., Wieclawek, W. (eds.) Information Technologies in Medicine 5th International Conference. Advances in Intelligent System and Computing, vol. 472, pp. 75–85. Springer, Cham (2016)
14. Nowakowska, K., Michnik, R., Jochymczyk-Woniak, K., Jurkojć, J., Kopyta, I.: Evaluation of locomotor function in patients with CP based on muscle length changes. In: Gzik, M., Tkacz, E., Paszenda, Z., Pietka, E. (eds.) Innovation in Biomedical Engineering. Advances in Intelligent System and Computing, vol. 526, pp. 161–168. Springer, Cham (2017)
15. Pierce, R., Orendurff, M., Sienko, T.S.: Gait parameters norms for children ages 6–14. Gait Posture **16**(Suppl. 1), 53–54 (2002)
16. Pietraszewski, B., Winiarski, S., Jaroszczuk, S.: Three-dimensional human gait pattern - reference data for normal men. Acta Bioeng. Biomech. **14**(3), 9–16 (2002)
17. Pinzone, O., Schwartz, M.H., Thomason, P., Baker, R.: The comparison of normative reference data from different gait. Gait Posture **40**(2), 286–290 (2014)
18. Romei, R., Galli, M., Motta, F., Schwartz, M., Crivellini, M.: Use of the normalcy index for the evaluation of gait pathology. Gait Posture **19**(1), 85–90 (2004)
19. Schutte, L.M., Narayanan, U., Stout, J.L., Selber, P., Gage, J.R., Schwartz, M.H.: An index for quantifying deviations from normal gait. Gait Posture **11**(1), 25–31 (2000)
20. Schwartz, M., Rozumalski, A.: The gait deviation index: a new comprehensive index of gait pathology. Gait Posture **28**(3), 351–357 (2008)
21. Stansfield, B.W., Hillman, S.J., Hazlewood, M.E., Robb, J.E.: Regression analysis of gait parameters with speed in normal children walking at self-selected speeds. Gait Posture **23**(3), 288–294 (2006)
22. Steinwender, G., Saraph, V., Scheiber, S., Zwick, E.B., Witz, C., Hackl, K.: Intra-subject repeatability of gait analysis data in normal and spastic. Child. Clin. Biomech. **15**(2), 134–139 (2000)

23. Syczewska, M.: Rehabilitation diagnostics of child's motor system. Standardy Medyczne **5**(9), 1254–1264 (2003). (in Polish)
24. Webber, J.T., Raichlen, D.A.: The role of plantigrady and heel-strike in the mechanics and energetics of human walking with implications for the evolution of the human foot. J. Exp. Biol. **219**, 3729–3737 (2016)
25. Winiarski, S., Czamara, A.: Evaluation of gait kinematics and symmetry during the first two stages of physiotherapy after anterior cruciate ligament reconstruction. Acta Bioeng. Biomech. **14**(2), 91–100 (2012)

The Long-Term Effects of Surgery in Patients with Myelomeningocele and Their Influence on the Parameteres of Gait – Preliminary Research

Katarzyna Jochymczyk-Woźniak[1]([✉]), Robert Michnik[1],
Katarzyna Nowakowska[1], Weronika Bartecka[2], Tomasz Koszutski[3],
and Agnieszka Pastuszka[4]

[1] Faculty of Biomedical Engineering, Department of Biomechatronics,
Silesian University of Technology, Roosevelta 40, Zabrze, Poland
Katarzyna.Jochymczyk-Wozniak@polsl.pl
[2] Student Research Group of Biomechatronics 'BIOKREATYWNI',
Faculty of Biomedical Engineering, Department of Biomechatronics,
Silesian University of Technology, Roosevelta 40, Zabrze, Poland
[3] Department of Children Surgery and Urology in Katowice Children's Hospital,
School of Medicine in Katowice, Medical University of Silesia, Katowice, Poland
[4] School of Medicine with Division of Dentistry in Zabrze,
Department of Descriptive and Topographic Anatomy,
Medical University of Silesia, Katowice, Poland

Abstract. The aim of the work was to assess locomotion functions and posture stability of patients who had undergone prenatal or postnatal surgery for myelomeningocele. The gait tests were conducted with BTS System and the stabilographic tests with the dynamographic platform by Zebris. Eight patients operated for myelomeningocele, 4 prenatally and 4 postnatally, have undergone the analysis. A thorough analysis was made of the set of space-time, kinematic parameters, values of the Gillette Gait Index and Gait Deviation Index. The patients' posture stability was assessed on the basis of the path length and the ellipse area. The obtained results were compared with the standard values. The conducted biomechanical examinations of indicate that regardless of the time when the closing of the myelomeningocele was done, the patients show biggest disorders in the motion of the pelvis. Posture stability of children with myelomeningocele is reduced when compared to a group of healthy children.

Keywords: Myelomeningocele · Gait analysis · GGI · GDI
Stabilography

1 Introduction

According to the Polish Register of Congenital Disorders, approximately 3% of children are born with at least one congenital disorder, which makes it a serious

© Springer International Publishing AG, part of Springer Nature 2019
E. Pietka et al. (Eds.): ITIB 2018, AISC 762, pp. 602–611, 2019.
https://doi.org/10.1007/978-3-319-91211-0_53

social problem. Myelomeningocele is one of the most often occurring congenital anomalies, the incidence of which is 0.3–5 per 1000 liveborn infants. The etiology of the anomaly is multifactorial and not fully known. The mother's folic acid deficiency in the preconception period and during pregnancy is mentioned as one of the main causes. The anomaly means that as a result of a defective closure of the neural tube and the spinal canal, a progressive damage to the spinal cord and nerves occurs, which consequently leads to irreversible disorders of the function of the motion, urinary and digestive systems.

In the past two decades, thanks to significant progress of prenatal diagnostics, the right diagnosis of the defect has been possible already in the first trimester of pregnancy. In the case of numerous congenital disorders, their early diagnosis enables the commencement of treatment already in the period of foetal life. Tests conducted on an animal model have proven unequivocally that a surgery of myelomeningocele while still in foetal life period results in a reduction or a complete recovery from neurological disorders caused by the damaged systems [4, 9]. The above results encouraged the first open uterus myelomeningocele surgery on a human foetus to be performed at the Children Hospital of Philadelphia, USA, in 1998 [1]. Nowadays, such operations are done in a few centers in the USA and two centers in Europe, Poland and Switzerland. The randomized results of pre- and postnatal myelomeningocele plasty have been presented in the work by A.S. Adzick [2]. The analysis proves unequivocally that prenatal myelomeningocele plasty lowers the risk of hydrocephalus and improves the children's motor functions of the lower limbs.

Gait, being one of the basic forms of locomotion, is a factor closely combined with a child's cognitive abilities. Thus, one of the main aims of treating patients with myelomeningocele is providing them with the opportunity to move independently which benefits a better development of the children. One of the methods to provide an acceptable level of functional walking by children with myelomeningocele is a proper selection of walking support devices. The choice of the devices depends on the level of the damage to the spinal cord. The rule being that the lower section of the spine was subject to the spina bifida, the better functional results can be obtained. The application of a 3-dimensional gait analysis making it possible to obtain space-time, kinetic and dynamic parameters enables us to demonstrate the existence of dependencies in the gait of children with myelomeningocele. The results obtained during such an analysis (test) allow an individual selection of the best possible orthopaedic equipment, which may significantly improve the motion system function and enable its better development [7, 8, 10].

Vankoski and co. assessed the kinematics of patients with myelomeningocele by using a system for a 3-dimensional gait analysis (VICON) [15]. The patients were divided into two groups on the basis of muscle power test results: group Ia – patients without orthoses, group Ib – patients moving about in orthoses. It was stated, on the basis of the conducted tests, that muscle power for the dorsi- and the plantar flexion of the foot, and abduction and adduction in the hip joint, were lower for Ib group than for Ia group, which may be related to a higher degree of the injury. In addition, it was observed that the dorsi- and plantar flexion of the foot as well as the straightening in the hip joint was weaker for Ib than for Ia.

Other tests of people with myelomeningocele have been presented by Gutierrez and co. [6]. The authors divided the patients into five groups depending on the scope of movement in the lower limb joints (some of the patients moved about in orthoses). The tested people were given a 3-dimensional gait test with the use of a motion analysis system, Motion Systems Vico (Newington's model), and a dynamometric platform, Kistler. The tests proved that the use of orthoses compensated for the lost powers of dorsi- and plantar flexors. This, however, was a cause of higher load exerted on the hip joint. Muscle weakness of children with myelomeningocele causes a change in the strategy of gait where it is necessary to recruit the stronger muscle groups in order to maintain independent gait.

Gabrieli A. and co. made a gait analysis of 20 people with myelomeningocele in order to determine whether surgical intervention was necessary or not to prevent unilateral dislocation or subluxation in the hip joint, which are a common complication in patients with the condition [5]. The patients were divided into two 10-person groups: the first group was made of people having problems with flexing the hip joint, while the second group was made of patients who experienced unilateral contractures during adduction and flexion in the hip joint. During the test, symmetry of the gait was assessed and special attention was paid to the movements of the pelvis and the hip joint. It was observed that most people from the first group had symmetrical movements, while only two people in the second group achieved the same result.

Biomechanical tests of people with myelomeningocele are not popular. In recent years, only few works have appeared on the subject of gait analysis of patients with myelomeningocele, and the authors mainly focused their attention on the assessment of gait from the point of view of the used orthopaedic equipment or the lack of such.

This work has attempted to assess and compare the locomotion functions and posture stability of patients who had undergone prenatal or postnatal surgery for myelomeningocele.

2   Materials and Methods

Eight children who had undergone myelomeningocele surgery took part in the tests, four of which had been operated on pre- and four postnatally. The age of the children was 7 ± 2.0 y.o., body mass: 23.4 ± 10.5 kg and body height: 116.38 ± 15.2 cm. The patients underwent a medical assessment (neuromuscular tests) and a biomechanical one (gait and posture stability test). The control group was composed of 56 healthy children at the age of 11 ± 3 y.o., body mass: 41.8 ± 13.2 kg and body height: 147 ± 17 cm.

The gait tests were conducted with the use of a system allowing a 3-planar gait analysis, BTS Smart, and a stabilographic platform, FDM Zebris. The BTS system consisted of six optoelectronic cameras allowing to record the location of passive markers in space. The frame rate of the cameras during the test was 250 Hz. The location of the markers complied with Helen Heyes protocol, and a model built in the BTS System was used for the calculations. Before the commencement of the gait test, the necessary anthropometric measurements were made in accordance with the Davis model, and then each child covered the measurement path ten times. All the passes were averaged in further analysis. During the tests, the children moved at their natural velocity. For the sake of further analysis, the children were divided into two groups depending on the timing of the operation: group I with prenatal – and group II with postnatal surgery.

On the basis of the recorded parameters, a series of space-time parameters and kinematic quantities was obtained. Furthermore, with the use of original applications written in Matlab environment, the following gait indices were determined: Gillette Gait Index (GGI) and Gait Deviation Index (GDI) [13,14]. A detailed analysis was made on a set of the following sixteen variables describing gait kinematics, on the basis of which the GGI index is made [7]: the percentage share of the support phase (1), the speed of gait standardized by the length of the lower limb (2), the stride frequency (3), the average anterior pelvic tilt in the sagittal plane (4), the scope of pelvic movement in the sagittal plane (5), the average pelvic rotation in the lateral plane (6), the minimal flexion of the hip joint in the sagittal plane (7), the scope of movement of the hip joint in the sagittal plane (8), the maximum abduction of the hip joint (9), the average rotation of the hip joint in the support phase (10), flexion of the knee joint at the beginning of floor contact (11), the time till the maximum knee flexion (12), the scope of flexion-extension of the knee joint (13), the highest dorsiflexion in the support phase (14), the highest dorsiflexion in the swing phase (15), the average foot angle to the line of progression in the support phase (16).

The obtained results were referred to the standard values determined for a group of 56 healthy children – control group (R.Michnik and co.) [7,10] and in order to interpret the obtained results correctly, scopes of classification were set for each of the obtained parameters. Four scopes were distinguished, the characteristics of which is presented in Fig. 1.

The range classification	Evaluation of the results	Compartment
very good	results in the norm	average of control group ± standard deviation
admissible	results beyond the norm	average of control group ± 2 x standard deviation
bad	results beyond the norm	average of control group ± 3 x standard deviation
very bad	results beyond the norm	≥ average of control group ± 3 x standard deviation

Fig. 1. Classification of results according to the scale adopted

The investigation of the body balance posture (the analysis of resultant force's application point of the components acting between feet and ground) was based on the Romberg's test assessing the balance during the free standing on both lower limbs with eyes open. Legs astride within the pelvis width, and arms arranged freely along the body. There were following quantities analysed: path length (the distance that GOP covers) and the ellipse area (COP displacement area).

3   Results

Within this work, gait analysis was made for two groups of patients, those after prenatal and those after postnatal surgery of myelomeningocele. The analysis included sixteen chosen space-time and kinematic parameters. For each of the groups, the GGI and the GDI were determined. The results are presented in Table 1. The patients' results were referred to standard values determined for a group of 56 healthy children [8] and they were classified according to an assumed scale (Fig. 1). On the basis of the conducted stabilogtaphic tests, the stance path length [mm] (Fig. 2) and the ellipse area [mm²] (Fig. 3) were determined. The values of the path length obtained in the initial tests were compared with the tests by Lebiedowska [11] where the tested group was made of healthy children, and with the tests by Baltich [3] where adults with no symptoms of gait anomalies were tested. The values of the ellipse area obtained in the initial tests were compared with the tests by Sobery [12] where the tested group was made of healthy children, and to the tests by Baltich [3] where adults with no symptoms of gait anomalies were tested.

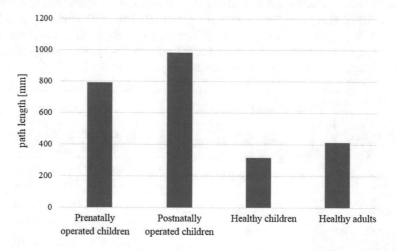

Fig. 2. Juxtaposition of path length for patients operated on pre- and postnatally and the values taken from literature [3, 11]

Table 1. Mean values of GDI, GGI and 16 parameters of GGI determined for two groups of patients according to the scale adopted [7]

	Prenatally operated children		Postnatally operated children		Healthy children
	Right	Left	Right	Left	
GDI	78.76	76.99	80.66	72.85	99.23±8.37
GGI	477.24	474.59	514.76	555.67	15.71±5.68
P1 [% of gait cycle]	60.50	59.75	59.75	60.83	58.92±1.5
P2	1.12	1.14	1.27	1.28	1.56±0.28
P3 [step/s]	1.96	1.96	2.25	2.25	2.06±0.24
P4 [°]	16.29	16.29	16.79	16.79	7.4±4.57
P5 [°]	8.74	8.74	13.48	13.48	4.01±1.07
P6 [°]	-18.75	-18.75	2.93	2.93	-0.88±2.13
P7 [°]	11.64	8.47	0.99	7.73	-9.75±7.78
P8 [°]	43.56	45.22	57.63	49.17	46.16±5.84
P9 [°]	-7.56	-11.13	-10.39	-13.08	-11.58±2.26
P10 [°]	-3.03	17.86	3.66	-8.75	3.68±7.69
P11 [°]	26.89	18.17	13.55	22.75	11.51±4.41
P12 [% of gait cycle]	73.33	68.89	71.70	73.35	70.46±1.16
P13 [°]	49.03	41.38	56.70	54.99	58.88±3.74
P14 [°]	32.69	20.80	21.48	20.04	13.29±3.64
P15 [°]	13.43	8.06	4.04	9.36	4.69±3.42
P16 [°]	-7.09	3.31	-21.18	-4.59	-11.17±4.68

4 Discussion

The high GGI values obtained for the research group are confirmed damage to the spinal cord and nerves occurs, which consequently leads to irreversible disorders of the function of the motion. The analysis of the results of gait tests was made on the basis of an interpretation of sixteen parameters making the GGI index. The obtained results unequivocally prove that children with myelomeningocele, both those operated on pre- and postnatally, achieved very weak results for the scope of pelvic movement in the sagittal plane (P5) and for the average rotation in the lateral plane (P6). A higher deviation from norm for the average value of the pelvic rotation in the lateral plane (P6) is revealed in the results of the prenatally operated children. The results for such parameters as: the percentage share of the support phase (P1), the speed of gait standardized by the length of the lower limb (P2), the scope of movement of the hip joint in the sagittal plane (P8), the maximum abduction of the hip joint (P9), the average rotation of the hip joint in the support phase (P10), and the average foot angle to the line of progression in the support phase (P16), range from the very good to acceptable scope for both limbs, both for the children operated pre- and postnatally. In the case of the determined gait indices, it can be observed that GDI for children with myelomeningocele is lower when compared to the norm (Table 1).

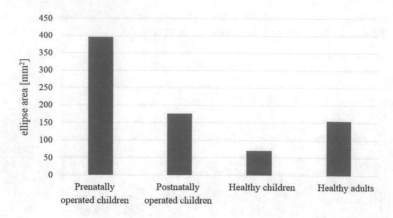

Fig. 3. Juxtaposition of ellipse area for patients operated on pre- and postnatally and the values taken from literature [3,12]

In Figs. 4 and 5, a distribution of the chosen gait parameters has been presented in percentage terms for the particular groups of patients. All the children operated on prenatally showed very weak results in the scope of the average pelvic rotation in the lateral plane (P6) and the highest dorsiflexion in the support phase (P14). However, the results for the following parameters: the percentage share of the support phase (P1), the maximum abduction of the hip joint (P9), and the average rotation of the hip joint in the support phase (10), were classified for most of the patients as very good. The results obtained for such parameters as: the speed of gait standardized by the length of the lower limb (P2), the stride frequency (P3), the average anterior pelvic tilt in the sagittal plane (P4), the time till the maximum knee flexion (P12), and the highest dorsiflexion in the swing phase (P15), were strongly varied with a few patients obtaining values from the very good scope while others being very weak. In the case of the average foot angle to the line of progression in the support phase (P16), most of the prenatally operated children obtained results being within the scope of the average for the norm $\pm 3\sigma$.

Most postnatally operated children obtained very weak results for such parameters as: the scope of pelvic movement in the sagittal plane (P5), the average pelvic rotation in the lateral plane (P6), the time till the maximum knee flexion (P12), and the average foot angle to the line of progression in the support phase (P16). The results for the maximum abduction of the hip joint (9) were mostly acceptable or very good. The values for the other parameters were of high variability (Fig. 5).

The results of stabilographic tests obtained during the initial tests of children with myelomeningocele show that people with this condition, regardless of the time of the surgery, obtained a much greater value of the path length than the scope considered as standard. What it means, is that postural reactions occurring in those children were activated later than in healthy children (Fig. 2). Moreover, a significant difference (220 mm^2) was observed between the average value of

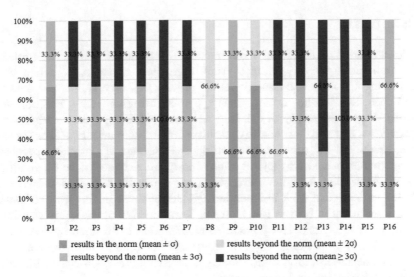

Fig. 4. Distribution, in percentage terms, of the obtained results of GGI parameters for a group of prenatally operated children

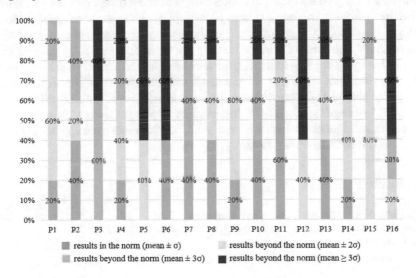

Fig. 5. Distribution, in percentage terms, of the obtained results of GGI parameters for a group of postnatally operated children

ellipse area obtained for the prenatally and postnatally operated children. It can be stated, that the stability of children operated postnatally is better and, additionally, its value is comparable to the value of the ellipse area obtained for adults (Fig. 3).

5   Summary

The conducted biomechanical examinations of patients who have undergone myelomeningocele surgery indicate that regardless of the time when closing the myelomeningocele was done, whether pre- or postnatally, the patients show biggest disorders in the motion of the pelvis (anterior pelvic tilt and pelvic rotation). Posture stability of children with myelomeningocele is reduced when compared to a group of healthy children. In the context of the obtained results, statistical information concerning the number of patients operated on for myelomeningocele and moving about independently seems to be significant. The data show that a higher percentage of prenatally operated patients with myelomeningocele can walk independently than of those in the group of patients operated postnatally. It is certain that the lower section of the spine was subject to the spina bifida, the better functional results can be obtained by the patients. The final decision on the method of treatment for a child with myelomeningocele should be made individually for each patient by a doctor who has all the necessary information and experience.

The conducted pilot tests aiming at a creation of a methodology of tests and examinations for patients with myelomeningocele constitute a point of reference for further research. In the next stage, it is planned to conduct gait tests and stabilography of a greater group of pre- and postnatally operated patients, which, in the authors' opinion, will unequivocally show the impact of the timing of the performed surgery for myelomeningocele onto the motor skill development of a child. The results of experimental research will be used to make simulations of loads in the skeletal and muscular system, and the obtained results will constitute a source of information about the functioning of the motion system of patients with myelomeningocele, which will translate into further therapy and selection of orthopaedic devices in the future.

References

1. Adzick, N.S., Sutton, L.N., Crombleholme, T.M., Flake, A.W.: Successful fetal surgery for spina bifida. Lancet 352(9141), 1675–1676 (1998)
2. Adzick, N.S., Thom, E.A., Spong, C.Y., et al.: A randomized trial of prenatal versus postnatal repair of myelomeningocele. N. 'Engl.' J. Med. 364(11), 993–1004 (2011)
3. Baltich, J., Tscharner, V., Zandiyeh, P., Nigg, B.: Quantification and reliability of center of pressure movement during balance tasks of varying difficulty. Gait Posture 40(2), 327–332 (2014)
4. Bouchard, S., Davey, M.G., Rintoul, N.E., et al.: Correction of hindbrain hernation and anatomy of the vermis after in utero repair of myelomeningocele in sheep. J. Pediatr. Surg. 38(3), 451–458 (2003)
5. Gabrieli, A., Vankoski, S., Dias, L., Milani, C., Lourenco, A., Filho, J., Novak, R.: Gait analysis in low lumbar myelomeningocele patients with unlitareral hip dislocation or subluxation. J. Pediatr. Orthop. 23(3), 330–334 (2003)
6. Gutierrez, E.M., Bartonek, A., Haglund, Y., Saraste, H.: Kinetics of compensatory gait in persons with myelomenigocele. Gait Posture 21(1), 12–23 (2005)

7. Michnik, R., Jochymczyk-Woźniak, K., Kopyta, I. (eds.): Use of engineering methods in gait analysis of children with cerebral palsy. Wyd. Politechniki Śląskiej, pp. 98–158 (2016). ISBN: 978-83-7880-398-0 (in Polish)
8. Michnik, R., Nowakowska, K., Jurkojć, J., Jochymczyk-Woźniak, K., Kopyta, I.: Motor functions assessment method based on energy changes in gait cycle. Acta Bioeng. Biomech. **19**(4), 63–75 (2017)
9. Mueli, M., Mueli-Simmen, C., Hutchins, G.M., et al.: The spinal cord lesion in human fetus with myelomeningocele: Implications for fetal surgery. J. Pediatr. Surg. **32**(3), 448–452 (1997)
10. Nowakowska, K., Michnik, R., Jochymczyk-Woźniak, K., Jurkojć, J., Mandera, M., Kopyta, I.: Application of gait index assessment to monitor the treatment progress in patients with cerebral palsy. In: Piętka, E., Badura, P., Kawa, J., Wieclawek, W. (eds.) Information Technologies in Medicine 5th International Conference, Advances in Intelligent System and Computing, vol. 472(2), pp. 75–85. Springer, Cham (2016)
11. Lebiedowska, M., Syczewska, M.: Invariant sway properties in children. Gait Posture **12**(3), 200–204 (2000)
12. Sobera M.: Charakteristics of a standing postural control process in children aged 2–7, Wrocław (2010). (in Polish)
13. Schutte, L.M., Narayanan, U., Stout, J.L., Selber, P., Gage, J.R., Schwartz, M.H.: An index for quantifying deviations from normal gait. Gait Posture **11**(1), 25–31 (2000)
14. Schwartz, M., Rozumalski, A.: The gait deviation index: a new comprehensive index of gait pathology. Gait Posture **28**(3), 351–357 (2008)
15. Vankoski, S.J., Sarwark, J.F., Moore, C., Dias, L.: Characteristic pelvic, hip and knee kinematic patterns in children with lumbosacral myelomeningocele. Gait Posture **3**, 51–57 (1995)

Author Index

© Springer International Publishing AG, part of Springer Nature 2019
E. Pietka et al. (Eds.): ITIB 2018, AISC 762, pp. 613–615, 2019.
https://doi.org/10.1007/978-3-319-91211-0

Printed in the United States
By Bookmasters